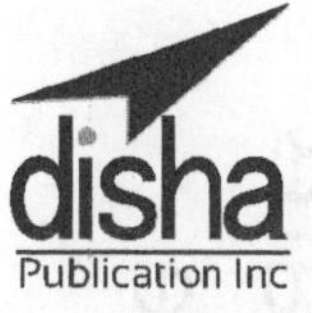

Master NEET BIOLOGY

with Matching & Assertion Reason Questions

Corporate Office

DISHA PUBLICATION
45, 2nd Floor, Maharishi Dayanand Marg, Corner Market, Malviya Nagar, New Delhi - 110017
Tel : 49842349 / 49842350

Typeset by Disha DTP Team

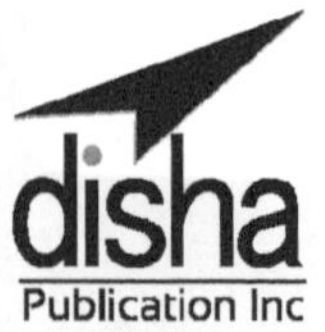

Write to us at feedback_disha@aiets.co.in

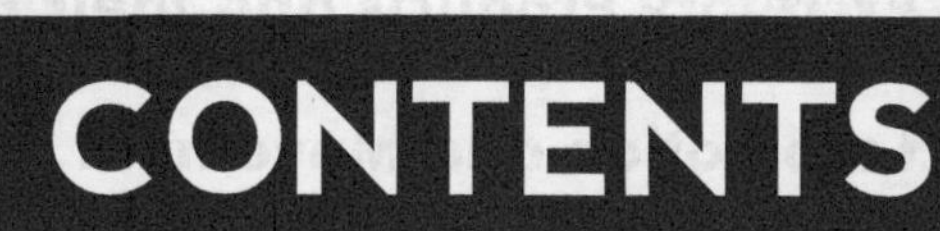

CONTENTS

CHAPTER

The Living World

1. Match the following columns.

Column I	Column II
A. Linnaeus	1. Living species of today
B. John Ray	2. Father of taxonomy
C. Synchronic species	3. Coined the term species
D. Neontological species	4. Species belonging to same time period

Codes

	A	B	C	D		A	B	C	D
(a)	2	3	4	1	(b)	1	3	2	4
(c)	4	3	2	1	(d)	1	2	3	4

2. Match the following columns.

Column I	Column II
A. Numerical taxonomy	1. Nuclear and chromosomal studies
B. Classical taxonomy	2. Number of shared characters
C. Practical taxonomy	3. Utility of organism
D. Karyotaxonomy	4. a-taxonomy

Codes

	A	B	C	D		A	B	C	D
(a)	2	4	3	1	(b)	1	3	2	4
(c)	4	2	3	1	(d)	1	2	4	3

3. Match the column I with column II :

Herbarium	Location
(A) Royal Botanical Garden	(i) Paris
(B) Conservation and Botanical Garden	(ii) St. Petersburg
(C) Herbarium of forest Reseach Institute	(iii) London
(D) British Museum of Natural History	(iv) Kolkata
(E) Museum of Natural History	(v) Kew
	(vi) Dehradun
	(vii) Geneva

(a) A-(v), B-(vii), C-(vi), D-(iii), E-(i)
(b) A-(ii), B-(iv), C-(v), D-(i), E-(iii)
(c) A-(vi), B-(v), C-(vii), D-(iii), E-(ii)
(d) A-(iii), B-(ii), C-(i), D-(iv), E-(vii)

4. Match the Coloumn I with Column II :

Museums	Locations
(A) Zoology Museum	(i) Mumbai
(B) Natural History Museum	(ii) Delhi
(C) Prince of klales Museum	(iii) Chicago (USA)
(D) National Museum of National History	(iv)
(E) Field Museum of Natural History	(v)
	(vi) London
	(vii) Amesterdam

(a) A-(vi), B-(vii), C-(ii), D-(i), E-(iv)
(b) A-(ii), B-(iii), C-(vii), D-(vi), E-(v)
(c) A-(iv), B-(vi), C-(iii), D-(i), E-(v)
(d) A-(vii), B-(vi), C-(i), D-(ii), E-(iii)

5. Match the following columns and select the correct option.

Column I	Column II
A. *Panthera tigris*	(i) Mango
B. *Mangifera indica*	(ii) Common Indian frog
C. *Musca domestica*	(iii) Cockroach
D. *Periplaneta americana*	(iv) Tiger
E. *Rana tigerina*	(v) House fly

(a) A-(ii), B-(v), C-(i), D-(iii), E-(iv)
(b) A-(iv), B-(i), C-(v), D-(iii), E-(ii)
(c) A-(ii), B-(v), C-(iii), D-(i), E-(iv)
(d) A-(iv), B-(i), C-(v), D-(ii), E-(iii)

6. Match each item in Column-I with one in Column-II and choose your answer from the codes given below:

Column-I Taxonomical Aid	Column-II Feature
I. Flora	1. Useful in providing information for identification of names of species found in an area
II. Manuals	2. Contains the actual account of habitat and distribution of plants of a given area.
III. Monographs	3. Contain information on any one taxon

	I	II	III		I	II	III
(a)	1	2	3	(b)	3	2	1
(c)	2	1	3	(d)	2	3	1

7. Match Column-I with Column-II for housefully classification and select the correct option using the codes given below:

Column-I	Column-II
A. Family	1. Diptera
B. Order	2. Arthropoda
C. Class	3. Muscidae
D. Phylum	4. Insecta

Codes

	A	B	C	D		A	B	C	D
(a)	3	1	4	2	(b)	3	2	4	1
(c)	4	3	2	1	(d)	4	2	1	3

8. Which of the following taxonomic categories are correctly matched to their standard termination of names with respect to biological classification of plants?

I. Division – phyta
II. Class – opsida
III. Order – ales
IV. Family – idae

(a) I, II, IV (b) II, III, IV
(c) II, III, IV (d) I, II, III, IV

9. The living organisms can be unexceptionally distinguished from the non-living things on the basis of their ability for:
(a) responsiveness to touch
(b) interaction with the environment and progressive evolution
(c) reproduction
(d) growth and movement

10. Herbarium sheet gives information about
(a) Date and place of collection only
(b) English and local names only
(c) Collector's name only
(d) Not a single option with correct information

11. Match Column-I with Column-II and choose the correct option

Column-I	Column-II
A. Ex-situ conservation	(i) Central National Herbarium
B. Quick referral system	(ii) Museum
C. Preserved plants and animals	(iii) Flora
D. Actual account of habitat and distribution of plants in a given area	(iv) Royal Botanical

(a) A-(ii), B-(iii), C-(iv), D-(i)
(b) A-(i), B-(iv), C-(ii), D-(iii)
(c) A-(iv), B-(i), C-(iii), D-(ii)
(d) A-(iv), B-(i), C-(ii), D-(iii)

12. Match Column-I with Column-II and select the correct option from the codes given below.

Column-I	Column-II
A. Binomial nomenclature	(i) Hippocrates
B. The Darwin of the 20th century	(ii) Earnst Mayr
C. Father of Botany	(iii) Linnaeus
D. Father of medicine	(iv) Theopharastus

(a) A-(iii), B-(ii), C-(iv), D-(i)
(b) A-(iii), B-(ii), C-(i), D-(iv)
(c) A-(i), B-(ii), C-(iii), D-(iv)
(d) A-(ii), B-(iii), (i) C-(iv), D-(i)

13. Which of the following is a mismatched pair of common name and biological name of an organism?
(a) Para rubber – *Hevea brasiliensis*
(b) Tea – *Thea chinesis*
(c) Earthworm – *Pheretima posthuma*
(d) Frog – *Bufo melanostictus*

14. Match Column-I with Column-II and select the correct option from codes given below.

Column-I	Column-II
A. John Ray	(i) Gave the concept of new systematics.
B. C. Linnaeus	(ii) First described species as a unit of classification
C. Aristotle	(iii) Father of Zoology
D. Julian Huxley	(iv) Introduced binomial nomenclature

(a) A-(i), B-(ii), C-(iii), D-(iv)
(b) A-(iv), B-(ii), C-(iii), D-(i)
(c) A-(ii), B-(iii), C-(i), D-(iv)
(d) A-(ii), B-(iv), C-(iii), D-(i)

15. Match Column-I with Column-II and select the correct option from the codes given below.

Column-I	Column-II
A. Ecology	(i) Relationships of organisms and environment
B. Herbarium	(ii) Original specimen cited by an author
C. Holotype	(iii) A hierarchical unit
D. Taxon	(iv) Collection of wild and domestic plants

(a) A-(i), B-(ii), C-(iii), D-(iv)
(b) A-(i), B-(ii), C-(iv), D-(iii)
(c) A-(i), B-(iv), C-(ii), D-(iii)
(d) A-(iv), B-(ii), C-(iii), D-(i)

16. Select the mismatched pair.

(a) *Panthera leo*	Belongs to class Mammalia
(b) *Musca domestica*	The common house lizard, a reptile
(c) *Entamoeba coli*	Commonly occurring protozoan in human intestine
(d) *Solanum tuberosum*	Adicotyledonous plant

17. Select the correct option to complete the given table:

Common name	Biological name	Phylum/ Division	Class	Order	Family	Genus
Man	*Homo sapiens*	Chordata	Mammalia	Primata	(i)	*Homo*
Housefly	*Musca domestica*	Arthropoda	Insecta	(ii)	Muscidae	*Musca*
Mango	*Mangifera indica*	Angiospermae	(iii)	Sapindales	Anacardiaceae	*Mangifera*
Wheat	*Triticum aestivum*	(iv)	Monocotyledonae	Poales	Poaceae	*Triticum*

(a) (i) – Hominidae, (ii) – Diptera, (iii) – Dicotyledonae, (iv) – Angiospermae
(b) (i) – Hominidae, (ii) – Dicotyledonae, (iii) – Diptera, (iv) – Angiospermae
(c) (i) – Hominidae, (ii) – Diptera, (iii) – Angiospermae, (iv) – Dicotyledonae
(d) (i) – Hominidae, (ii) – Dicotyledonae, (iii) – Angiospermae, (iv) – Diptera

18. Select the incorrect set from the following:
(a) Polymoniales – Convolvulaceae, Solanaceae.
(b) Primata – gorilla, gibbon
(c) Felidae – cat, dog
(d) Panthera – leopard, tiger

Solutions

1. (a) 2. (a) 3. (a) 4. (d) 5. (b)
6. (c) 7. (a) 8. (d) 9. (c) 10. (a)
11. (d) 12. (c)

13. (d) *Bufo melanostictus* is a biological name of toads. Bufo is a genus of true toads in the amphibian family Bufonidae.

14. (d)

15. (a) A particular specimen or illustration designated by the author to represent the type of a species is referred to as holotype. It is now essential to designate a holotype when publishing a new species.

16. (b) 17. (a)

18. (c) Cat belongs to family Felidae and dog belongs to Family Canidae.

CHAPTER

Biological Classification

1. Match the following Columns.

	Column I		Column II
A.	Artificial system	1.	AW Eichler
B.	Phylogenetic system	2.	Peter Sneath
C.	Phenetic system	3.	C Linnaeus
D.	*Systema Naturae*	4.	Theophrastus

Codes

	A	B	C	D		A	B	C	D
(a)	4	1	2	3	(b)	1	2	3	4
(c)	4	3	2	1	(d)	2	4	1	3

2. Match the following Columans.

	Column I		Column II
A.	Animalia	1.	Unicellular prokaryotes
B.	Monera	2.	Multicellular and prokaryotes
C.	Protista	3.	Unicellular eukaryotes
D.	Plantae	4.	Multicelluar ingestive heterotrophs

Codes

	A	B	C	D		A	B	C	D
(a)	4	3	1	2	(b)	4	1	3	2
(c)	1	2	4	3	(d)	2	3	1	4

3. Match the following Coumns.

	Column I		Column II
A.	Plant virus	1.	Potato spindle tuber disease
B.	Animal virus	2.	Kuru disease
C.	Viroid	3.	Tobacco necrosis disease
D.	Prions	4.	Polio

Codes

	A	B	C	D		A	B	C	D
(a)	2	1	3	4	(b)	3	4	1	2
(c)	4	3	2	1	(d)	1	2	3	4

4. Match the following Coumns.

	Column I		Column II
A.	Flex d'Herelle	1.	Bacteriophage
B.	Loeffler and Frosch	2.	Foot and mouth disease
C.	Robert Gallo	3.	Prions
D.	Stanley Prusiner	4.	HIV

Codes

	A	B	C	D		A	B	C	D
(a)	1	2	3	4	(b)	4	3	2	1
(c)	2	1	3	4	(d)	1	2	4	3

5. Match the following Coumns.

	Column I		Column II
A.	Filovirus	1.	Mumps
B.	Paramyxoviridae	2.	Ebola
C.	Deltaviridae	3.	Influenza virus
D.	Orthomyxoviridae	4.	Hepatitis-D

Codes

	A	B	C	D		A	B	C	D
(a)	2	1	4	3	(b)	3	4	1	2
(c)	1	2	3	4	(d)	2	3	4	1

6. Select the correct difference between bacteriophage and animal virus multiplication.

	Bacteriophage	Animal viruses
I.	Biosynthesis occur in cytoplasm.	Biosynthesis occur in nucleus (DNA viruses) or cytoplams (RNA viruses).

II.	Tail fibres attach to thecell wall proteins.	Attachment sites are plasma membrane proteins or glycoproteins.
III.	Uncoating is necesary.	Uncoating is not necessary.
IV.	Viral DNA enters into host cell endocytosis.	Viral DNA injected into host cell.

Choose the correct option from the codes given below.

(a) I and II (b) III and IV
(c) II, III and IV (d) I, II, III and IV

7. Consider the following given bacteria and classify them as Gram positive (+) and Gram negative (–) bacteria.

Choose the correct option from the codes that follow.

I. Acetobacter II. Escherichia
III. Vibrio IV. Salmonella
V. Streptococcus VI. Mycobacterium
VII. Enterocococus VIII. Pneumococcus

	Gram positive	Gram negative
(a)	V, VI, VII, VIII	I, II, III, IV
(b)	I, II, III, IV	V, VI, VII, VIII
(c)	II, IV, VIII	I, III, V, VI, VII
(d)	I, VIII, III, II	IV, V, VI, VII

8. In the following table identify the correct matching of the crop, its disease and the corresponding pathogen

	Crop	Disease	Pathogen
(a)	Citrus	Canker	*Pseudomonas rubrilineans*
(b)	Potato	Late blight	*Fusarium udum*
(c)	Brinjal	Root-knot	*Meloidogyne incogita*
(d)	Pigeon Pea	Seed gall	*Pytopthora infestons*

9. Match the following Columns.

Column I	Column II
A. *Nitrobacter*	1. Free-living aerobic nitrogen-fixer
B. *Clostridium*	2. Converts ammonia into nitrite
C. *Nitrosococcus*	3. Changes nitrite to nitrate
D. *Azotobacter*	4. Free-living anaerobic nitrogen-fixer

Codes

	A	B	C	D
(a)	2	4	3	1
(b)	3	4	2	1
(c)	4	2	1	3
(d)	1	2	3	4

10. Match the following Columns.

Column I	Column II
A. Actinomycin-D	1. Inhibits mRNA synthesis
B. Tetracycline	2. Inhibits 50S subunits of robosomes
C. Streptomycin	3. Inhibits binding of tRNA with ribosomes
D. Chloramphenicol	4. Alters 30S Subunits of ribosomes

Codes

	A	B	C	D
(a)	1	2	3	4
(b)	3	4	2	1
(c)	1	3	2	4
(d)	1	3	4	2

11.

Column I	Column II	Column III
A. Obligate aerobes	1. Respire anaerobically under normal condition, but can respire aerobically when oxygen is available	(i) *Bacillus subtilis*
B. Facultative anaerobes	2. Respire only anaerobically	(ii) Halophiles
C. Obligate anaerobes	3. Generally respire aerobically, but switch over to anaerobic mode of respiration if oxygen becomes deficient	(iii) *Clostridium botulinum*
D. Facultative aerobes	4. Respire only aerobically	(iv) Rhodopseudomonas

Codes

	A	B	C	D
(a)	4-(i)	3-(iii)	1-(iv)	3-(ii)
(b)	4-(i)	3-(ii)	2-(iii)	1-(iv)
(c)	1-(ii)	2-(i)	3-(iv)	4-(iii)
(d)	4-(iii)	3-(iv)	2-(i)	1-(ii)

12. Match the following Columns.

Column I	Column II
A. Mycoplasma	1. Ether linked lipids
B. Transduction	2. Sex pili
C. Conjugation	3. Requires virus
D. Thermophiles	4. Cell wall-less bacteria

Codes

	A	B	C	D
(a)	4	3	2	1
(b)	1	2	3	4
(c)	2	3	4	1
(d)	3	4	1	2

13. Match the following Columns.

Column I	Column II
A. Archaebacteria	1. Do not possess photosynthetic pigments
B. Mesosomes	2. Atrichous
C. Pili	3. More prominent in Gram negative bacteria
D. Cocci bacteria	4. One or two per cell
E. Chemosynthetic	5. Lack peptidoglycan in cell wall bacteria

Codes

	A	B	C	D	E
(a)	5	3	4	2	1
(b)	1	2	3	4	5
(c)	4	2	1	3	5
(d)	5	4	3	2	1

14. Match the type of flagellar arrangement in Column I with their correct names in Coulmn II and mark the right code.

Column I	Column II
A.	1. Cephalotrichous
B.	2. Lophotrichous
C.	3. Atrichous
D.	4. Peritrichous
E.	5. Amphitrichous

Codes

	A	B	C	D	E
(a)	4	2	5	3	1
(b)	4	1	5	3	2
(c)	4	3	5	1	2
(d)	4	1	5	2	3

15. Match the following Columns.

	Column I		**Column II**
A.	Syphilis	1.	*Acetobacter*
B.	Pathogen of Cattle	2.	*Agrobacterium*
C.	Crown gall of apple	3.	*Corynebacterium*
D.	Diphtheria	4.	*Mycobacterium*
		5.	*Treponema*

Codes

	A	B	C	D		A	B	C	D
(a)	3	1	4	2	(b)	5	4	2	3
(c)	5	3	2	1	(d)	2	4	5	3

16. Match the following Columns.

	Column I (Type of pseudopodia)		**Column II** (Protozoan species)
A.	Lobopodia	1.	Euglypha
B.	Filopodia	2.	*Globigerina* (Forminiferans)
C.	Reticulopodia	3.	Amoeba
D.	Axopodia	4.	*Actinophyrus*

Codes

	A	B	C	D		A	B	C	D
(a)	3	1	2	4	(b)	4	3	2	1
(c)	1	2	3	4	(d)	2	4	1	3

17. Match the following Columns.

	Column I **(Structures)**		**Column II** **(Features)**
A.	Magna form	1.	Precystic stage of Entamoeba.
B.	Minuta form	2.	Most active form of Entamoeba.
C.	Trophozoite	3.	Infective stage of *Entamoeba histolytica*.
D.	Tetranucleate cyst	4.	The normal trophozoites in *Entamoeba histolytica*.

Codes

	A	B	C	D
(a)	1	2	3	4
(b)	4	1	3	2
(c)	4	1	2	3
(d)	3	4	1	2

18. Match the following Columns.

	Column I		**Column II**
A.	Dinoflagellate	1.	*Dicyostelium*
B.	*Plasmodium*	2.	*Noctiluca*
C.	Myxomycota	3.	Slime mould
D.	Acrasiomycota	4.	*Fuligo*

Codes

	A	B	C	D		A	B	C	D
(a)	3	2	1	4	(b)	1	4	3	2
(c)	2	3	4	1	(d)	4	3	1	2

19. Match the following Columns.

	Column I		**Column II**
A.	*Entamoeba histolytic*	1.	Cytozoic parasite
B.	*Plamodium*	2.	Coelozoic parasite
C.	*Wuchereria*	3.	Rhabditiform larva
D.	Extraintestinal migration	4.	Monogenic parasite
		5.	Lymphadenitis

Codes

	A	B	C	D		A	B	C	D
(a)	4	2	1	3	(b)	4	1	5	3
(c)	5	1	2	3	(d)	4	2	5	1

20. Which of the following is not matched correctly?

(a) *Anabaena* – Cyanobacteria
(b) *Amoeba* – Protozoa
(c) *Gonyaulax* – Dinoflagellated
(d) *Thermoacidophiles* – Archaebacteria
(e) *Albugo* – Chrysophytes

21. Match the following Columns.

	Column I		**Column II**
A.	*E. histolytica*	1.	Kala-azar
B.	*E. gingivalis*	2.	Sleeping sickness
C.	*P. vivax*	3.	Amoebic dysentery
D.	*T. gambiense*	4.	Malaria
		5.	Pyorrhoea

Codes

	A	B	C	D
(a)	4	3	2	1
(b)	3	4	5	1
(c)	3	5	4	2
(d)	3	5	2	1

22. Match the following Columns.

Column I	Column II
A. A domain of plant-like,heterotrophic organims that work primarily as decompose	1. Lichen
B. The slender, reproductive structures of fungi	2. Dikaryotic
C. Indicator of SO_2	3. Hyphae
D. Cells with two nuclei	4. Fungi

Codes

	A	B	C	D		A	B	C	D
(a)	4	3	1	2	(b)	1	2	3	4
(c)	4	3	2	1	(d)	3	2	1	4

23. Match the following Columns.

Column I	Column II
A. Morels	1. Deuteromycetes
B. Smut	2. Ascomycetes
C. Bread mould	3. Basidiomycetes
D. Imperfect fungi	4. Phycomycetes

Codes

	A	B	C	D		A	B	C	D
(a)	3	4	1	2	(b)	2	3	4	1
(c)	4	1	2	3	(d)	3	4	2	1
(e)	2	1	4	3					

24. Match the following Columns.

Column I	Column II
A. *Rizopus*	1. Eurotiomycetes
B. *Penicillium*	2. Ustilaginomycetes
C. *Ustilago*	3. Deuteromycetes
D. *Alternaria*	4. Zygomycetes

Codes

	A	B	C	D		A	B	C	D
(a)	4	3	1	2	(b)	2	3	4	1
(c)	4	1	2	3	(d)	3	4	2	1
(e)	2	1	4	3					

25. Match the following Columns.

Column I	Column II
A. Eubacteria	1. *Trichoderma*
B. Dinoflagellates	2. *Albugo*
C. Phycomycetes	3. *Gonyaulax*
D. Deuteromycetes	4. *Anabaena*

Codes

	A	B	C	D		A	B	C	D
(a)	1	2	3	4	(b)	2	3	4	1
(c)	4	3	2	1	(d)	4	3	1	2

26. Which one of the following is incorrectly matched?

(a) Puccinia – Smut
(b) Root – Exarch protoxylem
(c) Cassia – Imbricate aestivation
(d) Root pressure – Guttation

27. Study the figures given below.

A B C

Choose the correct option.

	A	B	C
(a)	Monococcus	Diplococcus	Streptococcus
(b)	Bacillus	Diplococcus	Streptobacillus
(c)	Micrococcus	Bacillus	Streptobacillus
(d)	Streptococcus	Diplococcus	Bacillus

28. In Gram negative bacterial cell wall, the peptidoglycan chains are laterally linked by short chains of four amino acids which are constituted of

(a) L-Alanine; D-Glutamic acid; L-Lysine; D-alanine
(b) L-Alanine; D-Glutamic acid, diaminopimelic acid, D-Alanine
(c) L-Alanine; L-Lyisne; D-Alanine, diaminopimelic acid
(d) L-Alanine; D-Glutamic; L-Lyisne, diaminopimelic acid

29. Consider the following given bacteria and classify them as Gram positive (+) and Gram negative (–) bacteria.

Choose the correct option from the codes that follow.

I. Acetobacter II. Escherichia
III. Vibrio IV. Salmonella
V. Streptococcus VI. Mycobacterium
VII. Entercococus VIII. Pneumococcus

	Gram positive	Gram negative
(a)	V, VI, VII, VIII	I, II, III, IV
(b)	I, II, III, IV	V, VI, VII, VIII
(c)	II, IV, VIII	I, III, V, VI, VII
(d)	I, VIII, III, II	IV, V, VI, VII

30. Select the correct pair(s).

I. Methanogens – *Methanogenium, Methanothrix*
II. Halophiles–*Halococcus, Haloarchaea*
III. Themoacidophiles–*Sulfolobus, Desulphurococcus*

Choose the correct option.

(a) I and II (b) II and III
(c) I and III (d) All of these

31. Match the following Columns.

	Column I		Column II
A.	*Nitrobacter*	1.	Free-living aerobic nitrogen-fixer
B.	*Clostridium*	2.	Converts ammonia into nitrite
C.	*Nitrosococcus*	3.	Changes nitrite to nitrate
D.	*Azotobacter*	4.	Free-living anaerobic nitrogen-fixer

Codes

	A	B	C	D
(a)	2	4	3	1
(b)	3	4	2	1
(c)	4	2	1	3
(d)	1	2	3	4

32. Match the following Columns.

	Column I		Column II
A.	Actinomycin-D	1.	Inhibits mRNA synthesis
B.	Tetracycline	2.	Inhibits 50S subunits of robosomes
C.	Streptomycin	3.	Inhibits binding of tRNA with ribosomes
D.	Chloramphenicol	4.	Alters 30S Subunits of ribosomes

Codes

	A	B	C	D
(a)	1	2	3	4
(b)	3	4	2	1
(c)	1	3	2	4
(d)	1	3	4	2

33. **Column I :**

A. Obligate aerobes
B. Facultative anaerobes
C. Obligate anaerobes
D. Facultative aerobes

Column II :

1. Respire anaerobically under normal condition, but can respire aerobically when oxygen is available
2. Respire only anaerobically
3. Generally respire aerobically, but switch over to anaerobic mode of respiration if oxygen becomes deficient
4. Respire only aerobically

Column III :

(i) *Bacillus subtilis*
(ii) Halophiles
(iii) *Clostridium botulinum*
(iv) Rhodopseudomonas

Codes

	A	B	C	D
(a)	4-(i)	3-(iii)	1-(iv)	3-(ii)
(b)	4-(i)	3-(ii)	2-(iii)	1-(iv)
(c)	1-(ii)	2-(i)	3-(iv)	4-(iii)
(d)	4-(iii)	3-(iv)	2-(i)	1-(ii)

34. Read the following statements and mark them as True(T)/False(F).

I. The cell wall strengthening material in a bacterial cell is murein.
II. The food reserve present in a bacterial cell is starch and maltose.
III. The ribosomes present are of 70S type.
IV. The mesosome helps in sexual reproduction.

	I	II	III	IV		I	II	III	IV
(a)	T	F	T	F	(b)	F	T	T	F
(c)	T	T	F	T	(d)	F	T	T	F

35. Match the following Columns.

	Column I		Column II
A.	Actinomycetes	1.	*Streptomyces*
B.	Enterobacteria	2.	*Salmonella*
C.	Spirochaetes	3.	*Treponema*
D.	Chemoautotroph	4.	*Nitrosomonas*

Codes

	A	B	C	D
(a)	4	3	2	1
(b)	1	2	3	4
(c)	3	4	1	2
(d)	2	1	4	3

36. Match the following Columns.

	Column I		Column II
A.	Archaebacteria	1.	Do not possess photosynthetic pigments
B.	Mesosomes	2.	Atrichous
C.	Pili	3.	More prominent in Gram negative bacteria
D.	Cocci bacteria	4.	One or two per cell
E.	Chemosynthetic	5.	Lack peptidoglycan in cell wall bacteria

Codes

	A	B	C	D	E
(a)	5	3	4	2	1
(b)	1	2	3	4	5
(c)	4	2	1	3	5
(d)	5	4	3	2	1

37. Match the following Columns.

	Column I		Column II
A.	Syphilis	1.	*Acetobacter*
B.	Pathogen of Cattle	2.	*Agrobacterium*
C.	Crown gall of apple	3.	*Corynebacterium*
D.	Diphtheria	4.	*Mycobacterium*
		5.	*Treponema*

Codes

	A	B	C	D
(a)	3	1	4	2
(b)	5	4	2	3
(c)	5	3	2	1
(d)	2	4	5	3

38. Choose the incorrect match.
(a) Sarcomastigophora – *Euglena*
(b) Sporozoa – *Plasmodium*
(c) Cnidospora – *Myxidium*
(d) Ciliophora – *Monocystis*

39. Choose the correct option for the part labelled A-E of the given figure of *Trypanosoma*.

	A	*B*	*C*	*D*	*E*
(a)	Attached Flagella	Nucleus	Food granule	Endo-plasm	Endoplasm
(b)	Undulating membrane	Blepharoplast	Pellicle	Ecto-plasm	Kenetoplast
(c)	Free flagellum	Blepharoplast	Kinetoplast	Endo-plasm	Pellicle
(d)	Free flagellum	Nucleus	Kinetoplast	Pellicle	Food granule

40. Which is an incorrect combination?
(a) Haemocyanin – Prawn
(b) Haemocyanin – RBC
(c) Haemoglobin in plasma – *Pheretima*
(d) Haemozoin – *Plasmodium* cytoplasm

41. Choose the incorrect match
(a) *Trypanosoma rhodensia* – East African sleeping sickness
(b) *T. cruzi* – Chaga's disease
(c) *T. brucei* – South American sleeping sickness
(d) *T. evansi* – Surra disease

42. Match the following Columns.

	Column I		Column II
A.	Protozoan	1.	*Gonyaulax*
B.	Bacillariophyceae	2.	Diatoms
C.	Euglenoid	3.	*Paramecium*
D.	Dinoflagellates	4.	*Euglena*

Codes:

	A	B	C	D		A	B	C	D
(a)	2	3	4	1	(b)	4	2	3	1
(c)	1	3	2	4	(d)	3	2	4	1

43. Match the following Columns.

	Column I (Structures)		Column II (Features)
A.	Magna form	1.	Precystic stage of Entamoeba.
B.	Minuta form	2.	Most active form of Entamoeba.
C.	Trophozoite	3.	Infective stage of *Entamoeba histolytica*.
D.	Tetranucleate cyst	4.	The normal trophozoites in *Entamoeba histolytica*.

Codes

	A	B	C	D		A	B	C	D
(a)	1	2	3	4	(b)	4	1	3	2
(c)	4	1	2	3	(d)	3	4	1	2

44. Match the following Columns.

Column I (Type of pseudopodia)	Column II (Protozoan species)
A. Lobopodia	1. Euglypha
B. Filopodia	2. *Globigerina* (Forminiferans)
C. Reticulopodia	3. Amoeba
D. Axopodia	4. *Actinophyrus*

Codes

	A	B	C	D
(a)	3	1	2	4
(b)	4	3	2	1
(c)	1	2	3	4
(d)	2	4	1	3

45. Match the following Columns.

Column I	Column II
A. Dinoflagellate	1. *Dicyostelium*
B. *Plasmodium*	2. *Noctiluca*
C. Myxomycota	3. Slime mould
D. Acrasiomycota	4. *Fuligo*

Codes

	A	B	C	D
(a)	3	2	1	4
(b)	1	4	3	2
(c)	2	3	4	1
(d)	4	3	1	2

46. Match the following Columns.

Column I	Column II
A. *Entamoeba histolytic*	1. Cytozoic parasite
B. *Plamodium*	2. Coelozoic parasite
C. *Wuchereria*	3. Rhabditiform larva
D. Extraintestinal migration	4. Monogenic parasite
	5. Lymphadenitis

Codes

	A	B	C	D
(a)	4	2	1	3
(b)	4	1	5	3
(c)	5	1	2	3
(d)	4	2	5	1

47. Which of the following is not matched correctly?

(a) *Anobaena* – Cyanobacteria
(b) *Amoeba* – Protozoa
(c) *Gonyaulax* – Dinoflagellated
(d) *Thermoacidophiles* – Archaebacteria
(e) *Albugo* – Chrysophytes

48. Match the following Columns.

Column I	Column II
A. *E. histolytica*	1. Kala-azar
B. *E. gingivalis*	2. Sleeping sickness
C. *P. vivax*	3. Amoebic dysentery
D. *T. gambiense*	4. Malaria
	5. Pyorrhoea

Codes

	A	B	C	D
(a)	4	3	2	1
(b)	3	4	5	1
(c)	3	5	4	2
(d)	3	5	2	1

49. Match the Columns I with coloumn II & choose the correct option.

Column I	Column II
A. Rhizopus	(i) Basidiomyates
B. Penicillium	(ii) Euarotimyates
C. Ustilago	(iii) Deuteromyates
D. Alternaria	(iv) Phyomycetes

(a) A – (i); B–(ii); C–(i); D–(iii)
(b) A – (ii); B–(i); C–(iv); D–(iii)
(c) A – (iv); B–(i); C–(iii); D–(ii)
(d) A – (iii); B–(ii); C–(iv); D–(i)

Solutions

1. (a) **2.** (b) **3.** (b) **4.** (d) **5.** (a)
6. (a) **7.** (a) **8.** (c) **9.** (b) **10.** (d)
11. (b) **12.** (a) **13.** (a) **14.** (d) **15.** (b)
16. (a) **17.** (c) **18.** (c) **19.** (d) **20.** (e)
21. (c) **22.** (a) **23.** (b) **24.** (c) **25.** (c)
26. (a) **27.** (a) **28.** (b) **29.** (a) **30.** (d)
31. (b) **32.** (d) **33.** (b) **34.** (a) **35.** (b)
36. (a) **37.** (b) **38.** (d) **39.** (c) **40.** (d)
41. (c) **42.** (d) **43.** (c) **44.** (a) **45.** (c)
46. (d) **47.** (e) **48.** (c) **49.** (c)

CHAPTER

Plant Kingdom

1. Match the following Columns.

Column I	Column II
A. Largest ovules	1. *Cannabis sativa*
B. *Cuscutta*	2. *Papaver sominiferum*
C. *Drosera*	3. *Cycas*
D. Morphine	4. Carnivorous plant
E. Opium	5. Parasitic plant

Codes

	A	B	C	D	E
(a)	3	5	4	1	2
(b)	1	3	2	4	5
(c)	3	2	1	5	4
(d)	4	2	1	3	5

2. Match the following Columns.

Column I	Column II
A. Cycadales	1. Vesseles present
B. Cycadofilicales	2. *Zamia*
C. Ginkgoals	3. Extinct genera
D. Gnetales	4. Single living species

Codes

	A	B	C	D		A	B	C	D
(a)	2	3	4	1	(b)	3	2	1	4
(c)	4	2	3	1	(d)	1	2	3	4

3. Match the following Columns.

Column I	Column II
A. Protonema	1. Numerous neck canal cell in the capsule
B. Columella	2. Bryophyte of economic importance
C. Sphagnum	3. Haploid structrue of Funaria
D. Funaria	4. Middle sterile region in moss capsul

Codes

	A	B	C	D
(a)	1	2	3	4
(b)	3	4	2	1
(c)	1	2	4	3
(d)	3	2	1	4

4. Match the following column with correct combination.

Column I	Column II
A. Anthoceros	1. Alga
B. *Adiantum*	2. Hornwort
C. *Sargassum*	3. Gametophyte
D. Prothallus	4. Inferae
E. Asthallus	5. Walking fern

Codes

	A	B	C	D	E
(a)	2	5	1	3	4
(b)	5	4	3	2	1
(c)	5	1	2	4	3
(d)	3	2	1	5	4

5. Match the following Columns.

Column I	Column II
A. Liverworts	1. *Funaria*
B. Hornworts	2. *Anthoceros*
C. Mosses	3. *Riccia*
D. Gnetales	4. *Ephedra*

Codes

	A	B	C	D
(a)	4	1	2	3
(b)	3	1	2	4
(c)	3	2	1	4
(d)	2	1	3	4

6. Match each term with its definition and choose your answer from the codes given:

I. Isogamy	1. The union of two gametes
II. Syngamy	2. Two gametes, one larger than the other
III. Heterogamy	3. Two kinds of gametes, one motile and other non motile
IV. Anisogamy	4. Two kinds of morphologically distinct gametes
V. Oogamy	5. Both gametes morphologically indistinguishable

Codes

	I	II	III	IV	V
(a)	1	2	3	4	5
(b)	4	1	2	3	4
(c)	5	1	2	4	3
(d)	3	1	2	4	5

7. Match Column-I with Column-II and select the correct option from the codes given below.

Column-I	Column-II
A. Psilopsida	(i) ***Psilotum***
B. Lycopsida	(ii) ***Equisetum***
C. Sphenopsida	(iii) ***Selaginella***
D. Pteropsida	(iv) ***Dryopteris***

(a) A-(i), B-(ii), C-(iii), D-(iv)
(b) A-(i), B-(iv), C-(iii), D-(ii)
(c) A-(i), B-(iii), C-(ii), D-(iv)
(d) A-(i), B-(iii), C-(iv), D-(ii)

8. Select the mismatched pair.
(a) Smallest angiosperm – *Rafflesia*
(b) Tallest angiosperm – *Eucalyptus regnans*
(c) Marine angiosperms – *Zostera, Thalassia*
(d) Angiosperm with smallest seed – Orchid

9. Which is the correct combination ?

Column-I	Column-II
(A) Agar	(I) Single cell protein, use as food supplements by space travellers
(B) Algin	(II) Red algae
(C) Carrageen	(III) Brown algae
(D) *Chlorella and Spirullina*	(IV) *Gelidium, Gracilaria*

(a) A → I; B → II; C → III; D → IV
(b) A → IV; B → III; C → II; D → I
(c) A → II; B → I; C → III; D → IV
(d) A → III; B → II; C → I; D → IV

10. Match the following

Column-I (Classes)	Column-II (Examples)
(A) Psilotopsida	(I) *Dryopteris, Pteris, Adiantum*
(B) Lycopsida	(II) *Equisetum*
(C) Sphenopsida	(III) *Selaginella*
(D) Pteropsida	(IV) *Lycopodium*
	(V) *Psilotum*

(a) A → V; B → III; C → II; D → I
(b) A → I; B → II; C → III; D →! IV
(c) A → IV; B → III; C → II; D → I
(d) A → III; IV; B → V; C → I; D → II

11.

Column-I	Column-II
(A) Haplontic life cycle	(I) Bryophytes, Pteridophytes, *Ectocarpus, Polysiphonia*, kelps
(B) Diplontic life cycle	(II) Seed bearing plants (Gymnosperm and Angiosperm), *Fucus*
(C) Haplo-diplontic life cycle	(III) Many algae (*Volvox, Spyrogyra*, and some species of *Chlamydomonas*)

Which is the correct combination ?

(a) A → III; B → II; C → I

(b) A → I; B → II; C → III

(c) A → II; B → I; C → III

(d) A → III; B → I; C → II

12. Match items in Column I with those in Column II :

Column -I	Column -II
(I) Peritrichous flagellation	(J) *Ginkgo*
(II) Living fossil	(K) *Macrocystis*
(III) Rhizophore	(L) *Escherichia coli*
(IV) Smallest flowering plant	(M) *Selaginella*
(V) Largest perennial alga	(N) *Wolffia*

Select the correct answer from the following:

(a) I-L; II-J; III-M; IV-N; V-K;

(b) I-K; II-J; III-L; IV-M; V-N

(c) I-N; II-L; III-K; IV-N; V-J;

(d) I-J; II-K; III-N; IV-L; V-K

Solutions

1. (a) 2. (a) 3. (b) 4. (a) 5. (c)
6. (c) 7. (c) 8. (a) 9. (b) 10. (a)
11. (a) 12. (a)

CHAPTER

Animal Kingdom

1. Match the following Columns.

	Column I (Phylum)		**Column II** (Level of organisation)
A.	Porifera	1.	Cell tissue
B.	Protozoa	2.	Protoplasmic
C.	Cnidaria	3.	Organ system
D.	Chordata	4.	Cellular

Codes

	A	B	C	D
(a)	4	2	1	3
(b)	2	3	4	1
(c)	4	3	2	1
(d)	3	2	4	1

2. Match the follwoing Columns.

	Column I (Cells)		**Column II** (Functions)
A.	Epitheliomuscular cells	1.	Totipotent
B.	Glandular eclls	2.	Unique cells of phylum-Coelenterata
C.	Interstitial cells	3.	Main cells of epidermis with the ability of contraction
D.	Cnidoblats	4.	Secretion
E.	Sensory cells	5.	Condition of stimulus

Codes

	A	B	C	D	E
(a)	3	4	1	2	5
(b)	1	2	3	4	5
(c)	5	4	3	2	1
(d)	4	3	2	1	5

3. Match the following Columns.

	Column I		**Column II**
A.	10 hooked larva	1.	Sponges
B.	Acetabulum	2.	*Hydra*
C.	Stinging cells	3.	*Planaria*
		4.	*Ascaris*

Codes

	A	B	C
(a)	3	1	2
(b)	3	1	4
(c)	3	4	1
(d)	3	2	4

4. Match the following columns.

	Column I		**Column II**
A.	*Fasciola hepatica*	1.	Sheep liver fluke
B.	*Fasciola gigantica*	2.	Cattle liver fluke
C.	*Fasciolopsis buski*	3.	Intestinal fluke
D.	*Schistosoma mansoni*	4.	Human blood fluke

Codes

	A	B	C	D
(a)	1	4	3	2
(b)	1	2	3	4
(c)	4	1	2	3
(d)	3	2	1	4

5. Match the following Columns.

	Column I (Symmetry)		**Column II** (Phylum)
A.	Asymmetry	1.	Arthropoda
B.	Radial symmetry	2.	Ctenophora
C.	Biradila symmetry	3.	Cnidarai
D.	Bilateral symmetry	4.	Porifera

Codes

	A	B	C	D
(a)	4	2	3	1
(b)	2	3	4	1
(c)	3	2	4	1
(d)	4	3	2	1

6. Match the following Columns.

Column I (Phylum)	Column II (Body cavity)
A. Platyhelminthes	1. Enterocoel
B. Nematoda	2. No body cavity
C. Annelida	3. Pseudocoel
D. Echinodermata	4. Schizocoel

Codes

	A	B	C	D
(a)	4	2	3	1
(b)	2	3	4	1
(c)	4	3	2	1
(d)	3	2	4	1

7. Match the following Columns.

Column I	Column II
A. Mollusca	1. Prawn
B. Annelida	2. *Pila*
C. Arthropoda	3. Earthworm
D. Plathelminthes	4. *Fasciola*

Codes

	A	B	C	D		A	B	C	D
(a)	1	3	4	2	(b)	2	3	1	4
(c)	1	2	3	4	(d)	4	3	2	1

8. Match the following Columns.

Column I	Column II
A. Incomplete digetive system	1. Sponges
B. Cellular level of organisation	2. Coelentrates
C. Radial symmetry	3. Annelids
D. Pseudocoelomate	4. Platyhelminthes
E. Metamerism	5. Aschelminthes

Codes

	A	B	C	D	E
(a)	3	4	1	2	5
(b)	4	5	2	3	1
(c)	4	1	2	5	3
(d)	1	2	3	4	5
(e)	2	3	4	1	5

9. Match the Columns with reference to *Taenia*.

Column I	Column II
A. Mehlis' glands	1. Tegument formation
B. Vitelline gland	2. Osmoregulation and exceretion
C. Mesenchymal cells	3. Lubricate passage of capsules into uterus
D. Flame cells	4. Secretion of embryophore
	5. Capsule formation around zygote

Codes

	A	B	C	D		A	B	C	D
(a)	3	5	1	2	(b)	3	5	2	4
(c)	5	1	2	4	(d)	4	3	1	2

10. Match the following Columns.

Column I	Column II
A. Organ level	1. *Pheretima*
B. Cellular aggregate level	2. *Fasciola*
C. Tissue level	3. *Spongilla*
D. Organ system level	4. *Obelia*

Codes

	A	B	C	D		A	B	C	D
(a)	4	3	1	2	(b)	4	2	3	1
(c)	2	4	3	1	(d)	2	3	4	1

11. Match the following Columns.

Column I	Column II
A. *Physalia*	1. Sea anemone
B. *Meandrina*	2. Brain coral
C. *Gorgonia*	3. Sea fan
D. *Adamsia*	4. Portuguese man of war

Codes

	A	B	C	D		A	B	C	D
(a)	3	2	1	4	(b)	4	3	2	1
(c)	4	2	3	1	(d)	2	3	4	1
(e)	1	2	3	4					

12. Which one of the following phyla is correctly matched with its two general characteristics?

(a) Chordata – Notochord at some stages and separate anal and urinary openings to the outside

(b) Mollusca – Normally oviparous and development through a trochophore or veliger larva

(c) Arthropoda – Body divided into head, thorax and abdomen; and respiration by tracheae

(d) Echinodermata – Pentamerous radial symmetry and mostly internal fertilisation

13. Match the following Columns.

Column I	Column II
A. Nucleated RBCs	1. Aves
B. Sweat glands	2. Mammary glands
C. Carnivora	3. Dogs, cats, tigers
D. Cetacea	4. Aquatic mammals

Codes

	A	B	C	D
(a)	1	2	3	4
(b)	4	3	2	1
(c)	3	2	1	4
(d)	1	2	4	3

14. Match the following Columns.

Column I (Birds)	Column II (Type of beak)	Column III (Type of feet)
A. Duck	(i) Tearing and piercing	1. Raptorial
B. Sparrow	(ii) Water straining	2. Swimming
C. Owl	(iii) Seed eating	3. Perching
	(iv) Spatulate	4. Wading

Codes

	A	B	C
(a)	(iii), 3	(iv), 2	(ii), 4
(b)	(ii), 4	(iii), 3	(iv), 1
(c)	(i), 4	(iv), 1	(iii), 3
(d)	(ii), 2	(iii), 3	(i), 1

15. Identify and select the correct match in the Column I, II and III.

	Column I	Column II	Column III
(a)	Earthworm	Annelida	Superclass
(b)	Frog	Rana	Species
(c)	Lancelet	Vertebrata	Division
(d)	Walrus	Mammalia	Class

16. Match the following Columns.

Column I	Column II
A. Ostracodermi	1. Lobe finned fishes
B. Coelacanth	2. *Exocoetus*
C. Cyclostomes	3. Extinct jawless fibres
D. Osteichthyes	4. Hagfish

Codes

	A	B	C	D
(a)	3	1	4	2
(b)	2	3	1	4
(c)	1	3	2	4
(d)	3	2	4	1

17. Match the following list of animals with their level of organisation and choose the correct sequence.

Column I	Column II
A. Organ level	(p) *Pheretima*
B. Cellular aggregate level	(q) *Fasciola*
C. Tissue level	(r) *Spongilla*
D. Organ system level	(t) *Obleia*

(a) A-(s), B-(r), C-(p), D-(q)

(b) A-(s), B-(q), C-(r), D-(p)

(c) A-(q), B-(s), C-(r), D-(p)

(d) A-(q), B-(r), C-(s), D-(p)

18. Match the following and select the correct answer.

Column I	Column II
A. Choanocytes	1. Platyhelminthes
B. Cnidoblasts	2. Ctenophora
C. Flame cells	3. Porifera
D. Nephridia	4. Coelenterata
E. Comb plates	5. Annelida

(a) A-2, B-1, C-4, D-5, E-3
(b) A-2, B-4, C-1, D-5, E-3
(c) A-5, B-1, C-3, D-2, E-4
(d) A-3, B-4, C-1, D-5, E-2
(e) A-3, B-1, C-4, D-5, E-2

19. Match the following and choose the correct option.

(i) *Physalia*	A. Sea anemone
(ii) *Meandrina*	B. Brain coral
(iii) *Gorgonia*	C. Sea fan
(iv) *Adamsia*	D. Portuguese man-of-war

(a) (i)-C; (ii)-B; (iii)-A; (iv)-D
(b) (i)-D; (ii)-C; (iii)-B; (iv)-A
(c) (i)-D; (ii)-B; (iii)-C; (iv)-A
(d) (i)-B; (ii)-C; (iii)-A; (iv)-D
(e) (i)-A; (ii)-B; (iii)-C; (iv)-D

20. Match Column I with Column II and choose the correct answer.

Column I	Column II
I. Incomplete digestive system	A. Sponges
II. Cellular levle of organisation	B. Coelenterates
III. Radial symmetry	C. Annelids
IV. Pseudocoelomate	D. Platyhelminthes
V. Metamerism	E. Aschelminthes

(a) I - C, II - D, III - A, IV - B, V - E
(b) I - D, II - E, III - B, IV - C, V - A
(c) I - D, II - A, III - B, IV - D, V - C
(d) I - A, II - B, III - C, IV - D, V - E
(e) I - B, II - C, III - D, IV - A, V - E

21. Which one of the following groups of 3 animals each is correctly matched with their one characteristic morphological features?

Animals	Morphological features
(a) Centipede, Prawn, Sea urchin	– Jointed appendages
(b) Cockroach, Locust, *Taenia*	– Metameric segmentation
(c) Scorpion, Spider, Cockroach	– Ventral solid nerve cord
(d) Liver fluke, Sea anemone, Sea cucumber	– Bilateral symmetry

22. Choose the correct pair.

(a) Radial symmetry – Coelenterates
(b) Coelomates – Aschelminthes
(c) Metamerism – Molluscs
(d) Triploblastic – Sponges
(e) Metagenesis – Echinoderms

23. Match Column I with Column II and Column III. Choose the correct option.

Column I	Column II	Column III
1. Cnidocytes	A. *Ctenoplana*	(i) Balancing
2. Statocyst	B. *Fasciola*	(ii) Defence
3. Radula	C. *Pennatula*	(iii) Feeding
4. Flame cells	D. *Locusta*	(iv) Locomotion
5. Comb plates	E. *Pila*	(v) Osmo-regulation

(a) 1-A-(ii), 2-B-(v), 3-E-(iii), 4-C-(i), 5-D-(iv)
(b) 1-A-(iii), 2-B-(iv), 3-E-(v), 4-C-(ii), 5-D-(i)
(c) 1-A-(ii), 2-B-(i), 3-E-(iii), 4-C-(v), 5-D-(iv)
(d) 1-A-(i), 2-B-(ii), 3-E-(iv), 4-C-(iii), 5-D-(v)
(e) 1-A-(ii), 2-B-(v), 3-E-(iv), 4-C-(i), 5-D-(iii)

24. Match the following organisms with respective characteristics.

(A) *Pila* (i) Flame cells
(B) *Bombyx* (ii) Comb plates
(C) *Pleurobrachia* (iii) Radula
(D) *Taenia* (iv) Malpighian tubules

Select the correct option from the following.

	(A)	(B)	(C)	(D)
(a)	(iii)	(ii)	(iv)	(i)
(b)	(iii)	(ii)	(i)	(iv)
(c)	(iii)	(iv)	(ii)	(i)
(d)	(ii)	(iv)	(iii)	(i)

25.

Organ	Phylum	Function
Parapodia	Annelida	A
B	Ctenophora	Locomotion
C	Mollusca	Rasping organ
Malpighian tubules	Arthropoda	D
Cnidoblasts	Coelenterata	E

From the above table find out the missing organ or function - A, B, C, D and E respectively.

(a) A-swimming, B-comb plates, C-radula, D-excretion, E-defence
(b) A-defence, B-radula, C-comb plates, D-excretion, E-swimming
(c) A-protection, B-parapodia, C-visceral mass, D-locomotion, E-excretion
(d) A-swimming, B-parapodis, C-comb plates, D-anchorag, E-digestion

26. In which one of the following the genus name, its two characters and its phylum are not correctly matched, whereas the remaining three are correct?

	Genus	Characters	Phylum
(a)	*Pila*	(i) Body segmented (ii) Mouth with radula	Mollusca
(b)	*Asterias*	(i) Spiny skinned (ii) Water vascular system	Echinodermata
(c)	*Sycon*	(i) Pore bearing (ii) Canal system	Porifera
(d)	*Periplaneta*	(i) Jointed appendages (ii) Chitinous exoskeleton	Arthropoda

27. Match the following genera with their respective phylum.

(1) *Ophiura* (i) Mollusca
(2) *Physalia* (ii) Platyhelminthes
(3) *Pinctada* (iii) Echinodermata
(4) *Planaria* (iv) Coelenterata

Select the correct option.

(a) (1)-(iv), (2)-(i), (3)-(iii), (4)-(ii)
(b) (1)-(iii), (2)-(iv), (3)-(i), (4)-(ii)
(c) (1)-(i), (2)-(iii), (3)-(iv), (4)-(ii)
(d) (1)-(iii), (2)-(iv), (3)-(ii), (4)-(i)

28. Select the option that correctly matches characteristic features with the group of three animals.

(a) Skeleton of spicules - *Sycon, adamsia, spongilla*
(b) Excretion by flame - *Taenia, Fasciola, Ancylostoma*
(c) Mouth contains radula - *Dentalium, Octopus, Ophiura*
(d) Jointed appendages - *Limulus, Apis, Laccifer*

29. Some salient features and phyla of organisms are given below. Select the option which shows correct combination of organism, its phylum and salient features.

(a)	*Hydra*	Coelen-terata	Bilateral symmetry	Cnidoblasts present
(b)	*Planaria*	Platyhel-minthes	Bilateral symmetry	High regeneration capacity
(c)	*Ancylo-stoma*	Annelida	Bilateral symmetry	Elongated and worm shape
(d)	*Octopus*	Mollusca	Radial symmetry	External skeleton of shell present

30. Which one of the following matching pairs is wrong?
(a) Mollusca-Pseudocoel
(b) Cnidaria-Nematocyst
(c) Annelida-Chloragogan cells
(d) Echinodermata-Water vascular system

31. Column I contains larval stages and column II contains the groups to which they belong. Match them correctly and choose the right answer.

	Column I		Column II
A.	Planula	1.	Annelida
B.	Tornaria	2.	Mollusca
C.	Trochopore	3.	Arthropoda
D.	Bipinnaria	4.	Chordata
E.	Glochidium	5.	Echinodermata
		6.	Coelenterata

(a) A-6, B-4, C-1, D-5, E-2
(b) A-2, B-5, C-1, D-4, E-6
(c) A-5, B-4, C-3, D-2, E-1
(d) A-4, B-3, C-2, D-1, E-5

32. Find the wrongly matched pair.

	Animal	–	Excretory organ/ structure
(a)	*Balanoglossus*	–	Proboscis gland
(b)	Earthworm	–	Nephridia
(c)	Grasshopper	–	Malpighian tubules
(d)	Prawn	–	Flame cells
(e)	*Amphioxus*	–	Protonephridia

33. Match the name of the animal (column I), with one characteristic (column II), and the phylum/ class (column III) to which it belongs.

	Column I	Column II	Column II
(a)	*Limulus*	Body covered by chitinous exoskeleton	Pisces
(b)	*Adamsia*	Radially	Porifera
(c)	*Petromyzan*	Ectoparasite	Cyclostomata
(d)	*Ichthyophis*	Terrestrial	Reptilia

34. Match the following and select the correct option.

A.	Cyclostomes	(1)	Hemichordata
B.	Aves	(2)	Urochordata
C.	Tunicates	(3)	Agnatha
D.	*Balanoglossus*	(4)	Pisces
E.	Osteichtyes	(5)	Tetrapod

(a) A-1, B-2, C-3, D-4, E-5
(b) A-2, B-3, C-4, D-1, E-5
(c) A-3, B-5, C-2, D-1, E-4
(d) A-3, B-1, C-5, D-2, E-4
(e) A-5, B-3, C-2, D-1, E-4

35. Choose the correct option.
(a) Mammalia – *Ornithorynchus, Macropus, Betta*
(b) Aves – *Pteropus, Neophron, Aptenodytes*
(c) Amphibia – *Ichthyophis, Hyla, Salamandra*
(d) Reptilia – *Bangarus, Pristis, Crocodylus*

36. Identify the aquatic mammal(s) from the following.
(i) *Balaenoptera*
(ii) *Equus*
(iii) *Delphinus*
(iv) *Pteropus*
(v) *Felis*
(a) (i) and (iii)
(b) (ii) and (iv)
(c) (v) only
(d) (iv) and (v)

37. Which of the following is correct?
(a) *Macropus* – Ear pinna, body hari, 4 chambered heart
(b) *Pavo* – Long bones filled with bone marrow, forelimbs modified to wings
(c) *Ichtyophis* – Eyes lack eyelids, scales present on skin
(d) *Limulus* – Chitinous exoskeleton, respiration through coxal glands

38. Which one of the following animals is correctly matched with its one characteristic and the taxon?

	Animal	Characteristic	Taxon
(a)	Millipede	Ventral nerve cord	Arachnida
(b)	Sea Anemone	Triploblastic	Cnidaria
(c)	Silver fish	Pectoral and pelvic fins	Chordata
(d)	Duck-billed platypus	Oviparous	Mammalia

39. In which one of the following the genus name, its two characters and its class/phylum are correctly matched?

	Genus name	Two charcters	Class/ Phylum
(a)	*Ascaris*	(i) Body segmented	annelida
		(ii) Males and females distince	
(b)	*Salamandra*	(i) A tympanum represents ear	amphibia
		(ii) Fertilisation is external	
(c)	*Pteropus*	(i) Skin possess hair	Mammalia
		(ii) Oviparous	
(d)	*Aurelia*	(i) Cnidoblasts	
		(ii) Organ level of organisation	

40. Identify the Phylum X.

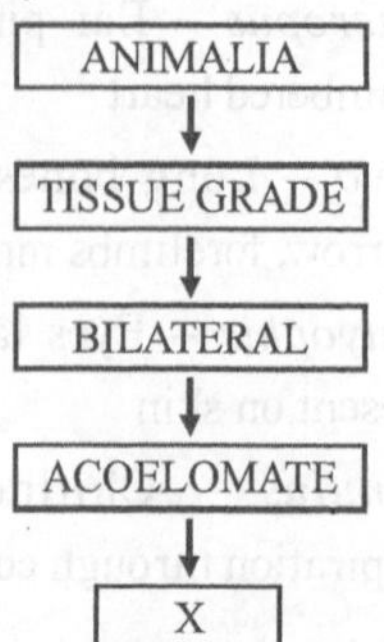

(a) Hemichordata
(b) Aschelminthes
(c) Platyhelminthes
(d) Ctenophora

41. Identify the correct sequence of classification of the following.

I. Eutheria
II. Mammalia
III. Tuhulidentata
IV. Lagomorpha
V. Hyracoidea

(a) II → IV → I → V → III
(b) II → I → IV → III → V
(c) II → I → IV → V → III
(d) I → V → III → II → IV

42. See the following figures and choose the correct option with their respective orders.

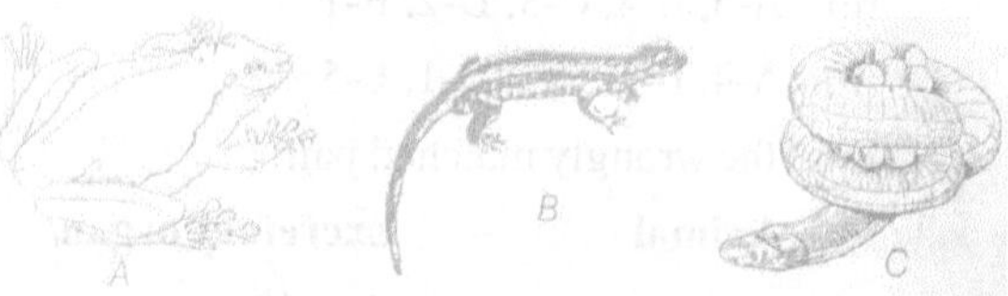

(a)	A-Caecilians	B-Caudata	C-Anura
(b)	A-Caudata	B-Anura	C-Caecilians
(c)	A-Anura	B-Caecilians	C-Caudata
(d)	A-Anura	B-Caudata	C-Caecilians

43. Choose the incorrect pair from the following.

(a) Emu-Flightless bird and confined to Australia
(b) Kiwi-National bird of New Zealand
(c) Ostrich-Wings modified into paddles (flippers)
(d) Dodo-Recently extinct bird

44. In most simple type of canal system of Porifera, water flows through which one of the following ways?

(a) Ostia → Spongocoel → Osculum → Exterior
(b) Spongocoel → Ostia → Osculum → Exterior
(c) Osculum → Spongocoel → Osita → Exterior
(d) Osculum → Ostia → Spongocoel → Exterior

Solutions

1. (a) 2. (a) 3. (a) 4. (b) 5. (a)
6. (b) 7. (b) 8. (c) 9. (a) 10. (d)
11. (c)
12. (b) Devil fish (*Octopus*) is a mollusc which can paralyse its prey by poisonous saliva. It feeds on prawns, crabs and small fishes.
13. (a) 14. (d)
15. (d) Out of the options given the correct one is walrus a large flippered marine mammal which belongs to class-Mammalia.

    Correct matches for the three options are

Earthworm	Annelida	Phylum
Frog	Rana	Genus
Lancelet	Vertebrata	Subphylum

16. (a) 17. (d) 18. (d) 19. (c) 20. (c)
21. (c) Scorpion, spider and cockroach belonging to Phylum Arthropoda, have annelidan type of nervous system which constists of a nerve ring and a solid double ventral nerve cord with gangila.
22. (a) 23. (c)
24. (c) The buccal cavity of *Pila* (apple snail) possess rasping organ, radula, with transverse row of teeth for cutting grass. *Bombyx* (silk moth), an insect has Malpighian tubules, as excretory organ. *Pleurobrachia* is a ctenophore having eight ciliary plates called comb plates. *Taenia* is a platyhelminth having flame cells for excretion and osmoregulation.
25. (a)
26. (a) *Pila* belongs to phylum Mollusca. The body of molluscs (soft bodied animals) is unsegmented, with a distinct head, muscular foot and visceral hump. Buccal cavity of *Pila*, contains a brownish, curved, ribbon - like structure called radula. Radula acts as a rasping organ.
27. (b)
28. (d) In poriferans, the body is supported by a skeleton made up of spicules or spongin fibres. *Sycon* and *Spongilla* are examples of poriferans, whereas *Adamsia* is a coelenterate. In platyhelminths, specialised cells called flame cells help in excretion. *Taenia* and *Fasciola* are platyhelminths whereas *Ancylostoma* is an aschelminth. In molluscs, mouth contains a file-like rasping organ for feeding called radula. *Dentalium* and *Octopus* are molluscs whereas *Ophiura* is an echinoderm. Arthropods have jointed appendages. *Limulus*, *Apis* and *Laccifer* all three are arthropods.
29. (b) *Hydra* shows radial symmetry, *Ancylostoma* is an aschelminth. *Octopus* shows bilateral symmetry and also lacks an external skeleton of shell.
30. (a) Molluscs coelomates, i.e., possess true coelom. In molluscs, coelom, a body cavity develops as a split in the mesoderm sheet and is filled with coelomic fluid.
31. **None of the options is correct.**

    Planula – Coelentrata

    Tornaria – Hemichordata

    (This was earlier considered as a sub-phylum under phylum chordata. But now it is placed as a separate phylum under non-chordata).

    Trochophore – Annelida

    Bipinnaria – Echinodermata

    Glochidium – Mollusca
32. (d) Prawn is an Arthropod and have green glands or Malpighian tubules as excretory organs. Flame cells are excretory organs of Platyhelminthes.
33. (c) *Limulus* belongs to Phylum Arthropoda. *Adamsia* belongs to Phylum Coelenterata. *Petromyzon* (lamprey) (Cyclostomata) is a sanguivorous ectoparasite of larger fishes. *Ichthyophis* is a limbless amphibian and belongs to class Amphibia.

34. **(c)**

35. **(c)** *Betta* belongs to Class Osteichthyes, *Pteropus* belongs to class Mammalia, *Pristis* belongs to class chondrichthyes and Bangarus belongs to class *Reptilia.*

36. **(a)** **37.** **(a)**

38. **(d)** Duck-billed platypus is oviparous and belongs to Class Mammalia. Millipede belongs to class Diplopoda. Sea anemone has two germ layers, *i.e.*, they are diploblastic. Silverfish (*Lepisma*) belongs to Non-chordata. It is an insect.

39. **None of the optios is correct**

Ascaris is member of Phylum Nemotoda, which are round worms. They do not have segmented body. In *Ascaris* female is longer than male.

Salamandra is member of amphibia. Salamanders do not have tympanum, although they have greatly reduced middle ears and fertilisation is usually internal in them.

Pteropus is member of Class Mammalia. They are viviparous a mantle of golden hair covers the head, neck and shoulders in *Pteropus*.

Aurelia is member of coelenterata, which has tissue level of organisation. Its epidermis contain cnidoblasts (stinging cells) for defence and offence purpose.

40. **None of the options is correct.**

Hemichordata, Aschelminthes and Platyhelminthes show organ system level of organisation, *i.e.*, organs get associated to form functional systems, each system concerned with a specific physiology function. Ctenophores have tissue grade level of organisation but are biradially symmetrical, *i.e.*, (radial + bilateral)

41. **(b)** **42.** **(d)** **43.** **(c)** **44.** **(a)**

CHAPTER

Morphology of Flowering Plants

1. Match the column A (type of root) with column B (example of plants)

Column A	Column B
I. Tap roots	1. Maize
II. Fibrous roots	2. Mustard
	3. Wheat
	4. Sugarcane
	5. Neem

(a) I-2, 4 and II-1, 3, 5
(b) I-2, 5 and II-1, 3, 4
(c) I-2, 5 and II-1, 3
(d) I-5 and II-1, 2, 3, 4

2. Match the column I with column II and choose the correct options

Column I	Column II
A. Storage roots	1. *Taeniophyllum*
B. Pneumatophores	2. *Avicennia*
C. Haustoria	3. Carrot
D. Prop roots	4. Cuscuta
E. Assimilatory roots	5. Banyan

(a) A-3, B-2, C-4, D-5, E-1
(b) A-2, B-3, C-4, D-5, E-1
(c) A-3, B-4, C-5, D-1, E-2
(d) A-3, B-1, C-2, D-5, E-4

3. Match the column and find out the correct combination:

A. Storage	1. *Taeniophyllum*
B. Pneumatophores	2. *Avicennia*
C. Haustoria	3. Carrot
D. Prop roots	4. *Cuscuta*
E. Assimilatory roots	5. Banyan

(a) A-3, B-2, C-4, D-5, E-1
(b) A-2, B-3, C-4, D-5, E-1
(c) A-3, B-4, C-5, D-1, E-2
(d) A-3, B-1, C-2, D-5, E-4

4. Match the following columns and choose the correct options:

	Position of modified root	Genus	Function
A.	Underground	Turnip	Photosynthesis
B.	Aerial	*Taeniophyllum*	Liliaceae
C.	Aerial	*Vanda*	Respiration
D.	Underground	*Asparagus*	Storage

(a) A and B
(b) B and C
(c) B and D
(d) A and C

5. Which of the following pair is not correct?

Column I	Column II
A. Stem tendril	(1) Grapes
B. Leaf bladder	(2) *Gloriosa*
C. Leaf tendril	(3) Pea
D. Phyllode	(4) *Australian acacia*

6. Match the columns and find out the correct combination:

A. Opuntia	1. Stem thorns
B. Asparagus	2. Phyllocaldes
C. Citrus	3. Cladodes

(a) A-1, B-2, C-3
(b) A-2, B-3, C-1
(c) A-3, B-2, C-1
(d) A-2, B-1, C-3

7. Match the columns and find out the correct combination:

A. Horizontally growing underground stem	1. *Amorphophallus*
B. Obliquely growing underground stem	2. *Curcuma*
C. Reduced disc like stem	3. *Allium cepa*
D. Vertically growing underground stem with special adventitious roots americana	4. *Chrysanthemum*
	5. *Agave americana*

(a) A-2, B-4, C-3, D-5
(b) A-1, B-2, C-3, D-5
(c) A-2, B-4, C-3, D-1
(d) A-1, B-4, C-3, D-2

8. Match the columns and find out the correct combination:

A.	*Pistia*	Single internodal branch	Offset
B.	*Oxalis*	Many nodes and internodes	Runner
C.	*Pistia*	Bulged internode	Stem tuber
D.	Sweet potato	Nodes bear eyes	Tuberous stem

(a) A & B (b) C & D
(c) B & C (d) A & B

9. Match the column I with column II and choose the correct option:

Column I	Column II
A. Largest flower	1. *Rafflesia*
B. Zygomorphic flower	2. *Brassica*
C. Actinomorphic flower	3. *Pisum*
D. Asymmetric flower	4. *Capsicum*
	5. *Cana*

	A	B	C	D		A	B	C	D
(a)	1	3	2	5	(b)	5	3	2	1
(c)	2	3	1	5	(d)	3	1	2	4

10. Which of the following option is correct?

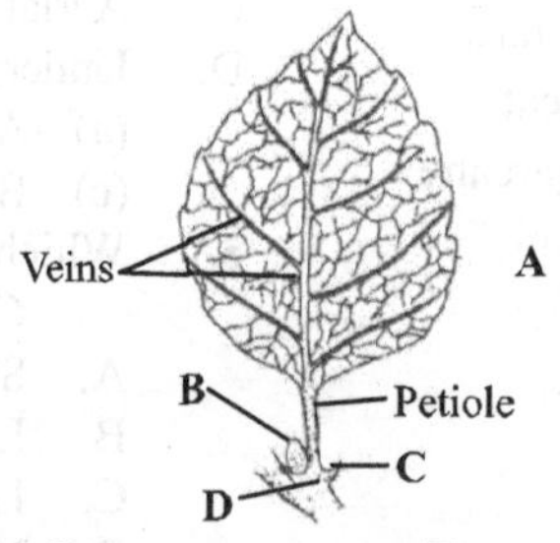

	A	B	C	D
(a)	Lamina	Axillary bud	Stipule	Leaf base
(b)	Lamina	Stipule	Axillary bud	Leaf base
(c)	Lamina	Axillary bud	Stipule	Pedicel
(d)	Leaflet	Axillary bud	Stipule	Leaf base

11. Chosse the correct combinations.

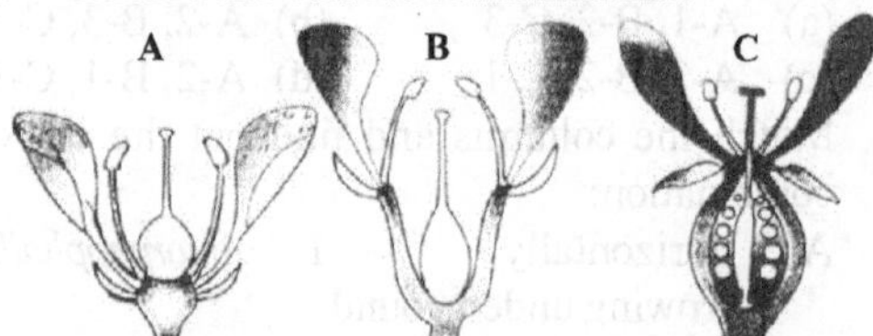

I. Hypogynous flower
II. Perigynous flower
III. Epigynous flower

(a) A-I, B-II, C-III
(b) A-I, B-III, C-II
(c) A-III, B-II, C-I
(d) A-III, B-I, C-II

12. Which is the correct combination?

Column I	Column II	Column III
A. Mariginal	I.	p. Sunflower, Marigold
B. Axile	II.	q. Dianthus, Primrose
C. Parietal	III.	r. Musatrd, Argemone

D. Free Central IV. 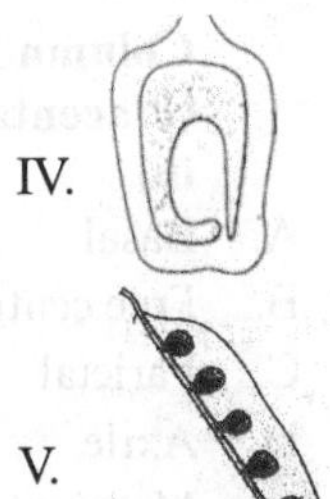 s. China rose, Tomato, Lemon

E. Basal V. t. Pea

(a) A- V, t; B -II, s; C -I, r; D -III, q; E -IV, p
(b) A - I, t; B - II, s; C - III, r; D - IV, p; E - V, q
(c) A - V, p; B - II, s; C - I, q; D - III, r; E - IV, t
(d) A - V, p; B - III, q; C - II, s; D - I, t; E - IV, r

13. Which one of the following option is correct?

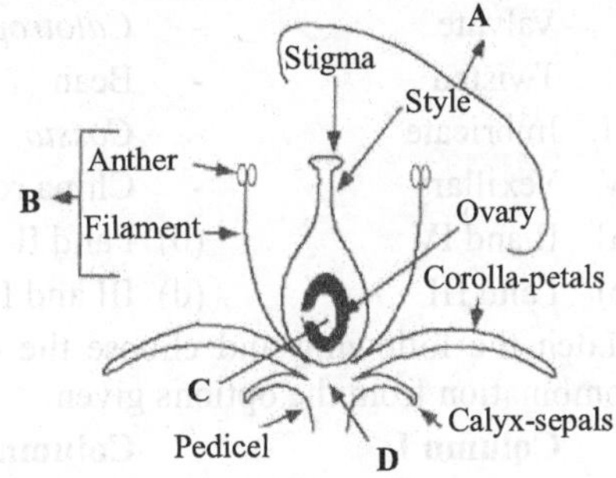

	A	B	C	D
(a)	Gynoecium	Megasporo-phyll	Ovule	Thalamus
(b)	Gynoecium	Stamen	Seed	Thalamus
(c)	Microsporo-phyll	Stamen	Ovule	Thalamus
(d)	Gynoecium	Stamen	Ovule	Thalamus

14. Matching the following and choose the correct option

	Column I		Column II
A.	Bud in the	I.	Pitcher plant axil of leaf and Venus fly trap
B.	Outer layer of	II.	Cacti seed coat
C.	Spines	III.	Testa (modified leaves)
D.	Leaves modiied	IV.	Simple leaf to catch insects
E.	Fleshy leaves	V.	Garlic and onion with stored food

	A	B	C	D	E
(a)	I	II	III	IV	V
(b)	V	IV	III	II	I
(c)	IV	III	II	I	V
(d)	IV	II	III	I	V

15. Choose the correct combinations.

	Column I		Column II
A.	Gamosepalous	I.	Flower of lily
B.	Polysepalous	II.	Sterile anther
C.	Gamopetalous	III.	Free petals
D.	Polypetalous	IV.	Free sepals
E.	Epiphyllous	V.	Fused petals
F.	Staminode	VI.	Fused sepals

	A	B	C	D	E	F
(a)	IV	V	III	I	VI	II
(b)	IV	V	III	I	II	VI
(c)	VI	IV	V	III	I	II
(d)	VI	IV	V	III	II	I

16. Matching the following and choose the correct option.

	Column I		Column II
A.	Coleorrhiza	I.	Grapes
B.	Food storing tissue	II.	Mango
C.	Parthenocarpic fruit	III.	Maize
D.	Single seeded fruit developing from monocarpellary superior ovary	IV.	Radicle
E.	Membranous seed coat	V.	Endosperm

(a) A - III, B-I, C -IV, D - II, E - V
(b) A - IV, B-II, C - V, D - I, E - III
(c) A - V, B-I, C - III, D - IV, E - II
(d) A - IV, B - V, C - I, D - II, E - III

17. Which is the correct combinations ?

	Column I (Members of Fabaceae)		Column II (Economic importance)
A.	Gram, sem, moong, soyabean	I.	Medicine
B.	Soyabean, groundnut	II.	Ornamental
C.	Indigofera	III.	Fodder
D.	Sunhemp	IV.	Fibres
E.	*Sesbania, Trifolium*	V.	Dye
F.	Lupin, Sweet potato	VI.	Edible oil
E.	*Mulaaithi*	VII.	Pulses

(a) A - I, B - II, C - III, D - IV, E - V, F - VI, G - VII
(b) A-VII, B - VI, C - V, D -IV, E - III, F - II, G-I
(c) A - II, B - IV, C - VI, D - I, E - III, F - V, G - VII
(d) A - I, B - III, C - V, D - VII, E - II, F - IV, G - VI

18. Match the following and choose the correct option

	List I	List II
I.	Acicular	(A) Grass
II.	Linear	(B) *Nerium*
III.	Lanceolate	(C) Banana
IV.	Oblong	(D) Pine

(a) I-D, II-A, III-B, IV-C
(b) I-D, II-A, III-C, IV-B
(c) I-D, II-B, III-C, IV-A
(d) I-D, II-C, III-B, IV-A

19. Match column I with II and choose the right option

Column I	Column II
1. *Artemisia*	A. Fibre
2. *Astragalus*	B. Insecticide
3. *Phormium*	C. Rat poison
4. *Chrysanthemum*	D. Medicine
5. *Withania*	E. Vermifuge
	F. Gum

(a) 1 - D, 2 - C, 3 - F, 4 - B, 5 - E
(b) 1 - B, 2 - E, 3 - D, 4 - C, 5 - A
(c) 1 - C, 2 - E, 3 - A, 4 - F, 5 - D
(d) 1 - E, 2 - F, 3 - A, 4 - B, 5 - D

20. Match the following and choose the correct combination from the options given below.

	Column I (Placentation in)		Column II (Represented Types)
A.	Basal	1	*Dianthus*
B.	Free central	2	Pea
C.	Parietal	3	Lemon
D.	Axile	4	Marigold
E.	Marginal	5	*Argemone*

(a) A – 1, B – 2, C – 3, D – 4, E – 5
(b) A – 2, B – 3, C – 4, D – 5, E – 1
(c) A – 4, B – 1, C – 5, D – 3, E – 2
(d) A – 4, B – 3, C – 5, D – 1, E – 2

21. Find out the pairs, which are correctly matched with respect to aestivation of petals.

I.	Valvate	-	*Calotropis*
II.	Twisted	-	Bean
III.	Imbricate	-	*Cassia*
IV.	Vexillary	-	China rose

(a) II and IV
(b) I and II
(c) I and III
(d) III and IV

22. Match the following and choose the correct combination from the options given.

	Column I (Family)		Column II (Androecium formula)
A.	Brassicaceae	1.	A_{3+3}
B.	Fabaceae	2.	$A_{(5)}$
C.	Solanaceae	3.	$A_{(9)+1}$
D.	Liliaceae	4.	A_{2+4}

(a) A – 4; B – 3; C – 2, D – 1
(b) A – 1; B – 2; C – 3, D – 4
(c) A – 2; B – 3; C – 4, D – 1
(d) A – 3; B – 4; C – 1, D – 2

23. Match the following and choose the correct combination from the options given.

Column I (Position of floral parts on thalamus)	Column II (Represented in)
(A) Hypogynous	(1) Ray florets of sunflower
(B) Perigynous	(2) Brinjal
(C) Epigynous	(3) Peach

(a) A-2, B-1, C-3
(b) A-1, B-2, C-3
(c) A-3, B-2, C-1
(d) A-2, B-3, C-1

24. Matching the following and choose the correct option

	Column – I		Column – II
A.	Tubercular storage roots	I.	*Tinospora*
B.	Pneumatophores	II.	*Heritiera*
C.	Haustoria	III.	*Asparagus*
D.	Prop-roots	IV.	*Viscum*
E.	Assimilatory roots	V.	*Screwpine*

(a) A–II, B–III, C–IV, D–V, E–I
(b) A–III, B–IV, C–V, D–I, E–II
(c) A–III, B–I, C–II, D–V, E–IV
(d) A–III, B–II, C–IV, D–V, E–I

25. Chosse the correct combinations

	List-I		List-II
(A)	Entire leaf modified into a spine	(i)	*Clematis*
(B)	Leaf except stipules modified into a tendril	(ii)	*Citrus*
(C)	Stipules modified into a tendril	(iii)	*Euphorbia*
(D)	First leaf of axillary bud modified into a spine	(iv)	*Lathyrus*

	A	B	C	D
(a)	(iii)	(iv)	(i)	(ii)
(b)	(iii)	(i)	(iv)	(ii)
(c)	(ii)	(iii)	(i)	(iv)
(d)	(iv)	(ii)	(i)	(iii)

26. Select the correct option

	List I		List II
A.	Spike	I.	*Bougainvillea*
B.	Capitulum	II.	*Coleus*
C.	Dichasial cyme	III.	*Adhatoda*
D.	Multiparous cyme	IV.	*Zinnia*
E.	Verticillaster	V.	*Asclepias*

(a) A – III, B – IV, C – I, D – V, E – II
(b) A – III, B – I, C – IV, D – V, E – II
(c) A – II, B – IV, C – I, D – V, E – III
(d) A – IV, B – II, C – V, D – I, E – III

27. Match the following and choose the correct combination.

	Column I		Column II
A.	Pollen grains	I.	Microsporangia
B.	Pollen sacs	II.	Microspores
C.	Stamens	III.	Microsporophylls

	A	B	C
(a)	I	II	III
(b)	II	I	III
(c)	III	I	II
(d)	I	III	II

28. Choose the correct option-

	Column I		Column II
A.	Apple	I.	Outer portion of receptacle
B.	Coconut	II.	Fleshy thalamus
C.	Jack fruit	III.	Thalamus & pericarp
D.	Guava	IV.	Endosperm
E.	Pineapple	V.	Bract, perianth & seeds

(a) A – II, B – III, C – IV, D – V, E – I
(b) A – V, B – III, C – I, D – IV, E – II
(c) A – II, B – III, C – I, D – V, E – IV
(d) A – II, B – IV, C – V, D – III, E – I
(e) A – V, B – IV, C – III, D – II, E – I

29. Match the following

	List-I		List-II
(1)	Spongy aril	(I)	*Jussiaea*
(2)	Multiple epidermis	(II)	*Pistia*
(3)	Respiratory roots	(III)	*Nerium*
(4)	Root pockets	(IV)	*Sagittaria*
		(V)	*Nymphaea*

	A	B	C	D
(a)	I	III	II	V
(b)	II	I	IV	III
(c)	IV	II	III	I
(d)	V	III	I	II

30. Match the following-

	List-I		List-II
(A)	Coleorhiza	(I)	Development of sporophyte directly from gametophyte without intervention of gametes

(B) Apogamy	(II) Development of gametophyte directly from sporophyte without the involvement of reduction division.
(C) Indusium	(III) An unbranched columnar stem with a crown of leaves.
(D) Caudex	(IV) Protective covering of radicle
	(V) Protective structure of a sorus.

	A	B	C	D
(a)	V	II	IV	I
(b)	IV	I	V	III
(c)	III	V	II	IV
(d)	II	III	I	V

Solutions

1.	(b)	2.	(a)	3.	(a)	4.	(c)	5.	(b)
6.	(b)	7.	(c)	8.	(b)	9.	(a)	10.	(a)
11.	(a)	12.	(a)	13.	(d)	14.	(c)	15.	(c)
16.	(d)	17.	(b)	18.	(a)	19.	(d)	20.	(c)
21.	(c)	22.	(a)	23.	(d)	24.	(d)	25.	(a)
26.	(a)	27.	(b)	28.	(d)	29.	(d)	30.	(b)

CHAPTER

Anatomy of Flowering Plants

1. Pair the species with the type of wood.

Species		Type of wood
A. *Tectona grandis*	I	Softwood
B. *Cedrus deodara*	II	Hardwood
C. *Shorea robusta*		
D. *Dalbergia sissoo*		

	A	B	C	D
(a)	I	II	II	I
(b)	I	I	II	II
(c)	II	I	II	II
(d)	II	I	I	II

2. Match the names of the structures listed under column-I with the functions given under column-II, choose the answer which gives the correct combination of the alphabets of the two columns :

Column-I (Structure)	Column-II (Function)
A. Stomata	(i) Protection of stem
B. Bark	(ii) Plant movement
C. Cambium	(iii) Secondary growth
D. Hydathode	(iv) Transpiration
	(v) Guttation

(a) A – (v), B – (iii), C – (i), D – (iv)
(b) A – (i), B – (iv), C – (v), D – (iii)
(c) A – (ii), B – (iv), C – (i), D – (iii)
(d) A – (iv), B – (i), C – (iii), D – (v)

3. Match the following and choose the correct option

A. Cuticle	i. guard cells
B. Bulliform cells	ii. outer layer
C. Stomata	iii. waxy layer
D. Epidermis	iv. empty colourless cell

(a) A–iii, B–iv, C–i, D–ii
(b) A–i, B–ii, C–iii, D–iv
(c) A–iii, B–ii, C–iv, D–i
(d) A–iii, B–ii, C–i, D–iv

4. Match the Column I with Column II and choose the correct combination

A. Radial vascular bundle	i. *Cucurbita pepo*
B. Collateral vascular bundle	ii. *Dracaena*
C. Bicollateral vascular	iii. Root of angiosperms
D. Bundle	iv. Sunflower stem
E. Amphivasal vascular bundle	v. Fern

(a) A–iii, B–iv, C–i, D–v, E–ii
(b) A–ii, B–iii, C–i, D–v, E–iv
(c) A–iii, B–iv, C–v, D–i, E–ii
(d) A–iv, B–v, C–i, D–ii, E–iii
(e) A–iii, B–i, C–ii, D–iv, E–v

5. Match the following and choose the correct combination

A. Xylem vessels	i. Store food materials
B. Xylem tracheids	ii. Obliterated lumen

C. Xylem fibre iii. Perforated plates

D. Xylem parenchyma iv. Chisel-like ends

(a) A–iv, B–iii, C–ii, D–i

(b) A–iii, B–ii, C–i, D–iv

(c) A–iii, B–iv, C–ii, D–i

(d) A–i, B–ii, C–iii, D–iv

6. Match the followings and choose the correct option.

A. Meristem i. Photosynthesis, storage

B. Parenchyma ii. Mechanical support

C. Collenchyma iii. Actively dividing cells

D. Sclerenchyma iv. Stomata

E. Epidermal tissue v. Sclereids

(a) A–i, B–iii, C–v, D–ii, E–iv

(b) A–iii, B–i, C–ii, D–v, E–iv

(c) A–ii, B–iv, C–v, D–i, E–iii

(d) A–v, B–iv, C–iii, D–ii, E–i

7. Match the followings and choose the right combination

A. Endodermis i. Companion cells

B. Stomata ii. Lenticels

C. Sieve tube iii. Palisade cells

D. Periderm iv. Passage cells

E. Mesophyll v. Accessory cells

(a) A–iv, B–v, C–ii, D–i, E–iii

(b) A–v, B–iii, C–i, D–ii, E–iv

(c) A–iv, B–v, C–i, D–ii, E–iii

(d) A–ii, B–v, C–iii, D–iv, E–i

8. Match Column I with Column II and choose the correct option.

Column I	Column II
(A) Bulliform cells	1. Initiation of lateral roots
(B) Pericycle	2. Root
(C) Endarch xylem	3. Grasses
(D) Exarch xylem	4. Dicot leaf
(E) Bundle sheath cells	5. Stem

(a) A-3, B-5, C-4, D-1, E-2

(b) A-2, B-5, C-1, D-3, E-4

(c) A-2, B-4, C-1, D-3, E-5

(d) A-3, B-1, C-5, D-2, E-4

(e) A-5, B-4, C-2, D-1, E-3

9.

Column-I	Column-II
A. Spring wood or early wood	I. Lighter in colour
B. Autumn wood or late wood	II. Density high
	III. Density low
	IV. Darker in colour
	V. Larger number of xylem elements
	VI. Vessels with wider cavity
	VII. Lesser number of xylem elements
	VIII. Vessels with small cavity

Which of the following combination is correct?

(a) A – II, IV, VII, VIII; B – I, III, V, VI

(b) A – I, II, VII, VIII; B – III, IV, V, VI

(c) A – I, III, V, VI; B – II, IV, VII, VIII

(d) A – I, III, VII, VIII; B – II, IV, V, VI

10. Select the option with correct identification of type of tissue from which the given structure is formed:

	Hypodermis in dicot stem	Medullary rays
(a)	Parenchyma	Parenchyma
(b)	Parenchyma	Parenchyma

(c)	Parenchyma	Sclerenchyma
(d)	Sclerenchyma	Collenchyma

11. During secondary growth in stellar region of a dicot stem, many changes come in the various tissues. Select the option in which is the particular tissue is incorrectly matched with its fate:

	Tissue	Fate during secondary growth
(a)	Secondary xylem	Produced in high amount
(b)	Primary phloem	Produced in low amount
(c)	Cambial ring	Cut off secondary permanent tissue on both side
(d)	Secondary phloem	Synthesized on outer side

12. Match the following columns:

	Column I		Column II
A.	Cuticle	1.	Guard cells
B.	Bulliform cells	2.	Single layer
C.	Stomata	3.	Waxy layer
D.	Epidermis	4.	Empty colourless cell

(a) A-3, B-4, C-1, D-2 (b) A-1,B-2,C-3,D-4
(c) A-3, B-2, C-4, D-1 (d) A-3,B-2,C-1,D-4

13. Match the columns and find out the correct combination:

A.	Xylem vessels	1.	Store food material
B.	Xylem trachieds	2.	Obliterated lumen
C.	Xylem fibre	3.	Perforated plates
D.	Xylem parenchyma	4.	Chisel-like ends

(a) A-4, B-3, C-2, D-2
(b) A-3, B-2,C-1, D-4
(c) A-2,B-1, C-4,D-3
(d) A-3, B-2, C-3, D-4
(e) A-3,A-4,C-2,D-1

14. Which of the following permanent tissue is incorrectly matched with its cell wall component and function?

(a)	Collenchyma	Cellulose, hemicelluloses and pectin	Mechanical support
(b)	Sclerenchyma	Lignin	Mechanical support
(c)	Xylem vessel	Suberin	Mechanical support and condition of water
(d)	Parenchyma	Cellulose	Photosynthesis and storage

15. Which of the following meristem is correctly

(a)	Apical meristem	Shoot and root apex	Elongation of stem and root
(b)	Intercalary meristem	In between the apical meristem	Growth in grasses
(c)	Intrafasicular cambium	In the vascular bundles	Increases the girth of stem/ root
(d)	Interfascicular cambium	In between vascular bundles	Increases the girth of stem/ root

Solutions

1.	**(c)**	**2.**	**(d)**	**3.**	**(a)**	**4.**	**(a)**	**5.**	**(c)**
6.	**(b)**	**7.**	**(c)**	**8.**	**(d)**	**9.**	**(c)**	**10.**	**(a)**
11.	**(b)**	**12.**	**(a)**	**13.**	**(a)**	**14.**	**(c)**	**15.**	**(a)**

CHAPTER

Structural Organisation in Animals

1. Match the following cell structure with its characteristic feature.

(A) Tight junctions	(i)	Cement neighbouring cells toghether to form sheet
(B) Adhering Junctions	(ii)	Transmit information through chemical to another cells
(C) Gap junctions	(iii)	Establish a barrier to prevent leakage of fluid across epithelial cells
(D) Synaptic junctions	(iv)	Cytoplasmic channels to facilitate communication between adjacent cells

Select correct option from the following.

	(A)	(B)	(C)	(D)
(a)	(ii)	(iv)	(i)	(iii)
(b)	(iv)	(ii)	(i)	(iii)
(c)	(iii)	(i)	(iv)	(iii)
(d)	(iv)	(iii)	(i)	(iii)

2. Match the following.

List I	List II
(i) Squamous epithelium	A. Bone
(ii) Dense regular connective tissue	B. skin
(iii) Glandular epithelium	C. Air sacs of lungs
(iv) Specialised connective tissue	D. Tendon
(v) Dense irregular Connective tissue	E. Goblet cells

(a) (i)-B, (ii)-E, (iii)-C, (iv)-D, (v)-A
(b) (i)-C, (ii)-E, (iii)-A, (iv)-B, (v)-D
(c) (i)-C, (ii)-D, (iii)-E, (iv)-A, (v)-B
(d) (i)-E, (ii)-A, (iii)-B, (iv)-D, (v)-C
(e) (i)-D, (ii)-C, (iii)-E, (iv)-B, (v)-A

3. Choose the correctly matched pair.

(a) Inner lining of salivary ducts - Ciliated epithelium
(b) Moist surface of buccal cavity - Glandular epithelium
(c) Tubular parts of nephrons - Cuboidal epithelium
(d) Inner surface of bronchioles - Squamous epithelium

4. Choose the wrongly matched pair regarding the position of reproductive structure in earthworm.

(a) Testes - 10th and 11th segments
(b) Spermathecae - 6th to 9th segments
(c) Male genital pore - 9th segments
(d) Ovaries - Inter segmental septum of 12th and 13th segments
(e) Female genital pore - 14th segment

5. Match the following regarding the morphology of cockroach and choose the correct option.

List-I	List-II
(i) Tergites	A. Forewings
(ii) Tegmina	B. Upper lip
(iii) Hypopharynx	C. Dorsal sclerite
(iv) Labium	D. Tongue
(v) Labrum	E. Lower lip

(a) (i)-D, (ii)-E, (iii)-C, (iv)-B, (v)-A
(b) (i)-B, (ii)-C, (iii)-E, (iv)-D, (v)-A
(c) (i)-E, (ii)-A, (iii)-C, (iv)-D, (v)-B
(d) (i)-C, (ii)-A, (iii)-D, (iv)-E, (v)-B
(e) (i)-C, (ii)-B, (iii)-E, (iv)-A, (v)-D

6. Match the columns.

	Column I		Column II
A.	Squamus	1.	Intestinal glands
B.	Cuboidal	2.	Trachea
C.	Columnar	3.	Ovary
D.	Ciliated	4.	Blood vessels
E	Pseudostratified	5.	Bronchioles

(a) A - 5, B - 4, C - 2, D - 1, E - 3
(b) A - 4, B - 3, C - 1, D - 5, E - 2
(c) A - 4, B - 3, C - 1, D - 2, E - 5
(d) A - 4, B - 5, C - 1, D - 2, E - 3

7. Match the following and select the correct option.

	Glands		Mode of secretion
A.	Merocrine	(i)	Entire cell disintegrates and is discharged as secretion.
B.	Apocrine	(ii)	Secretion is discharged by simple diffusion.
C.	Holocrine	(iii)	Apical part breaks off and is discharged as secretion.

(a) A-(i), B-(iii), C-(ii)
(b) A-(ii), B-(i), C-(iii)
(c) A-(ii), B-(iii), C-(i)
(d) A-(i), B-(ii), C-(iii)

8. Match the types of animal tissues listed under column I with the location given under column II. Choose the answer which gives the correct combination of the alphabets of the two columns.

	Column I (Tissues)		Column II (Location)
A.	Simple columnar epithelium	p.	Wall of heart
B.	Cardiac muscle	q.	Bone joint
C.	Adipose tissue	r.	Inner lining of stomach and intestince
D.	Hyaline cartilage	s.	Below the skin in the abdomen, buttocks, thighs and breasts
		t.	Diaphragm

(a) A - r, B - p, C - t, D - s
(b) A - r, B - t, C - q, D - s
(c) A - p, B - r, C - s, D - t
(d) A - r, B - p, C - s, D - q

9. Match the following Columns.

	Column I		Column II
A.	Neutrophil	1.	Single large nucleus
B.	Eosinophil	2.	Usually trilobed nucleus
C.	Basophil	3.	Kidney-shaped nucleus
D.	Lymphocyte	4.	Multilobed nucleus
E	Monocyte	5.	Bilobed nucleus

Codes

	A	B	C	D	E
(a)	4	1	3	5	2
(b)	2	5	1	4	3
(c)	4	5	2	1	3
(d)	2	4	5	3	1

10. Identify the pair that does not match.

(a) Sarcomere – Ultrastructural unit of striated muscle
(b) Copper containing respiratory pigment of Arachnida – Haemocyanim
(c) Osteoclast – Bone destroying cells
(d) Volkmann's canal – Which drain blood from bones

11. Match the following Columns.

	Column I		Column II
A.	Pseudostratified ciliated columner epithelium	1.	Trachea and large bronchi
B.	Stratified squamous epithelium	2.	Lining the oral cavity
C.	Transitional epithelium	3.	Wall of urinary bladder
D.	Simple ciliated columnar epithelium	4.	Lining the respiratory tract

Codes

	A	B	C	D
(a)	1	2	3	4
(b)	3	1	2	4
(c)	4	3	1	2
(d)	2	4	1	3

12. Match the following Columns.

	Column I		Column II
A.	Simple acinar gland	1.	Parotid gland
B.	Compound tubular glnad	2.	Seminal vesicle
C.	Compound tubulo-acinar gland	3.	Intestinal gland
D.	Simple tubular gland	4.	Liver
E.	Compound acinar gland	5.	Mammary gland

Codes

	A	B	C	D	E
(a)	2	3	4	1	5
(b)	4	2	1	3	5
(c)	3	1	2	4	5
(d)	5	4	3	2	1

13. Match the following Columns.

	Column I		Column II
A.	Adipose tissue	1.	Nose
B.	Stratified epithelium	2.	Blood
C.	Hyaline cartilage	3.	Skin
D.	Fluid connective tissue	4.	Fat storage

Codes

	A	B	C	D
(a)	1	2	3	4
(b)	4	3	1	2
(c)	3	1	4	2
(d)	2	1	4	3

14. Select the correctly matched pair.

(a) Chondroblast – Form chondrocyte in cartilage

(b) Elastic cartilage – Pubic symphysis

(c) Fibrous cartilage – Pinna of ear

(d) Hyaline cartilage – Intervertebral disc

15. Which word combination applies to stratified squamous epithelium?

(a) Mesoderm – Calcification

(b) Ectoderm – Keratinisation

(c) Mesoderm – Ossification

(d) Endoderm – Cornification

16. Select the option having all the correct characteristcs.

	Structure	Percentage of WBCs	Function
(a)	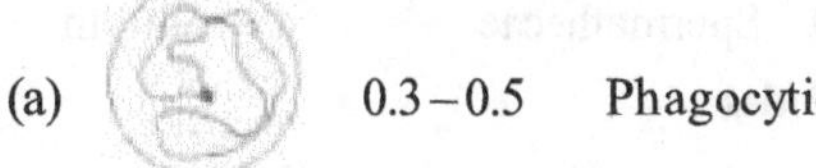	0.3 – 0.5	Phagocytic
(b)	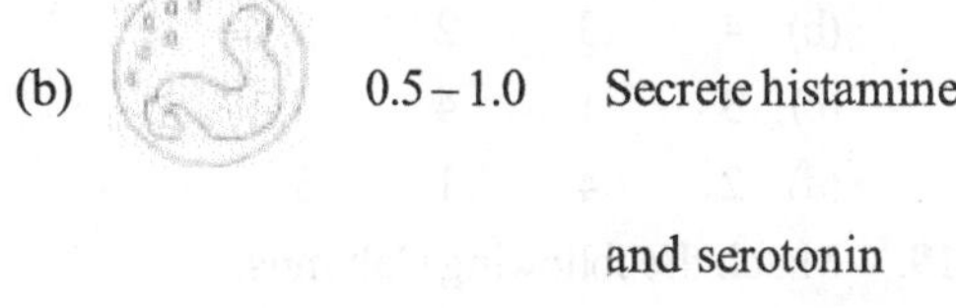	0.5 – 1.0	Secrete histamine and serotonin
(c)	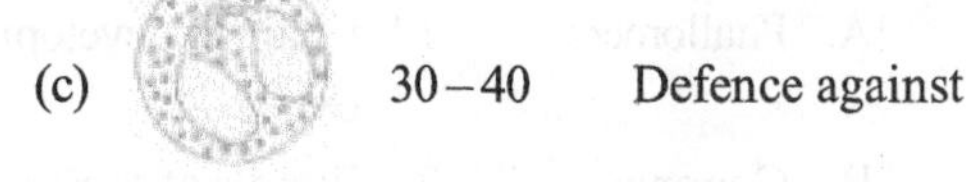	30 – 40	Defence against parasites
(d)	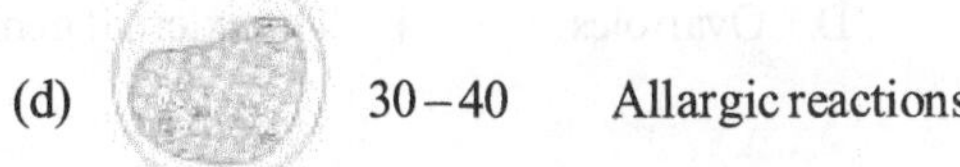	30 – 40	Allargic reactions

17. Match the following Columns.

Column I	Column II
A. Hermaphrodite	1. Produces blood cells and haemoglobin
B. Direct development	2. Testis and ovary in the same animal
C. Chemoreceptor	3. Larval form absent
D. Blood gland in earthworm	4. Sense of chemical substanes

Codes

	A	B	C	D
(a)	2	3	4	1
(b)	3	2	4	1
(c)	1	3	2	4
(d)	2	4	3	1

18. Match the following Columns.

Column I (Parts of reproductive system or earthworm)	Column II (Respective segments)
A. Testes	1. 10th-11th
B. Seminal vesicles	2. 11th-12th
C. Accessory gland	3. 17th-19th
D. Spermathecae	4. 6th-9th

Codes

	A	B	C	D
(a)	1	2	3	4
(b)	4	3	2	1
(c)	3	1	4	2
(d)	2	4	1	3

19. Match the following Columns.

Column I	**Column II**
A. Phallomere	1. Chain of developing ova
B. Gonopore	2. Bundls of sperm
C. Spermatophore	3. Opening of the ejaculatory duct
D. Ovarioles	4. The external genitalia

Codes

	A	B	C	D
(a)	3	4	2	1
(b)	4	3	2	1
(c)	4	2	3	1
(d)	2	4	3	1

20. Choose the correctly matched pair.

(a) Adipose tissue – Dense connective tissue
(b) Areolar tissue – Loose connective tissue
(c) Cartilage – Loose connective tissue
(d) Tendon – Specialised connective tissue

21. Match the column I with column II and choose the correct option:

Column I	**Column II**
A. Anal Cerci	(i) 4th and 6th segments
B. Tegmina	(ii) 10th segment
C. Testes	(iii) Forewings
D. Ommatidia	(iv) Sclerites
E. Exoskeleton	(v) Visual unit

	A	B	C	D	E
(a)	(ii)	(iii)	(i)	(v)	(iv)
(b)	(iv)	(iii)	(ii)	(v)	(i)
(c)	(iii)	(iv)	(v)	(ii)	(i)
(d)	(v)	(iv)	(iii)	(ii)	(i)

22. Match the column I with column II and choose the correct option:

Column I	**Column II**
A. Hermaphrodite	(i) Produces blood cells and haemoglobin
B. Direct development	(ii) Testis and ovary in the same animal
C. Chemoreceptor	(iii) Larval form absent
D. Blood gland in earthworm	(iv) Sense of chemical substances

	A	B	C	D
(a)	(ii)	(iii)	(iv)	(i)
(b)	(iii)	(ii)	(iv)	(i)
(c)	(i)	(iii)	(ii)	(iv)
(d)	(ii)	(iv)	(iii)	(i)

23. Match the following cell structure with its characteristic feature :

Column-I	Column-II
(a) Tight junctions	(i) Cement neighbouring cells together to form sheet.
(b) Adhering junctions	(ii) Transmit information through chemical to another cells.
(c) Gap junctions	(iii) Establish a barrier to prevent leakage of fluid across epithelial cells.
(d) Synaptic junctions	(iv) Cytoplasmic channels to facilitate communication between adjacent cells.

Select correct option from the following :

(a) (a)-(iv), (B)-(iii), (C)-(i), (D)-(ii)
(b) (a)-(ii), (B)-(iv), (C)-(i), (D)-(iii)
(c) (a)-(iv), (B)-(ii), (C)-(i), (D)-(iii)
(d) (a)-(iii), (B)-(i), (C)-(iv), (D)-(ii)

24. Which type of tissue correctly matches with its location ?

	Tissue	Location
(a)	Smooth muscle	Wall of intestine
(b)	Areolar tissue	Tendons
(c)	Transitional epithelium	Tip nose
(d)	Cuboidal epithelium	Lining of stomach

25. Given below is the diagrammatic sketch of a certain type of connective tissue. Identify the parts labeled A, B, C and D, and select the correct answer from the given option.

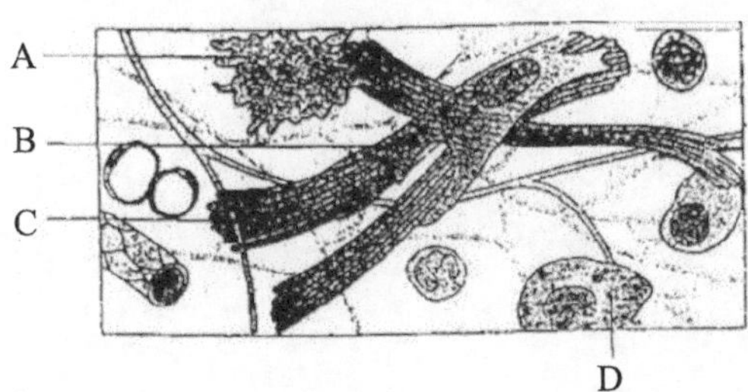

	Part-A	Part-B	Part-C	Part - D
(a)	Macro-phage	Fibro-blast	Collagenfibres	Mast cells
(b)	Mastcell	Macro-phage	Fibroblast	Collagenfibres
(c)	Macro-phage	Collagenfibres	Fibroblast	Mast cell
(d)	Mast cell	Collagenfibres	Fibroblast	Macrophage

26. The four sketches (1, 2, 3 and 4) given below, represent four different types of animal tissues. Which one of these is correctly identified in the options given, along with its correct location and function?

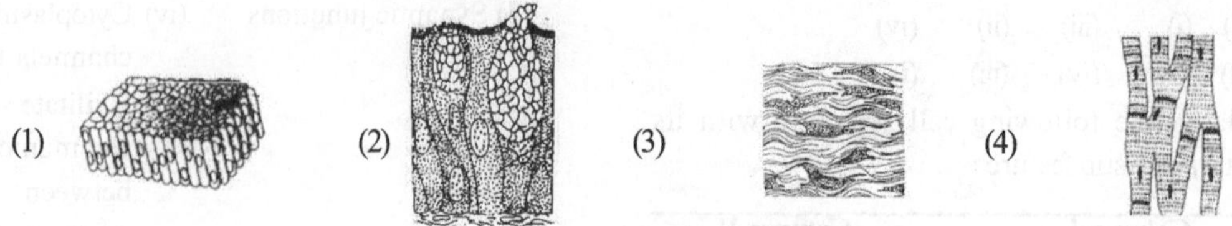

		Tissue	Location	Function
(a)	(2)	Glandular epithelium	Intestine	Secretion
(b)	(3)	Collagen fibres	Cartilage	Attach skeletal muscles to bones
(c)	(4)	Smooth muscle tissue	Heart	Heart contraction
(d)	(1)	Columnar epithelium	Nephron	Secretion and absorption

27. Which one of the following is correct pairing of a body part and the kind of muscle tissue that moves it?
(a) Biceps of upper arm–Smooth muscle fibres
(b) Abdominal wall–Smooth muscle
(c) Iris–Involuntary smooth muscle
(d) Heart wall–Involuntary unstriated muscle

Solutions

1. (c) 2. (c) 3. (c)

4. (c) Male genital pore is present in 18th segment.

5. (d) 6. (b) 7. (a) 8. (d) 9. (c)

10. (d) 11. (a) 12. (a) 13. (b) 14. (a)

15. (b) 16. (b) 17. (a) 18. (a) 19. (b)

20. (b) 21. (a) 22. (a)

23. (d) *Tight junctions* provide a barrier which prevents leakage of fluid across epithelial cells.

    Adherens junctions aid to cement adjacent cells to form a sheet.

    Gap junctions provide cytoplasmic channels to facilitate communication between adjacent cells.

    Synaptic junctions help in transmission of information through chemicals.

24. (a) Wall of intestine is made of smooth muscle. Tendons consist of dense regular connective tissue fascicles encased in dense irregular connective tissue sheaths. Tip of nose consists of squamous epithelium. Lining of epithelium is made of columnar epithelium.

25. (a) Connective tissue is the most diverse of the four tissue types with a wide variety of functions. Connective tissue is made up of cells and fibers in a "jelly-like" ground substance.

26. (a) Glandular epithelium invaginates epithelia into connective tissue which differentiate into secretory units. Examples include sebaceous glands of the skin and glands in the intestinal lining (exocrine glands), and many endocrine glands releasing hormones, such as the thyroid follicle.

27. (b) The structure of the abdominal wall is similar in principle to the thoracic wall. There are three layers, an external, internal and innermost layer. The vessels and nerves lie between the internal and innermost layers. The abdomen can be divided into quadrants or nine abdominal regions.

CHAPTER

Cell: The Unit of Life

1. Match the column I with column II.

Column I	Column II
A. Golgi appartus	(i) Synthesis of protein
B. Lysosomes	(ii) Trap waste and excretory products
C. Vacuoles	(iii) Formation of glycoproteins and glycolipids
D. Ribosomes	(iv) Digesting biomolecules

Choose the right match from options given below.

(a) A-(iii), B-(iv), C-(ii), D-(i)
(b) A-(iv), B-(iii), C-(i), D-(ii)
(c) A-(iii), B-(ii), C-(iv), D-(i)
(d) A-(i), B-(ii), C-(iv), D-(iii)

2. Match the following.

Column I	Column II
A. Protein	(i) SER
B. Lipid	(ii) Golgi body
C. Glycoprotein	(iii) Lysosome
D. Hydrolytic enzyme	(iv) RER

(a) A-(i), B-(ii), C-(iii), D-(iv)
(b) A-(iv), B-(ii), C-(i), D-(iii)
(c) A-(iv), B-(i), C-(ii), D-(iii)
(d) A-(i), B-(iii), C-(ii), D-(iv)

3. Match the columns and identify the correct option.

Column I	Column II
A. Thylakoids	(i) Disc-shaped sacs in Golgi appartus
B. Cristae	(ii) Condensed structure of DNA
C. Cisternae	(iii) Flat membranous sacs in stroma
D. Chromation	(iv) Infoldings in mitochondria

(a) A-(iii), B-(i), C-(iv), D-(ii)
(b) A-(iii), B-(iv), C-(ii), D-(i)
(c) A-(iv), B-(iii), C-(i), D-(ii)
(d) A-(iii), B-(iv), C-(i), D-(ii)

4. Which of these is wrongly matched?

(a) 70S ribosomes – Prokaryotes
(b) 80S ribosomes – Eukaryotes
(c) Axoneme – Cilia
(d) Centromere – Centrosome
(e) Thylakoids – Chloroplast

5. Given below are cell organelles and their functions. Select the incorrect match.

(a) Lysosome – Phagocytosis
(b) Centriole – Spindle formation
(c) Sphaerosomes – Storage and synthesis of fats
(d) Leucoplast – Photosynthesis

6. Match the column I with that of column II and choose the correct combination from the options given.

Column I Organelle	Column II Site for
A. Rough ER	(i) Synthesis of glycoproteins
B. Smooth ER	(ii) Aerobic respiration

C. Mitochondria (iii) Synthesis of lipid
D. Golgi appartus (iv) Protein synthesis

(a) A - (i), B - (ii), C - (iii), D - (iv)
(b) A - (ii), B - (iii), C - (iv), D - (i)
(c) A - (iii), B - (iv), C - (ii), D - (i)
(d) A - (iv), B - (iii), C - (ii), D - (i)
(e) A - (iv), B - (iii), C - (i), D - (ii)

7. Match the following and select the correct answer.

(A) Centriole (i) Infoldings in mitochondria
(B) Chlorophyll (ii) Thylakoids
(C) Cristae (iii) Nucleic acids
(D) Ribozymes (iv) Basal body of cilia or flagella

	A	**B**	**C**	**D**
(a)	(iv)	(ii)	(i)	(iii)
(b)	(i)	(ii)	(iv)	(iii)
(c)	(i)	(iii)	(ii)	(iv)
(d)	(iv)	(iii)	(i)	(ii)

8. Choose the matched ones.

(A) Vibrio - Rod like bacteria
(B) Mesosome - Helps in cell wall formation
(C) Smooth endoplasmic - synthesis of lipid reticulum
(D) Vacuoles - Rich in hydrolytic enzymes

(a) (B) and (C) only
(b) (A) and (D) only
(c) (A), (B) and (C) only
(d) (B) and (D) only
(e) (B), (C) and (D) only

9. Which of these is wrongly matched?

(a) Chloroplasts – Chlorophyll
(b) Elaioplasts – Starch
(c) Chromoplasts – Carotenoids
(d) Amyloplasts – Carbohydrates
(e) Aleuroplasts – Proteins

10. Match the following Columns.

Column I	**Column II**
A. Dictyosomes	1. Osmoregulation
B. Mitochondria	2. Photosynthesis
C. Vacuoles	3. Transort
D. Grana	4. Secretion
	5. Respiration

Codes

	A	B	C	D
(a)	4	5	1	2
(b)	3	4	2	1
(c)	4	5	3	2
(d)	4	3	1	2

11. Match the following Columns.

Column I	**Column II**
A. Karyolymph	1. Nucleolus
B. Ribonucleoprotein	2. Nucleus
C. Spindle fibre	3. DNA
D. Genes	4. Centrioles
E. Rough endoplasmic reticulum	5. Protein synthesis

Codes

	A	B	C	D	E
(a)	1	3	2	4	5
(b)	4	2	3	5	1
(c)	2	1	4	3	5
(d)	1	2	3	4	5

12. Analyse the following pairs and identify the correct options given

A. Chromoplasts - Contains pigments other than chlorophyll
B. Leucoplasts - Devoid of any pigments
C. Amyloplasts - Store proteins
D. Alueroplasts - Store oils and fats
E. Elaioplasts - Store carbohydrates

(a) B and C are correct
(b) C and D are correct

(c) D and E are correct
(d) A and B are correct

13. Match the following and choose the correct combination from the options given.

Column I Cell type	Column II Size
A. Viruses	(1) 1-2 mm
B. PPLO	(2) 10-20 mm
C. Eukaryotic cell	(3) About 0.1 mm
D. Bacterium	(4) 0.02 - 0.2 mm

(a) A-1, B-2, C-3, D-4
(b) A-4, B-3, C-2, D-1
(c) A-1, B-3, C-2, D-4
(d) A-4, B-2, C-3, D-1

14. Match the following and select the correct answer:

A. Centriole	(i) Infoldings in mitochondria
B. Chlorophyll	(ii) Thylakoids
C. Cristae	(iii) Nucleic acids
D. Ribozymes	(iv) Basal body cilia or fiagella

	A	B	C	D
(a)	(iv)	(ii)	(i)	(iii)
(b)	(i)	(ii)	(iv)	(iii)
(c)	(i)	(iii)	(ii)	(iv)
(d)	(iv)	(iii)	(i)	(ii)

15. Match the following and select the correct answer:

A. Centriole	(i) Infoldings in mitochondria
B. Chlorophyll	(ii) Thylakoids
C. Cristae	(iii) Nucleic acids
D. Ribozymes	(iv) Basal body cilia or fiagella

	A	B	C	D
(a)	(iv)	(ii)	(i)	(iii)
(b)	(i)	(ii)	(iv)	(iii)
(c)	(i)	(iii)	(ii)	(iv)
(d)	(iv)	(iii)	(i)	(ii)

16. Match the columns and identify the correct option.

Column-I	Column-II
A. Thylakoids	(i) Disc-shaped sacs in Golgi apparatus
B. Cristae	(ii) Condensed structure of DNA
C. Cisternae	(iii) Flat membranous sacs in stroma
D. Chromatin	(iv) Infoldings in mitochondria

	A	B	C	D
(a)	(iii)	(iv)	(i)	(ii)
(b)	(iii)	(i)	(iv)	(ii)
(c)	(iii)	(iv)	(ii)	(i)
(d)	(iv)	(iii)	(i)	(ii)

17. Match the items in column I with column II and choose the correct option.

Column I	Column II
A. Sap vacuole	1. Contain digestive enzyme
B. Contractile vacuole	2. Store metabolic gases
C. Food vacuole	3. Osmoregulation
D. Air vacuole	4. Store lipids
E. Spherosomes	5. Store and concentrate mineral salts and nutrients

	A	B	C	D	E
(a)	5	3	1	2	4
(b)	2	3	4	5	1
(c)	5	3	2	4	1
(d)	4	1	3	5	2

18. Which of the following four cell structures is correctly matched with the accompanying description ?

(a) Plasma membrane — Outer layer of cellulose or chitin

(b) Mitochondria — Bacteria like elements with inner membrane forming sacs containing chlorophyll, found in plant cell and algae

(c) Chloroplasts — Bacteria like elements with inner membrane highly folded

(d) Golgi apparatus — Stacks of flattened vesicles

19. Match column I and column II and select the correct option.

	Column I		Column II
A.	Endoplasmic recticulum	1.	Stack of cisternae
B.	Spherosome	2.	Store oils or fats
C.	Dictyosome	3.	Synthesis and storage of lipids
D.	Peroxisome	4.	Photorespiration
E.	Elaioplasts	5.	Detoxification of drugs

	A	B	C	D	E
(a)	5	3	1	4	2
(b)	2	3	2	4	1
(c)	2	3	1	4	5
(d)	3	5	1	4	2

20. Match List I and List II and select the correct answer

List I	List II
(i) Lysosome	A. Bacteria without walls
(ii) Mycoplasma	B. A virus that infects bacterial cells
(iii) Thylakoid	C. Flattened sacs in a chloroplast
(iv) Bacteriophage	D. A vesicle in which hydrolytic enzymes are stored

(a) (i) – C, (ii) – A, (iii) – B, (iv) – D

(b) (i) – D, (ii) – A, (iii) – C, (iv) – B

(c) (i) – B, (ii) – C, (iii) – D, (iv) – A

(d) (i) – A, (ii) – D, (iii) – B, (iv) – C

Solutions

1. (a) 2. (c) 3. (d)

4. (d) The two chromatids are attached to each other by a narrow area called centromere or primary constriction.

   The complex formed from centrioles and centrosphere is called centrosome.

5. (d) Leucoplasts take part in storage of various substances like starch (amyloplasts), fat(elaioplasts) and protein(aleuroplasts). These are colourless plastids that lack grana and photosynthetic pigments.

6. (d) 7. (a)

8. (a) Vibrio are comma shaped bacteria. Vacuolar sap contains mineral salts, sugars, amino acids, esters, proteins, waste products and water soluble pigments called anthocyanin. Lysosomes are rich in hydrolytic enzymes.

9. (b) Elaioplasts are colourless plastids which store lipids *e.g.*, tube rose.

10. (a) 11. (c) 12. (d) 13. (b) 14. (a)

15. (a) 16. (a) 17. (a) 18. (b) 19. (a)

20. (b)

CHAPTER

Biomolecules

1. Match the following Columns.

	Column I		Column II
A.	Cellulose	1.	Insulin
B.	Peptide	2.	Alkaline phosphatase
C.	Steroid	3.	Cotton fibres
D.	Phospholipid	4.	Diosgenin
E.	Enzymes	5.	Lecithin

Codes

	A	B	C	D	E
(a)	3	4	5	1	2
(b)	2	1	4	5	3
(c)	3	1	4	5	2
(d)	1	4	3	5	2

2. Match the following Columns.

	Column I		Column II
A.	Abrin	1.	Lectin
B.	GLUT-4	2.	Intercellular ground substcne
C.	Collagen	3.	Hormone
D.	Concanavalin	4.	Enables glucose transport into cells
		5.	Toxin

Codes

	A	B	C	D
(a)	3	4	2	1
(b)	5	4	2	1
(c)	3	4	2	5
(d)	3	5	2	1

3. Match the following Columns.

	Column I		Column II
A.	Oxidoreductase	1.	Linking of two copounds
B.	Isomerases	2.	Removal of group from sustrates
C.	Ligases	3.	Interconversion of isomers
D.	Lyases	4.	Dehydrogenases
		5.	Hydrolysis

Codes

	A	B	C	D
(a)	4	1	3	2
(b)	4	3	1	2
(c)	3	4	2	5
(d)	2	5	3	1

4. Identify the incorrect match between protein and its role.

(a) Keratin - Structural component of hair

(b) Immunoglobulins - Protection of body against diseases

(c) Haemoglobin - Transport of oxygen in muscles

(d) Thrombin - Blood clotting

5. Match the follwing Columns.

	Column I		Column II
A.	Nitrogen bae	1.	RNA
B.	Nucleoside	2.	Thymidylic acid
C.	Nucleotide	3.	Cytidine
D.	Nucleic acid	4.	Uracil

Codes

	A	B	C	D
(a)	1	2	3	4
(b)	1	3	2	4
(c)	4	3	2	1
(d)	4	1	2	3
(e)	4	2	3	1

6. Find out the wrongly matched pair.
   (a) Primary metabolite – Ribose
   (b) Secondary metabolite – Anthocyanin
   (c) Protein – Insulin
   (d) Chitin – Polyscharide
   (e) Cellulose – Heteropolymer

7. Match the following Columns.

	Column I		Column II
A.	Triglycerides	1.	Galactose
B.	Lactose	2.	Glycerol
C.	RNA	3.	Palmitic acid
D.	b-pleats	4.	Uracil
E.	Bee-wax	5.	Secondary structure

Codes

	A	B	C	D	E
(a)	4	1	5	2	3
(b)	5	1	4	2	3
(c)	3	1	4	5	2
(d)	2	1	4	5	3

8. Which one of the following biomolecules is correctley characterised?
   (a) Lecithin - a phophorylated glyceride found in cell membrane.
   (b) Palmitic acid - an unsaturated fatty acid wiht 18 carbon atoms.
   (c) Adenylic acide - adenosine with a glucose phosphate molecule.
   (d) Alanine amino acid - contains an amino group and an acidic group anywhere in the molecule.

9. Match the following and choose the correct combination from the options given.

	Column I (Organic Compound)		Column II (Example)
A.	Fattyacid	1.	Glutamic acid
B.	Phospholipid	2.	Tryptophan
C.	Aromatic amino acid	3.	Lecithin
D.	Acidic amino acid	4.	Palmitic acid

   (a) A-1, B-2, C-3, D-4 (b) A-4, B-3, C-2, D-1
   (c) A-2, B-3, C-4, D-1 (d) A-3, B-4, C-1, D-2
   (e) A-4, B-3, C-1, D-2

10. Match the following and choose the correct combination from the options given.

	Column I (Chemical compounds)		Column II (Examples)
A.	Nitrogen base	I.	RNA
B.	Nucleoside	II.	Thymidylic acid
C.	Nucleotide	III.	Cytidine
D.	Nucleic acid	IV.	Uracil

   (a) A-I, B-II, C-III, D-IV
   (b) A-I, B-III, C-II, D-IV
   (c) A-IV, B-III, C-II, D-I
   (d) A-IV, B-I, C-II, D-III
   (e) A-IV, B-II, C-III, D-I

11. Match the itemes in colum I with those in colum II and choose the correct answer.

	Column I (Biomolecules)		Column II (Examples)
A.	Carbohydrates	1.	Trypsin
B.	Protein	2.	Cholestrol
C.	Nucleic acid	3.	Insulin
D.	Lipid	4.	Adenylic acid

   (a) A-3; B-1: C-4; D-2
   (b) A-2; B-3 C-4; D-1
   (c) A-3; B-4 C-1; D-2
   (d) A-4; B-1; C-2; D-3
   (e) A-1; B-2; C-3; D-4

12. Match column I with column II and select the correct option from codes given below.

Column I	Column II
A. Pigments	(i) Abrin, ricin
B. Toxins	(ii) Concanavalin A
C. Alkaloids	(iii) Carotenoids
D. Lectins	(iv) Morphine, codeine

(a) A-(iv), B-(iii), C-(i), D-(ii)
(b) A-(ii), B-(iv), C-(i), D-(iii)
(c) A-(ii), B-(i), C-(iv), D-(ii)
(d) A-(i), B-(ii), C-(iii), D-(iv)

13. Which of the following secondary metabolites belong to the group drugs?

I. Morphine II. Curcumin
III. Codeine IV. Vinblastin
V. Abrin

(a) I and II only
(b) I and V only
(c) II and III only
(d) II and IV only
(e) III and IV only

14. Which of these is/are wrongly matched?

I. Alkaloid - Codeine
II. Lectin - Morphine
III. Toxic - Abrin
IV. Terpene - Curcumin

(a) I and II only
(b) II and III only
(c) II and IV only
(d) III and IV only
(e) I and IV only

15. Find out the wrongly matched pair.

(a) Primary metabolite - Ribose
(b) Secondary metabolite - Anthocyanins
(c) Protein - Insulin
(d) Chitin - Polysaccharide
(e) Cellulose - Heteropolymer

16. Match the following nutritional vitamin deficiencies in column I with the causes/ deficiencies in column II and choose the correct option from the answer key. **[Kerala '05]**

Column I	Column II
A. Kwashiorkar	p. Iron
B. General anaemia	q. Menadione
C. Dermatitis	r. Protein
D. Marasmus	s. Pyridoxine
E. Bleeding	t. Biotin

(1) A = p, B = t, C = q, D = r, E = s
(2) A = t, B = q, C = r, D = s, E = p
(3) A = t, B = r, C = s, D = p, E = q
(4) A = r, B = s, C = p, D = t, E = q

17. Match the items in column I with items in column II and choose the correct answer **[Kerala'06]**

Column I	Column II
a. triglyceride	1. animal hormones
b. membrane lipid	2. feathers and leaves
c. steroid	3. phospholipids
d. wax	4. fat stored in form of droplets

(1) a–4, b–3, c–1, d–2
(2) a–2, b–3, c–4, d–1
(3) a–3, b–4, c–1, d–2
(4) a–4, b–1, c–2, d–3

18. Match the column I and II and choose the correct combination from the options given.

Column I	Column II
A. Acidic amino acid	(i) Valine
B. Basic amino acid	(ii) Glutamic acid
C. Neutral amino acid	(iii) Phenylalanine
D. Aromatic amino acid	(iv) Lysine

(a) A-(ii), B-(iv), C-(i), D-(iii)
(b) A-(ii), B-(i), C-(iv), D-(iii)
(c) A-(iii), B-(ii), C-(i), D-(iv)
(d) A-(i), B-(iv), C-(iii), D-(ii)

19. Match the columns and find out the correct combination

Proteinaceous amino acids	R-group
A. Serine	1. Hydrogen
B. Glycine	2. Hydroxyl methyl
C. Alanine	3. Methyl group

(a) A-3, B-1, C-2 (b) A-2, B-2, C-1
(c) A-2, B-2, C-3 (d) A-2, B-1, C-3

20. Correctly match the column-I with column-II

Column I	Column II
A. Drugs	I. Gums, cellulose
B. Polymeric substances	II. Morphine, codeine
C. Alkaloids	III. Carotenoids, Anthocyanins
D. Pigments	IV. Vinblastin, curcumin

(a) A-c, B-a, C-b, D-d
(b) A-d, B-b, C-a, D-c
(c) A-d, B-a, C-b, D-c
(d) A-a, B-d, C-b, D-c

21. Which of the following polysaccharide is wrongly matched with its monomer?

(a) Starch — Glucose
(b) Chitin — N-acetyl glucosamine (NAG)
(c) Inulin — Mannose
(d) Mucopolysaccharide — Amino sugars and other chemically modified sugars

Solutions

1. (c) 2. (b) 3. (b) 4. (c) 5. (c)

6. (e) Cellulose is the most important structural component of the cell wall of plants. It is a linear polymer of β-D glucose units connected through β-1, 4-glycosidic linkage. The linear chains form microfibrillae or bundles of parallel chains held together by hydrogen bonds.

7. (d)

8. (a) Lecithin is a triglyceride lipid where one fatty acid is replaced by phosphoric acid which is linked to additional nitrogenous group called choline. It is a common membrane lipid. It is an amphipathic phospholipid having both hydrophilic polar and hydrophobic nonpolar groups.

9. (b) 10. (c) 11. (a) 12. (c)

13. (d) secondary metabolites are derivatives of primary metabolites. These metabolites are generally found in plant, fungal and microbial cells. These are organic compounds which are not involved in primary metabolism and seen to have no direct function in growth and development of plants. Curcumin and vinblastin are drugs, morphine and codeine are alkaloids and abrin is toxin.

14. (c) Morphine is an alkaloid and curcumin is a drug.

15. (e) Cellulose is a polysaccharide and a homopolymer that consists of a long unbranched chain of glucose units. It is the main constituent of the cell walls of all plants, many algae, and some fungi and is responsible for providing the rigidity of the cell wall.

16. (d) 17. (a) 18. (a) 19. (d) 20. (c)

21. (c)

CHAPTER

Cell Cycle and Cell Division

1. Identify the stage of mitosis with its characteristics.

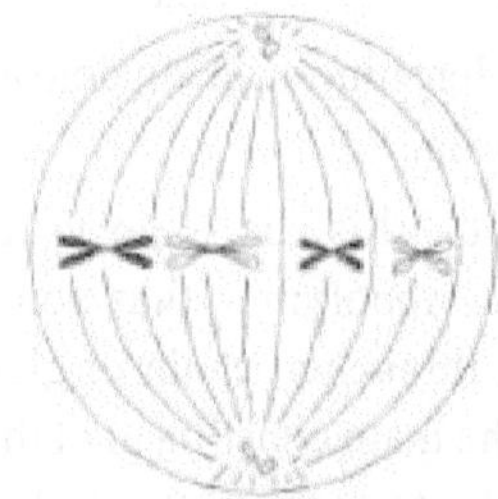

(a) Metaphase – Chromosomes move to spindle equator, chromosomes made up of two chromatids

(b) Anaphase – Centromeres split, chromatids separate and start moving away

(c) Late prophase – Chromosomes move to spindle equator

(d) Metaphase – Spindle fibres attached move to kinetochores, centromeres split and chromatids separate

2. Identify the pair which is a mismatch for plant cell division.

(a) Spindle – amphiaster

(b) Centrioles – absent

(c) Cytokinesis – by cell plate formation which grows centrigugally

(d) New cell membrane – endoplasmic reticulum

3. At which stage of mitosis, do these events occur?

	Spiralisation and condensation of DNA	**Nuclear envelope breakdown**	**centromeres split**
(a)	Interphase	Interphase	Metaphase
(b)	Interphase	Prophase	Metaphase
(c)	Prophase	Metaphase	Anaphase
(d)	Prophase	Prophase	Anaphase

4. Beads on string of *A* are seen in *B* which condense to form chromosomes in *C*-stage of cell division

	A	*B*	*C*
(a)	Chromonema	Chromatin	Metaphase
(b)	Chromation	Chromatid	Metaphase
(c)	Chromonema	Chromosome	Anaphase
(d)	Chromonema	Chromatid	Anaphase

5. Match the following Columns.

Column I		**Column II**
A. Interkinesis	1.	S-phase
B. Histone synthesis	2.	Cytokinesis
C. Colchicine	3.	Chromosome fibre
D. Terminalisation	4.	Spindle

Codes

	A	B	C	D
(a)	4	1	2	3
(b)	2	1	4	3
(c)	1	2	3	4
(d)	3	2	1	4

6. Match the following Columns.

	Column I		Column II
A.	Synapsis aligns homologous chromosomes	1.	Anaphase-II
B.	Synthesis of RNA and protein	2.	Zygotene
C.	Action of enzyme recombinase	3.	G_2 - phase
D.	Centromeres do not separate, but chromatids move towards opposite poles	4.	Anaphase-I
		5.	Pachytene

Codes

	A	B	C	D
(a)	2	1	3	4
(b)	2	3	5	4
(c)	1	2	5	4
(d)	2	3	4	5

7. Match of the item in Column I with those in Column II and the choose the correct answer.

Column I	Column II
A. Mitosis	1. Occurs in diploid cells only
B. Meiosis	2. Occurs in both haploid and diploid cells
	3. Daughter and parent cells have same chromosome numbers
	4. Synapsis of homologous chromosomes

Codes

	A	B		A	B
(a)	1	2	(b)	2	3
(c)	3	4	(d)	4	1

8. Match the following Columns.

Column I	Column II
A. G_1-phase	1. Replication of DNA
B. S-phase	2. Quiescent stage
C. G_2-phase	3. Condensation of chromatin
D. G_0-phase	4. Protein synthesis
	5. Interval between mitosis and initiation of DNA replication

Codes

	A	B	C	D
(a)	3	5	1	2
(b)	5	4	1	3
(c)	5	1	4	2
(d)	5	2	3	4

9. Match the following Columns.

	Column I	Column II
A.	Leptotene	1. Terminalisation of chiasms
B.	Zygotene	2. Crossing over and recombination
C.	Pachytene	3. Synapsis
D.	Diakinesis	4. Visibility of chromosomes

Codes

	A	B	C	D
(a)	1	2	3	4
(b)	1	3	2	4
(c)	4	3	2	1
(d)	4	1	2	3
(e)	4	2	3	1

10. Match the stages of meiosis in column I to their characteristics features in column II and select the correct option using the codes given below.

	Column I		Column II
A.	Pachytene	(i)	Pairing of homologous chromosomes
B.	Metaphase I	(ii)	Terminalisation of chiasmata
C.	Diakinesis	(iii)	Crossing-over takes place
D.	Zygotene	(iv)	Chromosomes aligh at equatorial plate

(a) A-(iii), B-(iv), C-(ii), D-(i)
(b) A-(i), B-(iv), C-(ii), D-(iii)
(c) A-(ii), B-(iv), C-(iii), D-(i)
(d) A-(iv), B-(iii), C-(ii), D-(i)

11. Match the items in column I with those in column II, and choose the correct answer.

	Column I		Column II
P.	Mitosis	(i)	Occurs in diploid cells only
Q.	Meiosis	(ii)	Occurs in both haploid and diploid cells.
		(iii)	Daughter and parent cells have same chromosome numbers
		(iv)	Synapsis of homologous chromosomes

(a) P-(i), Q-(ii) (b) P-(ii), Q-(iii)
(c) P-(iii), Q-(iv) (d) P-(iv), Q-(i)

12. Match the sub-stage of prophase I of meiosis in column I and the events in column II and choose the right option.

	Column I		Column II
A.	Leptotene	I.	Terminalisation of chiasma
B.	Zygotene	II.	Crossing over and recombination
C.	Pachytene	III.	Synapsis
D.	Diakinesis	IV.	Visibility of chromosomes

(a) A-I, B-II, C-III, D-IV
(b) A-I, B-III, C-II, D-IV
(c) A-IV, B-III, C-II, D-I
(d) A-IV, B-I, C-II, D-III
(e) A-IV, B-II, C-III, D-I

13. Find the correctly matched pairs and choose the correct option.

A. Leptotene – The chromosomes become invisible
B. Zygotene – Pairing of homlogous chromosomes
C. Pachytene – Dissolution of the synaptonemal complex takes place
D. Diplotene – Bivalent chromosomes appear as tetrads
E. Diakinesis – Terminalisation of chiasmata takes place.

(a) A and B are correct.
(b) B and D are correct.
(c) B and E are correct.
(d) B and C are correct.
(e) C and D are correct.

14. Select the correct match.

(A) S phase – DNA replication
(B) Zygotene – Synapsis
(C) Diplotene – Crossing over
(D) Meiosis – Both haploid and diploid cells
(E) Gap 2 phase – Quiescent stage

(a) nuclease
(b) RNA polymerase
(c) recombinase
(d) DNA polymerase.

15. Identify the correct stage in cell division with its characteristics.

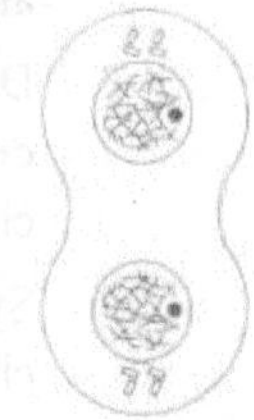

(a) Telophase – Endoplasmic reticulum and nucleolus not reformed yet
(b) Telophase – Nuclear envelop reforms, Golgi complex reforms
(c) Late anaphase – Chromosomes move away from equatorial plate, Golgi complex not present

(d) Cytokinesis – Cell plate formed, mitochondria distributed between two daughter cells

16. Match the following and choose the correct option.

	Column I	Column II
I.	Chromosomes are moved to spindle equator	(A) Pachytene
II.	Centromere splits and chromatids apart	(B) Zygotene
III.	Pairing between homologous chromosomes takes place	(C) Anaphase
IV.	Crossing between homologous chromosomes	(D) Metaphase

	I	II	III	IV
(a)	A	B	C	D
(b)	B	C	D	A
(c)	D	C	B	A
(d)	C	A	D	B

17. Match the following and choose the correct option.

	Column I		Column II
I.	Terminalization of chiasmata	A.	Zygotene
II.	Synapsis	B.	Diplotene
III.	Crossing over	C.	Metaphase I
IV.	Dissolution of Synaptonemal complex	D.	Diakinesis
V.	Best stage for the study of chiasmata	E.	Pachytene
VI.	Nuclear membrane and nucleolus disappear		
VII.	Tetrads are arranged on equatorial line		

(a) A - II, B - V, C - VII, D - I, IV, VI, E - III

(b) A - II, B - III, C - VII, D - I, IV, VI, E - V

(c) A - II, B - VII, C - III, D - I, IV, V, E - VI

(d) A - II, B - I, C - IV, D - V, III, E - VI

18. Find the correctly matched pairs and choose the correct option.

A.	Leptotene	-	The chromosomes become invisible
B.	Zygotene	-	Pairing of homologous chromosomes
C.	Pachytene	-	Dissolution of the complex synaptonemal takes place
D.	Diplotene	-	Bivalent chromosomes appear as tetrads
E.	Diakinesis	-	Terminalization of chiasmata takes place

(a) A and B are correct

(b) B and D are correct

(c) B and E are correct

(d) B and C are correct

19. A stage in cell division is shown in the figure. Select the answer which gives correct identification of the stage with its characteristics.

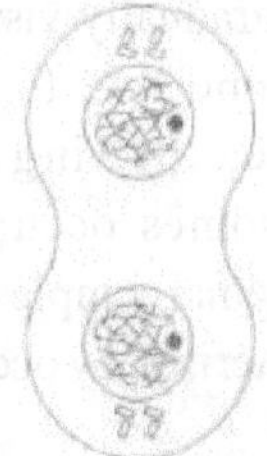

(a)	Late anaphase	Chromosomes move away from equatorial plate, Golgi complex not present
(b)	Cytokinesis	Cell plate formed, mitochondria distributed between two daughter cells
(c)	Telophase	Endoplasmic reticulum and nucleolus not reformed yet
(d)	Telophase	Nuclear envelop reforms, golgi complex reforms

20. Select the correct option :

	I	II
A	"Synapsis aligns homologous chromosomes"	(i) Anaphase-II
B	"Synthesis of RNA and protein"	(ii) Zygotene
C	"Action of enzyme recombinase"	(iii) G2-phase
D	"Centromeres do not separate but chromatids move towards opposite poles"	(iv) Anaphase-I
		(v) Pachytene

	A	B	C	D
(a)	(ii)	(iii)	(v)	(iv)
(b)	(i)	(ii)	(v)	(iv)
(c)	(ii)	(iii)	(iv)	(v)
(d)	(ii)	(i)	(iii)	(iv)

Solutions

1. (a) 2. (a) 3. (d) 4. (d) 5. (b)
6. (b) 7. (c) 8. (c) 9. (c) 10. (a)
11. (c) 12. (c)
13. (c) Prophase I of meiosis consists of 5 stages: leptotene, zygotene, pachytene, diplotene and diakinesis. Leptotene is the initial stage of prophase. During this, chromosomes become gradually visible under the light microscope due to condensation. In zygotene, pairing of homologous chromosomes occur by formation of synaptonemal complexes. Next, pachytene is characterised by occurrence of crossing over. Bivalent chromosomes now clearly appears as tetrads. Diplotene follows pachytene and involves dissolution of synaptonemal complex. Terminalisation of chaiasmata is observed in diakinesis.
14. (a) During S phase DNA replication takes place. During zygotense synapsis occurs. The process of attachment of the homologous chromosomes is called synapsis.
15. (b) 16. (c) 17. (a) 18. (c) 19. (d)
20. (a)

CHAPTER

Transport in Plants

1. The table below shows the comparison of different transport process. Identify the correct comparison.

	Property	Simple Diffusion	Facilitated Diffusion	Active Transport
(a)	Needs carrier protein	Yes	Yes	Yes
(b)	Uphill transport	No	Yes	Yes
(c)	Transport saturates	No	No	No
(d)	Needs ATP energy	No	No	Yes

2. During osmosis, water moves through a membrane

	From	To
(a)	Low water potential	High water potential
(b)	High solute concentration	Low solute concentration
(c)	High osmotic potential	Low osmotic potential
(d)	A hypotonic solution (less solute)	A hypertonic solution (more solute)

3. Match the name of the activities listed under column I with the description of activity given under column II.

Column I	Column II
A. Transpiration	I. Anaerobic respiration in yeast
B. Guttation	II. Active absorption of water
C. Exudation	III. Loss of water vapour from plant parts
D. Fermentation	IV. Loss of liquid water from leaves.
	V. Loss of water from injured plant parts.

(a) A-I; B-II; C-III; D-V
(b) A-II; B-I; C-IV; D-III
(c) A-III; B-IV; C-V; D-I
(d) A-IV; B-V; C-II; D-III

4. Match the theories given in column I with the name of scientists listed in column II. Choose the answer which gives the correct combination of the alphabet.

Column I	Column II
(A) Relay Pump Theory	(I) Stocking
(B) Transpiration Cohesion Theory	(II) Sir J. C. Bose
(C) Mass Flow Theory	(III) Godlewski
(D) Pulsation Theory	(IV) Dixon and Jolly
	(V) Ernest Munch

(a) A–III,B–II,C–V,D–I
(b) A–II,B–I,C–V,D–III
(c) A–III,B–IV,C–V,D–II
(d) A–IV,B–III,C–I,D–II

5. Match the following

Column I	Column II
(A) Hypotonic	(I) Water
(B) Hypertonic	(II) Sucrose
(C) Solute	(III) Lower tonicity
(D) Solvent	(IV) Higher tonicity

(a) A–I,B–II,C–III,D–IV
(b) A–III,B–II,C–I,D–IV
(c) A–III,B–IV,C–II,D–I
(d) A–III,B–II,C–IV,D–I

6. The value of osmotic potential (π) and pressure potential (p) of cells a, b, c, d are given below

Cells

Cells	π	P
A	– 1.0	0.5
B	– 0.6	0.3
C	– 1.2	0.6
D	– 0.8	0.4

Identify the correct sequence that shows the path of movement of water from the following

(a) $D \rightarrow C \rightarrow A \rightarrow B$
(b) $B \rightarrow D \rightarrow A \rightarrow C$
(c) $B \rightarrow C \rightarrow D \rightarrow A$
(d) $C \rightarrow B \rightarrow A \rightarrow D$

7. Match List – I with List – II and find out the correct answer from the code given below.

List – I	List – II
(A) Diffusion	(i) hydrophoilic substances
(B) Osmosis	(ii) shrinkage of protoplasm
(C) Imbibition	(iii) semipermeable membrane
(D) Plasmolysis	(iv) free movement of ions and gases

(a) A – (II), B – (I), C –(IV), D – (III)
(b) A – (IV), B – (III). C – (I), D – (II)
(c) A – (III), B – (I), C – (IV), D – (II)
(d) A – (II), B – (III), C – (IV), D – (I)

8. The osmotic potential and pressure potential of three cells (A, B, C) located in different parts of an actively transpiring plant are given below.

Cell	Osmotic Potential (Mpa)	Pressure Potential (MPa)
A	–0.87	0.44
B	–0.92	0.34
C	–0.68	0.27

Identify these three cells as root hair, root cortical and leaf mesophyll cells respectively.

(a) A, B, C
(b) A, C, B
(c) C, A, B
(d) B, C, A

9. Match the terms of column I with the appropriate terms of column II.

Column I	Column II
(i) K^+ pump theory	(A) Semi-permeable membrane
(ii) Plasmolysis	(B) Hydathodes
(iii) Imbibition	(C) Stomatal movement
(iv) Guttation	(D) Exosmosis
(v) Osmosis	(E) Hydrophilic colloids

(a) (I)-(C); (II)-(D); (III)-(E); (IV)-(B); (V)-(A)
(b) (I)-(A); (II)-(B); (III)-(C); (IV)-(D); (V)-(E)
(c) (I)-(B); (II)-(C); (III)-(E); (IV)-(A); (V)-(D)
(d) (I)-(D); (II)-(E); (III)-(B); (IV)-(C); (V)-(A)

10. The graph shows the relationship between ψ (water potential), ψ_s(solute potential) and ψ_p (pressure potential) for a plant cell placed in pure water.

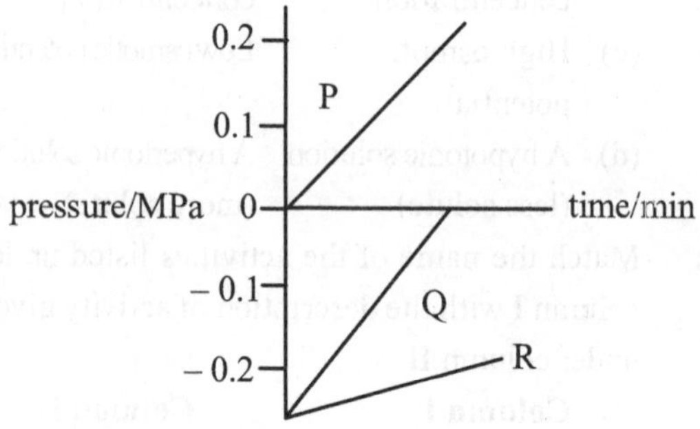

What are the correct labels for the graph?

	P	Q	R
(a)	ψ	ψ_p	ψ_s
(b)	ψ	ψ_s	ψ_p
(c)	ψ_p	ψ	ψ_s
(d)	ψ_p	ψ_s	ψ

11. In cells A, B, C, D potentials are as given below.

Cell	Solute potential	Pressure potential
A	– 15.0 bars	5.0 bars
B	– 25.0 bars	15.0 bars
C	– 30.0 bars	20.0 bars
D	– 35.0 bars	25.0 bars

Water will move from

(a) A to B

(b) B to A

(c) A to B to C to D

(d) Remain stationary

12. Match the columns and find out the correct combination:

A.	Simultaneous transport of two types of molecules	1.	Uniport
B.	Co-transport of two molecules across the membrane in same direction	2.	Co-transport
C.	Co-transport of two molecules across the membrane in opposite directions	3.	Symport
D.	Transport of a molecule across a membrane, independent of other molecules	4.	Antiport
		5.	Passive transport

(a) A-5, B-2, C-1,D-3

(b) A-2,B-3, C-1,D-4

(c) A-2, B-3,C-4,D-1

(d) A-5,B-1,C-2,D-4

13. Find the wrongly match pair:

(a)	Guttation	Loss of impure water
(b)	Transpiration	Account for the majority of water transport
(c)	Girdling	Pholem is responsible for translocation of food
(d)	Unloading of minerals at the fine vein endings	Through active transport

14. Match the columns and find out the correct combinations:

A.	Potential gradient between root and leaf	1.	Helps in gaseous exchange
B.	Organic solute gradient between source and sink	2.	Helps in ascent of sap
C.	Positive hydrostatic pressure near roots	3.	Helps in guttation
D.	Negative hydrostatic pressure near leaf	4.	Helps in bulk flow of photosynthates
		5.	Helps in transpiration pull (tension)

(a) A-5, B-4, C-3, D-2

(b) A-5, B-3, C-4, D-1

(c) A-3, B-2, C-1, D-4

(d) A-3, B-2, C-4, D-5

Solutions

1. (b) 2. (a) 3. (c) 4. (c) 5. (c)

6. (b) 7. (b)

8. (c) Water potentials of the given cells are

$\Psi w = \Psi s + \Psi p$

A = – 0.87 + 0.44 = – 0.43

B = – 0.92 + 0.34 = – 0.58

C = –0.68 + 0.27 = – 0.41

As water moves from greater water potential to less, root hair, root cortical and leaf mesophyll cells are C,A,B respectively.

9. (a)

10. (c) Pure water has the highest water potential as zero. As water enters the cells, solute potential becomes less negative and the pressure potential is usually positive. As water enters the cell, the volume of protoplast increases, causing the pressure potential to rise from zero MPa.

11. (d) Water potentials of all the four cells are equal.

12. (c) 13. (d) 14. (a)

CHAPTER

Mineral Nutrition

1. Select incorrect match with respect to mineral and the function:
   (a) Zinc — Synthesis of auxin
   (b) Chlorine — Photolysis of water
   (c) Copper — Activator of alcohol dehydrogenase
   (d) Molybednum — Nitrogen metabolism

2. Find out correctly matched pair:

	Nutrients	Functions
(a)	Zinc	Helps to maintain ribosome structure
(b)	Magnesium	Needed during formation of mitotic spindle
(c)	Potassium	Plays a role in opening and closing of stomata
(d)	Calcium	Needed in splitting of water to liberate oxygen during photosynthesis.

3. Match the columns and choose the correct combination:

A.	Phosphorus	1.	Cell wall formation
B.	Potassium	2.	Activation of RuBisCo
C.	Calcium	3.	Phosphorylation
D.	Magnesium	4.	Take part in electron transport
		5.	Closing and opening of stomata

   (a) A-1, B-5, C-3,D-2
   (b) A-3,B-5, C-1,D-2
   (c) A-2,B-5,C-1,D-3
   (d) A-3,B-5,C-2,D-1

4. Match the columns and choose the correct options:

Disease	Deficiency of Minerals
(A) Khaira Disease	(i) Mn
(B) Marsh spot of Pea	(ii) Zn
(C) Brown rot disease	(iii) Mo
(D) Whip tail of cauliflower	(iv) B

   (a) A-ii , B-i, C-iii, D-iv
   (b) A-ii, B-i, C-iv, D-iii
   (c) A-i, B-ii, C-iii, D-iv
   (d) A-i, B-ii, C-iv, D-iii

5. Match the columns-I and column-II and choose the correct option:

Column I	Column II
1. Micronutrients	A. Fe, Mn
2. Macronutrients	*B. Nitrosomonas*
3. Nitrification	C. K, S
4. Denitrification	*D. Thiobacillus*

   (a) 1-C, 2-A, 3-D,4-B
   (b) 1-C,2-A,3-B,4-D
   (c) 1-A, 2-C,3-D, 4-B
   (d) 1-A,2-C,3-B,4-D

6. Match the columns:

Column I	Column II
A. Hydroponics	1. Zinc
B. Trace elements	2. Fe
C. Activation of catalase	3. Julius von sachs
D. Dark reaction	4. Calvin

   (a) A-3, B-2,C-1,D-4
   (b) A-4,B-3,C-2,D-1

7. Match the column-I with column-II

Column-I		Column-II
(A) Mg	p.	Found in some amino acids
(B) S	q.	Structural component of chlorophyll
(C) I	r.	Not important for plants
(D) Mn	s.	Required for photolysis of water

(a) A-q, B-p, C-r, D-s (b) A-p, B-q, C-r, D-s
(c) A-p, B-r, C-s, D-q (d) A-q, B-r, C-p, D-s

8. Match the Column-I containing minerals with the functions given in Column-II.

Column-I		Column-II
I. K	A.	Stomatal opening
II. Mo	B.	Constituent of cell membrane
III. P	C.	Photolysis of water
IV. Mn	D.	Free ion
	E.	Component of nitrogenase and nitrate reductase

	I	II	III	IV
(a)	A, D	E	B	C
(b)	A, E	D	C	B
(c)	A, E	D	B	C
(d)	D	A	C	B, E

9. Refer the figure given below and select the option which gives correct words for all the four blanks A, B, C and D.

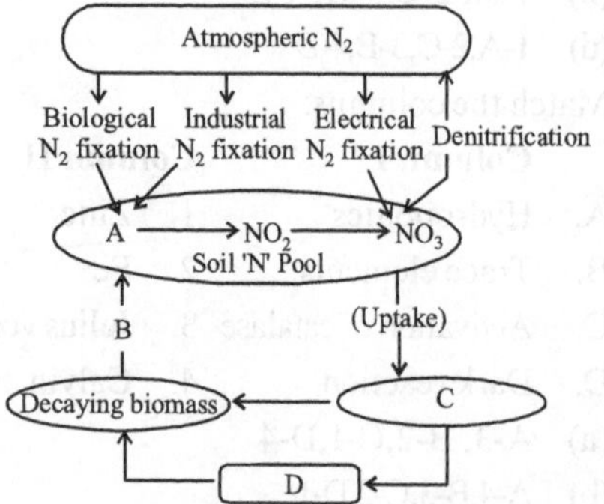

	A	B	C	D
(a)	K	Ammonification	Animal biomass	Plant biomass
(b)	NH_3	Ammonification	Plant biomass	Animal biomass
(c)	CO_2	Denitrification	Animal biomass	Plant biomass
(d)	CHO	Nitrification	Plant biomass	Animal biomass

10. A small aquatic plant was put in each of the petridishes -X, Y & Z, containing different culture solutions. After six weeks the plant in dish X had the same number of leaves as it had previously & were all small and yellowish. Plant in dish Y had more leaves of normal size and dark green colour. Plants in dish Z had more leaves of normal size but very pale. Which of the following show the element missing in the culture?

	X	Y	Z
(a)	Magnesium	Phosphorus	Nitrogen
(b)	Phosphorus	Magnesium	Nitrogen
(c)	Phosphorus	Nitrogen	Magnesium
(d)	Magnesium	Nitrogen	Phosphorus

11. Match the words of column I with the phrases in column II. Choose the answer which gives the correct combination.

Column I	Column II
(1) Magnesium	(p) Found in some amino acids
(2) Sulphur	(q) Not important for plants
(3) Iodine	(r) Structural component of chlorophyll
(4) Manganese	(s) Component of sugar
	(t) Required for enzyme activity

(a) (1) – (r), (2) – (s), (3) – (q), (4) – (p)
(b) (1) – (r), (2) – (p), (3) – (q), (4) – (s)
(c) (1) – (r), (2) – (p), (3) – (q), (4) – (t)
(d) (1) – (s), (2) – (r), (3) – (p), (4) – (t)

12. Match the following and choose the correct combination from the options given.

Column I	Column II
A. Potassium	I. Constituent of ferredoxin
B. Sulphur	II. Involved in stomatal movement
C. Molybdenum	III. Needed in the synthesis of auxin
D. Zinc	IV. Component of nitrogenase

(a) A-II, B-I, C-IV, D-III
(b) A-I, B-II, C-III, C-IV
(c) A-IV, B-III, C-II, D-I
(d) A-I, B-III, C-IV, D-II

13. Which of the following option shows correct co-relation between Column-I, II and III.

Calumn-I	Column-II	Column-III
(A) Calcium	(I) Required for ionic-balance.	(i) Grey blot on leaves.
(B) Boron	(II) Essential for constitution of nucleic acid	(ii) Fruit-yield decreases.
(C) Phosphorus	(III) Required for absorption of calcium.	(iii) Red blots on leaves.
(D) Chlorine	(IV) Required to activate respiratory enzyme.	(iv) Fruit-size diminishes.
(E) Manganese	(V) Required for synthesis of bipolar spindle.	(v) Young root tip begin to die.

(a) (A-I-iv), (B-II-v), (C-III-iii), (D-IV-i), (E-V-ii)
(b) (A-V-v), (B-IV-iv), (C-III-i), (D-III-iii), (E-I-ii)
(c) (A-IV-iii), (B-I-iv), (C-V-v), (D-III-ii), (E-II-i)
(d) (A-V-v), (B-III-iv), (C-II-iii), (D-I-ii), (E-IV-i)

14. Study the following lists.

List I	List II
(A) Photolysis of water	(i) Zinc
(B) Diazotrophy	(ii) Copper
(C) Cytochrome 'c' oxidase	(iii) Manganese
(D) Biosynthesis of IAA	(iv) Molybdenum
	(v) Boron

Identify the correct match.

(a) A – iii, B – iv, C – ii, D – i
(b) A – v, B – ii, C – iii, D – iv
(c) A – iii, B – ii, C – i, D – iv
(d) A – iv, B – i, C – iii, D – ii

15. Match the following and choose the correct combination from the options given.

Column I	Column II
(A) Sulphur	I. Chlorophyll
(B) Zinc	II. Nitrogenase
(C) Magnesium	III. Methionine
(D) Molybdenum	IV. Auxin

(1) A – I, B – II, C – III, D – IV
(2) A – III, B – IV, C – I, D – II
(3) A – III, B – I, C – II, D – IV
(4) A – II, B – IV, C – I, D – III

19. Match column-I and Column-II and choose the correct option given below the columns.

Column-I (Element)	**Column-II (Function)**
A. Calcium	1. Required for ionic-balance.
B. Boron	2. Essential for constitution of nucleic acid
C. Phosphorus	3. Required for absorption of calcium.
D. Chlorine	4. Required to activate respiratory enzyme.
E. Manganese	5. Required for synthesis of mitotic spindle.

(a) $A \to 1$; $B \to 2$; $C \to 3$; $D \to 4$; $E \to 5$
(b) $A \to 5$; $B \to 4$; $C \to 3$; $D \to 2$; $E \to 1$
(c) $A \to 4$; $B \to 1$; $C \to 5$; $D \to 3$; $E \to 2$
(d) $A \to 5$; $B \to 3$; $C \to 2$; $D \to 1$; $E \to 4$

20. The given diagram shows a typical setup for hydroponic technique. Select the option which gives correct labelling for A, B and C.

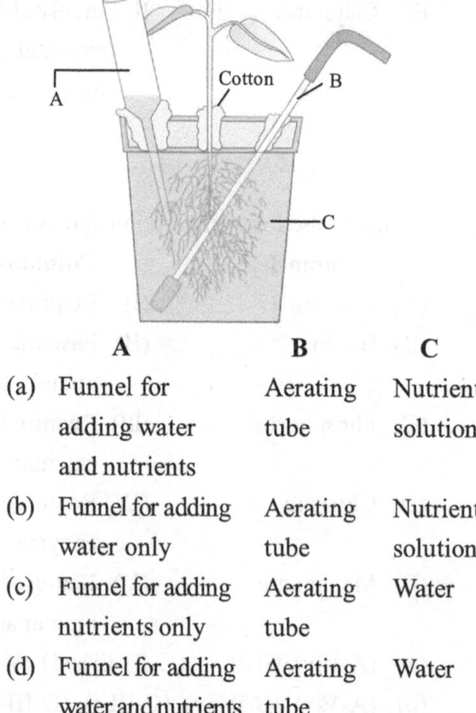

	A	B	C
(a)	Funnel for adding water and nutrients	Aerating tube	Nutrient solution
(b)	Funnel for adding water only	Aerating tube	Nutrient solution
(c)	Funnel for adding nutrients only	Aerating tube	Water
(d)	Funnel for adding water and nutrients	Aerating tube	Water

Solutions

1.	**(c)**	**2.**	**(c)**	**3.**	**(b)**	**4.**	**(b)**	**5.**	**(d)**
6.	**(c)**	**7.**	**(a)**	**8.**	**(a)**	**9.**	**(b)**	**10.**	**(a)**
11.	**(c)**	**12.**	**(a)**	**13.**	**(d)**	**14.**	**(a)**	**15.**	**(b)**
19.	**(a)**	**20.**	**(a)**						

CHAPTER

Photosynthesis

1. The rate of photosynthesis of a freshwater plant is measured using five spectral colours. Which sequence of colours would give an increasing photosynthetic response?

Smallest → Largest response

(a) Blue Green Yellow Orange Red
(b) Green Yellow Orange Red Blue
(c) Red Orange Yellow Green Blue
(d) Yellow Green Orange Blue Red

2. Which one of the following correctly identifies X and Y and shows their functions?

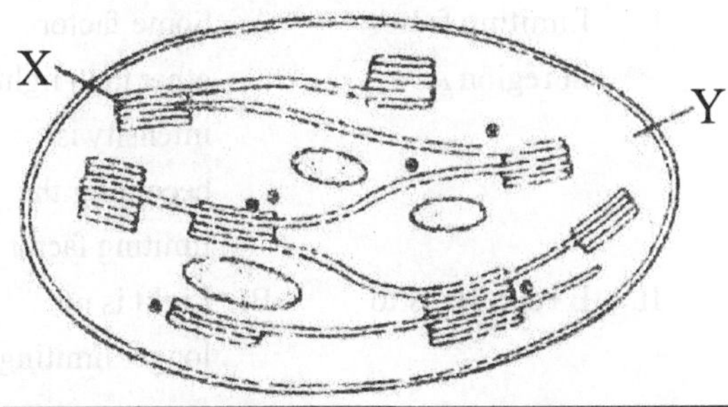

	X		Y	
	Structure	Function	Structure	Function
(a)	Grana	Photolysis of water	Stroma	CO_2 fixation
(b)	Grana	CO_2 fixation	Stroma	Photolysis of water
(c)	Stroma	Photolysis	Grana	CO_2 fixation
(d)	Grana	CO_2 fixation	Lamellae	Photolysis of water

3. Which of the following changes in concentration of chemicals (RuBP & GP) would occur if an illuminated green plant cell's source of carbon dioxide were removed?

	Ribulose bisphosphate	Glycerate phosphate
(a)	increase	increase
(b)	decrease	decrease
(c)	increase	decrease
(d)	decrease	increase

4. Which of the following with respect to early experiments of photosynthesis is wrongly matched?

(a) Joseph Priestley - Showed that plants release O_2
(b) Jan Ingenhousz - Showed that sunlight is essential for photosynthesis
(c) Julius von Sachs - Proved that plants produce glucose when they grow.
(d) T. W. Engelmann - Showed that the green substance is located within special bodies in plants

5. Which of following ratio is correct for the production of one molecule of glucose through 6 round of Calvin cycle?

	CO_2	:	ATP	:	$NADPH_2$
(a)	1	:	2	:	2
(b)	6	:	18	:	12
(c)	6	:	12	:	18
(d)	5	:	6	:	9

6. Which one is correct for C_4-plants?

	Mesophyll		Bundle Sheath	
(a)	PEPcase	C_4-Cycle	RuBisCO	C_3-Cycle
(b)	PEPcase	Calvin Cycle	RuBisCO	C_4-Cycle
(c)	RuBisCO	C_4-Cycle	PEPcase	C_3-Cycle
(d)	RuBisCO	C_2-Cycle	PEPcase	C_3-Cycle

7. The given diagram shows the ultrastructure of a chloroplast as seen in section. What are the functions of A, B and C?

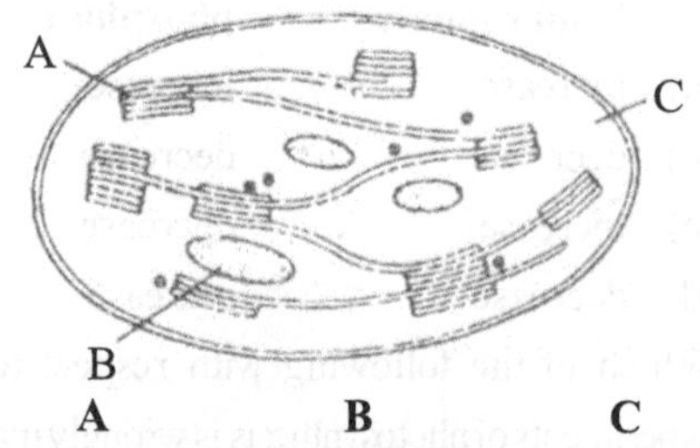

	A	B	C
(a)	Carbohydrate storage	Carbohydrate synthesis	Light reaction
(b)	Light reaction	Carbohydrate synthesis	Carbohydrate storage
(c)	Light reaction	Carbohydrate storage	Carbohydrate synthesis
(d)	Light absorption	Carbohydrate synthesis	Carbohydrate storage

8. The diagram below shows the movement of substances into in and out of a chloroplast with labelling A, B, C & D.

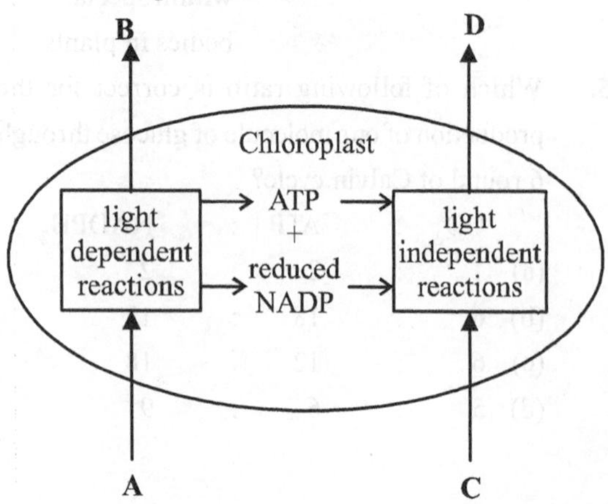

What do labels A to D represent ?

	A	B	C	D
(a)	CO_2	ATP	H_2O	Starch
(b)	CO_2	H_2O	Sugars	O_2
(c)	H_2O	O_2	CO_2	Sugar
(d)	Sugar	H_2O	ATP	O_2

9. Study the figure showing graph of light intensity on the rate of photosynthesis. Choose the correct option by matching the column I with column II

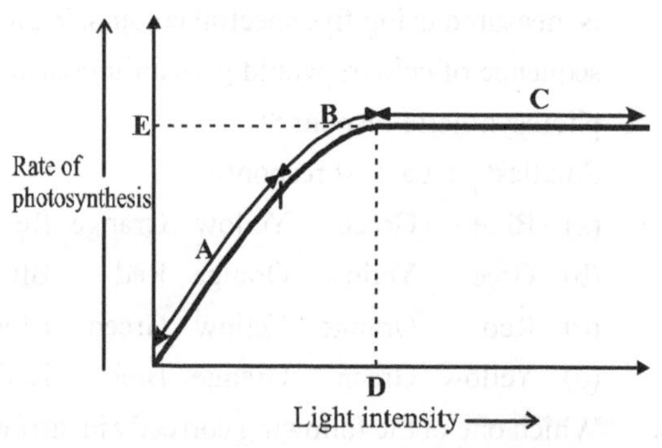

	Column - I		Column - II
I.	Limiting factor in region A	A.	Some factor other than light intensity is becoming the limiting factor
II.	B represents to	B.	Light is no longer limiting factor
III.	C represents to	C.	Light intensity
IV.	D represents to	D.	Maximum rate of photosynthesis
V.	E represents to	E.	Saturation point for light intensity

The correct option is -

(a) I - A, II - B, III - C, IV - D, V - E
(b) I - C, II - A, III - B, IV - E, V - D
(c) I - D, II - B, III - E, IV - C, V - A
(d) I - E, II - D, III - C, IV - B, V - A

10. The diagram below shows the Calvin cycle.

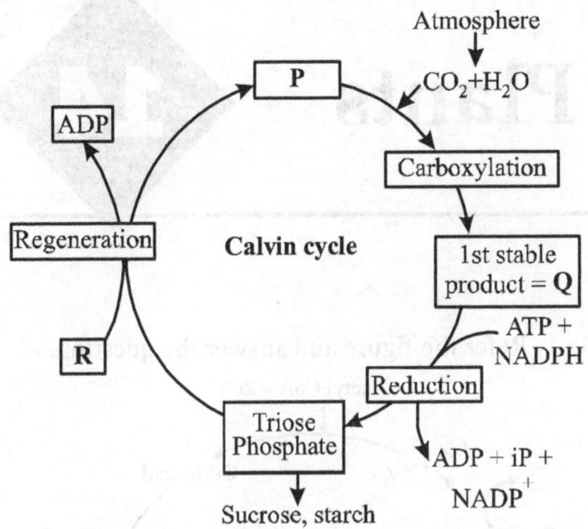

Identify P, Q and R

	P	Q	R
(a)	ATP	3PGA	RuBP
(c)	3PGA	ATP	Sugar
(b)	RuBP	3-PGA	ATP
(d)	Sugar	RuDP	NADPH

11. Two groups of isolated thylakoids are placed in an acidic bathing solution so that H^+ diffuses into the thylakoids. They are then transferred to a basic bathing solution, and one group is placed in the light, while the other group is kept in the dark. Select the choice given below that describes what you expect each group of thylakoids to produce.

	In Light	In Dark
(a)	ATP only	Nothing
(b)	ATP, O_2	ATP only
(c)	ATP, O_2, glucose	ATP, O_2
(d)	ATP, O_2	O_2

12. Make column I with column II.

Column-I	Column-II
(A) Emerson effect	(I) C_4 cycle
(B) Hill reaction	(II) Photolysis
(C) Calvin's cycle	(III) C_3 cycle
(D) Hatch and Slack cycle	(IV) Photosystem-I and II

(a) AI, BII, CIII, DIV
(b) AI, BIII, CIV, DI
(c) AIII, BIV, CI, DII
(d) AIV, BII, CIV, DI

Solutions

1.	(b)	2.	(a)	3.	(c)	4.	(d)	5.	(b)
6.	(a)	7.	(c)	8.	(c)	9.	(b)	10.	(c)
11.	(b)	12.	(d)						

CHAPTER

Respiration in Plants

1. Choose the correct combination between respiratory substrates and their respective RQs.

	Carbohydrate	Fat	Protein
(a)	2	1	1
(b)	0	1	1
(c)	1	0.7	0.9
(d)	0.5	0.5	0.5

2. Refer the figure showing major pathway of anaerobic respiration.

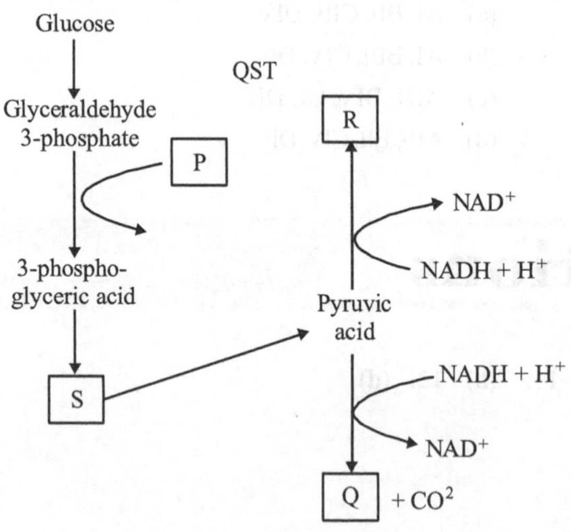

Identify P, Q, R and S in the above.

	P	Q	R	S
(a)	NAD^+	Ethanol	Lactic acid	PEP
(b)	Ethanol	NAD^+	Lactic acid	ATP
(c)	Lactic acid	Ethanol	Glucose	ADP
(d)	NAD	Lactic acid	Ethanol	DHAP

3. Refer the figure and answer the question.

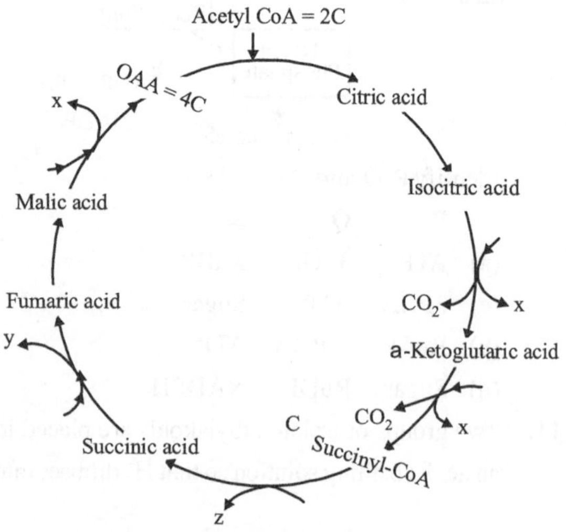

Identify X, Y and Z.

	X	Y	Z
(a)	GTP	$NADH_2$	CO_2
(b)	$FADH_2$	$NADH_2$	GTP
(c)	$NADH_2$	$FADH_2$	GTP
(d)	CO_2	$NADH_2$	ADP

4. The expressions given below shows the summary equations.

(i) Pyruvate $\xrightarrow{NADH + H^+ \;\rightarrow\; NAD^+}$ $C_2H_5OH + CO_2$

(i) $C_6H_{12}O_6 + NAD^+ + 2ADP + 2\ iP \rightarrow 2C_3H_4O_3 + 2ATP + 2NADH + 2H^+$

(iii) Pyruvic acid $+ 4NAD^+ + FAD^+ + 2H_2O + ADP + Pi \rightarrow 3CO_2 + 4NADH + 4H^+ + ATP + FADH_2$

Categorise the summary equations under respective phases.

	I	II	III
(a)	Krebs' cycle	Glycolysis	Fermentation
(b)	Glycolysis	Krebs' cycle	Fermentation
(c)	Fermentation	Krebs' cycle	Glycolysis
(d)	Fermentation	Glycolysis	Krebs' cycle

5. Match the number of carbon atoms given in List - I with that of the compounds given in List - II and select the correct option.

	List - I		List - II
A.	4C Compound	I.	Acetyl CoA
B.	2C Compound	II.	Pyruvate
C.	5C Compound	III.	Citric acid
D.	3C Compound	IV.	α-ketoglutaric acid
		V.	Malic acid

(a) A-II, B-V, C-III, D-I
(b) A-V, B-I, C-IV, D-II
(c) A-III, B-I, C-IV, D-II
(d) A-V, B-III, C-I, D-II

6. Match the column I with column II

Column I		Column II
(A) EMP pathway	I.	Mitochondrial matrix
(B) TCA cycle	II.	Cytoplasm
(C) ETC	III.	Inner mitochondrial membrane

	A	B	C
(a)	I	II	III
(b)	II	I	III
(c)	II	III	I
(d)	III	II	I

7. Match the sites in column I with processes in column II and choose the correct combination from the options.

Column I	Column II
(A) Grana of chloroplast	(i) Krebs cycle
(B) Stroma of chloroplast	(ii) Light reaction
(C) Cytoplasm	(iii) Dark reaction
(D) Mitochondrial matrix	(iv) Glycolysis

(a) A – (iv), B – (iii), C – (ii), D – (i)
(b) A – (i), B – (ii), C – (iv), D – (iii)
(c) A – (ii), B – (i), C – (iii), D – (iv)
(d) A – (ii), B – (iii), C – (iv), D – (i)

8. Choose the correct combination of labelling the number of carbon compounds in the substrate molecules, involved in the citric acid cycle.

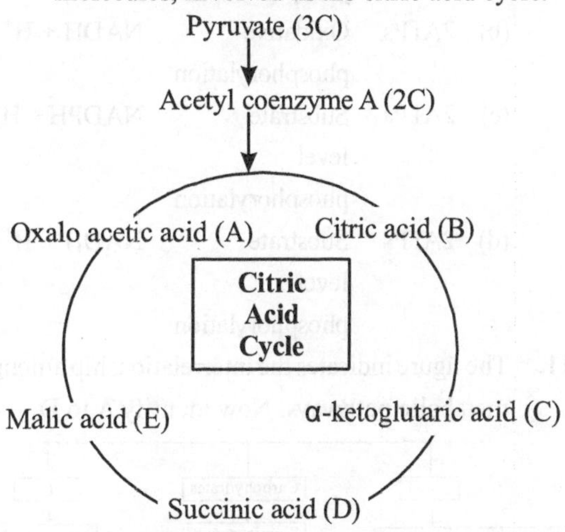

(a) (A) 4C, (B) 6C, (C) 5C, (D) 4C, (E) 4C
(b) (A) 6C, (B) 5C, (C) 4C, (D) 3C, (E) 2C
(c) (A) 2C, (B) 5C, (C) 6C, (D) 4C, (E) 4C
(d) (A) 4C, (B) 6C, (C) 4C, (D) 4C, (E) 5C

9. Match the compounds given in Column I with the number of carbon atoms present in them which are listed under Column II. Choose the answer which givens the correct combination of alphabets of the two column.

	Column-I		Column-II
A.	Oxaloacetate	p.	6-C compound
B.	Phosphoglycrealdehyde	q.	5-C compound
C.	Isocitrate	r.	4-C compound
D.	α-ketoglutarate	s.	3-C compound
		t.	2-C compound

	A	B	C	D
(a)	s	t	q	r
(b)	r	s	p	q
(c)	r	t	p	q
(d)	q	s	p	t

10. At the end of glycolysis X is the net energy gain from one molecule of glucose *via* Y, but there is also energy stored in the form of Z. Identify X, Y and Z from the given options.

	X	Y	Z
(a)	1ATP	Oxidative phosphorylation	$NADH + H^+$
(b)	2ATPs	Oxidative phosphorylation	$NADH + H^+$
(c)	2ATPs	Substrate level phosphorylation	$NADPH + H^+$
(d)	2ATPs	Substrate level phosphorylation	$NADH + H^+$

11. The figure indicates the interrelationship among metabolic pathways. Now identify A to D.

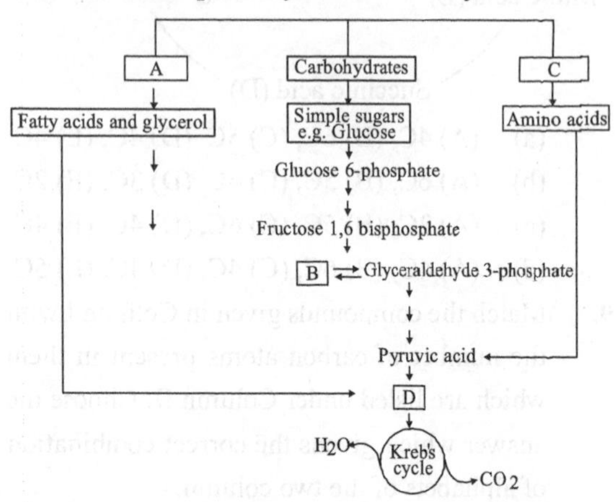

	A	B	C	D
(a)	Protein	Acetyl CoA	Fat	DHAP
(b)	Fat	DHAP	Protein	Acetyl CoA
(c)	Acetyl CoA	Fat	DHAP	Protein
(d)	Fat	DHAP	Acetyl CoA	Protein

12. The diagram shows stalked particles on part of a crista membrane in a mitochondrion.

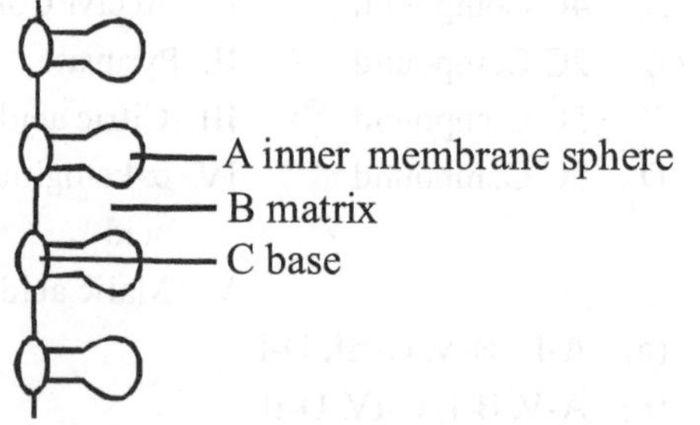

What occurs in each of the numbered regions?

	A	B	C
(a)	ADP synthesis	Electron transport	Krebs cycle
(b)	ADP synthesis	Glycolysis	Krebs cycle
(c)	ATP synthesis	Krebs cycle	Electron transport
(d)	ATP synthesis	Krebs cycle	Glycolysis

Solutions

1. (c) 2. (a) 3. (c) 4. (d) 5. (b)
6. (b) 7. (d) 8. (a) 9. (b) 10. (d)
11. (b)
12. (c) The electron transport system occurs in 3, and is coupled to proton transport across the inner membrane (1), generating the proton-motive force, powering ATP synthesis. Krebs cycle occurs in the matrix, where two molecules of acetyl CoA are oxidized.

CHAPTER

Plant Growth and Development

1. Refer the functions of the growth hormones given below.

I. Cell division
II. Cell enlargement
III. Pattern formation
IV. Tropic growth
V Flowering
VI. Fruiting
VII. Seed germination
VIII. Response to wound
IX. Response to stresses of biotic and abiotic origin

Identify the functions of growth promoters and growth inhibitors from the above.

	Functions of growth promoters	Functions of growth inhibitor
(a)	I, II, VII, IX	III, IV, V, VI, VII
(b)	VIII, IX	I, II, III, IV, V, VI, VII
(c)	I, II, III, IV, V, VI, VII	VIII, IX
(d)	I, II, III, IV, V, VI, VII, IX	VIII

2. Match the column A (Scientists) with column B (Discovery).

Column-A	Column-B
I. C. Darwin and F. Darwin	A. Cytokinin
II. Miller and Skoog	B. ABA
III. F.W. Went	C. C_2H_4
IV. Kurosawa	D. Auxin
	E. GA

	I	II	III	IV
(a)	D	A	C	E
(b)	D	A	E	B
(c)	C	A	B	D
(d)	E	D	A	C

3. Refer the statements given below.

Statement-I :
Confirmation of the release of volatile substance from ripened oranges that hastened the ripening of stored unripe bananas.

Statement-II :
Callus formation takes place from internodal segments of tobacco stem with the auxin and the nutrient medium containing extracts of vascular tissues/yeast/coconut milk/ DNA. Later, cytokinesis promoting substance was identified, crystallized and named as Kinetin.

Statement-III :
Reporting of appearance of symptoms of bakane/foolish seedling disease caused by fungus, Gibberella fujikuroi, in uninfected seedling when they were treated with sterile filtrates of the fungus. The active substances were later identified as GA.

Choose the correct option.

	I	II	III
(a)	Miller + Skoog	Cousins	Kurosawa
(b)	Kurosawa	Cousins	Miller + Skoog
(c)	Cousins	Kurosawa	Miller + Skoog
(d)	Cousins	Miller + Skoog	Kurosawa

4. The picture below shows three different types of plants (marked as P-I, P-II and P-III) which flower on the basis of their critical photoperiod. Now identify these plants (P-I, II and III).

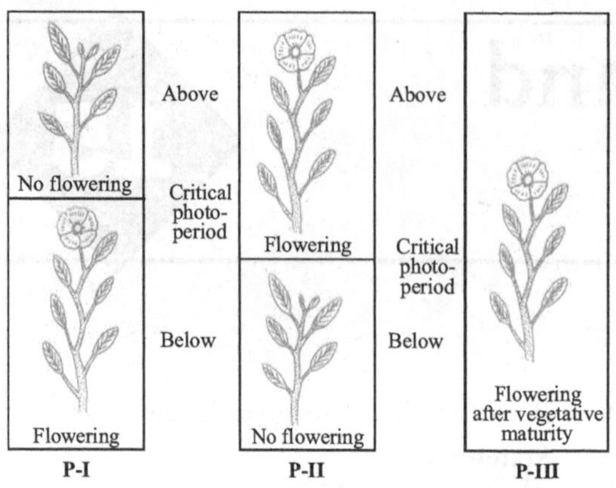

(a) P-I = Long day plant; P-II = Short day plant; P-III = Day neutral plant
(b) P-I = Short day plant; P-II = Long day plant; P-III = Day neutral plant
(c) P-I = Short day plant; P-II = Short day plant; P-III = Day neutral plant
(d) P-I =Long day plant; P-II = Long day plant; P-III = Day neutral plant

5. The picture below shows a graph drawn on the parameters of growth versus time. A, B, C respectively represent

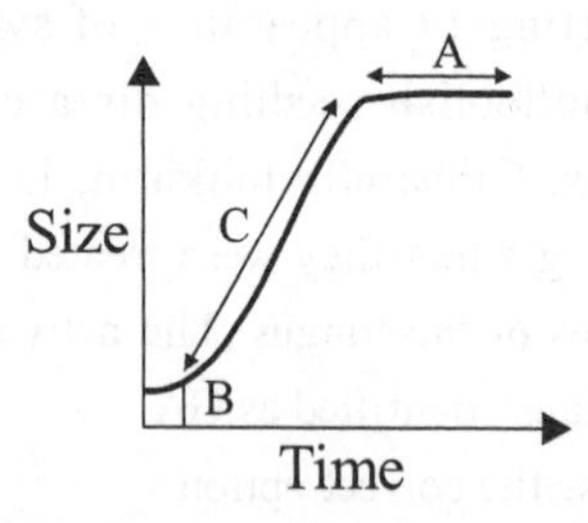

	A	B	C
(a)	Exponential phase	Log phase	Steady state phase
(b)	Steady state phase	Lag phase	Log phase
(c)	Log phase	Steady state phase	Logarithmic phase
(d)	Log phase	Lag phase	Steady state phase

6. Refer the diagram which shows the stages of seed germination.

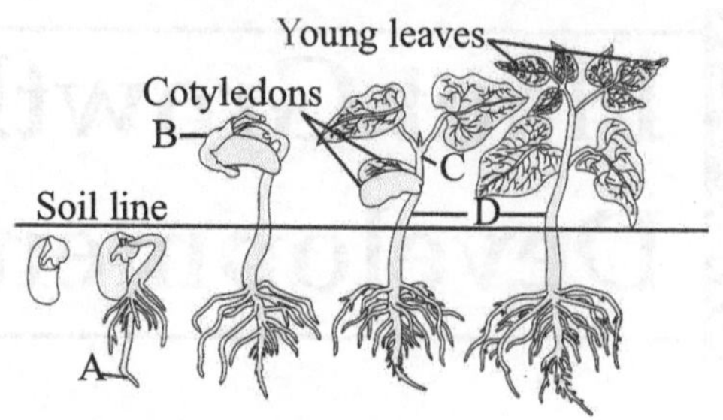

Identify A, B, C and D.

	A	B	C	D
(a)	Plumule	Cotyledons	Hypocotyl	Epicotyl
(b)	Radicle	Seed coat	Epicotyl	Hypocotyl
(c)	Hypocotyl	Cotyledons	Epicotyl	Root hair
(d)	Root hair	Cotyledons	Plumule	Hypocotyl

7. Match the plant hormones listed in column-I with their major role listed in column-II. Select the correct option from the codes given below.

Column-A	Column-B
(A) Auxin	(I) Fruit ripening
(B) Cytokinins	(II) Phototropism
(C) Abscisic acid	(III) Antagonist to GAs
(D) Ethylene	(IV) Stomatal opening and closing
	(V) Growth of lateral buds

(a) A-IV; B-V; C-III; D-I
(b) A-II; B-IV; C-III, IV; D-I
(c) A-I; B-V; C-III, IV; D-I
(d) A-III, IV; B-V; C-II; D-I

8. Match the growth regulators in column-I with the processes in column-II and choose the correct combination.

Column-I	Column-II
(A) Auxin	(i) Colouring test in lemon
(B) Gibberellin	(ii) Cell division test in plants
(C) Cytokinin	(iii) Avena curvature test
(D) Ethylene	(iv) Dwarf corn test

(a) (A) – (iii), (B) – (iv), (C) – (ii), (D) – (i)
(b) (A) – (i), (B) – (iv), (C) – (ii), (D) – (iii)
(c) (A) – (iv), (B) – (iii), (C) – (i), (D) – (ii)
(d) (A) – (ii), (B) – (i), (C) – (iv), (D) – (iii)

9. Which of the following is **incorrectly** matched?
(a) Explant – Excised plant part used for callus formation
(b) Cytokinins – Root initiation in callus
(c) Somatic embryo – Embryo produced from a vegetative cell
(d) Anther culture – Haploid plants

10. Match list I and list II and select the correct option.

List-I	**List-II**
(A) Auxin	(I) Herring sperm DNA
(B) Cytokinin	(II) Inhibitor of growth
(C) Gibberellin	(III) Apical dominance
(D) Ethylene	(IV) Epinasty
(E) Abscisic acid	(V) Induces amylase synthesis

(a) A-III, B-I, C-V, D-IV, E-II
(b) A-IV, B-V, C-I, D-III, E-II
(c) A-II, B-I, C-V, D-III, E-IV
(d) A-III, B-I, C-V, D-II, E-IV

11. Match the following and choose the correct combination

Column I	**Column II**
(1) Zeatin	1. Flowering hormone
(2) Florigen	2. Synthetic auxin
(3) IBA	3. Cytokinin
(4) NAA	4. Natural auxin

(a) A – 3, B – 4, C – 1, D – 2
(b) A – 2, B – 1, C – 4, D – 3
(c) A – 1, B – 2, C – 3, D – 4
(d) A – 3, B – 1, C – 4, D – 2

12. Which one of the following pairs, is not correctly matched?
(a) Abscisic acid — Stomatal closure
(b) Gibberellic acid — Leaf fall
(3) Cytokinin — Cell division
(4) IAA — Cell wall elongation

13. Which one of the following pairs is incorrectly matched?
(a) Adenine derivative - kinetin
(b) Carotenoid derivative - ABA
(c) Terpenes - IAA
(d) Indole compounds - IBA

14. Match the following and choose the correct combination from the options given.

Column I (Growth Regulator)	**Column II (Action)**
(A) Abscisic acid	1. Delays leaf senescence
(B) Ethylene	2. Inhibits seed germination
(C) Cytokinin	3. Herbicide
(D) Auxin	4. Hastens fruit ripening

(a) A-2, B-4, C-1, D-3
(b) A-1, B-2, C-3, D-4
(c) A-2, B-3, C-4, D-1
(d) A-2, B-1, C-3, D-4

15. Match the following columns and choose the correct combination

Column A	**Column B**
(A) Zeatin	(i) Flowering hormone
(B) Florigen	(ii) Natural auxin
(C) IBA	(iii) Cytokinin
(D) NAA	(iv) Synthetic auxin

	A	**B**	**C**	**D**
(a)	iii	i	iv	ii
(b)	iii	iv	i	ii
(c)	ii	i	iv	iii
(d)	i	ii	iii	iv

Solutions

1.	**(c)**	**2.**	**(a)**	**3.**	**(d)**	**4.**	**(b)**	**5.**	**(b)**
6.	**(b)**	**7.**	**(c)**	**8.**	**(a)**	**9.**	**(b)**	**10.**	**(a)**
11.	**(d)**	**12.**	**(b)**	**13.**	**(c)**	**14.**	**(a)**	**15.**	**(a)**

CHAPTER

Digestion and Absorption

1. Match the entities of Column I with Column II and choose the right option from the codes given below.

	Column I	Column II
A.	Cardiac sphincter	1. Hepatopancreatic duct
B.	Pyloric sphincter	2. Join gall bladder to common bile duct
C.	Sphincter of Oddi	3. Opening of stomach into duodenum
D.	Cystic ducts	4. Opening of oesophagus into stomach

Codes

	A	B	C	D
(a)	4	3	1	2
(b)	4	3	2	1
(c)	3	4	1	2
(d)	2	1	3	4

2. Match the following Columns.

	Column I	Column II
A.	Kupffer's cells	1. Islets of Langerhans
B.	β - cells	2. Liver sinusoids
C.	Bruch border cells	3. Thyroid gland
D.	Paneth cells	4. Proximal convoluted tubule
		5. Small intestine

Codes

	A	B	C	D
(a)	3	1	4	2
(b)	4	5	1	2
(c)	2	1	4	5
(d)	3	5	4	1

3. Match the following Column.

Column I	Column II
A. Vitamin - B_1	1. Thiamin
B. Vitamin - B_3	2. Niacin
C. Vitamin - A	3. Retinol
D. Vitamin - B_2	4. Riboflavin

Codes

	A	B	C	D
(a)	1	2	3	4
(b)	1	3	4	2
(c)	3	4	2	1
(d)	4	3	2	1

4. Match the following Column.

	Column I	Column II
A.	Retinol	1. Inhibits oxidation of unsaturated fatty acids
B.	Tocoferol	2. Absorption of calcium ions
C.	Calciferol	3. Essential for maintenance of epithelial tissue
D.	Ascorbic acid	4. Required for amino acid metabolism

Codes

	A	B	C	D
(a)	3	2	4	1
(b)	2	3	1	4
(c)	3	1	2	4
(d)	4	1	2	3

5. Match the enzyme with their rrespective substrates and choose the right one among options given.

Column I	Column II
A. Lipase	1. Dipeptides
B. Nuclease	2. Fats
C. Carboxypeptidase	3. Nucleic acids
D. Dipeptidases	4. Proteins, peptones and proteoses

Codes

	A	B	C	D
(a)	2	3	1	4
(b)	3	4	2	1
(c)	3	1	4	2
(d)	2	3	4	1

6. Match column I with column II and select the correct option from the given codes.

Column I (Types of cell)	Column II (Secretions)
A. Peptic cells	(i) Mucus
B. Oxyntic cells	(ii) Alkaline fluid
C. Goblet cells	(iii) Pro-enzymes
	(iv) HCl

(a) A-(ii), B-(iii), C-(i)
(b) A-(iii), B-(ii), C-(i)
(c) A-(i), B-(ii), C-(iii)
(d) A-(ii), B-(i), C-(iii)

7. Match column I with column II and select the correct option from the given codes.

	Column I	Column II
A.	Van Kupffer cells	(i) Islets of Langerhans
B.	β-cells	(ii) Liver sinusoids
C.	Oxyntic cells	(iii) Thyroid gland
D.	Crypts of Lieberkuhn	(iv) Stomach
		(v) Small intestine

(a) A-(iv), B-(v), C-(i), D-(ii)
(b) A-(iii), B-(i), C-(iv), D-(ii)
(c) A-(iv), B-(v), C-(iii), D-(i)
(d) A-(ii), B-(i), C-(iv), D-(v)

8. Column I contains names of the sphincter muscles of the alimentary canal and Column II contains their locations. Match them properly and choose the correct answer.

	Column I		Column II
A.	Sphincter of ani internus	1.	Opening of hepato-pancreatic duct into duodenum
B.	Cardiac sphincter	2.	Between duodenum and posterior stomach
C.	Sphincter of Oddi	3.	Guarding the terminal part of alimentary canal
D.	Ileocaecal	4.	Between oesophagus sphincter and anterior stomach
E.	Pyloric sphincter	5.	Between small intestine and bowel

(a) A – 3, B –2, C – 4, D – 1, E – 5
(b) A – 2, B – 5, C – 1, D – 4, E – 3
(c) A – 3, B – 4, C – 1, D – 5, E – 2
(d) A – 4, B – 3, C – 1, D – 2, E – 5

9. Match the column I with column II and column III. Choose the correct option.

	Column I (Substrate)	Column II (Enzyme)	Column III (Product)
1.	Lactose	A. Lipase	I. Galactose
2.	Monoglycerides	B. Trypsin	II. Maltose
3.	Starch	C. Lactase	III. Fatty acid
4.	Peptones	D. Amylase	IV. Dipeptides

(a) 1-A-I; 2-C-II; 3-B-III; 4-D-IV
(b) 1-D-I; 2-A-II; 3-B-III; 4-C-IV
(c) 1-C-I; 2-A-III; 3-D-II; 4-B-IV
(d) 1-C-I; 2-A-II; 3-D-III; 4-B-IV
(e) 1-D-I; 2-D-II; 3-C-III; 4-A-IV

10. Match column I with column II and choose the correct option.

Column I		Column II
A. Goblet cells	1.	Antibacterial agent
B. Lysozyme	2.	Mucus
C. Saliva	3.	HCl
D. Oxyntic cells	4.	Sublingual gland

(a) A-3, B-1, C-4, D-2
(b) A-1, B-3, C-4, D-2
(c) A-2, B-3, C-1, D-4
(d) A-4, B-1, C-2, D-3
(e) A-2, B-1, C-4, D-3

11. Match the items given in column I with those in column II and choose the correct option.

Column I	Column II
A. Rennin	(i) Vitamin B_{12}
B. Enterokinase	(ii) Facilitated transport
C. Oxyntic cells	(iii) Milk proteins
D. Fructose	(iv) Trypsinogen

(a) A-iii, B-iv, C-ii, D-i
(b) A-iv, B-iii, C-i, D-ii
(c) A-iv, B-iii, C-ii, D-i
(d) A-iii, B-iv, C-i, D-ii

12. Select the correct match of the digested products in humans given in column I with their absorption site and mechanism in column II.

	Column I	Column II
(a)	Glycerol, fatty acids	Duodenum, move as chylomicrons
(b)	Cholesterol, maltose	Large intestine, active absorption
(c)	Glycine, glocose	Small intestine, active absorption
(d)	Fructose, Na^+	Small intestine, passive absorption

13. Match column I with column II.

Column I		Column II
A. Vitamin B1	1.	Accumulation of fat
B. Gastric juice	2.	Loss of fat
C. Starvation	3.	Pepsin
D. Obesity	4.	Beri-beri

(a) P-(iii), Q-(iv), R-(ii), S-(i)
(b) P-(iii), Q-(iv), R-(i), S-(ii)
(c) P-(iv), Q-(iii), R-(ii), S-(i)
(d) P-(iv), Q-(ii), R-(iii), S-(i)

14. Which one of the following four secretions is correctly matched with its source, target and nature of action ?

	Secretion	Source	Target	Action
(1)	Gastrin	Stomach lining	Oxyntic cells	Production of HCl
(2)	Inhibin	Sertoli cells	Hypotha-lamus	inhibition of secretion of ganadotropin releasing hormone
(3)	Entero-kinase	Duode-num	Gall bladder	Release of bile juice
(4)	Atrial Natriuretic factor (ANF)	Sinu atrial node(SAN) M-cells of Atria	Juxta-glomerular apparatus (JGA)	Inhibition of release of renin

15. Find out the correct matching between the cells of gastric gland and their respective secretory products:

	Column I		Column II
A.	Neck cells	I.	HCl, Intrinsic factor
B.	Peptic/ Chief cells	II.	Mucus
C.	Parietal/ Oxyntic cells	III.	Pepsinogen

(a) A-II, B-III, C-I
(b) A-III, B-II, C-I
(c) A-I, B-II, C-III
(d) A-I, B-III, C-II

16. Match the following structures with their respective location in organs

A.	Crypts of Lieberkuhn	i.	Pancreas
B.	Glisson's Capsule	ii.	Duodenum
C.	Islets of Langerhans	iii.	Small intestine
D.	Brunner' glands	iv.	Liver

Select the correct option from the following

	(A)	(B)	(C)	(D)
(a)	(iii)	(i)	(ii)	(iv)
(b)	(ii)	(iv)	(i)	(iii)
(c)	(iii)	(iv)	(i)	(ii)
(d)	(iii)	(ii)	(i)	(iv)

17. Read the following table carefully and choose the incorrectly matched option

	Enzyme	State of	Substrate Function	Products
(a)	Ptyalin	Mouth	Starch	Disaccharides
(b)	Pepsin	Stomach	Protein	Large peptides
(c)	Lipase	Small Intestine	Triglycerides	Fatty acids
(d)	Nucleotidase	Large Intestine	Nucleotidase	Nucleosides phosphoric acid

18. Match the following

	Column I		Column II
A.	Mucosa	(i)	Bases of villi
B.	Villi	(ii)	Small intestine
C.	Submucosa	(iii)	Villi and rugae
D.	Crypts	(iv)	Nerves, blood and lymphatic vessels

(a) A-(ii), B-(iii), C-(i), D-(iv)
(b) A-(i), B-(iv), C-(ii), D-(iii)
(c) A-(iii), B-(ii), C-(iv), D-(i)
(d) A-(ii), B-(iii), C-(iv), D-(i)

Solutions

1. (a) 2. (c) 3. (a) 4. (c) 5. (d)

6. (d) Gastic glands are numerous, microscopic, simple tubular glands present in the wall of the stomach. They have three common types of gland cell : (i) Peptic (= chief or zymogen) cells that are usually basal in location and secrete digestive enzymes pepsinogen and proprennin (proenzymes) and small amounts of gastric amylase and gastric lipase. (ii) Parietal (= oxyntic) cells secrete HCl and Castle's intrinsic factor. (iii) Mucous (= Goblet) cells secrete mucus.

7. (d) 8. (c) 9. (a) 10. (e) 11. (d)

12. (c) Glycerol and fatty acids are absorbed in jejunum by diffusion into intestinal cells where thy are converted into chylomicrons. Cholesterol is also absorbed by simple diffusion in small intestine. Maltose is broken into glucose and galactose which are absorbed by active transport into small intestine. Fructose is absorbed by facilitated diffusion. Amino acids are also absorbed in small intestine, some by active transport and some by facilitated diffusion.

13. (c) 14. (d) 15. (a) 16. (c) 17. (d)
18. (c)

CHAPTER

Breathing and Exchange of Gases

1. Match the items listed under column I with those given under column II. Choose the appropriate option from the given choices.

Column I	Column II
(a) Residual volume (RV)	p. 4000mL - 4600 mL
(b) Inspiratory Reserve Volume (IRV)	q. 1100mL-1200 mL
(c) Vital capacity (VC)	r. 1000mL - 1100 mL
(d) Expiratory Reserve Volume (ERV)	s. 3000mL - 3500 mL
(e) Inspiratory capacity (IC)	t. 2500mL - 3000 mL

	A	B	C	D	E
(a)	t	q	s	r	p
(b)	q	r	s	t	p
(c)	q	t	p	r	s
(d)	r	t	p	q	s

2. Listed below are four respiratory capacities (i-iv) and four jumbled respiratory volumes of a normal human adult.

Respiratory capacities	Respiratory volumes
(i) Residual volume	2500 mL
(ii) Vital capacity	3500 mL
(iii) Inspiratory reserve volume	1200 mL
(iv) Inspiratory capacity	4500 mL

Which one oif the following is the correct matching of two capacities and volumes?

(a) (ii) 2500 mL, (iii) 4500 mL
(b) (iii) 1200 mL, (iv) 2500 mL
(c) (iv) 3500 mL, (i) 1200 mL
(d) (i) 4500 mL, (ii) 3500 mL

3. Match the columns and select the corect option from the codes given below.

A.	TV + ERV	1.	Expiratory capacity
B.	RV + ERV + TV + IRV	2.	Total lung capacity
C.	ERV + RV	3.	Functional residual capacity

(a) A-(i), B-(ii) C-(iii)
(b) A-(iii), B-(i) C-(ii)
(c) A-(iii), B-(ii) C-(i)
(d) A-(ii), B-(iii) C-(i)

4. Read the following statements with regard to oxyhaemoglobin dissociation curve.

I. The curve is ___*A*___ shaped under normal conditions.

II. ___*B*___ has an affinity to bind with deoxygenated haemoglobin by producing conformational changes in it.

III. The Curve is ___*C*___ in the presence of weak electrolytes. Identify *A*, *B* and *C*.

	A	*B*	*C*
(a)	sigmoid,	Carbon monoxide,	sigmoid
(b)	sigmoid,	2, 3-DPG,	hyperbolic
(c)	sigmoid,	Oxygen	hyperbolic
(d)	sigmoid,	Carbon monoxide,	straight

6. Match the following Columns.

	Column I		Column II
A.	Tiny air sacs in the lungs	1.	Internal respiration
B.	Gas diffusion between alveoli and blood in lungs	2.	Haemoglobin
C.	Gas exchange between blood and interstitial fluid	3.	Alveoli
D.	Molecule specialised for oxygen transprot	4.	External respiration

Codes

	A	B	C	D
(a)	3	4	1	2
(b)	1	2	3	4
(c)	4	3	2	1
(d)	2	1	4	3

7. Match the following Columns.

	Column I		Column II
A.	Bronchial tree	1.	Passage way for air from nasal cavity to larynx and food from mouth cavity to oesophagus
B.	Larynx	2.	Conducts air from trachea to the alveoli to its mucous lining continues to filter air
C.	Trachea	3.	Passage way for air, prevents foreign objects from entering trachea and houses vocal cords
D.	Pharynx	4.	Flexible tube, which connects larynx with bronchial tree

Codes

	A	B	C	D
(a)	1	2	3	4
(b)	2	3	4	1
(c)	4	3	2	1
(d)	3	2	1	4

8. Match the following Columns.

	Column I	Column II
A.	pO_2 of alveoli lungs	1. 40 mm Hg
B.	pO_2 of atmospheric air	2. 95 mm Hg
C.	pO_2 of deoxygenated blood	3. 104 mm Hg
D.	pO_2 of oxygenated blood	4. 159 mm Hg

Codes

	A	B	C	D
(a)	2	4	1	3
(b)	3	4	1	2
(c)	3	2	1	4
(d)	2	4	3	1

9. The correct match for kind of respiration is

	Animal		*Respiration*
A.	Earthworm	1.	Pulmonary
B.	Human	2.	Branchial
C.	Prawn	3.	Tracheal
D.	Insects	4.	Cutaneous

(a) 1-A, 2-B, 3-C, 4-D
(b) 4-A, 2-B, 1-C, 3-D
(c) 4-A, 1-B, 2-C, 3-D
(d) 3-A, 2-B, 4-C, 1-D

10. Match the disorders given in column I with symptoms under column II. Choose the answer which gives the correct combination of alphabets with numbers.

	Column I		Column II
A.	Asthma	1.	Inflammation of nasal tract

B.	Bronchitis	2. Spasm of bronchial muscles
C.	Rhinitis	3. Fully blown out alveoli
D.	Amphysema	4. Inflammation of bronchi
		5. Cough with blood strained sputum

(a) A = 4, B = 2, C = 5, D = 1
(b) A = 5, B = 3, C = 2, D = 1
(c) A = 3, B = 1, C = 5, D = 4
(d) A = 2, B = 4, C = 1, D = 3

11. Listed below are four respiratory capacities (a-d) and four jumbled respiratory volume of a normal human adult:

Respiratory capacities	***Respiratory volumes***
(a) Residual volume	2500 mL
(b) Vital capacity	3500 mL
(c) Inspiratory reserve volume	1200 mL
(d) Inspiratory capacity	4500 mL

12. Identify the wrong differences between inspiration and expiration:

	Inspiration	Expiration
(A)	EICM	Contract Relax
(B)	Size of thoracic cavity	Increases Decreases
(C)	Shape of diaphragm	Flat Dome shaped
(D)	Movement of air	Atmosphere to lungs Lungs to atmosphere

(a) A, B (b) B,C
(c) B,D (d) C,D

13. Match the items given in column I with column II and choose the correct option:

	Column I		Column II
A.	Hypocapnia	(i)	Destroy the alveolar wall
B.	Anoxia	(ii)	Difficulty in breathing
C.	Tachypnoea	(iii)	Decrease CO_2 concentration in blood
D.	Asthma	(iv)	To stop O_2 supply in tissue
E.	Emphysema	(v)	To increase breathing rate
F.	Dyspnoea	(vi)	Spasm in respiratory tubules

	A	B	C	D	E	F
(a)	(v)	(i)	(iii)	(ii)	(vi)	(iv)
(b)	(iii)	(iv)	(v)	(vi)	(i)	(ii)
(c)	(iii)	(iv)	(v)	(i)	(vi)	(ii)
(d)	(iv)	(v)	(vi)	(ii)	(iii)	(i)

Solutions

1. **(c)**

2. **(c)**

Respiratory capacities	Respiratory volumes
Residual volume	1200 mL
Vital capacity	4500 mL
Inspiratory reserve volume	2500 mL
Inspiratory capacity	3500 mL

3. **(a)** **4.** **(b)** **6.** **(a)** **7.** **(b)** **8.** **(b)**
9. **(c)** **10.** **(d)** **11.** **(d)** **12.** **(b)** **13.** **(b)**

CHAPTER

Body Fluids and Circulation

1. A red blood cell, entering the right side of the heart passes by or through the following structures.

1. Atrioventricular valves
2. Semilunar valves
3. Right atrium
4. Right ventricle
5. SAN

Which of the following options represents the correct sequence?

(a) $2 \rightarrow 3 \rightarrow 1 \rightarrow 4 \rightarrow 5$

(b) $3 \rightarrow 1 \rightarrow 5 \rightarrow 2 \rightarrow 4$

(c) $3 \rightarrow 5 \rightarrow 1 \rightarrow 2 \rightarrow 4$

(d) $5 \rightarrow 3 \rightarrow 1 \rightarrow 4 \rightarrow 2$

2. Identify the components labelled (A-D) in the given flow chart of the blood clotting process.

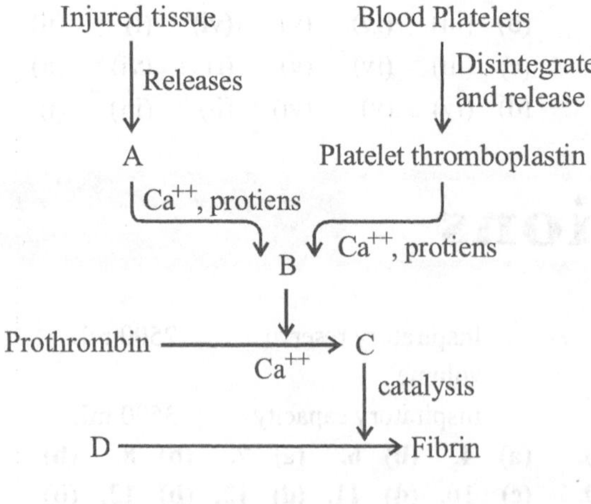

	A	B	C	D
(a)	Thrombo-plastin	Prothrom-binase	Thrombin	Fibrinogen
(b)	Fibrinogen	Thrombin	Prothrom-binase	Thrombo-plastin
(c)	Prothrom-binase	Fibrinogen	Thrombo-plastin	Thrombin
(d)	Thrombin	Thrombo-plastin	Fibrinogen	Prothrom-binase

3. Match the column I and column II and select the appropriate option with the given code.

	Column I		Column II
(a)	Coronary sinus	(i)	Mitral valve
(b)	Base of systemic aorta	(ii)	Eustachian valve
(c)	Left atrioventricular valve	(iii)	Semilunar valves
(d)	Opening of inferior vena cava	(iv)	Thebesian valve

(a) P-(iv); Q-(iii), R-(i), S-(ii)

(b) P-(iii); Q-(iv), R-(ii), S-(i)

(c) P-(ii); Q-(i), R-(iv), S-(iii)

(d) P-(i); Q-(ii), R-(iii), S-(iv)

4. Match the items given in column I with those in column II and select the correct option given below.

	Column-I		Column-II
A.	Tricuspid valve	(i)	Between left atrium and left ventricle
B.	Bicuspid valve	(ii)	Between right ventricle and pulmonary artery
C.	Semilunar valve	(iii)	Between right atrium and right ventricle

	A	B	C
(a)	(iii)	(i)	(ii)
(b)	(i)	(iii)	(ii)
(c)	(i)	(ii)	(iii)
(d)	(ii)	(i)	(iii)

5. Choose the correctly matched pair.
   (a) CAD - Atherosclerosis
   (b) Tetany - Disorder of neuromuscular junction
   (c) Gout - Rapid spasms in muscles
   (d) Goitre - Hyperthyroidism
   (e) Asthma - Alveolar wall are damaged
6. The given diagram shows the human heart.

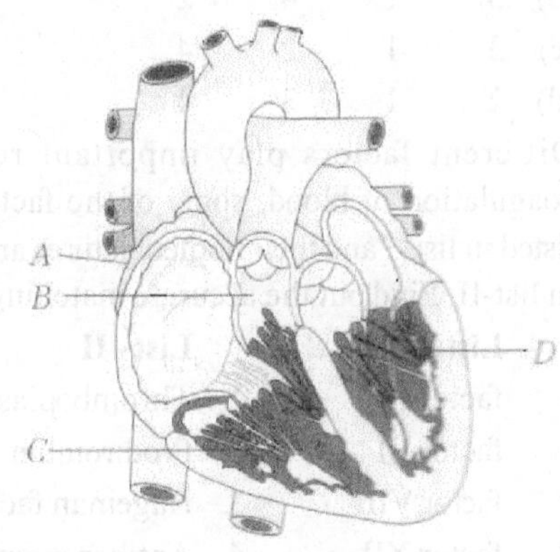

Which site represents the generation of action potential in human heart?
(a) D (b) C
(c) B (d) A
7. In diagram of the vertical section of human heart given here, certain parts have been indicated by alphabets. Choose the answer in which these alphabets have been correctly matched with the parts they indicate.

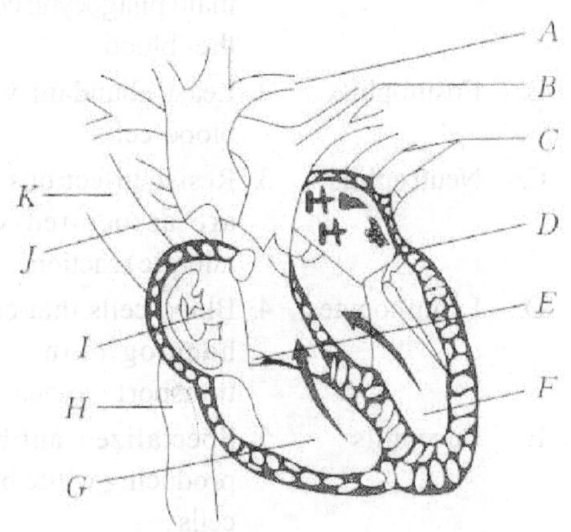

(a) *A-Aorta*, *B*-Pulmonary vein, *C*-Pulmonaryarteries, *D*-Left ventricle, *E*-Semilunar valves, *F-Left* auricle, *G*-Right auricle, *H*-Superior vena cava, *I-Right* ventricle, *J*-Tricuspid valves, *K*-Inferior vena cava
(b) *A-Aorta, B*-Pulmonary artery, *C*-Pulmonary veins, *D*-Left auricle, *E*-Tricuspid valves, *F-Left* ventricle, *G*-Right ventricle, *H*-Inferior vena cava, *I*-Right auricle, *J*-Semilunar valves, *K*-Superior vena cava
(c) *A-Aorta, B*-Superior vena cava, *C*-Inferior vena cava, *D*-Right ventricle, *E*-Tricuspid valves, *F-Right* auricle, *G*-Left auricle, *H*-Pulmonary vein, *I-Left* ventricle, *J*-Semilunar valves, *K*-Pulmonary artery
(d) *A-Aorta, B*-Superior vena cava, *C*-Inferior vena cava, *D*-Left ventricle, *E*-Semilunar valves, *F-Left* auricle, *G*-Right auricle, *H*-Pulmonary artery, *I*-Right ventricle, *J*-Tricuspid valves, *K*-Pulmonary vein
8. Identify the correct match wrt clotting factors and their specific characters.
   (a) Prothrombin – Lipoprotein synthesised in liver by vitamin K
   (b) Fibrinogen – Glycoprotein deficiency causes haemophilia-A
   (c) Hageman factor – Glycoprotein deficiency causes delayed blood clotting
   (d) Fibrin stabilising factor – Lipoprotein deficiency causes haemophilia-B
9. In which one of the following pairs of terms both represent one and the same thing?
   (a) Plasma – Serum
   (b) Atrioventricular node – Pacemaker
   (c) Leucocytes – Lymphocytes
   (d) Mitral valve – Bicuspid valve

10. Match the following columns.

Column-I	Column-II
A. P-wave	1. Atrial depolarisation
B. First heart sound	2. Ventricular depolarisation
C. Second heart sound	3. Ventricular repolarisation
D. QRS complex	4. Closure of the AV valves at the onset of systole
E. T-wave	5. Closure of the semilunar valves at the onset of diastole

Codes :

	A	B	C	D	E
(a)	1	4	5	2	3
(b)	1	2	3	4	5
(c)	5	4	3	2	1
(d)	3	5	1	2	4

11. Match the following columns.

Column-I	Column-II
A. Tricuspid valve	1. On the opening of inferior vena cava
B. Pulmonary valve	2. On the entrance of aorta
C. Eustachian valve	3. Between right atrium and right ventricle
D. Coronary valve	4. Entrance of pulmonary artery
	5. Over the opening of coronary sinus

Codes :

	A	B	C	D
(a)	3	5	4	1
(b)	3	4	1	5
(c)	4	2	1	5
(d)	4	3	1	3

12. Match the following columns.

Column-I	Column-II
A. Lymphatic system	1. Carries oxygenated blood
B. Pulmonary vein	2. Immune response
C. Thrombocytes	3. To drain back the tissue fluid to the circulatory system
D. Lymphocytes	4. Coagulation of blood

Codes :

	A	B	C	D
(a)	2	1	3	4
(b)	3	1	4	2
(c)	3	1	2	4
(d)	2	1	3	4

13. Different factors play important roles in coagulation of blood, some of the factors are listed in list -I and their nomenclatures are given in list-II. Find out the accurate matching

	List -I	List - II
a	factor II	1. Thromboplastin
b	factor III	2. Prothrombin
c	factor VIII	3. Hageman factor
d	factor XII	4. Antiheaemophilic globulin

(a) a : 2, b : 1, c : 4, d : 3
(b) a : 1, b : 2, c : 3, d : 4
(c) a : 3, b : 4, c : 2, d : 1
(d) a : 4, b : 4, c : 2, d : 1

14. Match the following columns and choose the correct answer from the options given below:

Column I	Column II
A. Erythrocytes	1. Most abundant white blood cells and the main phagocytic cell of the blood.
B. Eosinophils	2. Least abundant white blood cells
C. Neutrophils	3. Resist infections and are associated with allergic reaction
D. Lymphocytes	4. Blood cells that count haemoglobin and transport oxygen
E. Basophils	5. Specialized antibody producing white blood cells

	A	B	C	D	E
(a)	4	3	1	5	2
(b)	1	2	3	4	5
(c)	2	3	1	5	4
(d)	4	1	2	3	4

15. Match the items given in column I with those in column II and select the correct option given below:

Column I	Column II
A. Fibrinogen	(i) Osmotic balance
B. Globulin	(ii) Blood clotting
C. Albumin	(iii) Defence mechanism

(a) A-(iii), B-(ii), C-(i)
(b) A-(i), B-(ii), C-(iii)
(c) A-(i), B-(iii), C-(ii)
(d) A-(ii), B-(iii), C-(i)

16. Which of the following option is correctly matched with its category?

	Group	Type of Circulation	Blood is Oxygenated by
(a)	Fish	Single circulation	Skin
(b)	Amphibia	Double circulation	Gills
(c)	Reptilies	Incomplete double circulation	Lungs
(d)	Bird	Incomplete double circulation	Lungs

17. Match the blood vessels of human heart listed under column I with the functions given under column II and choose the answer.

Column I (Blood vessel)	Column II (Function)
A. Superior vena cava	1. Carries deoxygenated blood to lungs
B. Inferior vena cava	2. Carries oxygenated blood to lungs
C. Pulmonary artery	3. Brings oxygenated blood from lower parts of the body to the right atrium
D. Pulmonary vein	4. Brings oxygenated blood to the left atrium
	5. Brings deoxygenated blood from upper parts of the body into the right atrium

(a) A-5, B-1, C-3, D-2
(b) A-5, B-3, C-1, D-4
(c) A-4, B-5, C-3, D-1
(d) A-5, B-1, C-2, D-3

18. Match the column I with column II and choose the correct combination from the options given.

Column I	Column II
A. Eosinophils	(i) Coagulation
B. RBC	(ii) Universal recipient
C. AB group	(iii) Resist infection
D. Platelets	(iv) Contraction of heart
E. Systole	(v) Gaseous exchange

(a) A-(iii), B-(v), C-(ii), D-(i), E-(iv)
(b) A-(v), B-(i), C-(iii), D-(iv), E-(ii)
(c) A-(iii), B-(i), C-(ii), D-(v), E-(iv)
(d) A-(iii), B-(v), C-(ii), D-(iv), E-(i)

19. Match the column I blood (components) with column II (their specific functions) and choose the correct option:

Column I	Column II
A. Globulin protein	- Involved in defense mechanism of body
B. Fibrinogen protein	- Needed for clotting of blood
C. Albumin protein	- Role is transport of gases
D. Basophils	- Involved in inflammatory reactions
E. Eosinophils	- Help in osmotic balance
F. Lymphocytes	- Responsible for immune responses of the body

How many are correctly matched

(a) Four (b) Three
(c) Five (d) Six

20. Match the terms given under column I with their functions given under column II and select the answer from the options given below:

Column I	Column II
A. Lymphatic system	1. Carries oxygenated blood
B. Pulmonary vein	2. Immune response
C. Thrombocytes	3. To drain back the circulatory system
D. Lymphocytes	4. Coagulation of blood

(a) A-2, B-1, C-3, D-4
(b) A-3, B-1, C-4, D-2
(c) A-3, B-1, C-2, D-4
(d) A-2, B-1,C-3, D-4

Solutions

1. (d) Red blood cell (blood) will first meet SAN in the right atrium. Then from the right atrium it passes into right ventricle through atrio ventricular valve. From the right ventricle it enters into pulmonary artery through semilunar valve.

2. (a) 3. (a) 4. (a) 5. (a) 6. (d)
7. (b) 8. (c) 9. (d) 10. (a) 11. (b)
12. (b) 13. (a) 14. (a) 15. (d) 16. (c)
17. (b) 18. (a) 19. (a) 20. (b)

CHAPTER

Excretory Products and their Elimination

1. Select the correct combinations.
   I. Dysuria – Painful urination
   II. Pyuria – WBCs or pus in the urine
   III. Fructosuria – Absence of glucose in urine
   IV. Albumin-uria – Absence of ketone bodies in urine

   Choose the correct answer.
   (a) Only I
   (b) II and III
   (c) I and II
   (d) None of these

2. Match the following Columns.

	Column I		Column II
A.	Loop of Henle	1.	Carries blood into the kidney
B.	Renal artery	2.	Area, where a considerable amount of reabsorption takes place
C.	Proximal convoluted tubule	3.	Main area of secretion
D.	Glomerulus	4.	Filtration of blood
E.	Distal convoluted tubule	5.	Plays a role in concentration of urine

Codes

	A	B	C	D	E
(a)	1	2	3	4	5
(b)	5	4	3	2	1
(c)	5	1	2	4	3
(d)	4	3	1	5	2

3. Match the following Columns.

	Column I		Column II
A.	Uremia	1.	Excess of protein level in urine
B.	Haematuria	2.	The presence of high ketone bodies in urine
C.	Ketonuria	3.	The presence of blood cells in urine
D.	Glycosuria	4.	The presence of glucose in urine
E.	Proteinuria	5.	The presence of excess urea in urine

Codes

	A	B	C	D	E
(a)	5	3	2	4	1
(b)	4	5	3	2	1
(c)	5	3	4	2	1
(d)	3	5	2	1	4

4. Find the incorrectly matched pair of animal and its excretory structure.
   (a) *Balanoglossus* – Proboscis gland
   (b) Earthworm – Nephridia
   (c) Grasshopper – Malpighian tubules
   (d) Prawn – Flame cells
   (e) *Amphioxus* – Protonephridia

5. The correct match is
   I. DCT – Secretion of H^+ and K^+ ions.
   II. Henle's loop – Reabsorption of glucose, water and Na^+ ions.

III. Podocytes – Attached to parietal layer of Bowman's capsule.

IV. JGA – Rise in glomerular blood pressure activates it to release renin.

(a) Only III (b) Only II

(c) Only I (d) Only IV

6. Select the option which shows correct matching of animals with its excretory organ and excretory product.

	Animals	Excretory organ	Excretory product
(a)	Labeo (Rohu)	Nephridial tubes	Ammonia
(b)	Salamander	Kidneys	Urea
(c)	Peacock	Kidneys	Urea
(d)	Housefly	Renal tubules	Uric acid

7. Which one of the following options gives the correct categorisation of six animals according to the types of nitrogenous waste they give out?

	Ammonotelic	Ureotelic	Uricotelic
(a)	Pigeon, humans	Aquatic amphibia, lizards	Cockroach, frog
(b)	Frog, lizards	Aquatic amphibia, humans	Cockroach, Pigeon
(c)	Aquatic amphibia	Frog, human	Pigeon, lizards, cockroach
(d)	Aquatic amphibia	Cockroach, humans	Frog, pigeon, lizards

8. In which one of the following organisms its excetory organs are correctly stated?

(a) Humans – Kidneys, sebaceous glands and tear glnads

(b) Earthworm – Pharyngeal, integumentary and septal nephridia

(c) Cockroach – Malpighian tubules and enteric caeca

(d) Frog – Kidneys, skin and buccal epithelium

9. Match column I with column II regarding human excretory system. Choose the correct option.

Colum II		Column II	
I.	Epithelial cells of Bowman's capsule	A.	Juxtamedullary nephron
II.	Extension of cortex between the medullary pyramids as renal columns	B.	Vasa recta
III.	Nephrons with long loop of henle running deep into the medulla	C.	Juxtaglomerular Apparatus
IV.	A fine vessel of the periubular cappilaries running parallel to Henle's loop	D.	Podocytes
V.	A special sensitive regionin the DCT and afferent arteriole at the location of their contact	E.	Columns of Bertin
		F.	Cortical nephron

(a) I - C, II - B, III - A, IV - D, V - E

(b) I - E, II - A, III - B, IV - C, V - D

(c) I - D, II - C, III - F, IV - E, V - A

(d) I - D, II - E, III - A, IV - B, V - C

(e) I - B, II - D, III - F, IV - A, V - C

10.

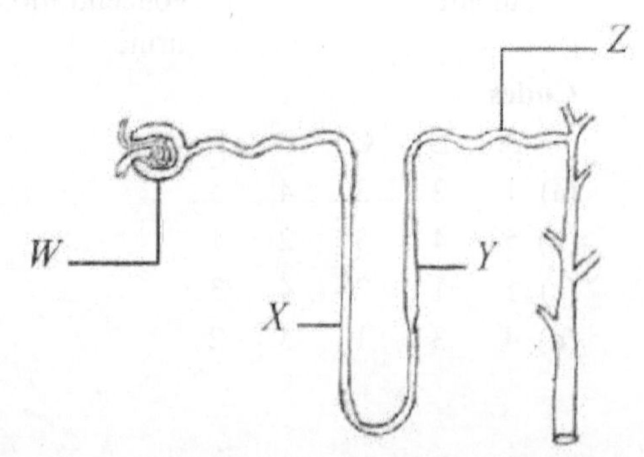

In the given diagram, water absorption does not occur in part labelled as ______.

(a) *W* (b) *X*
(c) *Y* (d) *Z*

11. Match the items given in column I with those in column II and select the correct options given below.

Column I (Function)	Column II (Part of excretory system)
A. Ultrafiltration	(i) Henle's loop
B. Concentration of urine	(ii) Ureter
C. Transport of urine	(iii) Urinary bladder
D. Storage of urine	(iv) Malpighian corpuscle
	(v) Proximal convoluted tubule

	A	B	C	D
(a)	(iv)	(v)	(ii)	(iii)
(b)	(iv)	(i)	(ii)	(iii)
(c)	(v)	(iv)	(i)	(ii)
(d)	(v)	(iv)	(i)	(iii)

12. Match the items given in column I with those in column II and select the correct options given below.

Column I	Column II
A. Glycosuria	(i) Accumulation of uric acid in joints
B. Gout	(ii) Mass of crystallised salts within the kidney
C. Renal calculi	(iii) Inflammation in glomeruli
D. Glomerular nephritis	(iv) Presence of glucose in urine

	A	B	C	D
(a)	(iii)	(ii)	(iv)	(i)
(b)	(i)	(ii)	(iii)	(iv)
(c)	(ii)	(iii)	(i)	(iv)
(d)	(iv)	(i)	(ii)	(iii)

13. Match the animals with their corresponding excretory structures

Animal	Excretory structure
1. Amphioxus	A. Pronephros kidney
2. Cockroach	B. Protonephridia
3. Prawn	C. Metanephridia
4. Earthworm	D. Green glands
	E. Malpighian tubules
	F. Antennal glands

(a) 1–B, 2–E, 3–D, 4–C
(b) 1–A, 2–C, 3–D, 4–B
(c) 1–B, 2–E, 3–F, 4–C
(d) None of these

14. Match the column I with the column II

Column I	Column II
A. Earthworm	I. Malpighian tubules
B. Cockroach	II. Green glands
C. Amphioxus	III. Solenocytes
D. Prawn	IV. Holonephridia
	V. Coxal glands

(a) A-IV, B-I, C-III, D-II
(b) A-I, B-V, C-IV, D-II
(c) A-IV, B-I, C-V, D-II
(d) A-III, B-I, C-II, D-V

15. Match the column-I with column-II and choose the correct option.

Column-I (Excretory organs)	Column-II (Animals)
A. Nephridia	I. Hydra
B. Malpighian tubules	II. Leech
C. Protonephridia	III. Shark
D. Kidneys	IV. Round worms
	V. Cockroach

(a) A-II, B-V, C-IV, D-III
(b) A-IV, B-II, C-I, D-V
(c) A-V, B-II, C-IV, D-III
(d) A-II, B-IV, C-V, D-I

16. A single load of insulin is injected into the bloodsteam. If the urine flow is constant, which graph best expresses the relationship between urine-insulin concentration and time?

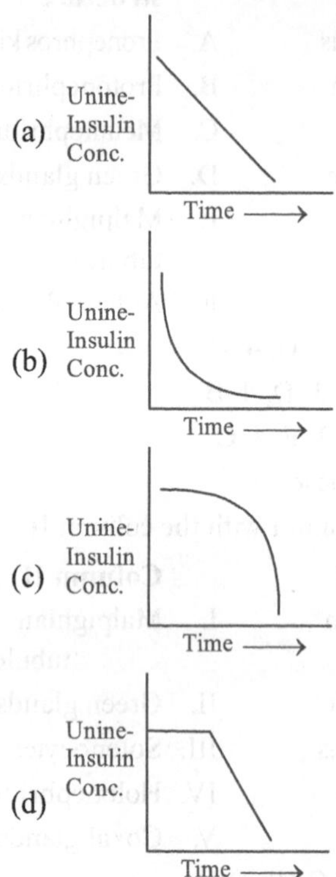

17. Select the correct match of the types of organs gives in column-I with their role in excretion given in column-II.

Column-I	Column-II
A. Lungs	I. Secretes bile contaiing substances like bilirubin, biliverdin, cholesterol, degraded steroid hormones, vitamins and drugs.
B. Liver	II. Eliminates water and salts in sweat and substances like sterols, hydrocarbons and waxes through sebum.
C. Skin	III. Remove large amounts of CO_2 (18 litres/day) and also significant quantities of water everyday.
D. Kidney	IV. Remove wastes (metabolic by products and regulate pH, ion concentration, volume and osmolarity of blood.

(a) A-I, B-II, C-III, D-IV
(b) A-III, B-I, C-II, D-IV
(c) A-III, B-I, C-IV, D-II
(d) A-IV, B-II, C-III, D-I

18. Which of the following hormone/enzyme is/are correctly paired with its function?

(i) Renin - Enzyme that catalyses the formation of angiotensin I.

(ii) Aldosterone ? Regulates water reabsorption at the distal convoluted tubule.

(iii) Anti-diuretic hormone (ADH) - It is a powerful vasoconstrictor that stimulates the secretion of aidosterone.

(iv) Angiotensin II ? Promotes reabsorption of sodium at distal convoluted tubule.

(a) Only (i)
(b) Only (iii)
(c) (i), (ii) and (iii)
(d) (ii), (iii) and (iv)

19. Match the column-I with column-II and choose the correct option.

Column-I	Column-II
A. Delivers blood	I. Proximal convoluted tubules
B. Carries urine to pelvis	II. Renal artery
C. Collects nitrate from Bowman's capsule	III. Collecting duct
D. Loop of Henie	IV. Ascending and descending limb

(a) A-IV, B-III, C-II, D-I
(b) A-I, B-II, C-III, D-IV
(c) A-II, B-III, C-IV, D-I
(d) A-II, B-III, C-I, D-IV

20. Match column-I with column-II regarding human excretory system and choose the correct option given below.

Column-I	Column-II
A. Epithelial cells of Bowman's capsule	I. Juxtamedullary nephron
B. Extension of cortex between the medullary pyramids as rental columns	II. Vasa recta
C. Nephrons with long loop of Henle running deep into the medulla	III. Juxtaglomerular Apparatus
D. A fine vessel of the peritubular capillaries running parallel to Henles loop	IV. Podocytes
E. A special sensitive region in the DCT and afferent arteriole at the location of their contact	V. Columns of Bertini

(a) A-III, B-II, C-I, D-IV, E-V
(b) A-V, B-I, C-II, D-III, E-IV
(c) A-IV, B-III, C-I, D-II, E-V
(d) A-II, B-IV, C-VI, D-I, E-III

21. Match the following parts of a nephron with their function :

Column-I	**Column-II**
(A) Descending limb of Henle's loop	(i) Reabsorption of salts only
(B) Proximal convoluted tubule	(ii) Reabsorption of water only
(C) Ascending limb of Henle's loop	(iii) Conditional reabsorption of sodium ions and water
(D) Distal convoluted tubule	(iv) Reabsorption of ions, water and organic nutrients

Select the correct option from the following :
(a) (A)-(iv), (B)-(i), (C)-(iii), (D)-(ii)
(b) (A)-(i), (B)-(iii), (C)-(ii), (D)-(iv)
(c) (A)-(ii), (B)-(iv), (C)-(i), (D)-(iii)
(d) (A)-(i), (B)-(iv), (C)-(ii), (D)-(iii)

22. Match the items given in Column I with those in Column II and select the correct option given below :

Column I	**Column II**
A. Glycosuria	I. Accumulation of uric acid in joints
B. Gout	II. Mass of crystallised salts within the kidney
C. Renal calculi	III. Inflammation in glomeruli
D. Glomerular	IV. Presence of in nephritis glucose urine

	A	**B**	**C**	**D**
(a)	III	II	IV	I
(b)	I	II	III	IV
(c)	IV	I	II	III
(d)	II	III	I	IV

Solutions

1. (c) 2. (c) 3. (a) 4. (d) 5. (c)
6. (b) In salamander, kidneys (mesonepheric) are the excretory organs and the excretory matter is urea. In *Labeo*, kidney is the excretory organ and is mesonephric. Excretion is ammonotelic. Peacock has metanephric kidneys with excretory matter being uric acid. In housefly, excretion takes place by Malpighian tubules. Excretory waste is uric acid chief.
7. (c)
8. (b) Nephridia is the excretory organ of the earthworm. Earthworms have three types of nephridial structures called as septal, integumentary and pharyngeal nephridia. These three nephridial structures are present on different positions in the body and also vary in structures. Septal and pharyngeal nephridia are both enteronephric *i.e.*, nitrogen products are expelled in gut. Integumentary nephridia is exonephric *i.e.*, nitrogen waste products are directly discharged outside.
9. (d)
10. (c) *W* represents the glomerulus where ultrafiltration occurs. It is permeable to water and low molecular weight substancs. Water is reabsorbed by osmosis in PCT, DCT (*Z*) and descending limb of loop of Henle (*X*) except ascending limb of loop of Henle (*Y*).
11. (b) 12. (d) 13. (c) 14. (a) 15. (a)
16. (c) 17. (b) 18. (a) 19. (d) 20. (d)
21. (c) 22. (c)

CHAPTER

Locomotion and Movement

1. Which one of the following pairs of chemical substances, is correctly categorised?
(a) Calcitonin and thymosin – Thyroid hormones
(b) Pepsin and prolactin – Two digestive enzymes secreted in stomach
(c) Troponin and myosin – Complex proteins in striated muscles
(d) Secretin and rhodopsin – Polypeptide hormones

2. Choose the wrongly matched pair.
(a) Portion of myofibril between two - Sarcomere 'Z' lines
(b) Isotropic band - Actin
(c) Anisotropic band - Myosin
(d) Central part of I-band - M-line
(e) Central part of A-band - H-zone

3. Select the correct matching of the type of the joint with the example in human skeletal system.

Type of joint	Example
(a) Cartilaginous joint –	Between frontal and parietal
(b) Pivot joint –	Between third and fourth cervical vertebrae
(c) Hinge joint –	Between humerus and pectoral girdle
(d) Gliding joint –	Between carpals

4. Match the following joints with the bones involved.
(1) Gliding joint (i) Between carpal and metacarpal of thumb
(2) Hinge joint (ii) Between atlas and axis
(3) Pivot joint (iii) Between the carpals
(4) Saddle joint (iv) Between humerus and ulana

select the correct option from the following.
(a) (1)-(iii), (2)-(iv), (3)-(ii), (4)-(i)
(b) (1)-(iv), (2)-(i), (3)-(ii), (4)-(iii)
(c) (1)-(iv), (2)-(ii), (3)-(iii), (4)-(i)
(d) (1)-(i), (2)-(iii), (3)-(ii), (4)-(iv)

5. Select the correct match pair.
(a) Abductor – Triceps extending forearm
(b) Adductor – Biceps bending forearm towards upper arm
(c) Elevator – Latissimus dorsi
(d) Rotator – Pyriformis that raises thigh

6. Select the correct match pair.
(a) Synarthrosis – Movable joints
(b) Amphiarthrosis – Slighly movable joints
(c) Shoulder joint – Between humerus and glenoid cavity
(d) Gliding joint – Monoaxial joint

7. Match the following Columns.

	Column I		Column II
A.	Ball and socket joint	1.	Radius and ulna
B.	Hinge joint	2.	Metacarpals of thumb
C.	Gliding joint	3.	Glenoid cavity of pectoral girdle
D.	Saddle joint	4.	Between radius and carpals at wrist
E.	Condyloid joint	5.	Phalanges of digits

Codes

	A	B	C	D	E
(a)	3	5	1	2	4
(b)	1	2	3	4	5
(c)	4	3	1	2	5
(d)	5	2	3	1	4

8. Match the following Columns.

Column I (skeleton)	Column II (Number of bones)
A. Sternum	1. 14
B. Ribs	2. 1
C. Pelvis	3. 24
D. Face	4. 3

Codes

	A	B	C	D
(a)	2	3	4	1
(b)	2	4	1	3
(c)	1	3	4	2
(d)	4	1	2	3

9. Match the following Columns.

Column I	Column II
A. Fast muscle fibres	1. Myoglobin
B. Slow muscle fibres	2. Lactic acid
C. Actin filament	3. Contractile unit
D. Sarcomere	4. I-band

Codes

	A	B	C	D
(a)	1	2	4	3
(b)	2	1	3	4
(c)	2	1	4	3
(d)	3	2	4	1

10. Match the following Columns.

Column I	Column II
A. Sternum	1. Synovial fluid
B. Glenoid cavity	2. Vertebrae
C. Freely movable joint	3. Pectoral girdle
D. Cartilaginous joint	4. Flat bones

Codes

	A	B	C	D
(a)	2	1	3	4
(b)	4	3	1	2
(c)	2	1	4	3
(d)	4	1	2	4

11. Match the following Columns.

Column I	Column II
A. Zygomatic bone	1. Keystone bone of cranium
B. Lacrimal bone	2. Cheek bone of cranium
C. Parietal bone	3. Smallest bone of face
D. Sphenoid	4. Root of crranium
	5. Floor of cranium

Codes

	A	B	C	D
(a)	1	3	5	2
(b)	2	4	5	1
(c)	2	4	1	3
(d)	2	3	4	5

12. Match the bones of column A with their corresponding number in column B

Column A	Column B
A. True ribs	a. 14
B. Cervical vertebrae	b. 12
C. Cranium bones	c. 8
D Vertebrochondral ribs	d. 6

(a) Ab, Be, Ca, Dd (b) Aa, Be, Cc, Dd
(c) Ab, Bc, Cd, Dc (d) Aa, Bc, Cb, Dd

13. Which one of the following pairs of structures is correctly matched with their correct description ?

	Structures		Description
(a)	Tibia and fibula	–	Both form parts of knee joint
(b)	Cartilage and cornea	–	No blood supply but do require oxygen for respiratory need
(c)	Shoulder joint and elbow joint	–	Ball and socket type of joint
(d)	Premolars and molars	–	20 in all and 3–rooted

14. Which of the following pairs, is correctly matched?

(a) Hinge joint - between vertebrae
(b) Gliding joint - between zygapophyses of the successive vertebrae
(c) Cartilaginous joint - skull bones
(d) Fibrous joint - between phalanges

15. Which one of the following is the correct matching of three items and their grouping category ?

	Items		**Group**
(a)	cytosine, uracil, thiamine	–	pyrimidines
(b)	malleus, incus, cochlea	–	ear ossicles
(c)	ilium, ischium,	–	coxal bones of pelvic girdle
(d)	actin, myosin, rhodopsin	–	muscle proteins

16. Which one of the following pairs of structures is correctly matched with their correct description?

	Structures		**Description**
(a)	Tibia and fibula	–	Both form parts of knee joint
(b)	Cartilage and cornea	–	No blood supply but do require oxygen for respiratory need
(c)	Shoulder joint and elbow joint	–	Ball and socket type of joint
(d)	Premolars and molars	–	20 in all and 3–rooted

17. Three of the following pairs of the human skeletal parts are correctly matched with their respective inclusive skeletal category and one pair is not matched. Identify the non-matching pair.

	Pairs of skeletal parts	**Category**
(a)	Humerus and ulna	Appendicular skeleton
(b)	Malleus and stapes	Ear ossicles
(c)	Sternum and Ribs	Axial skeleton
(d)	Clavicle and Glenoid cavity	Pelvic girdle

18. The characteristics and an example of a synovial joint in humans is

	Characteristics	**Examples**
(a)	Fibrous cartilage between two bones, limited movements	Knee joint
(b)	Fluid filled between two joints, provides cushion	Skull bones
(c)	Fluid filled synovial cavity between two bones	Joint between atlas and axis
(d)	Lymph filled between two bones, limited movement	Gliding joint between carpals

19. Match the locomotory structure of column I with the name of phylum in column II

	Column I		**Column II**
A.	Parapodia	I.	Mollusca
B.	Muscular foot	II.	Echinodermata
C.	Pseudopodia	III.	Protozoa
D.	Tube feet	IV.	Annelida
		V.	Arthropoda

(a) A-V, B-IV, C-III, D-II
(b) A-IV, B-I, C-III, D-II
(c) A-V, B-I, C-III, D-II
(d) A-IV, B-II, C-III, D-V

Solutions

1. **(c)**
2. **(d)** In a myofibril the dark bands (A bands) and light bands (I bands) are present alternately. At the centre of A band a comparatively lass dark H zone is present. In the centre of H zone is the M line. Each I band has at its centre a dark membrane called Z line. The part of myofibril between two successive Z lines is called a sarcomere.
3. **(d)** Cartilaginous joint – Between the adjacent vertebae in vertebral column

   Pivot joint – Between atlas and axis.

   Hinge joint – Knee joint

4. **(a)** 5. **(d)** 6. **(a)** 7. **(a)** 8. **(a)**
9. **(c)** 10. **(b)** 11. **(d)** 12. **(b)** 13. **(b)**
14. **(b)** 15. **(c)** 16. **(b)** 17. **(d)** 18. **(c)**
19. **(b)**

CHAPTER

Neural Control and Coordination

1. Select the answer with correct matching of the structure, its location and function

	Structure	Location	Function
(a)	Eustachian tube	Anterior part of internal ear	Equalizes air pressure on either sides of tympanic membrane
(b)	Cerebellum	Mid brain	Controls respiration and gastric secretions
(c)	Hypothalamus	Fore brain	Controls body temperature, urge for eating and drinking
(d)	Blind spot	Near the place where optic nerve leaves the eye	Rods and cones are present but inactive here

2. Column I lists the parts of the human brain and colum II lists the functions. Match the two columns and identify the correct choice from those given.

	Column I		Column II
A.	Cerebrum	p.	controls the pituitary
B.	Cerebellum	q.	controls vision and hearing
C.	Hypothalamus	r.	controls the rate of heart beat
D.	Midbrain	s.	seat of intelligence
		t.	maintains body posture

(a) A – t; B – s; C – q; D – p
(b) A – s; B – t; C – r; D – p
(c) A – t; B – s; C – r; D – q
(d) A – t; B – t; C – p; D – q

3. Match the following human spinal nerves in column I with the number of pairs in column II and choose the correct options

	Column I		Column II
A.	cervical nerves	1.	5 pairs
B.	thoracic nerves	2.	1 pair
C.	lumbar nerves	3	12 pairs
D.	coccygeal nerves	4.	8 pairs

(a) A - 2, B - 4, C - 1, D - 3
(b) A - 4, B - 3, C - 1, D - 2
(c) A - 3, B - 1, C - 2, D - 4
(d) A - 4, B - 1, C - 2, D - 3

4. Given below is a table comparing the effects of sympathetic and parasympathetic nervous system for four features (1–4). Which one feature is correctly described?

	Feature	Sympathetic nervous system	Parasympathetic nervous system
1.	Salivary glands	stimulates secretion	inhibits secretion
2.	Pupil of eye	dilates	constricts
3.	Heart rate	decreases	increases
4.	Intestinal peristalsis	stimulates secretion	inhibits secretion

5. Match the entries in column I with those in column II and choose the correct combination from the options given.

Column I		Column II
(A) diencephalon	1.	cerebellum
(B) telencephalon	2.	medulla
(C) myelencephalon	3.	amygdala
(D) metencephalon	4.	thalamus

(a) A–4, B–3, C–1, D–2
(b) A–3, B–4, C–1, D–2
(c) A–4, B–3, C–2, D–1
(d) A–1, B–2, C–3, D–4

6. Which one of the following is the correct difference between rod cells and cone cells of our retina.

		Rod Cells	Cone Cells
(a)	Distribution	More concentrated in centre of retina	Evenly distributed all over retina
(b)	Visual acuity	High	Low
(c)	Visual pigment contained	Iodopsin	Rhodopsin
(d)	Over all function	Vision in poor light	Colour vision and detailed vision in bright light

7. Choose the incorrect pair w.r.t conduction of nerve impulse through a nerve fibre:
(a) Depolarisation- Opening of Na+ channels and rapid influx of Na+ ions
(b) Polarisation- Ionisation gradient is maintained by Na+ -K- pump which transport Na+ outwards for 2K+ into the cell
(c) Depolarisation - High permeability of the axon membrane for K+
(d) Repolarisation - High permeability of the membrane for K+ and rapid influx of K+ ions.

8. Match the column I with column II and choose the correct options:

	Column I		Column II
A.	Electrical synapse	1.	Membranes of pre-and post-synaptic neurons are separated by fluid filled space
B.	Chemical synapse	2.	Membranes of pre- and post-synaptic neurons are in very close proximity
C.	Receptors	3.	Chemicals filled in the vesicle of axon terminals
D.	Neurotransmitter	4.	Sites where neurotransmitters bind
		5.	Adrenergic or cholinergic

	A	B	C	D
(a)	2	1	4	3
(b)	2	3	5	4
(c)	2	5	4	3
(d)	2	1	4	3

9. Match the columns and find out the correct combination:

A.	Resting phase	1.	Activation gates of Na+ open
B.	Depolarising phase	2.	Inactivation gates of Na+ open only
C.	Repolarising phase	3.	Inactivation gate and activation gate of Na+ is closed
D.	Hyperpolarising phase	4.	Both gates of Na+ open

	A	B	C	D
(a)	2	1	4	3
(b)	2	3	4	1
(c)	2	1	3	4
(d)	2	4	1	3

10. Match the column I with column II and choose the correct option:

	Column I		Column II
A.	Cerebrum	1.	Controls the pituitary
B.	Cerebellum	2.	Controls vision and hearing
C.	Hypothalamus	3.	Controls the rate of heart beat
D.	Midbrain	4.	Seat of intelligence
		5.	Maintains body posture

(a) A-5, B-4, C-2, D-1
(b) A-4, B-5, C-2, D-1
(c) A-5, B-4, C-1, D-2
(d) A-4, B-5, C-1, D-2

11. Match the column I and column II and choose the correct option.

A.	Fovea	1.	Provides opening for entry of light
B.	Iris	2.	Transduces RGB light
C.	Pupil	3.	Transmits information to CNS
D.	Lens	4.	Controls amount of light entering
E.	Optic nerve	5.	Focuses light on the retina

(a) A-2, B-4, C-1, D-5, E-3
(b) A-1, B-2, C-3, D-4, E-5
(c) A-5, B-1, C-4, D-3, E-2
(d) A-3, B-1, C-4, D-5, E-2

12. Find out the correct labelling for A, B, C and D in diagram:

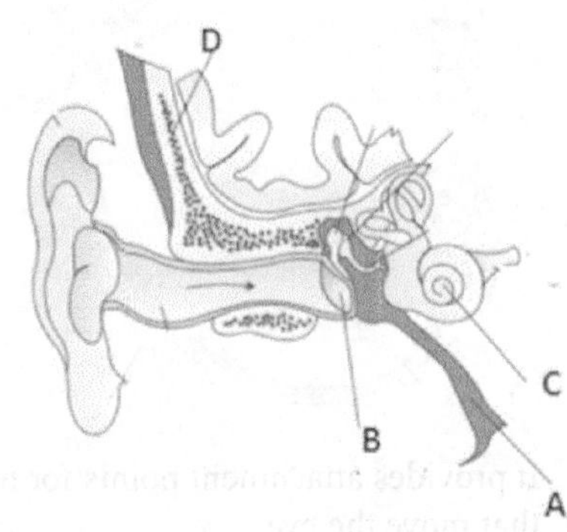

	A	B	C	D
(a)	External auditory Meatus	Tympanic membrane	Cochlea	Temporal bone
(b)	Temporal bone	Tympanic membrane	Cochlear nerve	Eustachian tube
(c)	Eustachian tube	Tympanic membrane	Cochlea	Temporal bone
(d)	Cochlea	Tympanic membrane	Auditory meatus	Temporal bone

13. Match the column I (various phase of an action potential) with column II (ionic activity associated) and choose the correct option.

Column I		Column II	
A.	Resting stage of a neuron	I.	Opening and then closing of the sodium channels
B.	Depolarization phase in the generation of an action potential.	II.	All voltage gated sodium and potassium channels are closed.
C.	Repolarization phase in the generation of action potential	III.	The sodium channels remain opened.
D.	Absolute refractory potassium phase.	IV.	Opening of gates and the rushing of potassium

(a) A – II, B – I, C – IV, D – III
(b) A – I, B – II, C – III, D – IV
(c) A – III, B – IV, C – I, D – II
(d) A – IV, B – II, C – III, D – I

14. Which of the following options correctly represents the name of 1, 2, 3 and 4 is the given diagram of neuron?

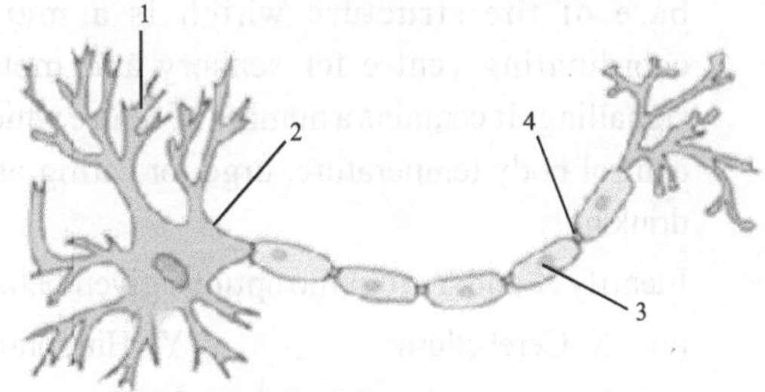

(a) 1- Axon, 2- Dendrites, 3- Node of Ranvier, 4- Myelin sheath
(b) 1- Dendrites, 2- Axon, 3- Node of Ranvier, 4- Myelin sheath
(c) 1- Dendrites, 2- Cell body, 3- Myelin sheath, 4- Node of Ranvier
(d) 1- Axon, 2- Cell body, 3- Dendrites, 4- Node of Ranvier

15. Unmyelinated nerve fibre is enclosed by an 'X' that does not form a myelin sheath around the 'Y', and is commonly found in 'Z' and the somatic neural systems. Identify 'X', 'Y' and 'Z'.

	X	Y	Z
(a)	Schwann cells	Axon	Autonomous
(b)	Nodes of Ranvier	Cell body	Synaptic knob
(c)	Synapse	Dendrites	Sympathetic
(d)	Meninges	Nerve impulse	Peripheral

16. Given below is a table comparing the effects of sympathetic and parasympathetic nervous system for four features (a – d). Which of the following feature is correctly described?

	Feature	Sympathetic nervous system	Parasympathetic nervous system
(a)	Salivary glands	Stimulates secretion	Inhibits secretion
(b)	Pupil of eye	Dilates	Constricts
(c)	Heart rate	Decreases	Increases
(d)	Intestinal peristalsis	Stimulates secretion	Inhibits secretion

17. 'X' is an important part of 'Y' which lies at the base of the structure which is a major coordinating centre for sensory and motor signalling. It contains a number of centre which control body temperature, urge for eating and drinking.

Identify X and Y from the options given below

(a) X-Cerebellum ; Y-Hindbrain
(b) X-Hypothalamus ; Y-Forebrain
(c) X-Corpora quadrigemina ; Y-Midbrain
(d) X-Pituitary gland ; Y-Forebrain

18. Given below is a diagrammatic cross section of a single loop of human cochlea with few part labelled as A, B, C & D.

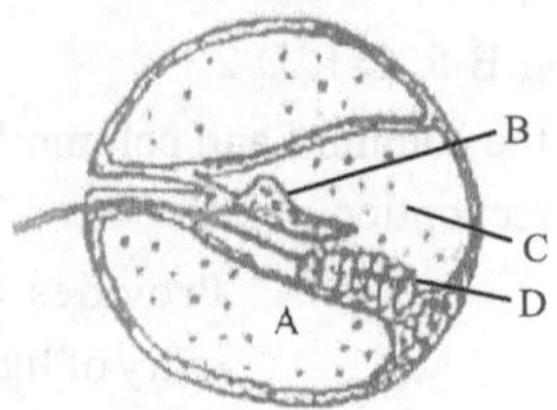

Which one of the following options correctly represents the name of three different parts?

(a) A: Perilymph, B: Tectorial membrane C: Endolymph
(b) B: Tectorial membrane, C:Perilymph, D: Secretory cells
(c) C: Endolymph, D: Sensory hair cells, A: Serum
(d) D: Sensory hair cells, A: Endolymph B: Tectorial membrane

19. Which of the following statements is/are functions of structure labelled as 'X' in the given diagram of eye?

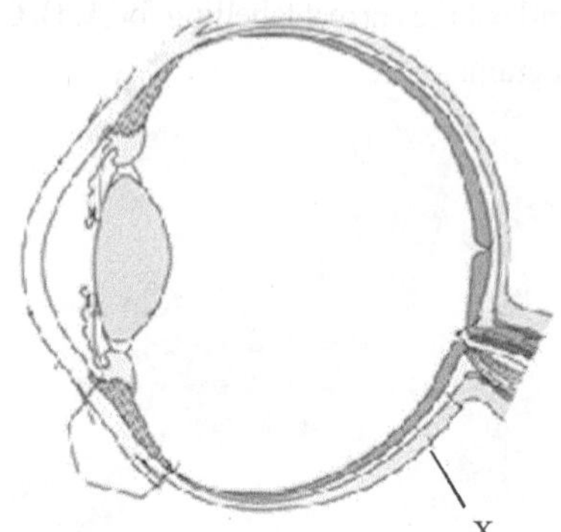

I. It provides attachment points for muscles that move the eye.
II. It maintains the shape of the eye ball.
III. It helps during accomodation.
IV. It is responsible for eye colour.

(a) I and II (b) I, II and IV
(c) II, III and IV (d) All of these

Solutions

1. (c) 2. (d) 3. (b) 4. (b) 5. (c)
6. (d) 7. (c) 8. (a) 9. (d) 10. (d)
11. (a) 12. (c) 13. (a)

14. (c) In the given diagram of neuron, the part marked as I, II, III and IV are respectively dendrites, cell body, myelin sheath and nodes of Ranvier. Neuron is a specialized, impulse-conducting cell that is the functional unit of the nervous system, consisting of the cell body and its processes, the axon and dendrites.

15. (a) Unmyelinated nerve fibre is enclosed by an Schwann cells that does not form a myelin sheath around the axon, and is commonly found in autonomous and the somatic neural systems.

16. (b)

	Features	Sympathetic nervous system	Parasympathetic nervous system
(a)	Salivary glands	Inhibits secretions	Stimulates secretions
(b)	Pupil of eye	Dilates	Constricts
(c)	Heart rate	Increases strength and rate of heart beat	Decreases strength and rate of heart beat
(d)	Intestinal peristalsis	Inhibits secretions	Stimulates secretions

17. (b) Hypothalamus is an important part of forebrain which lies at the base of the structure which is a major coordinating center for sensory and motor signaling. It contains a number of centers which control body temperature, urge for eating and drinking.

18. (a) In the given figure of cochlea, the correct labelling of A, B, C and D are respectively perilymph, tectorial membrane, endolymph and organ of corti.

The cochlea is the auditory portion of the inner ear. It is a spiral-shaped cavity in the bony labyrinth and receives sound in the form of vibrations, which cause the stereocilia to move. The stereocilia then convert these vibrations into nerve impulses which are taken up to the brain to be interpreted. Two of the three fluid sections are canals and the third is a sensitive 'organ of Corti' which detects pressure impulses which travel along the auditory nerve to the brain. The two canals are called the vestibular canal and the tympanic canal.

19. (b) The label X represents sclera. The white of the eye is called sclera. Choroid is responsible for eye colour. Ciliary muscles alters the shape of the lens during accomodation.

CHAPTER

Chemical Co-ordination and Integration

1. Identify A, B, C and D in the given flow chart and select the correct option.

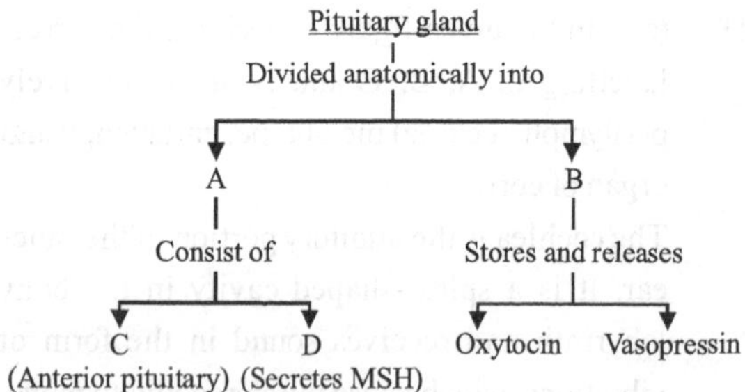

	A	B	C	D
(a)	Neuro-hypophysis	Adeno-hypophysis	Pars distalis	Pars intermedia
(b)	Adeno-hypophysis	Neuro-hypophysis	Pars intermedia	Pars distalis
(c)	Adeno-hypophysis	Neuro-hypophysis	Pars distalis	Pars intermedia
(d)	Neuro-hypophysis	Adeno-hypophysis	Pars intermedia	Pars distalis

2. Identify the parts labelled A, Band C in the given figure and select the correct option (second figure is the cross section of 'A').

	A	B	C
(a)	Adrenal gland	Cortex	Medulla
(b)	JGA	Cortex	Medulla
(c)	Adrenal gland	Medulla	Cortex
(d)	Adrenal gland	Pars distalis	Pars intermedia

3. Match column I with column II and select the correct option from the codes given below.

	Column I		Column II
A.	Thyroid	(i)	Acts on the renal tubules
B.	Adrenal	(ii)	Regulates blood calcium level
C.	Pituitary	(iii)	Maintains diurnal rhythm of our body
D.	Pineal	(iv)	Acts on the melanocytes

(a) A-(iv), B-(iii), C -(ii), D-(i)
(b) A-(iii), B-(iv), C -(i), D-(ii)
(c) A-(iv), B-(ii), C -(iii), D-(i)
(d) A-(ii), B-(i), C -(iv), D-(iii)

4. Match column I with column II and select the correct option from the given codes.

	Column I		Column II
A.	FSH	(i)	Transported axonally to neurohypophysis from hypothalamus
B.	MSH	(ii)	Acts on melanocytes and regulates pigmentation of skin
C.	Vasopressin (ADH)	(iii)	Stimulates the growth and development of ovarian follicles in female
D.	Pars intermedia	(iv)	In human, it is almost merged with pars distalis

(a) A-(iii), B-(ii), C -(i), D-(iv)
(b) A-(i), B-(ii), C -(iii), D-(iv)
(c) A-(iv), B-(iii), C -(ii), D-(i)
(d) A-(iii), B-(ii), C-(iv), D-(i)

5. Match the entries in Column - I with those of Column - II and choose the correct answer given below.

	Column-I		Column-II
(A)	FSH	(p)	Normal growth
(B)	GH	(q)	Ovulation
(C)	Prolactin	(r)	Parturition
(D)	Oxytocin	(s)	Water diuresis
		(t)	Milk secretion

(a) A - (q), B - (p), C - (t), D - (r)
(b) A - (q), B - (P), C - (t), D - (s)
(c) A - (P), B - (t), C - (r), D - (q)
(d) A - (q), B - (t), C - (s), D - (r)

6. Match the source gland with its respective hormone and function and select the correct option.

	Source gland	Hormone	Function
(a)	Anterior pituitary	Oxytocin	Contraction of uterus muscles during child birth
(b)	Posterior pituitary	Vasopressin	Stimulates resorption of water in the distal tubules in the nephron
(c)	Corpus luteum	Estrogen	Supports pregnancy
(d)	Thyroid	Thyroxine	Regulates blood calcium level

7. Match the hormones secreted by various endocrine structures and choose the correct option.

I.	Hypothalamus	A.	Melanocyte stimulating hormone
II.	Pars intermedia	B.	Aldosterone
III.	Pineal gland	C.	Gonadotrophin releasing hormone
IV.	Adrenal medulla	D.	Melatonin
V.	Adrenal cortex	E.	Catecholamines

(a) I - E, II - A, III - D, IV - B, V - C
(b) I - E, II - D, III - A, IV - B, V - C
(c) I - B, II - D, III - A, IV - C, V - E
(d) I - C, II - A, III - D, IV - B, V - E
(e) I - C, II - A, III - D, IV - E, V - B

8. Match Column I (hormone) with Column II (endocrine gland) and Column III (function).

	Column I	Column II		Column III
I.	Melatonin	A. Thyroid	i.	Acts on the renal tubules
2.	MSH	B. Adrenal	ii.	Regulates blood calcium levels
3.	Aldosterone	C. Pituitary	iii.	Maintains diurnal rhythm of our body
4.	TCT	D. Pineal	iv.	Acts on the melanocytes

(a) 4-A-iv; 3-D- iii; 1-B-ii; 2-C-i
(b) 1-D-iii; 2-C-iv; 3-B-i; 4-A-ii
(c) 1-B-i; 4-A-iii; 3-C-ii; 2-D-iv
(d) 2-D-ii; 1-B-i; 4-C-iv; 3-C-iii
(e) 2-C-iv; 3-A-ii; 1-D-iii; 4-B-i

9. Select the correct matching of a hormone, its source and function.

	Hormone	Source	Function
(a)	Vasopressin	Posterior pituitary	Increases loss of water through urine
(b)	Norepinephrine	Adrenal medulla	Increases heart beat, rate of respiration and alertness
(c)	Glucagon	Beta-cells of Islets of Langerhans	Stimulates glycogenolysis
(d)	Prolactin	Posterior pituitary	Regulates growth of mammary glands and milk fonnation in females

10. Select the option which correctly matches the endocrine gland with its hormone and its function.

	Endocrine gland	Hormone	Function
(a)	Placenta	Estrogen	Initiates secretion of the milk
(b)	Corpus luteum	Estrogen	Essential for maintenance of endometrium
(c)	Leydig's cells	Androgen	Initiates the production of sperms
(d)	Ovary	FSH	Stimulates follicular development and the secretion of estrogens

11. Match the Column I with Column II and select the correct option.

Column I		Column II	
A.	ANF	1.	Regulates blood calcium levels
B.	MSH	2.	Decreases blood pressure
C.	GIP	3.	Pigmentation
D.	TCT	4.	Inhibits gastric secretion

(a) A-4, B-1, C-2, D-3
(b) A-2, B-1, C-4, D-3
(c) A-4, B-1, C-3, D-2
(d) A-3, B-2, C-4, D-1
(e) A-2, B-3, C-4, D-1

11. In the given figure, what is indicated as 'X?

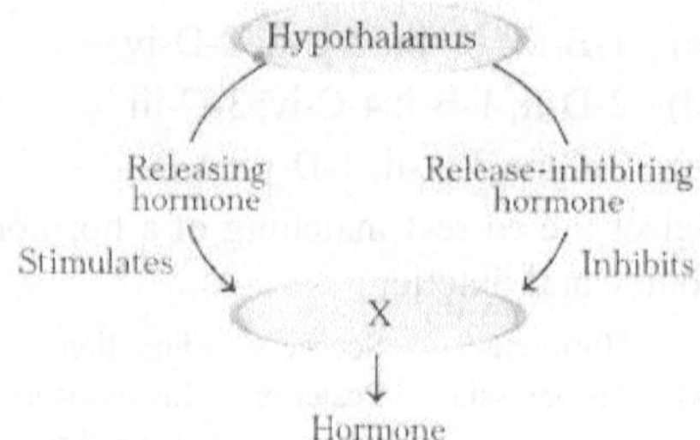

(a) Thyroid
(b) Parathyroid
(c) Anterior pituitary
(d) Gonads

12. Find out the correct labelling of the given figure.

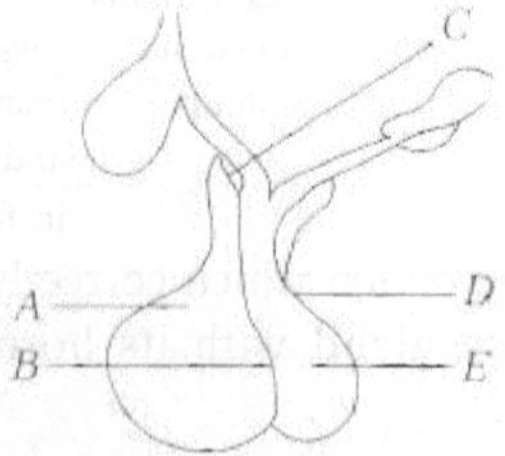

(a) A-Adenohypophysis, *B-Pars* intermedia, C-Hypothalamus, D-Infundibulum, E-Neurohypophysis
(b) A-Neurohypophysis, *B-Pars* intermedia, C-Hypothalamus, D-Infundibulum, *E*-Adenohypophysis
(c) A-Adenohypophysis, B-Infundibulum, C-Hypothalamus, D-Pars intermedia, E-Neurohypophysis
(d) A-Neurohypophysis, B-Infundibulum, C-Hypothalamus, D-Pars intermedia, *E*-Adenohypophysis

13. Which one of the following pairs is the correctly matched pair of the organ and the hormone it secretes?
(a) Thyroid – Epinephrine
(b) Alpha cells of pancreas – Glucagon
(c) Anterior pituitary – Adrenaline
(d) Stomach epithelium – Secretin

14. Identify the hormones, labelled as *A*, Band C in the following figure.

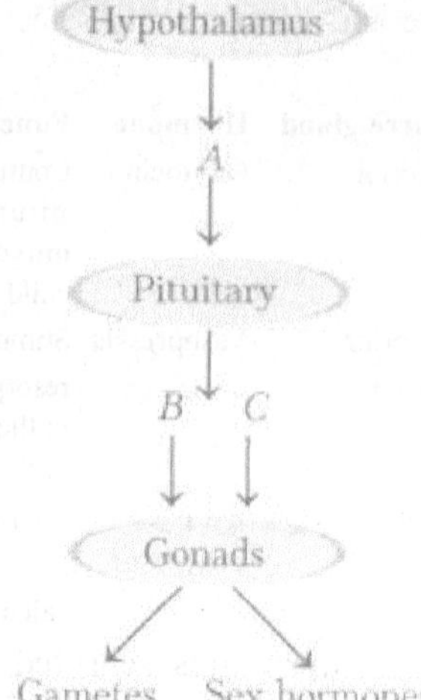

(a) *A*-GH, B-*FSH*, C-LH
(b) *A*-GnRH, *B*-FSH, C-LH
(c) *A*-GH, *B*-GnRH, C-PRT
(d) *A*-GnRH, *B*-GH, C-PRT

15. Match the source gland with its respective hormone and function.

	Source gland	Hormone	Function
(a)	Anterior piturity	Oxytocin	Contaction of uterus muscles during child birth
(b)	Posterior piturity	Vasopressin	Stimulates reabsoption of water in the distal tubules in nephron
(c)	Corpus luteum	Oestrogen	Supports pregnancy
(d)	Thyroid	Thyroxine	Reguulates blood calcium level

16. Match the following Columns.

	Column I		Column II
A.	Calcitonin	1.	Diabetes mellitus
B.	Gonadotrophin	2.	Rickets
C.	Erythropoietin	3.	Diabetes insipidus
D.	Insulin	4.	Formation of erythrocytes
E.	ADH	5.	Infertility

Codes

	A	B	C	D	E
(a)	3	1	4	2	5
(b)	3	2	1	5	4
(c)	4	3	2	1	5
(d)	2	5	4	1	3

17. Match the following Columns.

Column I	Column II
A. Pineal	1. Epinephrine
B. Thyroid	2. Melatonin
C. Ovary	3. Oestrogen
D. Adrenal medulla	4. Tetraiodothyromine

Codes

	A	B	C	D
(a)	4	2	1	3
(b)	2	4	1	3
(c)	3	2	1	4
(d)	2	4	3	1

18. Match the following Columns.

Column I	Column II
A. Epinephrine	1. Regulates blood calcium levels
B. Testosterone	2. Decreases blood pressure
C. Glucagon	3. Pigmentation
D. Atrial natriuretric factor	4. Increase heartbeat

Codes

	A	B	C	D
(a)	2	1	3	4
(b)	4	1	3	2
(c)	1	2	3	4
(d)	1	4	2	3

19. Given below is an incomplete table about certain hormones, their source glands and one major effect of each on the body in humans. Identify the correct option for the three blanks *A*, Band C.

Gland	Secretion	Effect on Body
A	Oestrogen	Maintance of secondary sexual characters
Alpha cells of islets Of Langerhans	B	Raises blood sugare level
Anterior pituitary	C	Over secretion leads to gigantism

	A	B	C
(a)	Placentra	Insulin	Vasopressin
(b)	Ovary	Insulin	Calcitonin
(c)	Placenta	Glucagon	Calcitonin
(d)	Ovary	Glucagon	Growth hormone

20. Identify the hormones A, B and C that are labelled in the given flowchart.

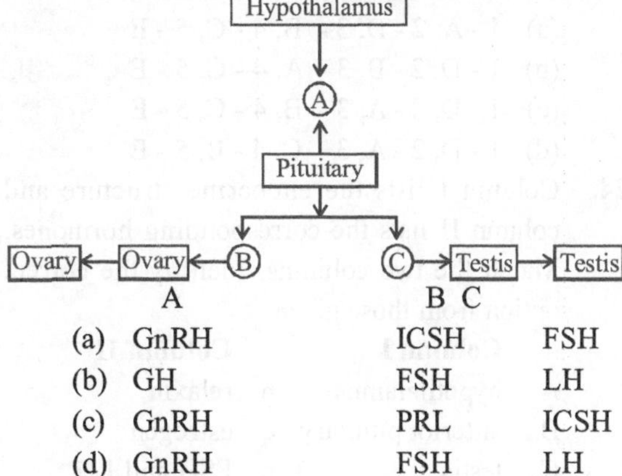

	A	B	C
(a)	GnRH	ICSH	FSH
(b)	GH	FSH	LH
(c)	GnRH	PRL	ICSH
(d)	GnRH	FSH	LH

21. Select the *correct* matching of a hormone, its source and function.

	Hormone	Source	Function
(a)	Vasopressin	Posterior pituitary	Increases loss of water through urine
(b)	Norepinephrine	Adrenal medulla	Increases heart beat, rate of respiration and alertness
(c)	Glucagon	Beta-cells of Islets of langerhans	Stimulates glycogenolysis
(d)	Prolactin	Posterior Pituitary	Regulates growth of mammary glands and milk formation in females

22. Match the list -I with list II

List - I	List -II
(a) adenohypophysis	(1) epinephrine
(b) adrenal medulla	(2) somatotropin
(c) parathyroid gland	(3) thymosin
(d) thymus gland	(4) calcitonin

(a) a : 3, b : 1, c : 4, d : 2
(b) a : 1, b : 2, c : 3, d : 4
(c) a : 2, b : 1, c : 4, d : 3
(d) a : 4, b : 3, c : 2, d : 1

23. Match item in column A with those given in column B

Column A	Column B
1. ADH	A. pituitary
2. ACTH	B. mineralocorticoid
3. alsosterone	C. diabetes mellitus
4. insulin	D. diabetes insipidus
5. adrenaline	E. vasodilator

(a) 1 - A, 2 - D, 3 - B, 4 - C, 5 - E
(b) 1 - D, 2 - B, 3 - A, 4 - C, 5 - E
(c) 1 - D, 2 - A, 3 - B, 4 - C, 5 - E
(d) 1 - D, 2 - A, 3 - C, 4 - B, 5 - E

24. Column I lists the endocrine structure and column II lists the corresponding hormones. Match the two columns. Identify the correct option from those given

Column I	Column II
A. hypothalamus	p. relaxin
B. anterior pituitary	q. estrogen
C. testis	r. FSH and LH
D. ovary	s. testosterone
	t. gonadotropin releasing hormone

(a) A = t, B = r, C = s, D = q
(b) A = t, B = r, C = q, D = s
(c) A = p, B = q, C = s, d = r
(d) A = r, B = t, C = s, D = q.

25. Given below is an incomplete table about certain hormones, their source glands and one major effect of each on the body in humans. Identify the correct option for the three blanks A, B and C

GLANDS	SECRETION	EFFECT ON BODY
A	Oestrogen	Maintenance of secondary sexual characters
Alpha cells of Islets of LangerhansAnterior pituitary	BC	Raises blood sugar levelOver secretion leads to Gigantism

Options:

	A	B	C
(a)	Placenta	Glucagon	Calcitonin
(b)	Ovary	Glucagon	Growth hormone
(c)	Placenta	Insulin	Vasopressin
(d)	Ovary	Insulin	Calcitonin

26. Mark the correct matching of the hormone and the endocrine cells

I. C-Cell	A Inhibin
II. b-cell	B Calcitonin
III. Leydig cell	C Insulin
IV. Sertoli cells	D Testosterone

(a) I-A, II-C, III-D, IV-B
(b) I-C, II-B, III-D, IV-A
(c) I-A, II-C, III-B, IV-D
(d) I-B, II-C, III-D, IV-A

Solutions

1. (c) 2. (a) 3. (d) 4. (a) 5. (a)
6. (b) 7. (e) 8. (b)
9. (b) Vasopressin reduces water loss through urine by stimulating resorption of water by the distal tubules of the kidney. Glucagon is released from a-cells. Prolactin is produced from anterior pituitary.
10. (c) Leydig's cells are present in between the seminiferous tubules which secrete androgens (*e.g.,* testosterone) that initiate the production of sperms. Theplacenta secretes into the mother's blood many hormones, such as estrogens and progesterone and these hormones supplement the hormones of same name produced by the ovary. Progesterone is secreted by corpus luteum. It brings about most of the pregnancy changes such as development of uterine lining and mammary glands, formation of placenta and also maintains pregnancy. Ovaries secrete two types of hormones - estrogens and progesterone.
11. (e)

ANF pressure	→	Decreases blood
MSH	→	Pigmentation
GIP	→	Inhibits gastric secretion
TCT	→	Regulates blood calcium levels

11. (c) 12. (a) 13. (b) 14. (b) 15. (b)
16. (d) 17. (d) 18. (b) 19. (d) 20. (d)
21. (b) 22. (c) 23. (c) 24. (a) 25. (b)
26. (d)

CHAPTER

Reproduction in Organisms

1. Match the column I with column II

	Column I		Column II
A.	Animals which give birth to young one	I.	*Hydra*
B.	Animal which produces bud	II.	*Planaria*
C.	An animal which shows regeneration	III.	Viviparous
D.	Provides nutrition to the developing embryo from the mother	IV.	Placenta

(a) A-I, B-III, C-II, D-IV
(b) A-III, B-I,C-II, D-IV
(c) A-III, B-II, C-IV, D-I
(d) A-III,B-IV, C-I, D-II

2. Match the column I with column II and choose the correct option:

A.	Root tubers	1.	*Curcuma* (Turmeric)
B.	Sucker	2.	*Chrysanthemum*
C.	Rhizome	3.	Sweet potato
D.	Corm	4.	*Colocasia*

Codes

	A	B	C	D		A	B	C	D
(a)	2	3	4	1	(b)	3	1	2	4
(c)	3	2	1	4	(d)	1	3	4	2

3. Match the columns and find out the correct combination:

A.	Rose	1.	2 weeks
B.	Pinus	2.	5+ years
C.	*Wolffia*	3.	300+ years
D.	Banana	4.	1 year
		5.	About 2 year

(a) A-2, B-3, C-4, D-5
(b) A-3, B-2, C-1, D-5
(c) A-2, B-3,C-1, D-4
(d) A-2, B-3,C-1,D-5

4. Match the column I with column II and choose the correct option:

	Column I		Column II
A.	Endothecium	1.	Starting cell of male gametophyte
B.	Tapetum	2.	Hypodermis in anther wall
C.	Microspore mother cell	3.	Nutritive tissue of female gametophyte
D.	Pollen grain	4.	Meiocytes
		5.	More than one nucleus

(a) A-2, B-5, C-4, D-1
(b) A-2, B-3, C-4, D-1
(c) A-3, B-5, C-2, D-1
(d) A-3, B-2, C-1, D-5

5. Which form of reproduction is correctly matched?

(a) *Euglena* $\rightarrow$ transverse binary fission
(b) *Paramecium* $\rightarrow$ longitudinal binary fission
(c) *Amoeba* $\rightarrow$ multiple fission
(d) *Plasmodium* $\rightarrow$ binary fission

6. Match the items in column I with those in column II and choose the correct option.

	Column I		Column II
A.	Binary fission	I.	Algae
B.	Zoospore	II.	*Amoeba*
C.	Conidium	III.	*Hydra*
D.	Budding	IV.	*Penicillium*
E.	Gemmules	V.	Sponge

(a) A – I; B – IV; C – V; D – III; E – II
(b) A – II; B – I; C – IV; D – III; E – V
(c) A – II; B – IV; C – III; D – V; E – I
(d) A – I; B – IV; C – III; D – II; E – V

7. Match column I with column II and select the correct option.

Column I (Name of the organism)	Column II (Haploid chromosome number in gamete)
A. *Ophioglossum*	I. 23
B. Rice	II. 24
C. Potato	III. 12
D. Man	IV. 630

(a) A – I; B – II; C – III; D – IV
(b) A – II; B – III; C – IV; D – I
(c) A – III; B – IV; C – II; D – I
(d) A – IV; B – III; C – II; D – I

8. Match list I with list II and select the correct option.

List I	List II
A. Gemmules	I. *Agave*
B. Leaf-buds	II. *Penicillium*
C. Bulbil	III. Water hyacinth
D. Offset	IV. Sponges
E. Conidia	V. *Bryophyllum*

(a) A – IV; B – V; C – I; D – III; E – II
(b) A – IV; B – III; C – II; D – I; E – V
(c) A – III; B – V; C – IV; D – II; E – I
(d) A – IV; B – I; C – V; D – III; E – II

9. Match the following and choose the correct combination from the options given.

Column I (Organism)	Column II (Approximate life span)
A. Butterfly	I. 60 years
B. Crow	II. 140 years
C. Parrot	III. 15 years
D. Crocodile	IV. 1 – 2 years

(a) A – I; B – II; C – III; D – IV
(b) A – IV; B – III; C – I; D – II
(c) A – II; B – III; C – IV; D – I
(d) A – IV; B – III; C – II; D – I

10. Match the following and choose the correct combination from the options given.

Column I (Name of the organism)	Column II (Chromosome number in meiocyte (2*n*))
A. Housefly	I. 20
B. Fruit fly	II. 34
C. Apple	III. 8
D. Maize	IV. 12

(a) A – I; B – II; C – III; D – IV
(b) A – II; B – III; C – IV; D – I
(c) A – III; B – IV; C – II; D – I
(d) A – IV; B – III; C – II; D – I

11. Examine the figures given below and select the right options out of (1 - 4); in which all the 4 items A, B, C and D are identified correctly

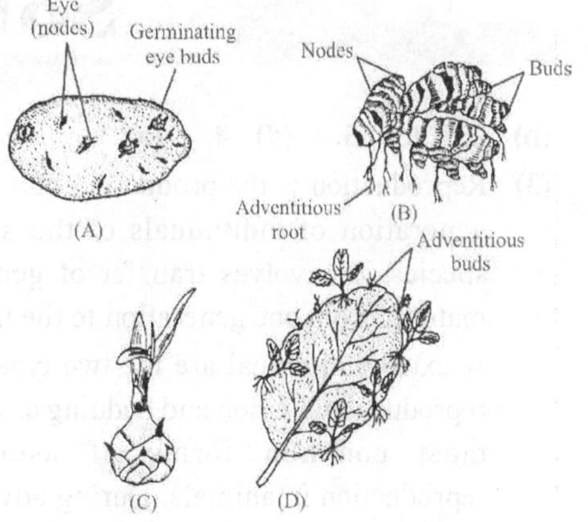

	(A)	(B)	(C)	(D)
(a)	Tuber	Rhizome	Bulb	Leaf buds
(b)	Offset	Sucker	Stolon	Leaf buds
(c)	Offset	Sucker	Stolon	Leaf buds
(d)	Tuber	Rhizome	Bulbil	Leaf buds

12. Pick the correct set

Column I	Column II
A. Bamboos	I. Bronchial allergy
B. Microspore	II. Die after flowering
C. Cleistozamous	III. Orchids
D. Micropropa- gation	IV. flowers which never open

(a) A–I; B–II; C–III; D–IV
(b) A–II; B–I; C–IV; D–III
(c) A–IV; B–II; C–III; D–I
(d) A–I; B–IV; C–II; D–III

13. Match the following and mark the correct set

Column I	Column II
A. Arum	I. Vegetative reproduction
B. Micropropagation	II. Fly-trap mechanism
C. Heterothallic	III. Entomophilly
D. Coloured petal and nectar	IV. Sexual reproduction

(a) A–I; B–II; C–III; D–IV
(b) A–II; B–I; C–IV; D–III
(c) A–III; B–II; C–IV; D–I
(d) A–I; B–III; C–IV; D–II

14. Match the columns

Column I	Column II
A. Phanerophytes	I. Buds are situated close to the ground
B. Chamaephytes	II. Buds completely hidden in the soil
C. Crytophytes	III. Buds naked or covered with scale
D. Therophytes	IV. Seasonal plants completing their life cycle in a single favourable season

(a) A – I; B–II; C–III; D–IV
(b) A–III; B–I; C–II; D–IV
(c) A–III; B–II; C–I; D–IV
(d) A–I; B–III; C–II; D–IV

Solutions

1. (b) **2.** (c) **3.** (d) **4.** (a)

5. (3) Reproduction is the production of a new generation of individuals of the same species. It involves transfer of genetic material from one generation to the next. Asexual and sexual are the two types of reproduction. Fission and budding are two most common forms of asexual reproduction in animals. During adverse conditions, amoeba reproduces by multiple fission that gives rise to many amoeba. *Euglena* reproduces by longitudinal binary fission, *Paramecium* reproduces by transverse binary fission and *Plasmodium* reproduces by multiple fission.

6. (b) **7.** (d) **8.** (a) **9.** (d) **10.** (d)

11. (d) **12.** (b) **13.** (b) **14.** (b)

CHAPTER

Sexual Reproduction in Flowering Plants

1. Match the items in column I with those in column II and choose the correct answer.

Column-I	Column-II
1. Funicle	A. Small opening of ovule
2. Integuments	B. Stalk of ovule
3. Chalaza	C. Protective envelopes of ovule
4. Hilum	D. Junction part of ovule and stalk
5. Micropyle	E Basal part of the ovule

(a) 1-B; 2-C; 3-E; 4-D; 5-A
(b) 1-A; 2-C; 3-B; 4-D; 5-E
(c) 1-B; 2-C; 3-A; 4-D; 5-E
(d) 1-B; 2-D; 3-E; 4-A; 5-C
(e) 1-C; 2-D; 3-E; 4-A; 5-B

2. Match the entries in Column I with those of Column II and choose the correct answer.

Column I	Column II
A. Cleistogamy	m. Insect pollination
B. Geitonogamy	n. Bud pollination
C. Entomophily	o. Pollination between flowers in the same plant
D. Xenogamy	p. Wind pollination
	q. Cross pollination

(a) A-o, B-m, C-q, D-n
(b) A-m, B-q, C-n, D-o
(c) A-n, B-o, C-m, D-q
(d) A-q, B-p, C-o, D-n

3. Match the column I with column II and select the correct answer from the given codes.

Column I	Column II
A. Parthenocarpy	(i) Seed formation without fertilisation
B. Polyembryony	(ii) More than one embryo in same seed
C. Apomixis	(iii) Seedless fruits without fertilisation
D. Somatic	(iv) Embryo develops from embryogenesis a somatic cell

(a) A - (iv), B - (ii), C - (iii), D - (i)
(b) A - (iii), B - (ii), C - (i), D - (iv)
(c) A - (i), B - (iv), C - (iii), D - (ii)
(d) A - (ii), B - (iii), C - (i), D - (iv)

4. Identity the parts labbled A, B, C and D in the given figure and select the correct option.

	A	B	C	D
(a)	Chalaza	Female gametophyte	Embryo sac	Micropyle
(b)	Chalaza	Nucellus	Embryo sac	Micropyle
(c)	Micropyle	Egg	Embryo sac	Chalaza
(d)	Micropyle	Nucellus	Embryo sac	Chalaza

5. Select the mismatched pair.

(a) Storage of pollen grains – 196ºC
(b) Pollen allergy – Carrot grass
(c) Chasmogamous flowers – Exposed anthers and stigmas
(d) Xenogamy – Self pollination

6. Match column I with column II and select the correct option from the given codes.

Column I	Column II
A. Anemophily	(i) Grasses, Date palm
B. Hydrophily	(ii) Rose, Jasmine
C. Entomophily	(iii) *Butea, Bignonia*
D. Ornithophily	(iv) *Vallisneria, Ceratophyllum*

(a) A-(i), B-(iv), C-(ii), D-(iii)
(b) A-(i), B-(iv), C-(iii), D-(ii)
(c) A-(ii), B-(iii), C-(i), D-(iv)
(d) A-(ii), B-(i), C-(iii), D-(iv)

7. Match column I with column II and select the correct option from the given codes.

Column I	Column II
A. Tallest flower	(i) Maize
B. *Pronuba* moth	(ii) *Amorphophallus*
C. Anemophily	(iii) *Salvia*
D. Entomophily	(iv) *Yucca*

(a) A-(ii), B-(iv), C-(i), D-(iii)
(b) A-(ii), B-(iv), C-(iii), D-(i)
(c) A-(iii), B-(ii), C-(i), D-(iv)
(d) A-(iv), B-(iii), C-(ii), D-(i)

8. Match column I with column II and select the correct . option from the given codes.

Column I	Column II
A. Monoecious	(i) *Primula*
B. Dioecious	(ii) Maize
C. Cleistogamous	(iii) Date palm
D. Heterostyly	(iv) *Commelina*

	A	B	C	D
(a)	(iii)	(ii)	(iv)	(i)
(b)	(ii)	(iii)	(iv)	(i)
(c)	(ii)	(iii)	(i)	(iv)
(d)	(i)	(ii)	(iii)	(iv)

9. Given below are the events that are observed in an artificial hybridisation programme. Arrange them in the correct sequential order and select the correct option.

1. Re-bagging
2. Selection of parents
3. Bagging
4. Dusting the pollen on stigma
5. Emasculation
6. Collection of pollen from male parent

(a) 2 → 3 → 5 → 6 → 4 → 1
(b) 2 → 5 → 3 → 6 → 4 → 1
(c) 5 → 2 → 3 → 6 → 1 → 4
(d) 2 → 3 → 6 → 4 → 5 → 1

10. Match column I with column II and select the correct option from the given codes.

Column I	Column II
A. Ovary	(i) Groundnut, mustard
B. Ovule	(ii) Guava, orange, mango
C. Wall of ovary	(iii) Pericarp
D. Fleshy fruits	(iv) Seed
E. Dry fruits	(v) Fruit

	A	B	C	D	E
(a)	(v)	(iv)	(iii)	(ii)	(i)
(b)	(i)	(ii)	(iii)	(iv)	(v)
(c)	(i)	(iii)	(ii)	(iv)	(v)
(d)	(v)	(iv)	(i)	(ii)	(iii)

11. Choose the correct match.

(a) Microspore – Pollen
(b) Megasporangium – Ovule
(c) Microsporangium – Anther lobes
(d) None of the above

12. Match the following Columns.

	Column I		Column II
A.	*Arum maculatum*	1.	Mosaic endosperm
B.	*Zea mays*	2.	Longest endosperm
C.	*Echinocystis lobata*	3.	Highest ploidy level of endosperm
D.	*Annona squamosa*	4.	Ruminate endosperm

Codes

	A	B	C	D
(a)	4	2	1	3
(b)	2	3	1	4
(c)	4	2	3	1
(d)	3	1	2	4

13. Match the following Columns.

	Column I		Column II
A.	Place where pollen grains land	1.	Spores
B.	The site, where the seeds develop	2.	Stigma
C.	Reproductive cells that have exactly the same number of chromosomes as the parent *plant*	3.	Microspore mother cells
D.	Meiotically dividing cells in the male reproductive tissues that make four microspores	4.	Ovary

Codes

	A	B	C	D
(a)	1	2	3	4
(b)	2	4	1	3
(c)	3	4	1	2
(d)	4	3	2	1

14. Match the following Columns.

Column I	Column II
A. *Salvia*	1. *Pronuba*
B. *Yucca*	2. Moth
C. *Arisaema*	3. Insect
D. *Ophrys*	4. Snail

Codes

	A	B	C	D
(a)	1	2	3	4
(b)	1	3	2	4
(c)	3	1	4	2
(d)	4	2	1	3

15. Macth column I with column II and selcet the correct option using the codes given below.

Column I	Column II
A. Pistils fused together	1. Gametogenesis
B. Formation of gametes	2. Pistillate
C. Hyphae of higher ascomycetes	3. Syncarpous
D. Unisexual female flower	4. Dikaryotic

Codes

	A	B	C	D
(a)	4	3	2	1
(b)	2	1	4	3
(c)	1	2	4	3
(d)	3	1	4	2

16. Which one of the following is mismatched in angiosperm?

(a) Pollen grains – Haploid
(b) Megaspore – Diploid
(c) Synergid – Haploid
(d) Endosperm – Triploid

17. Choose the mismatched option.

(a) Wind – *Cannabis* – Anemophily
(b) Water – *Zoostera* – Hydrophily
(c) Insects – *Salvia* – Entomophily
(d) Birds – *Adansonia* – Ornithophily
(e) Bats – *Kigelia* – Cheiropterophily

18. Match the following ovular structure with postfertilisation structure and select the correct alternative.

Column I	Column II
A. Ovule	1. Endosperm
B. Funiculus	2. Aril
C. Nucellus	3. Seed
D. Polar nuclei	4. Perisperm

Codes

	A	B	C	D
(a)	2	3	4	1
(b)	2	3	1	4
(c)	3	2	4	1
(d)	3	2	1	4

19. Match the following ovular structure with post-fertilisation structure and select the correct alternative.

Column I	Column II
A. Ovule	1. Endosperm
B. Funiculus	2. Aril
C. Nucellus	3. Seed
D. Polar nuclei	4. Perisperm

Codes

	A	B	C	D
(a)	2	3	4	1
(b)	2	3	1	4
(c)	3	2	4	1
(d)	3	2	1	4

(a) 4000 (b) 10000
(c) 24000 (d) 48000

20. Match the following and choose the correct option

	Column I		Column II
A.	Ovary	I.	Groundnut, mustard
B.	Ovule	II.	Guava, orange, mango
C.	Wall of ovary	III.	Pericarp
D.	Fleshy fruits	IV.	Seed
E.	Dry fruits	V.	Fruit

(a) A-V ; B-IV ; C-III ; D-II ; E-I
(b) A-I ; B-II ; C-III ; D-IV ; E-V
(c) A-I ; B-III ; C-II ; D-IV ; E-V
(d) A-V ; B-IV ; C-I ; D-II ; E-III

21. Match the following and choose the correct option.

	Column I		Column II
A.	Funicle with in ovule	I.	Mass of cells with more food
B.	Hilum	II.	Basal part of ovule
C.	Integument	III.	One or two protective layers of ovule
D.	Chalazal end	IV.	Region where body of ovules fuses with funicle
E.	Nucellus	V.	Stalk of ovule

(a) A-I ; B-II ; C-III ; D-IV ; E-V
(b) A-V ; B-IV ; C-III ; D-II ; E-I
(c) A-IV ; B-II ; C-I ; D-III ; E-V
(d) A-I ; B-III ; C-V ; D-II ; E-IV

22. Match the following and choose the correct option.

	Column I		Column II
A.	Megasporogenesis	I.	Monosporic development
B.	Megagametogenesis	II.	Fatty substance
C.	Sporopollenin	III.	Embryo sac formation
D.	Typical embryo & ac	IV.	Megaspore formation

(a) A-I ; B-II ; C-III ; D-IV
(b) A-IV ; B-III ; C-II ; D-I
(c) A-IV ; B-I ; C-II ; D-III
(d) A-III ; B-II ; C-I ; D-IV

23. Match the following columns.

Column I		Column II
A. Calyx	I.	Female gamete
B. Corolla	II.	Protection
C. Stamen	III.	Attraction
D. Carpel	IV.	Male gamete

Codes

(a) A-I; B-II; C-III; D-IV
(b) A-II; B-III; C-IV; D-I
(c) A-IV; B-III; C-II; D-I
(d) A-I; B-II; C-IV; D-III

Solutions

1. **(a)** 2. **(c)** 3. **(b)**

4. **(d)** Given figure represents an anatropous ovule where A, B, C and D represent micropyle, nucellus, embryo sac and chalaza respectively.

5. **(d)** Xenogamy or cross pollination is the transfer of pollen grains from the anther of one flower to the stigma of a genetically different flower. Cross pollination is performed with the help of an ecternal agency.

6. **(a)**	**7.** **(a)**	**8.** **(b)**	**9.** **(b)**	**10.** **(a)**
11. **(d)**	**12.** **(d)**	**13.** **(b)**	**14.** **(c)**	**15.** **(d)**
16. **(b)**	**17.** **(c)**	**18.** **(c)**	**19.** **(c)**	**20.** **(a)**
21. **(b)**	**22.** **(b)**	**23.** **(b)**		

CHAPTER

Human Reproduction

1. The given table shows differences between spermatogenesis and spermiogenesis. Select the incorrect option.

	Spermatogenesis	Spermiogenesis
(a)	Process of formation of spermatozoa.	Process of differentiatin of spermatozoon form a spermatid.
(b)	It changes a haploid stucture into another haploid structure.	It involves conversion of a diploid structure into haploid structure.
(c)	Growth and divisions occur.	Divisions and growth are absent.
(d)	A spermatogonium forms four spermatozoa.	A spermatid forms a single spermatozoon.

2. Match column I with column II and select the correct option from the codes given below.

Column I	Column II
A. Acrosome	(i) Rudimentary erectile tissue
B. Endometrium	(ii) Uterus
C. Polar body	(iii) Oogenesis
D. Clitoris	(iv) Spermatozoon

(a) A-(ii), B-(i), C-(iv), D-(iii)
(b) A-(iv), B-(ii), C-(iii), D-(i)
(c) A-(iv), B-(iii), C-(ii), D-(i)
(d) A-(iv), B-(iii), C-(i), D-(ii)

3. Which of the following options is correct?

	Haploid	Diploid
(a)	Secondary oocyte	Primary spermatocyte
(b)	Secondary spermatocyte	Secondary oocyte
(c)	Primary oocyte	Secondary spermatocyte
(d)	Ovum	Spermatid

4. Match column I with column II and select the correct option from the codes given below.

Column I	Column II
A. Cleavage	(i) Fertilisation
B. Morula	(ii) Mitotic divisions
C. Polyspermy	(iii) Endometrial
D. Implantation	(iv) Little mulberry

(a) A-(ii), B-(iv), C-(i), D-(iii)
(b) A-(i), B-(iv), C-(ii), D-(iii)
(c) A-(iv), B-(ii), C-(i), D-(iii)
(d) A-(ii), B-(iv), C-(iii), D-(i)

5. Match column I with column II and select the correct option from the codes given below.

Column I	Column II
A. Fertilisation	(i) Isthmus of oviduct
B. Cleavage	(ii) Later part of oviduct
C. Morula	(iii) Cervix
D. Blastocyst	(iv) Ampulla of oviduct
E. Parturition	(v) Uterine wall

(a) A-(iv), B-(i), C -(ii), D-(iii), E-(v)
(b) A-(ii), B-(i), C -(iv), D-(iii), E-(v)
(c) A-(ii), B-(i), C -(v), D-(iv), E-(iii)
(d) A-(iv), B-(i), (-(ii), D-(v), E-(iii)

6. Match column I (terms) with column II (definitions) and select the correct option from the codes given below.

Column I	Column II
A. Parturition	(i) Attachment of embryo to endometrium
B. Gestation	(ii) Release of egg from Graafian follicle
C. Ovulation	(iii) Delivery of baby from uterus
D. Implantation	(iv) Duration between pregnancy and birth
E. Conception	(v) Formation of zygote by fusion of the egg and sperm
	(vi) Stoppage of ovulation and menstruation

(a) A-(ii), B-(iv), C-(i), D-(v), E-(vi)
(b) A-(iv), B-(iii), C-(i), D-(v), E-(ii)
(c) A-(v), B-(vi), C-(ii), D-(iii), E-(iv)
(d) A-(iii), B-(iv), C-(ii), D-(i), E-(v)

7. Match column I with column II and select the correct option from the codes given below.

Column I	Column II
A. Hypothalamus	(i) Sperm lysins
B. Acrosome	(ii) Estrogen
C. Graafian follicle	(iii) Relaxin
D. Leydig's cells	(iv) GnRH
E. Parturition	(v) Testosterone

(a) A-(iv), B-(i), C-(ii), D-(iii), E-(v)
(b) A-(ii), B-(i), C-(iv), D-(iii), E-(v)
(c) A-(ii), B-(i), C-(v), D-(iv), E-(iii)
(d) A-(iv), B-(i), C-(ii), D -(v), E-(iii)

8. Match column I with column II and select the correct option from the codes given below.

Column I	Column II
A. Hyaluronidase	(i) Acrosomal reaction
B. Corpus luteum	(ii) Morphogenetic movements
C. Gastrulation	(iii) Progesterone
D. Capacitation	(iv) Mammary gland
E. Colostrum	(v) Sperm activation

(a) A-(v), B-(ii), C-(iv), D-(i), E-(iii)
(b) A-(i), B-(iii), C-(ii), D-(v), E-(iv)
(c) A-(iii), B-(ii), C-(v), D-(iv), E-(i)
(d) A-(i), B-(ii), C-(iii), D-(iv), E-(v)

9. Select the correct match.

Column I	Column II
(A) Seminal fluid	(i) Corpus spongiosum
(B) Prostate gland	(ii) Membranous urethra
(C) Ejaculatory duct	(iii) Clitoris
(D) Erectile tissues	(iv) Fructose
	(v) Prostaglandins

(a) (A)-(iv) (b) (B)-(v)
(c) (C)-(i) (d) (D)-(ii)

10. Match the items given in column I with those in column II and select the correct option given below.

Column I	Column II
A. Proliferative phase	(i) Breakdown of endometrial lining
B. Secretory phase	(ii) Follicular phasse
C. Menstruation	(iii) Luteal phase

	A	B	C
(a)	(iii)	(ii)	(i)
(b)	(i)	(iii)	(ii)
(c)	(ii)	(iii)	(i)
(d)	(iii)	(i)	(ii)

11. Column I contains terms and column II contains definitions. Match them correctly and choose the right answer.

Column I	Column II
A. Parturition	1. Attachment of zygote to endometrium
B. Gestation	2. Release of egg from Graffian follicle
C. Ovulation	3. Delivery of baby from uterus
D. Implantation	4. Duration between pregnancy and birth
E. Conception	5. Formation of zygote by fusion of the egg and sperm
	6. Stoppage of ovulation

(a) A - 2, B - 4, C - l, D - 5, E - 3
(b) A - 4, B - 3, C - 1, D - 5, E - 2
(c) A - 5, B - 1, C - 2, D - 3, E - 4
(d) A - 3, B - 4, C - 2, D - 1, E - 5

12. Which is the correctly matched pair among the following?

I. Colostrum	–	Secretion found in seminal fluid
II. Areola	–	Pigmented circular area around the nipple
III. Sexual intercourse	–	Coitus
IV. Bartholin's gland	–	Erectile body in female homologous to glans penis of male.

Codes

(a) II and III
(b) III and IV
(c) I and IV
(d) II and IV

13. Match the following Columns.

Column I	Column II
A. Male reproductive organ	1. Semen
B. Site of sperm maturation and strage	2. Seminiferous tubules
C. Unit of tests	3. Testis
D. Substance containig sperm and other secretions	4. Epididymis

Codes

	A	B	C	D
(a)	3	1	2	4
(b)	1	2	3	4
(c)	3	4	2	1
(d)	4	3	1	2

14. Match the following Columns.

Column I	Column II
A. A hollow ball of cells	1. Cleavage
B. Outer germ layer	2. Seminiferous
C. Cavity within a blastula	3. Blastocoel
D. Division of embryo	4. Ectoderm

Codes

	A	B	C	D
(a)	2	4	3	1
(b)	1	4	3	2
(c)	4	3	2	1
(d)	3	1	4	2

15. Match the following Columns.

Column I	Column II
A. The process of start of menstrual cycle in the life of a human female.	1. Capacitation

B. The process of maturation of sperms — 2. Luteal phase

C. The process of transformation of ruptured Graafian follicle into corpus luteum. — 3. Sperminogenesis

D. The process of activation of sperms in female reproductive system after their ejaculation inot it — 4. Menarche

Codes

	A	B	C	D
(a)	4	3	2	1
(b)	1	2	3	4
(c)	2	1	3	4
(d)	3	1	2	4

16. Which one of the following is the correct matching of the events occurring during menstrual cycle?

(a) Ovulation – FH and FSH attain peak level and sharp fall in the secretion of progesterone

(b) Proliferative – Rapid regeneration of myometrium and maturation of Graafian follicle

(c) Development of corpus luteum – Secretory phase and increased secretion of progesterone

(d) Menstruation – Breakdown of myometrium and ovum not fertilised

17. Match the hormones listed under column I with their functions listed under column II choose the answer, which gives the correct combination of the alphabets of the two columns.

Column I	**Column II**
A. Oxytocin	1. Stimulates ovulation
B. Prolactin	2. Implantation and maintenance of pregnancy
C. Luteinising hormone	3. Lactation after child birth
D. Progesterone	4. Uterine conraction ding labour
	5. Reabsorption of water by nephrons

Codes

	A	B	C	D		A	B	C	D
(a)	4	2	3	5	(b)	5	3	1	4
(c)	4	3	1	2	(d)	2	3	1	4

18. Match the following with correct combination.

A. hyaluronidase	p. acrosomal reaction
B. corpus luteum	q. morphogenetic movements
C. gastrulation	r. progesterone
D. capacitiation	s. mammary gland
E. colostrum	t. sperm activation

(a) A - t, B - q, C - s, D - p, E - r

(b) A - p, B - r, C - q, D - t, E - s

(c) A - r, B - q, C - t, D - s, E - p

(d) A - p, B - q, C - r, D - s, E - t

19. Match column I with column II and select the correct option using the code given below

Column I	**Column II**
A. Mons pubis	I. Embryo formation
B. Antrum	II. Sperm
C. Trophectoderm	III. Female external genitalia
D. Nebenkern	IV. Graafian follicle

(a) A–I; B–IV; C–III; D–II

(b) A–III; B–IV; C–II; D–I

(c) A–III; B–IV; C–I; D–II

(d) A–III; B–I; C–IV; D–II

20. In the given columns, column I contain structures of male reproductive system and column II contains its feature. Select the correct match from the options given below.

	Column I (Structure of Male Reproductive System)		Column II (Features)
A.	Seminiferous tubule	I.	Network of seminiferous tubule
B.	Rete testis	II.	Secondary sexual characters
C.	Leydig cells	III.	Meiosis and sperm formation occurs
D.	Prepuce	IV.	Place of implantation
		V.	Terminal skin of penis

(a) A – I; B – II; C – III; D – V
(b) A – III; B – I; C – II; D – V
(c) A – III; B – I; C – IV; D – II
(d) A – II; B – IV; C – III; D – V

21. In the given columns, column-I contain structures of female reproductive system and column-II contain its feature. Select the correct match from the option given below.

	Column-I (Structures of female reproductive system)		Column-II (Features)
A.	Ampulla	I.	It undergoes cyclical changes during menstrual cycle.
B.	Labia majora	II.	It helps in collection of ovum after ovulation.
C.	Oviduct	III.	Wider part of fallopian tube where fusion of male and female gametes takes place.
D.	Fimbriae	IV.	Larger hairy folds which extend down from the mons pubis and surrounds the vaginal opening.
E.	Endometrium	V.	Also called fallopian tubes, which extend from the periphery of each ovary to the womb.

(a) A – I; B – II; C – III; D – V; E – IV
(b) A – III; B – I; C – II; D – V; E – IV
(c) A – III; B – IV; C – V; D – II; E – I
(d) A – II; B – IV; C – III; D – V; E – I

22. The given figure shows the diagrammatic sectional view of female reproductive system with few structures marked as A, B, C, D, E and F.

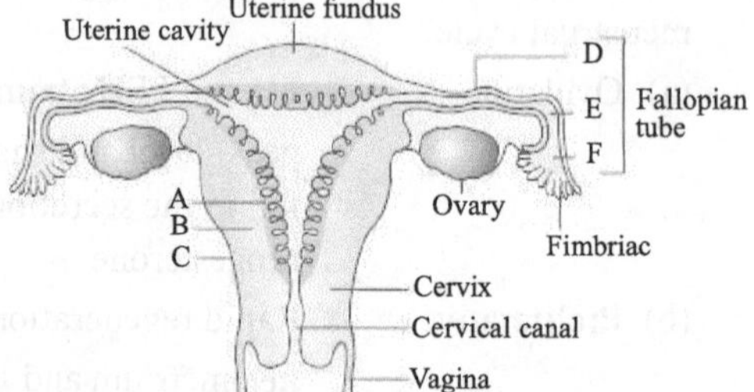

Which of the following options shows the correct labeling of A–F?

(a) A→Myometrium, B→Isthmus, C→Endometrium, D→Perimetrium, E→Ampulla, F→Infundibulum
(b) A→Infundibulum, B→Perimetrium, C→Endometrium, D→Myometrium, E→Ampulla, F→Isthmus
(c) A→Endometrium, B→Myometrium, C→Perimetrium, D→Isthmus, E→Ampulla, F→Infundibulum
(d) A→Perimetrium, B→Endometrium, C→Isthmus, D→Infundibulum, E→Ampulla, F→Myometrium

23. Refer the figure of mammary gland with few structures marked as A, B, C and D. Identify the marked structures.

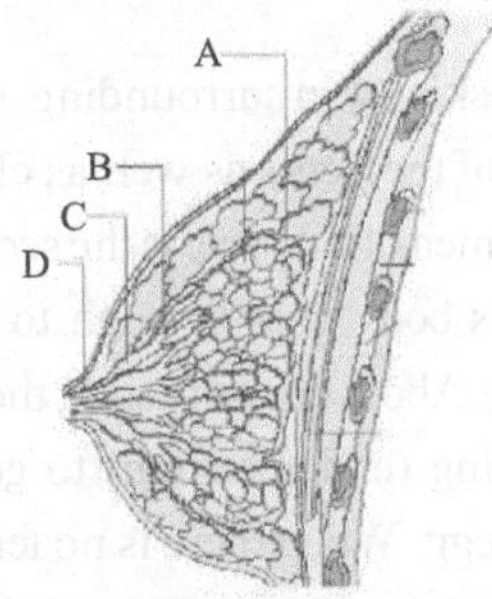

(a) Mammary lobe, mammary duct, ampulla and lactiferous duct.
(b) Ampulla, mammary duct, lactiferous duct and mammary lobe.
(c) Lactiferous duct, mammary lobe, mammary lobe and ampulla.
(d) Mammary duct, mammary lobe lactiferous duct and ampulla.

24. The figure given below shows the structure of sperm. Identify the correct feature corresponding to the marked structure A, B, C and D.

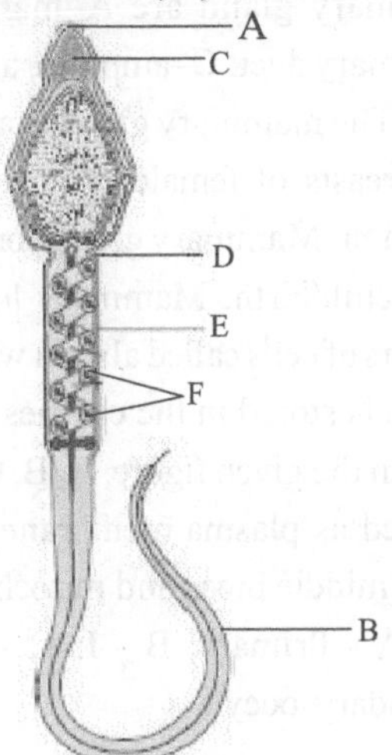

(a) A - plasma membrane, B - tail, C - Acrosome, D - Neck, E - middle piece and F - Mitochondria.
(b) A - middlepiece, B - plasma membrane, C - Neck, D - Mitochondria, E - tail and F - Acrosome.
(c) A - Mitochondria, B - tail, C - Neck, D - plasma membrane, E - Acrosome and F - middle piece.
(d) A - Acrosome, B - middle piece, C - mitochondria, D - tail, E - plasma membrane and F - Neck.

25. The given figure shows the diagrammatic representation of oogenesis. Identify the option which shows the correct label marked as A, B, C and D.

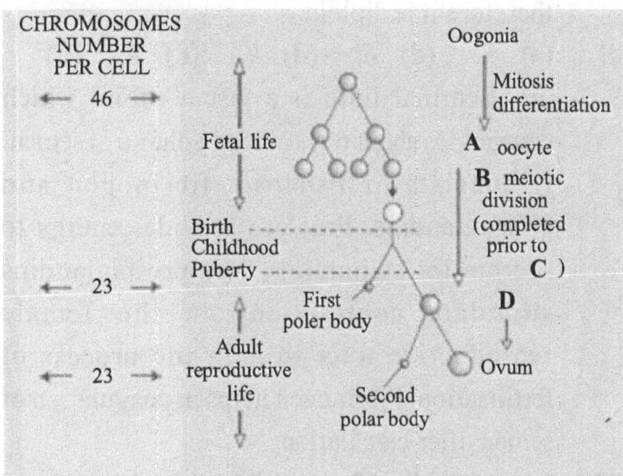

(a) A: Tertiary; B: I; C: Fertilization; D: Primary oocyte.
(b) A: Primary; B: II; C: Ovulation; D: Secondary oocyte.
(c) A: Secondary; B: II; C: Fertilization; D: Primary oocyte.
(d) A: Primary; B: I; C: Ovulation; D: Secondary oocyte.

Solutions

1. **(b)** Spermatogenesis involves conversion of a diploid structure (spermatogonia) into haploid structures (spermatozoa). Spermiogenesis changes a haploid structure (spermatid) into another haploid structure (spermatozoon).
2. **(b)**
3. **(a)** Secondary oocyte is formed by meiotic division of primary oocyte *(2n),* therefore, it is haploid. Primary spermatocyte is formed by mitotic division of spermatogonium *(2n),* therefore it is diploid.
4. **(a)** **5. (d)** **6. (d)** **7. (d)** **8. (b)**
9. **(a)** Seminal fluid is a viscous fluid which contributes about 60% of total volume of semen. It consists of fructose, fibrinogen and prostaglandins. Fructose provides energy to sperms for swimming. The prostaglandins stimulate contractions in the female reproductive tract to help the process of fertilisation. Fibrinogen helps in coagulation of semen after ejaculation.
10. **(c)** **11. (d)** **12. (a)** **13. (c)** **14. (a)**
15. **(a)** **16. (c)** **17. (c)** **18. (b)** **19. (c)**
20. **(b)** Seminiferous tubules are located in the testes, which are the specific location of meiosis, and the subsequent formation of sperms. Rete testis is a network of small tubules found in the part of the testicle that carries sperm. Leydig cells or interstitial cells of Leydig produce the hormone called testosterone which contributes to male secondary sexual characters. Prepuce is the foreskin, skin surrounding and protecting the head of the penis as well as clitoris.
21. **(d)** The menstrual cycle is the series of changes a woman's body goes through to prepare for a pregnancy. About once a month, the uterus grows a new lining (endometrium) to get ready for a fertilized egg. When there is no fertilized egg to start a pregnancy, the uterus sheds its lining. This is the monthly menstrual bleeding (also called menstrual period).
22. **(c)** In the given figure of female reproductive system, the marked structures (A to F) are the parts of uterus and fallopian tube. A to F are respectively endometrium, myometrium, perimetrium, isthmus, ampulla and infundibulum.
23. **(a)** The structures marked in the figure of mammary gland are A–mammary lobe, B–mammary duct, C–ampulla, and D–lactiferous duct. The mammary gland is a gland located in the breasts of females that is responsible for lactation. Mammary glands only produce milk after childbirth. Mammary lobe (A) contains clusters of cells called alveoli which secrete milk which is stored in the cavities of alveoli.
24. **(a)** In the given figure, A, B, C, D, E and F are marked as plasma membrane, tail, acrosome, neck, middle piece and mitochondria.
25. **(d)** A - Primary; B - I; C - Ovulation; D - Secondary oocyte

CHAPTER

Reproductive Health

1. Given below are four methods (A-D) and their modes of action (i-iv) in achieving contraception. Select their correct matching from the four options that follow.

Method	Mode of Action
A. Oral pill	(i) Prevents sperms reaching cerbix
B. Condom	(ii) Suppresses sperm motelity
C. Vasectomy	(iii) Prevents ovulation
D. Copper T	(iv) Semen contains on sperms

(a) A-(ii), B-(iv), C-(i), D-(ii)
(b) A-(ii), B-(iii), C-(i), D-(iv)
(c) A-(iii), B-(i), C-(iv), D-(ii)
(d) A-(iv), B-(i), C-(ii), D-(iii)

2. Match the contraceptive methods given under column I with their examples given under column II and select the correct option form the given codes.

Column I	Column II
A. Chemical	(i) Tubectomy and vasectomy
B. IUDs	(ii) Copper T and loop
C. Barriers	(iii) Condom and cervical cap
D. Sterilisation	(iv) Spermicidal jelly and foam
	(v) Coitus interruptus and calendar method

(a) A-(iv), B-(ii), C-(iii), D-(i)
(b) A-(iv), B-(v), C-(ii), D-(iii)
(c) A-(i), B-(iii), C-(ii), D-(v)
(d) A-(iv), B-(ii), C-(v), D-(i)

3. Which of the following contraceptive method correcty matches with its mode of action?

Contraceptive method	Mode of aciton
(a) Tubectomy	Makes the uterus unsuitable for implantation
(b) Oral pills	Inhibit ovulation and implantation
(c) Diaphragms	Spermicidal and increases phagocytosis of sperms within the uterus
(d) IUDs	Blocks gamete transport

4. Match column I with column II and select the correct option from the given codes.

Column I	Column II
A. Natural methods	(i) Coitus interruptus
B. IUDs	(ii) LNG - 20
C. Barrier methods	(iii) Diaphragms
D. Surgical methods	(iv) Multiload 375
E. Oral contraceptives	(v) Saheli
	(vi) Nirodh
	(vii) Sterilisation
	(viii) Vasectomy
	(ix) CuT

(a) A-(i), B-(ii); (iv); (ix) C-(iii);(vi), D-(vii); (viii), E- (v)
(b) A-(i), B-(ii); (iv), C-(iii);(vi); (ix), D-(vii);(viii), E-(v)
(c) A-(i), B-(ii); (iv), C-(iii);(ix), D-(vii); (viii), E-(v); (vi)
(d) A-(i), B-(iv); (ix), C-(ii);(iii); (vi), D-(vii); (viii), E-(v)

5. Match column I with column II and select the correct option from the given codes.

Column I	Column II
A. Syphilis	(i) Huaman papilloma virus
B. Chancroid	(ii) *Haemophilus ducreyi*
C. AIDS	(iii) *Treponema pallidum*
D. Genital warts	(iv) HIV

	A	B	C	D
(a)	(iii)	(ii)	(iv)	(i)
(b)	(ii)	(i)	(iii)	(iv)
(c)	(iv)	(ii)	(i)	(iii)
(d)	(i)	(iv)	(iii)	(ii)

6. Which of the following approaches does not give the defined action of contraceptive?

(a) Hormonal contraceptives	Prevent/retard entry of sperms, prevent ovulation and fertilisation
(b) Vasectomy	Prevents spermatogenesis
(c) Barrier methods	Prevent fertilisation
(d) Intra uterine	Increase phagocytosis of sperms, suppress sperm motility and fertilising capacity of sperms

7. Match the following.

List I	List II
A. Contraceptive pill	(i) Prevents sperms reaching the female reproductive tract
B. Condom	(ii) Inhibits ovulation and implantation
C. Vasectomy	(iii) Increases phagocytosis of sperms
D. Copper T	(iv) Block gamete transport

(a) A-(iv), B-(i), C-(ii), D-(iii)
(b) A-(i), B-(ii), C-(iii), D-(iv)
(c) A-(ii), B-(i), C-(iii), D-(iv)
(d) A-(iv), B-(iii), C-(i), D-(ii)
(e) A-(ii), B-(i), C-(iv), D-(iii)

8. Given below are four methods (A-D) and their modes of action (i-iv) in achieving contraception. Select their correct matching from the four options that follow.

Method	Mode of action
A. The pilll	(i) Pevents sperms reaching cervix
B. Condom	(ii) Prevents implantation
C. Vasectomy	(iii) Prevents ovulation
D. Copper T	(iv) Semen contains no sperms

(a) A-(ii), B-(iii), C-(i), D-(iv)
(b) A-(iii), B-(i), C-(iv), D-(ii)
(c) A-(iii), B-(iv), C-(i), D-(ii)
(d) A-(iv), B-(i), C-(ii), D-(iii)

9. Match the contraceptive methods given under column I with their examples given under column II. Select the correct choice from those given below.

Column I	Column II
A. Chemical	q. Tubectomy and Vasectomy
B. IUDs	q. Copper T and Loop
C. Barriers	r. Condom and Cervical cap
D. Sterilisation	s. Spermicidal jelly and foam
	t. Coitus interruptus and calendar method

(a) A-s, B-q, C-r, D-p (b) A-s, B-t, C-q, D-r
(c) A-p, B-r, C-q, D-t (d) A-s, B-q, C-t, D-p

10. Match the following sexully transmitted diseases (column I) with their causative agent (column II) and select the correct option.

Column I	Column II
(a) Gonorrhoea	(i) HIV
(b) Syphilis	(ii) *Neisseria*
(c) Genital warts	(iii) *Treponema*
(d) AIDS	(iv) Human papilloma virus

	A	B	C	D		A	B	C	D
(a)	(iii)	(iv)	(i)	(ii)	(b)	(iv)	(ii)	(iii)	(i)
(c)	(iv)	(iii)	(ii)	(i)	(d)	(ii)	(iii)	(iv)	(i)

11. Match the following Columns.

Column I	Column II
A. IUD	1. Intra Uterine Device
B. Spermicids	2. In vitro fertilisation
C. Temperature method	3. Kills the sperms
D. IVF	4. Natural birth control method

Codes

	A	B	C	D		A	B	C	D
(a)	1	3	4	2	(b)	2	1	3	4
(c)	4	3	1	2	(d)	3	2	1	4

12. Match the following Columns.

Column I	Column II
A. Gonorrhoea	1. HSV -1 and SHV-2 viruses
B. Syphilis	2. HIV virus
C. Chlamydia	3. *Treponema pallidum*
D. IVF	4. *Neisseria gonorrhoeae*
E. Herpes	5. *Chlamydia trachomatis*

Codes

	A	B	C	D	E
(a)	4	3	2	1	5
(b)	4	3	5	2	1
(c)	3	5	1	2	4
(d)	1	2	4	3	5

13. Which of the following approaches does not give the defined aciton of contraceptive?

(a) Intrauterine devices	–	Incrrease phagocytosis of sperms suppress sperm motility and fertilising capacity of sperms
(b) Hormonal	–	Prevent/retard entry of sperms, prevent ovulation and fertilisation
(c) Vasectomy	–	Prevents spermatogenesis
(d) Barrier methods	–	Prevents fertilisation

14. Match the following Columns.

Column I	Column II
A. Syphilis	1. Human papilloma virus
B. Genital warts	2. HBV
C. Hepatits-B	3. *Treponema pallidum*
D. Gonorrhoea	4. HSV (Herpes Simplex Virus)
	5. *Neisseria*

Codes

	A	B	C	D
(a)	2	1	4	5
(b)	3	1	4	2
(c)	3	1	2	5
(d)	2	3	4	5

15. Match the following Columns I, II with III.

Column I	Column II	Column III
A. Trichomoniasis	1. *Herpes simplex*	(i) Pain in lower abdomen
B. Syphilis	2. *Neissieria gonorrhoeae*	(ii) Inflammation and itching in and around vagina
C. Gonorrhoea	3. *Treponema pallidum*	(iii) Patchy hair loss
D. Genital herpes	4. *Trichomonas vaginalis*	(iv) Feelling of uneasiness

Codes

	A	B	C	D
(a)	1-(iii)	2-(ii)	4-(iv)	3-(i)
(b)	4-(ii)	1-(iii)	2-(i)	3-(iv)
(c)	4-(i)	1-(iv)	2-(ii)	3-(iii)
(d)	4-(ii)	3-(iii)	2-(i)	1-(iv)

16. Given below are four methods (A-D) and their modes of action (I - IV) in achieving contraception.
Select their correct matching from the four options that follow :

Method	Mode of Action
A. The pill	I. Prevents sperms reaching cervix
B. Condom	II. prevents implantation
C. Vasectomy	III. prevents ovulation
D. Copper T	IV. Semen contains no sperms

(a) A – II; B – III; C – I; D – IV

(b) A – III; B – I; C – IV; D – II

(c) A – IV; B – I; C – II; D – III

(d) A – III; B – IV; C – I; D – II

17. Match the following and choose the correct option

Column I	Column II
A. Non-medicated IUDs	I. Lippes loop
B. Hormone releasing IUDs	II. Multiload 375
C. Copper releasing IUDs	III. CuT

IV. Cu7

V. LNG - 20

VI. Progestasert

(a) A – I; B– II,VI; C – III, IV, V

(b) A– I; B – V, VI; C – II, III, IV

(c) A – I; B – V, VI; C – I, III, IV

(d) A – II; B – I, VI; C – III, IV, V

18. Match the following and choose the correct option

Column-I	Column-II
A. Hepatitis B	I. Vitamin E
B. Saheli	II. 7'April, 1948
C. Normal functioning	III. CDRI, Lucknow of reproductive organs
D. World Health organisation	IV. Detection of antibody/antigen
E. ELISA technique	V. Hepatitis B virus

(a) A – V; B – III; C – I; D – II; E – IV

(b) A – V; B – II; C – I; D – III; E – IV

(c) A – V; B – III; C – IV; D – II; E – I

(d) A – V; B – II; C – IV; D – III; E – I

Solutions

1. **(c)** **2.** **(a)**

3. **(d)**

Tubectomy	–	Blocks gamete transport
Oral pills	–	Inhibit ovulaiton and implantation
Diaphragms	–	Prevent sperms from reaching an ovum
IUDs	–	Increase phagocytosis of sperms within the uterus

4. **(a)** **5.** **(a)** **6.** **(b)** **7.** **(e)** **8.** **(b)**

9. **(a)** **10.** **(d)** **11.** **(a)** **12.** **(b)** **13.** **(c)**

14. **(c)** **15.** **(d)** **16.** **(b)** **17.** **(b)** **18.** **(a)**

CHAPTER

Principles of Inheritance and Variation

1. Match the following and choose the correct option–

	Column-I		Column-II
A.	Linkage	I.	Recombination of genes
B.	Mutation	II.	More than two sets of chromosome
C.	Crossing over	III.	Morgan
D.	Polyploidy	IV.	Hugo de Vries

(a) A – II; B – III; C –I; D – IV
(b) A– III; B – IV; C–I; D – II
(c) A – II; B – IV; C – III; D –I
(d) A – II; B – IV; C –I; D – III

2. Match the following and choose the correct option –

	Column – A		Column – B
A.	ABO blood groups	I.	Dihybrid cross
B.	Law of segregation	II.	Monohybrid cross
C.	Law of Independent assortment	III.	Base pairs substitution
D.	Gene mutation	IV.	Multiple allelism

(a) A – II; B – I; C – IV; D – III
(b) A – IV; B – I; C – II; D – III
(c) A – IV; B – II; C – I; D – III
(d) A – II; B – III; C – IV; D – I

3. Match the terms in Column- I with their description in Column- II and choose the correct option

	Column- I		Column- II
A.	Dominance	I.	Many genes govern a single character
B.	Co-dominance	II.	In heterozygous only one allele expresses itself
C.	Pleiotropy	III.	In heterozygous organism both alleles express themselves
D.	Polygenic Inh.	IV.	Single gene influences many characters

(a) A–IV; B–III; C–I; D–II
(b) A–II; B–I; C–IV; D–III
(c) A–II; B–III; C–IV; D–I
(d) A–IV; B–I; C–II; D–III

4. Match the terms in column I with their description in column II and choose the correct option

	Column I		Column II
A.	Dominance	(i)	Many genes govern a single character
B.	Co- dominance	(ii)	In a heterozygous organism only one allele expresses itself

C. Pleiotropy	(iii) In a heterozygous organism both alleles express themselves fully
D. Polygenic inheritance	(iv) A single gene influences many characters

(a) A-(ii), B-(i), C-(iv), D-(iii)
(b) A-(iv), B-(iii), C-(iv), D-(iv)
(c) A-(iv), B-(i), C-(ii), D-(iii)
(d) A-(iv), B-(iii), C-(i), D-(ii)

5. Match the columns and find out the correct combination:

	Column I		Column II
A.	G.J Mendel	1.	Chromosomal theory of inheritance
B.	Sturtevant	2.	Discovered linkage in Drosophila
C.	T. H Morgan	3.	Prepared chromosome maps
D.	Sutton & Boveri	4.	Proposed laws of heredity

(a) A-4, B-3, C-2, D-1
(b) A-1, B-2, C-3, D-4
(c) A-2, B-3, C-4, D-1
(d) A-4, B-1, C-2, D-3

6. Match the columns and find out the correct combination:

	Column I		Column II
A.	Pod shape	1.	Wrinkled
B.	Pod colour	2.	Yellow
C.	Seed shape	3.	Constricted
D.	Seed colour	4.	Green
		5.	Grey

(a) A-4, B-5, C-2, D-1
(b) A-3, B-2, C-1, D-4
(c) A-2, B-3, C-1, D-4
(d) A-1, B-2, C-4, D-3

7. Match the following Column - I with Column -II.

	Column - I		Column - II
A.	Complementary ratio	I.	9 : 7
B.	Supplementary ratio	II.	9 : 3 : 4
C.	Epistatic ratio (Masking)	III.	12 : 3 :1
D.	Inhibitory ratio	IV.	13 : 3

(a) A – IV; B – I; C – III; D – II
(b) A – I; B – II; C – III; D – IV
(c) A – IV; B – I; C – II; D – III
(d) A – I; B – III; C – II; D – IV

8. Which one of the following pair is not correct?
(a) Mongolian idiocy - 21st chromosome
(b) Patau syndrome - 13th chromosome
(c) Cri-Du-Chat - 11th chromosome
(d) Edward syndrome - 18th chromosome

9. Select the correct match
(a) Phenylketonuria – Autosomal dominant trait
(b) Sickle cell anaemia – Autosomal recessive trait, chromosome-11
(c) Thalassemia – X linked
(d) Haemophilia – Y linked

10. Match the items of Column-I with Column-II :

	Column-I		Column-II
(A)	XX-XO method	(i)	Turner's syndrome of sex determination
(B)	XX-XY method	(ii)	Female heterogametic of sex determination
(C)	Karyotype-45	(iii)	Grasshopper
(D)	ZW-ZZ method of sex	(iv)	Female homogametic determination

Select the correct option from the following :
(a) (A)-(iv), (B)-(ii), (C)-(i), (D)-(iii)
(b) (A)-(ii), (B)-(iv), (C)-(i), (D)-(iii)
(c) (A)-(i), (B)-(iv), (C)-(ii), (D)-(iii)
(d) (A)-(iii), (B)-(iv), (C)-(i), (D)-(ii)

11. Which of the following is correct match?
(a) Down's syndrome — 21st chromosome
(b) Sickle cell anaemia — X-chromosome
(c) Haemophila — Y-chromosome
(d) Parkinson disease — X & Y chromosome

12. Match the column I with column II and select the correct option from the given codes.

	Column I	Column II
A.	Dihybrid test cross	(i) 9:3:3:1
B.	Law of segregation	(ii) Dihybrid cross
C.	Law of independent assortment	(iii) 1:1:1:1
D.	ABO blood group	(iv) Purity of gametes in man
		(v) Multiple allelism

(a) A-(iii), B-(iv), C-(ii), D-(v)
(b) A-(i), B-(iv), C-(ii), D-(v)
(c) A-(iii), B-(ii), C-(iv), D-(v)
(d) A-(ii), B-(v), C-(iii), D-(i)

13. Match the column I with column II and select the correct option from the given codes.

	Column I	Column II
A.	Multiple allelism	(i) Tt x tt
B.	Back cross	(ii) Tt x TT
C.	Test cross	(iii) Human blood groups
D.	Crossing over	(iv) Non-parental combination
E.	Recombination	(v) Non-sister chromatids

(a) A-(iii), B-(i), C-(ii), D-(v), E-(iv)
(b) A-(iii), B-(ii), C-(i), D-(v), E-(iv)
(c) A-(iii), B-(ii), C-(i), D-(iv), E-(v)
(d) A-(iv), B-(ii), C-(i), D-(v), E-(iii)

14. Match the column I with column II and select the correct option from the given codes.

	Column I	Column II
A.	Gregor J. Mendel	(i) Chromosomal theory of inheritance
B.	Sutton and Boveri	(ii) Laws of inheritance
C.	Henking	(iii) Drosophila
D.	Morgan	(iv) Discovered X-body

(a) A-(ii), B-(i), C-(iv), D-(iii)
(b) A-(iv), B-(i), C-(ii), D-(iii)
(c) A-(iv), B-(ii), C-(i), D-(iii)
(d) A-(ii), B-(iii), C-(iv), D-(i)

15. Match the column I with column II and select the correct option from the given codes.

	Column I	Column II
A.	Sickle cell anaemia	(i) 7th chromosome
B.	Phenylketonuria	(ii) 4th chromosome
C.	Cystic fibrosis	(iii) 11th Chromosome
D.	Huntington's disease	(iv) X-chromosome
E.	Colourblindness	(v) 12th chromosome

(a) A-(iii), B-(v), C-(ii), D-(i), E-(iv)
(b) A-(iii), B-(v), C-(i), D-(ii), E-(iv)
(c) A-(v), B-(iv), C-(ii), D-(iii), E-(i)
(d) A-(iv), B-(ii), C-(iii), D-(i), E-(v)

16. Match column I with column II and select the correct option from the given codes.

	Column I	Column II
A.	Autopolyploidy	(i) 2n+1
B.	Trisomy	(ii) AAAA
C.	Allopolyploidy	(iii) AABB
D.	Nullisomy	(iv) 2n-2

(a) A-(ii), B-(i), C-(iii), D-(iv)
(b) A-(iv), B-(i), C-(ii), D-(iii)
(c) A-(ii), B-(iv), C-(iii), D-(i)
(d) A-(ii), B-(i), C-(iv), D-(iii)

17. Match the column I with column II and select the correct option from the given codes.

	Column I	Column II
A.	Autosomal recessive trait	(i) Down'ssyndrome or mongolism
B.	Sex-linked recessive trait	(ii) Phenylketonuria
C.	Metabolic error linked to autosomal recessive trait	(iii) Haemophilia
D.	Additional 21st chromosome	(iv) Sickle cell anaemia

(a) A-(ii), B-(i), C-(iv), D-(iii)
(b) A-(iv), B-(i), C-(ii), D-(iii)
(c) A-(iv), B-(iii), C-(ii), D-(i)
(d) A-(iii), B-(iv), C-(i), D-(ii)

18. Which of the following is mismatched pair of disease and its related symptom?

	Disease	Symptom
(a)	Phenylketonuria	Urine turns black on exposure to air
(b)	Down's syndrome	Physical and mental retardation
(c)	Klinefelter's syndrome	Sterile males
(d)	Turner's syndrome	Sterile female

19. Find out the mismatch pair:
(a) Haemophilia - Sex linked recessive
(b) Cystic fibrosis - Autosomal recessive
(c) Down' s syndrome - Trisomy 21
(d) Turner's syndrome - Y-linked

20. Match the column I and column II and select the correct option from the given codes.

	Column I	Column II
A.	Chromosomal aberration	(i) An additional sex chromosome
B.	Down's syndrome	(ii) Inversion
C.	Klinefelter's syndrome	(iii) Presence of an extra chromosome
D.	Turner's syndrome	(iv) Absence of sex chromosome

(a) A-(ii), B-(iv), C-(i), D-(i)
(b) A-(ii), B-(iv), C-(iii), D-(i)
(c) A-(ii), B-(iii), C-(i), D-(iv)
(d) A-(iii), B-(iv), C-(i), D-(ii)

Solutions

1. (b) 2. (c) 3. (c) 4. (b) 5. (c)
6. (b)
7. (b) Epistasis is an interaction between two or more genes to control a single phenotype. Dominant epistasis has a ratio 12 : 3 : 1 in the F_2 phenotype. Supplementary genes or recessive epistasis has a ratio of 9 : 3 : 4.
8. (c) Cri-Du-Chat (Cat Cry) syndrome was first described by Lejeune n 1963 in France. The affected newborn cries-like meowing of a cat. This condition appears due to a deletion in the short arm of the chromosome number 5.
9. (b) Phenylketonuria is an inborn error of metabolism is also inherited as the autosomal recessive trait. Sickle cell anemia is an autosomes linked recessive trait that can be transmitted from parents to the offspring when both the partners are carrier for the gene (or heterozygous). Thalassemia is an inherited blood disorder that causes your body to have less hemoglobin than normal. Hemoglobin enables red blood cells to carry oxygen. Thalassemia can cause anemia, leaving you fatigued. Haemophilia is a sex linked recessive disease, which shows its transmission from unaffected carrier female to some of the male progeny.

10. (d) XX- XO type of sex determination is seen in crickets, grasshoppers, and some other insects. In all these organisms the female is XX and is the homogametic sex. The male is the heterogametic sex but only has one sex chromosome. The male in XX-XO systems produce gametes with (X) or without (O) a sex chromosome.

In XX -XY method of sex determination, the sex of an individual is determined by a pair of sex chromosomes. Females typically have two of the same kind of sex chromosome (XX), and are called the homogametic sex. Males typically have two different kinds of sex chromosomes (XY), and are called the heterogametic sex.

Turner's syndrome is also known as 45, X or 45, X,. It is a condition that affects only females, and results when one of the X chromosme (sex chromosomes) is missing or partially missing. ZW-ZZ method of sex determination can be seen in some birds, butterflies, moths, and other organisms. Instead of X and Y chromosomes, they have Z and W chromosomes. The female is the heterogametic sex. In all these organisms female has a pair of dissimilar ZW chromosomes and male has two similar ZZ chromosomes.

11. (c) 12. (a) 13. (b) 14. (a) 15. (b)
16. (a) 17. (c) 18. (a) 19. (d) 20. (c)

CHAPTER

Molecular Basis of Inheritance

1. Match the following and choose the correct option –

Column I	Column II
A. Helicase	(I) Joining of nucleotides
B. Gyrase	(II) Opening of DNA
C. Primase	(III) Unwinding of DNA
D. DNA polymerase III	(IV) RNA priming

(a) A – II; B – I; C – III: D – IV
(b) A – II; B – I; C – IV; D – III
(c) A – IV; B – III; C – I; D – II
(d) A – II; B – III; C – IV; D – I

2. Match the enzyme in column I with its function in column II and choose the correct option.

Column I	Column II
A. β-galactosidase	I. Joining of DNA fragments
B. Permease	II. Peptide bond formation
C. Ligase	III. Hydrolysis of lactose
D. Ribozyme	IV. Increases permeability to β-galactosidase

(a) A – II; B – I; C – IV; D – III
(b) A – III; B – II; C – I; D – IV
(c) A – II; B – IV; C – I; D – III
(d) A – I; B – II; C – IV; D – III

3. Match the following columns.

Column I	Column II
A. Topoisomerase	I. Relieves strain of unwinding by DNA helicase this is a specific type of topoisomerase
B. DNA gyrase	II. Relaxes the DNA from its super-coiled nature
C. DNA ligase	III. Provides a starting point of RNA or DNA for DNA polymerase to begin synthesis of the new DNA strand.
D. Primase	IV. Re-anneals the semi conservative strands and joins Okazaki fragments of the lagging strand.
E. Telomerase	V. Lengthens telomeric DNA by adding repetitive nucleotide sequences to the ends of eukaryotic chromosomes.

(a) A–I; B–II; C–V; D–IV; E–III
(b) A–I; B–II; C–III; D–V; E–IV
(c) A–V; B–IV; C–III; D–II; E–I
(d) A–II; B–I; C–IV; D–III; E–V

4. Match the following:

	Column I		Column II
A.	Lactose permease	I.	Z gene
B.	Galactoside-transacetylase	II.	Y gene
C.	Peptidyl transferase	III.	A gene
D.	β-Galactosidase		

(a) D-I, A-I, B-III (b) A-II, B-III, C-I
(c) A-II, B-I, D-III (d) A-III, B-II, C-I

5. Match the enzyme in column I with its function in column II and choose the correct option.

	Column I		Column II
A.	β-galactosidase	I.	Joining of DNA fragments
B.	Permease	II.	Peptide bond formation
C.	Ligase	III.	Hydrolysis of lactose
D.	Ribozyme	IV.	Increases permeability to β-galactosidase

(a) A – II; B – I; C – IV; D – III
(b) A – III; B – II; C – I; D – IV
(c) A – II; B – IV; C – I; D – III
(d) A – I; B – II; C – IV; D – III

6. Select the correct option.

	Direction of RNA synthesis	Direction of reading of the template strand
(a)	5′→3′	3′→5′
(b)	3′→5′	5′→3′
(c)	5′→3′	5′→3′
(d)	3′→5′	3′→5′

7. Match the codons given in column-I with their respective amino acids given in column-II and choose the correct answer.

	Column-I (Codons)		Column-II (Amino acids)
A.	UUU	I.	Serine
B.	GGG	II.	Methionine
C.	UCU	III.	Phenylalanine
D.	CCC	IV.	Glycine
E.	AUG	V.	Proline

(a) A – III; B – IV; C – I; D – V; E – II
(b) A – III; B – I; C – IV; D – V; E – II
(c) A – III; B – IV; C – V; D – I; E – II
(d) A – II; B – IV; C – I; D – V; E – III

8. Match column-I to the column-II and select the option having correct matching.

	Column-I		Column-II
A.	Bacteriophage nucleotides	(I)	5386
B.	*E.coli*	(II)	3.3×10^9 bp
C.	Human genome	(III)	4.6×10^6 bp
D.	$\phi \times 174$	(IV)	48502 bp

(a) A – (IV), B – (III), C – (II), D – (I)
(b) A – (III), B – (II), C – (I), D – (IV)
(c) A – (IV), B – (III), C – (I), D – (II)
(d) A – (IV), B – (I), C – (II), D – (III)

9. Select the correct match
(a) Alec Jeffreys - *Streptococcus pneumoniae*
(b) Alfred Hershey and Martha Chase - TMV
(c) Francois Jacob and Jacques Monod - *Lac* operon
(d) Matthew Meselson and F. Stahl - *Pisum sativum*

10. Match the following genes of the Lac operon with their respective products:

(A)	i gene	(i)	β-galactosidase
(B)	z gene	(ii)	Permease
(C)	a gene	(iii)	Repressor
(D)	y gene	(iv)	Transacetylase

Select the **correct** option.

	(A)	(B)	(C)	(D)
(a)	(i)	(iii)	(ii)	(iv)
(b)	(iii)	(i)	(ii)	(iv)
(c)	(iii)	(i)	(iv)	(ii)
(d)	(iii)	(iv)	(i)	(ii)

11. Select the correct option:

	Direction of RNA synthesis the template	Direction of reading of DNA strand
(a)	5′—3′	3′—5′
(b)	3′—5′	5′—3′
(c)	5′—3′	5′—3′
(d)	3′—5′	3′—5′

12. Study the following table to identify the correct combination.

	Type of nitrogen base	Group	Systemic chemical name
I.	Adenine	Pyrimidine	6 aminopurine
II.	Guanine	Purine	2-amino-6-oxypurine
III.	Cytosine	Purine	6 amino-2-oxypurine
IV	Thymine	Pyrimidine	5 methyle-2, 4-dioxypyrimidine

(a) II and IV (b) I and IV
(c) III and IV (d) I and IV

13. Match the following:

Column I	Column II
A. Fredrick Griffith	1. A sequence of three nucleotides codes for single amino acid
B. Gamow	2. Double helical structures
C. Watson and Crick	3. Induced mutation
D. Meselson and Stahl	4. Semiconservation replication of DNA
	5. Phenomenon of transformation.

(a) A-5, B-1, C-2, D-4
(b) A-1, B-5, C-4, D-2
(c) A-1, B-2, C-3, D-4
(d) A-5, B-1, C-4, D-2

14. Study the following table and choose the correct combination

	Scientist	Proved	By Using
I.	Hershey and Chase	Proved that DNA is the genetic material	Bacteriophage
II.	Watson and Crick	Double helix model for the structure of DNA	X-ray diffraction
III.	Avery, Macleod and McCarty	Genetic material through a protein	Virus
IV.	Griffith	Transformation in bacteria	*Streptococcus pneumonia*

(a) I and III only
(b) II, III and IV only
(c) I, II and IV only
(d) All of these

15. Match the column-I with column-II and select the correct answer:

Column-I	Column-II
(A) Replication	(i) RNA → DNA
(B) Transcription	(ii) mRNA→protein
(C) Translation	(iii) DNA → RNA
(D) Reverse transcription	(iv) DNA → DNA
(E) Ribosome	(v) mRNA + protein
	(vi) DNA + protein
	(vii) t-RNA
	(viii) r-RNA
	(ix) SnRNA + protein
	(x) rRNA + protein

(a) A-(i), B-(ii), C-(iii), D-(iv), E-(v)
(b) A-(ii), B-(i), C-(iii), D-(iv), E-(vi)
(c) A-(iii), B-(iv), C-(ii), D-(i), E-(vii)
(d) A-(iv), B-(iii), C-(ii), D-(i), E-(x)

16. Match the columns and find out the correct combination:

A.	Reverse transcription	1.	Protein
B.	At 5' end of polynucleotide chain	2.	Splicing
C.	Removal of introns and joining of exons	3.	Phosphate group is attached
D.	Exon helps in synthesis of	4.	Fatty acids
		5.	RNA dependent DNA polymerase

(a) A-5, B-1, C-2, D-3
(b) A-5, B-1, C-3, D-2
(c) A-1, B-2, C-3, D-4
(d) A-5, B-3, C-2, D-1

17. The given figure shows *lac* operon and its functioning. Select the option which correctly labels A, B, X, Y and Z.

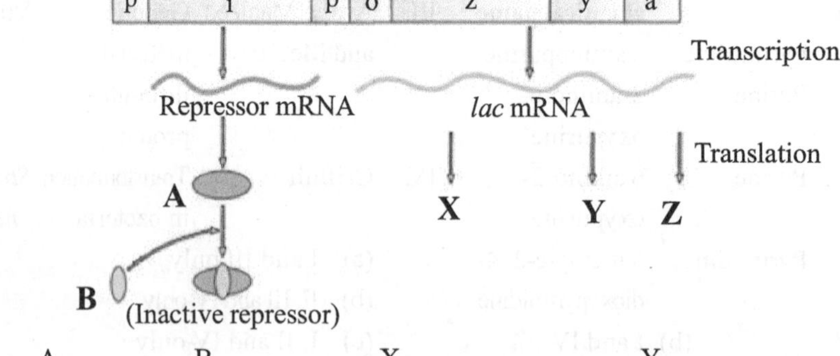

	A	B	X	Y	Z
(a)	Repressor	Inducer	Permease	Beta-galactosidase	Transacetylase
(b)	Inducer	Repressor	Beta-galactosidase	Permease	Transacetylase
(c)	Inducer	Repressor	Beta-galactosidase	Transacetylase	Permease
(d)	Repressor	Inducer	Beta-galactosidase	Permease	Transacetylase

18. Given diagram represent the components the components of a transcription unit. Select the correct answer regarding it.

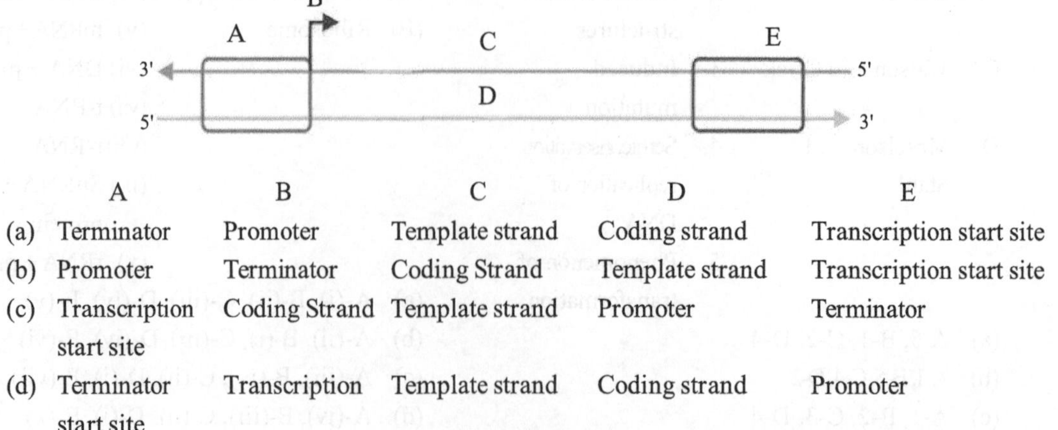

	A	B	C	D	E
(a)	Terminator	Promoter	Template strand	Coding strand	Transcription start site
(b)	Promoter	Terminator	Coding Strand	Template strand	Transcription start site
(c)	Transcription start site	Coding Strand	Template strand	Promoter	Terminator
(d)	Terminator	Transcription start site	Template strand	Coding strand	Promoter

19. Which of the following is/are correct matching(s)?

	Codon	**Amino acid**
(i)	5' AUG 3'	Serine
(ii)	5' AUC 3'	Tyrosine
(iii)	5' AUG 3'	Methionine
(iv)	5' GUG 3'	Valine

(a) (i) and (iii) (b) All of these
(c) (ii), (iii) and (iv) (d) (i), (ii) and (iii)

20. Match column-I with column-II and select the correct answer using the codes given below:

Column-I	**Column-I**
A. Operator site	I. Binding site for RNA polymerase
B. Promoter site	II. Binding site for repressor molecule
C. Structural gene	III. Codes for enzyme protein
D. Regulator gene	IV. Codes for repressor molecules

(a) A-II, B-I, C-III, D-IV
(b) A-II, B-I, C-IV, D-III
(c) A-IV, B-III, C-I, D-II
(d) A-II, B-III, C-I, D-IV

21. Identify the labels A, B, C and D in the given structure of tRNA and select the correct option.

	A	**B**	**C**	**D**
(a)	Anticodon loop	TψC loop	AA binding site	DHU loop
(b)	AA binding site	TψC loop	Anticodon loop	DHU
(c)	AA binding site	DHU loop	Anticodon loop	TψC loop
(d)	AA binding	DHU loop	TψC loop	Anti-codon loop

22. Match the enzymes given in column-I with its function given in column-II and select the correct option.

Column-I	**Column-II**
A. β-galactosidase	I. Joining of DNA fragments
B. Permease	II. Peptide bond formation
C. Ligase	III. Hydrolysis of lactose
D. Ribozyme	IV. Increase permeability of galactosidase

(a) A-II, B-I, C-IV, D-III
(b) A-III, B-IV, C-I, D-II
(c) A-II, B-IV, C-I, D-III
(d) A-I, B-II, C-IV, D-III

23. Match column-I with column-II and select the correct answer using the codes given below:

Column-I	**Column-II**
A. Helicase	I. Joining of nucleotides
B. Gyrase	II. Opening of DNA
C. Primase	III. Unwinding of DNA
D. DNA polymerase	IV. RNA priming

(a) A-II, B-I, C-III, D-IV
(b) A-II, B-I, C-IV, D-III
(c) A-IV, B-III, C-I, D-II
(d) A-II, B-III, C-IV, D-I

24. Match column-I with column-II and choose the correct option.

Column-I	**Column-II**
A. Exon	I. Coding sequence
B. Intron	II. Cistron
C. Genetic code	III. Triplet bases on mRNA

D.	DNA packaging	IV.	Nucleosome
		V.	Non-codding sequence

(a) A-I, B-III, C-II, D-V
(b) A-I, B-IV, C-II, D-III
(c) A-I, B-V, C-III, D-IV
(d) A-IV, B-I, C-V, D-III

25. Choose the sequence in which the following enzymes take part in DNA replication.
(i) Helicase
(ii) Primase
(iii) SSB
(iv) DNA polymerase
(v) DNA ligase
(a) (i) → (v) → (iv) → (iii) → (ii)
(b) (i) → (ii) → (iii) → (iv) → (v)
(c) (i) → (iii) → (ii) → (iv) → (v)
(d) (i) → (iv) → (iii) → (ii) → (v)

26. Match column-I with column-II and select the correct combination from the given options.

	Column-I		Column-II
A.	Sigma factor	I.	5'-3'
B.	Capping	II.	Initiation
C.	Tailing	III.	Termination
D.	Codding strand	IV.	5' end
		V.	3' end

(a) A-III, B-V, C-IV, D-II
(b) A-II, B-IV, C-V, D-I
(c) A-II, B-IV, C-V, D-III
(c) A-III, B-V, C-IV, D-I

27. Match column-I with column-II and select the correct answer using the codes given below.

	Column-I		Column-II
A.	Termination	I.	Aminoacyl tRNA synthetase
B.	Translation	II.	Okazaki fragments
C.	Transcription	III.	GTP dependent release factor
D.	DNA replication	IV.	RNA polymerase

(a) A-II, B-I, C-III, D-IV
(b) A-III, B-I, C-IV, D-II
(c) A-IV, B-III, C-I, D-II
(d) A-II, B-III, C-I, D-IV

Solutions

1. (d)
2. (b) β-gal is primarily responsible for the hydrolysis of the disaccharide lactose into its monomeric units, galactose and glucose. It is coded by Z structural gene.
3. (d) 4. (a)
5. (b) β-gal is primarily responsible for the hydrolysis of the disaccharide lactose into its monomeric units, galactose and glucose. It is coded by Z structural gene.
6. (a) Synthesis of RNA exhibits several features that are synonymous with DNA replication. RNA synthesis requires accurate and efficient initiation, elongation proceeds in the 5'→3' direction (i.e., the polymerase moves along the template strand of DNA in the 3'→5' direction), and RNA synthesis requires distinct and accurate termination. Transcription exhibits several features that are distinct from replication.
7. (a) UUU – Phenylalanine
   GGG – Glycine
   UCU – Serine
   CCC – Proline
   AUG – Methionine
8. (a)
9. (c) Francois Jacob and Jacque Monod proposed the model of gene regulation known as operon model/lac operon. Alec Jeffreys gave DNA fingerprinting technique. Matthew Meselson and F. Stahl gave semi-conservative DNA replication in E.coli. Alfred Hershey and Martha Chase proved DNA as genetic material not protein.
10. (c) Lac operon consist of one regulatory genes (*i* gene) and three structural genes (*z, y*, and *a)*.
    - *i* gene codes for Repressor.
    - *z* gene codes for Beta-galactosidase.
    - *y* gene codes for Permease.
    - *a* gene codes for Transacetylase.
11. (a) Synthesis of RNA exhibits several features that are synonymous with DNA replication. RNA synthesis requires accurate and efficient initiation, elongation proceeds in the 5'→3' direction (i.e. the polymerase moves along the template strand of DNA in the 3'→5' direction), and RNA synthesis requires distinct and accurate termination.
12. (a) 13. (a) 14. (d) 15. (d) 16. (d)
17. (d) 18. (d) 19. (c) 20. (a)
21. (b) tRNA or transfer RNA is a single stranded molecule and takes the shape of a clover leaf. In the process of transcription tRNA brings amino acid and reads the genetic code and acts as an adapter molecule. In the given structure of tRNA, the labels A, B, C and D are respectively AA binding site (amino acid binding site), TψC loop, anticodon loop (codon recognition site) and DHU loop (amino acid recognition site).
22. (b) 23. (d) 24. (c) 25. (c) 26. (b)
27. (c)

CHAPTER

Evolution

1. Match the following column I with column II

Column I	Column II
A. Darwin	I. Use and disuse theory
B. Lamarck	II. Origin of species
C. Hugo De Vries	III. Origin of life
D. A. I. Oparin	IV. Mutation theory

(a) A – I; B – II; C – III; D – IV
(b) A – II; B -A; C – III; D – IV
(c) A – IV; B – I; C – II; D – III
(d) A – II; B – I; C – IV; D – III

2. Match the following

Column-I	Column-II
A. Mesozoic	I. First land vertebrates
B. Devonian	II. Proliferation of reptiles
C. Palaeocene	III. Raise of modern mammals
D. Permian	IV. Radiation of primitive mammals
	V. 160 million years

(a) A–V; B–IV; C–III; D–II
(b) A–V; B–I; C–IV; D–II
(c) A–V; B–I; C–II; D–V
(d) A–V; B–I; C–IV; D–III

3. Match the following

Column-I	Column-II
A. Pliocene	I. *Sinanthropus pekinensis*
B. Richard leaky	II. *Australopithecus*
C. Mid pleistocene	III. *Homo neanderthalensis*
D. Dussel Dorf	IV. *Homo habilis*
E. Raymond Dart	V. *Oreopithecus*

(a) A–V; B – IV; C – I; D – III; E – II
(b) A– V; B – I; C – IV; D – III; E – II
(c) A– V; B – IV; C – I; D – II; E – III
(d) A– V; B – IV; C – III; D – I; E – II

4. Which one of the following pairs of items correctly belongs to the category of organs mentioned against it?

(a) Wings of honey bee and wings of crow - Homologous organs
(b) Thorn of *Bougainvillea* and tendrils of Cucurbita - Analogous organs
(c) Nictitating membrane and blind spot in human eye - Vestigial organs
(d) Nephridia of earthworm and malpighian tubules of Cockroach - Excretory organs

5. Which one of the following scientist's name is correctly matched with the theory put forth by him?

(a) Mendel – Theory of Pangenesis
(b) Weismann – Theory of continuity of Germplasm
(c) Pasteur – Inheritance of acquired characters
(d) de Vries – Natural selection

6. Which one of the following scientists name is correctly matched with the theory put forth by him?

(a) Weismann - Theory of continuity of germplasm

(b) Pasteur - Inheritance of acquired characters

(c) De Vries - Natural selection

(d) Mendel - Theory of Pangenesis

7. Match the columns

	Column-I		Column-II
A.	Hugo de Vries	1.	Inheritcance of acquired characters
B.	Julian Huxley	2.	Multiplication of individual species in geographical proportion
C.	Jean Baptiste	3.	Mutation theory of evolution

	A	B	C
(a)	1	2	3
(b)	2	3	1
(c)	3	1	2
(d)	3	2	1

8. Which one of the following options gives one correct example each of convergent evolution and divergent evolution?

	Convergent evolution	Divergent evolution
(a)	Eyes of octopus and mammals	Bones of forelimbs and vertebrates
(b)	Thorns of Bougainvillea and tendrils of Cucurbita	Wings of butterflies and birds
(c)	Bones of forelimbs of vertebrates	Wings of butterfly and birds
(d)	Thorns of Bougainvillea and tendrils of Cucurbita	Eyes of octopus and mammals

9. Identify the incorrectly matched pair:

(a) Ramapithecus — More man like ape like

(b) Homo habilis — First human like being, the hominid

(c) Homo erectus — Probably did not eat meat

(d) Neanderthal — Buried their dead

10. Match column-I with column-II and select the correct option.

	Column-I		Column-II
A.	Saltation	I.	Darwin
B.	Formation of life was preceded	II.	Louis Pasteur
C.	Reproductive fitness	III.	De Vries
D.	Life comes from pre-existing life	IV.	Oparin and haldance

(a) A-III, B-IV, C-I, D-II

(b) A-IV, B-III, C-II, D-I

(c) A-II, B-III, C-I, D-IV

(d) A-I, B-IV, C-III, D-II

11. Match the evolution concepts given in column-I with their description given in column-II and select the correct answer.

	Column-I		Column-II
A.	Mutation	I.	Change in populations allele frequencies due to chance alone.
B.	Gene flow	II.	Differences is survival and reproduction among variant individuals.
C.	Natural selection	III.	Immigration, emigration change allele frequencies.
D.	Genetic drift	IV.	Source of new alleles.

(a) A-I, B-II, C-III, D-IV

(b) A-IV, B-II, C-III, D-I

(c) A-III, B-I, C-IV, D-II

(d) A-IV, B-III, C-II, D-I

12. Match the column-I with column-II and select the correct option.

Column-I (Name of the Scientist)	Column-II (Contributions)
A. Charles Darwin	I. Mutation theory
B. Lamarck	II. Germ plasm theory
C. Hugo De Vries	III. Philosophie Zoologique
D. Ernst Haeckel	IV. The Origin of species
E. August Weismann	V. Biogenetic law
	VI. Essay on population

(a) A-IV, B-III, C-I, D-V, E-II
(b) A-IV, B-III, C-V, D-I, E-VI
(c) A-IV, B-VI, C-V, D-III, E-I
(d) A-II, B-III, C-I, D-V, E-II

13. Which one of the following scientists name is correctly matched with the theory put forth by him?
(a) Weismann - Theory of continuity of germplasm
(b) Pasteur - Inheritance of acquired characters
(c) De Vries - Natural selection
(d) Mendel - Theory of Pangenesis

14. Match the hominids with their **correct** brain size:

(A) *Homo habilis*	(i) 900 cc
(B) *Homo neanderthalensis*	(ii) 1350 cc
(C) *Homo erectus*	(iii) 650 - 800 cc
(D) *Homo sapiens*	(iv) 1400 cc

Select the **correct** option.

	(A)	(B)	(C)	(D)
(a)	(iii)	(i)	(iv)	(ii)
(b)	(iii)	(ii)	(i)	(iv)
(c)	(iii)	(iv)	(i)	(ii)
(d)	(iv)	(iii)	(i)	(ii)

15. Which one of the following scientists name is correctly matched with the theory put forth by him?
(a) Weismann - Theory of continuity of Germplasm
(b) Pasteur - Inheritance of acquired characters
(c) De Vries - Natural selection
(d) Mendel - Theory of Pangenesis

16. Identify the correct match from column-I and column-II

Column-I	Column-II
A. Origin of universe	1. 3 bya
B. Origin of Earth	2. 20 bya
C. Origin of first cellular form of life	3. 20 bya
D. Origin of first noncellular form of life	4. 2 bya

(a) A-1, B-2, C-3, D-4
(b) A-2,B-3,C-4,D-1
(c) A-2,B-4,C-3,D-1
(d) A-1,B-3,C-2,D-4

17. Which two periods are correctly matched with the dominance of organisms in that particular period?
(a) (A) Jurassic – Amphibians
(B) Carboniferous- Fishes
(b) (A) Jurassic – Amphibians
(B) Devonian – Amphibians
(c) (A) Devonian – Amphibians
(B) Jurassic –Dinosaurs
(d) (A) Devonian –fishes
(B) Jurassic – Dinosaurs

18. Match column I with column II and select the correct option from the codes given below.

	Column I	Column II
A.	Edward Lewis	(i) Australopithecus
B.	L.S.B Leakey	(ii) *Homo neanderthalensis*
C.	C. Fuhlrott	(iii) *Homo habilis*
D.	Raymond Dart	(iv) *Ramapithecus*

(a) A-(iv), B-(iii), C-(ii), D-(i)
(b) A-(ii), B-(i), C-(iv), D-(iii)
(c) A-(iii), B-(ii), C-(i), D-(iv)
(d) A-(i), B-(ii), C-(iii), D-(iv)

19. Match column I with column II and select the correct option from the given codes.

	Column I	Column II
A.	Wallace	(i) Essay of population
B.	Malthus	(ii) Biston
C.	Hardy-Weinberg law	(iii) $p^2+q^2+2pq=1$
D.	Industrial melanism	(iv) Co-proposer of Natural selection

(a) A-(iii), B-(iv), C-(ii), D-(i)
(b) A- (ii), B-(i), C-(iv), D-(iii)
(c) A-(iv), B-(i), C-(ii), D-(iii)
(d) A-(iv), B-(i), C-(iii), D-(ii)

20. Match column I with column II and select the correct option from the codes given below.

	Column I	Column II
A.	Francesco Redi	(i) Theory of chemical evolution of life
B.	L. Pasteur	(ii) Disproval of spontaneous generation
C.	Richter	(iii) Swan necked flask experiment
D.	Oparin	(iv) Mutation
		(v) Panspermia

(a) A- (v), B-(i), C-(iv), D-(ii)
(b) A-(ii), B-(iii), C-(v), D-(i)
(c) A-(v), B-(iv), C-(ii), D-(i)
(d) A-(i), B-(ii), C-(iii), D-(iv)

21. Match column I (containing list of scientists) with column II (their contributions) and choose the correct option.

	Column-I (Name of the Scientist)		Column-II (Contributions)
A.	Charles Darwin	I.	Mutation theory
B.	Lamarck	II.	Germ plasm theory
C.	Hugo de Vries	III.	Philosophie Zoologique
D.	Ernst Haeckel	IV.	The Origin of species
E.	August Weismann	V.	Biogenetic law
		VI.	Essay on population

(a) A – IV; B – III; C – I; D – V; E – II
(b) A – IV; B – III; C – V; D – I; E – VI
(c) A – IV; B – VI; C – V; D – III; E – I
(d) A – II; B – III; C – I; D – V; E – II

22. Following is the diagrammatic representation of the operation of natural selection of different traits. Which of the following options correctly identifies all the three graphs A, B and C?

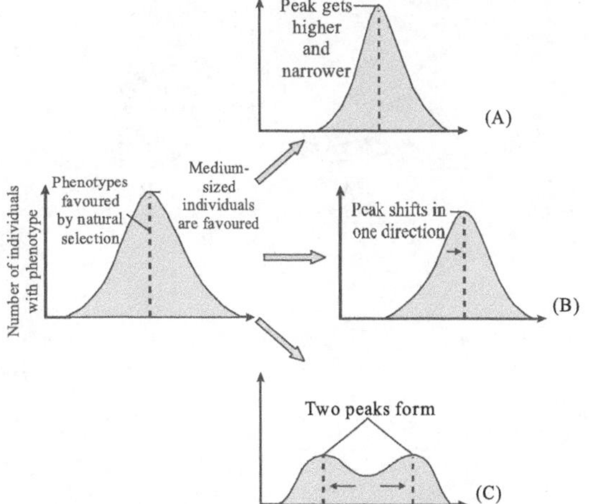

	A	B	C
(a)	Directional	Stabilizing	Disruptive
(b)	Stabilizing	Directional	Disruptive
(c)	Disruptive	Stabilizing	Directional
(d)	Directional	Disruptive	Stabilizing

23. Following is the diagrammatic representation of evolutionary history of vertebrates through geological periods. Identify the geological periods (A, B, C and D) and select the correct option.

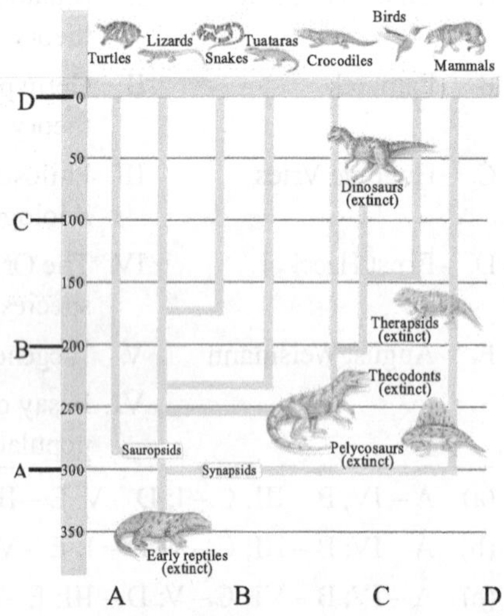

	A	B	C	D
(a)	Carboniferous	Triassic	Cretaceous	uaternary
(b)	Jurassic	Permian	Tertiary	retaceous
(c)	Permian	Jurassic	Quaternary	Tertiary
(d)	Cretaceous	Quaternary	Carboniferous	Jurassic

24. Identify the mammals from the diagrams of their respective skulls given below.

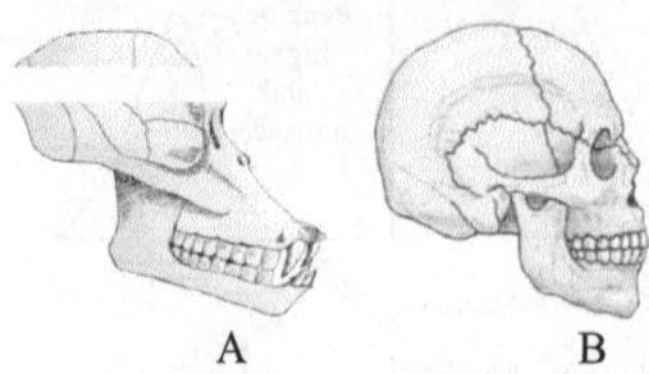

(a) Skull A : Human; Skull B : Old world monkey

(b) Skull A : Old world monkey; Skull B : Human

(c) Skull A : Ape; Skull B : Human

(d) Skull A : Human; Skull B : Ape

25. The diagram given below represents Miller's experiment. Choose the correct combination of labelling.

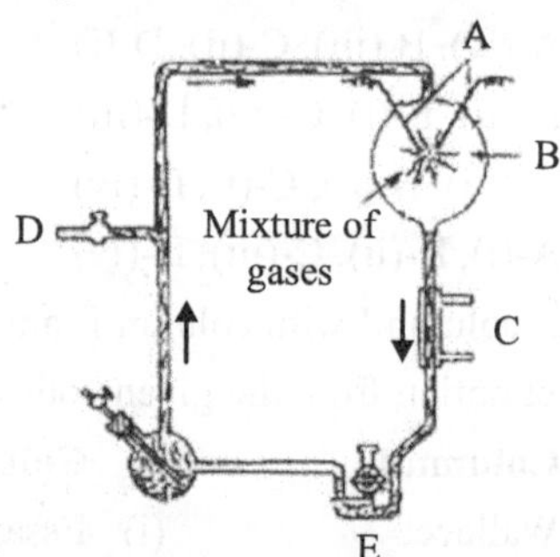

(a) A–electrodes, B– $NH_3 + H_2 + H_2O + CH_4$, C–cold water, D–vacuum, E–U trap

(b) A–electrodes, B–$NH_4 + H_2 + CO_2 + CH_3$, C–hot water, D–vacuum, E–U trap

(c) A–electrodes, B–$NH_3 + H_2O$, C–hot water, D–tap, E–U trap

(d) A–electrodes, B–$NH_3 + H_2 + H_2O + CH_4$, C–steam, D– vacuum, E–U trap

26. Match the name of scientists listed under column I with the ideas listed under column II.

Column I		Column II	
A.	Darwin	I.	Abiogenesis
B.	Oparin	II.	Use and disuse of organs
C.	Lamarck	III.	Continental drift theory
D.	Wagner	IV.	Evolution by natural selection

(a) A – I, B – IV, C – II, D – III

(b) A – IV, B – I, C – II, D – III

(c) A – II, B – IV, C – III, D – I

(d) A – IV, B – III, C – II, D – I

Solutions

1. (d) 2. (b) 3. (a) 4. (d) 5. (b)
6. (a) The theory of the continuity of the germplasm was published by August Weismann (1834-1914) in 1886. It proposes that the contents of the reproductive cells (sperms and ova) are passed on unchanged from one generation to the next, unaffected by any changes undergone by the rest of the body. It thus rules out any possibility of the inheritance of acquired characteristics, and has become fundamental to Neo-Darwinian theory.
7. (d) 8. (a) 9. (c) 10. (a) 11. (d)
12. (a)
13. (a) The theory of the continuity of the germplasm was published by August Weismann (1834-1914) in 1886. It proposes that the contents of the reproductive cells (sperms and ova) are passed on unchanged from one generation to the next, unaffected by any changes undergone by the rest of the body. It thus rules out any possibility of the inheritance of acquired characteristics, and has become fundamental to Neo-Darwinian theory.
14. (c) The correct match of the hominids and their brain sizes are:
Homo habilis – 650 - 800 c.c.
Homo neanderthalensis –1400 c.c.
Homo eractus –900 c.c.
Homo sapiens –1350 c.c.
15. (a) The theory of the continuity of the germplasm published by August Weismann (1834-1914) in 1886. It proposes that the contents of the reproductive cells (sperms and ova) are passed on unchanged from one generation to the next, unaffected by any changes undergone by the rest of the body. It thus rules out any possibility of the inheritance of acquired characteristics, and has become fundamental to Neo-Darwinian theory.
16. (b) 17. (d) 18. (a) 19. (d) 20. (b)
21. (a)
22. (b) The graph A, B and C shows stabilizing, directional and disruptive traits of natural selection. In stabilizing selection, the median phenotype is selected during natural selection and which does not tilt the bell curve in any way. Instead, it makes the peak of the bell curve even higher than what would be considered normal. Directional selection of natural selection derives its name from the shape of the approximate bell curve that is produced when all individuals' traits are plotted. Instead of the bell curve falling directly in the middle of the axes on which they are plotted, it tilts either to the left or the right by varying degrees. Hence, it has moved in one direction or the other. In disruptive selection instead of the bell curve having one peak in the middle, it has two peaks with a valley in the middle of them.
23. (a) In the given diagrammatic representation of the evolutionary history of vertebrates through geological periods, the geological periods marked as A, B, C and D are respectively carboniferous, triassic, cretaceous and quaternary. A geologic period is a sub-division of geologic time enabling cross-referencing of rocks and geologic events from place to place.
24. (c) The diagrams of two skulls of two different mammals show that skull A is of an ape and skull B is of human.
25. (a)
26. (b) Darwin is related with evolution by natural selection. According to the theory in the struggle for existence, the individuals which have more favourable variations will survive and reproduce, while others, which have less favourable or unfavourable variations will not puripetuate.
Oparin : Put forth abiogenesis theory.
According to abiogenesis : Life is originated from the non-living things spontaneously.
Lamarck : Use and disuse of organs is one of the important principle of Lamarckism.
Wagner : Proposed continental drift theory.

CHAPTER

Human Health & Disease

1. Match the column I with column II and choose the correct option:

	Column I		Column II
A.	IgE	(i)	Can cross placenta to provide passive immunity to the foetus
B.	IgM	(ii)	Provides passive immunity to the infant
C.	IgD	(iii)	Produced early in the primary immune response and Antigen receptor cells are present on B-cells
D.	IgA	(iv)	Activates B-cells
E.	IgG	(v)	Mediate immediate hypersensitivity reaction and also provide host defense against helminths infection.

	A	B	C	D	E
(a)	(v)	(iii)	(iv)	(ii)	(i)
(b)	(iii)	(iv)	(ii)	(i)	(v)
(c)	(v)	(iv)	(i)	(ii)	(iii)
(d)	(iv)	(v)	(iii)	(i)	(ii)
(e)	(i)	(iii)	(iv)	(v)	(ii)

2. Match the disease in column I with column II and choose the correct option:

	Column I		Column II
A.	Amoebiasis	(i)	*Treponema pallidum*
B.	Diphtheria	(ii)	use only clean and sterilized food as well as water
C.	Cholera	(iii)	DPT vaccine
D.	Syphilis	(iv)	Use oral dehydration therapy

	A	B	C	D
(a)	A-(ii)	B-(i)	C-(iii)	D-(iv)
(b)	A-(ii)	B-(iii)	C-(iv)	D-(i)
(c)	A-(i)	B-(ii)	C-(iii)	D-(iv)
(d)	A-(ii)	B-(iv)	C-(i)	D-(iii)

3. Choose the correct option about given above:

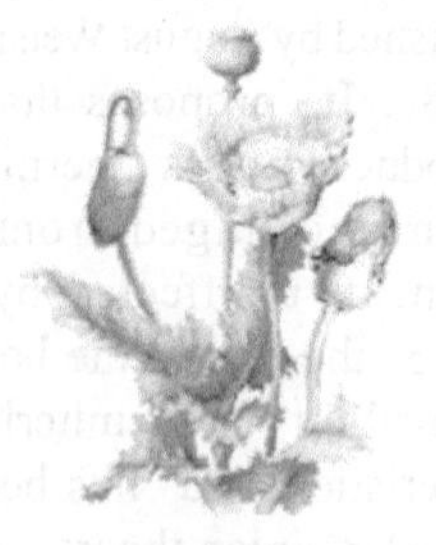

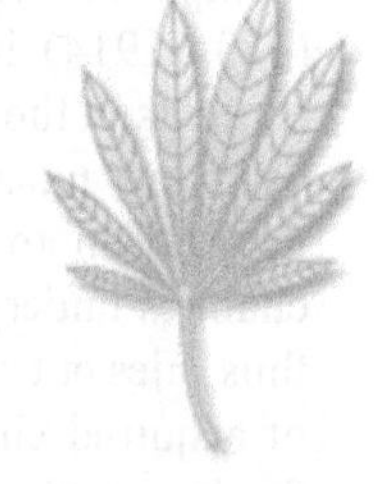

	(A)	(B)
(a)	Hallucinogen	Depressant
(b)	Morphine	Datura
(c)	Heroine	Bhang
(d)	Datura	Morphine

4. Match the column I with column II and select the correct option:

	Column I		Column II
A.	Charas	(i)	*Claviceps purpuria*
B.	Cocaine	(ii)	Euphoria
C.	L.S.D	(iii)	Stimulant
D.	Amphetamine	(iv)	*Cannabis sativa*

	A	B	C	D
(a)	(iv)	(ii)	(iii)	(i)
(b)	(iv)	(ii)	(i)	(iii)
(c)	(iv)	(i)	(ii)	(iii)
(d)	(iii)	(iv)	(iv)	(ii)

5. Match the column I with column II and choose the correct option:

	Column I		Column II
A.	Histamine	(i)	Organ transplant
B.	Attract phagocytes to antigen	(ii)	Autoimmune disease
C.	Immunosuppression	(iii)	AIDS
D.	Reduction in helper T-lymphocytes	(iv)	Active immunity
E.	Myasthenia gravis	(v)	Killer T-cells
F.	Infection or Vaccination	(vi)	Inflammatory responses

(a) A-(vi), B-(v), C-(i), D-(iii), E-(iv), F-(ii)
(b) A-(vi), B-(v), C-(i), D-(iii), E-(ii), F-(iv)
(c) A-(vi), B-(v), C-(iv), D-(iii), E-(ii), F-(i)
(d) A-(i), B-(ii), C-(iv), D-(iii), E-(vi), F-(v)

6. Match the column I with column II and select the correct option.

	Column I		Column II
A.	Saliva in mouth and acid in the stomach	(i)	Cytokine barriers
B.	Mucus coating of the epithelium lining of the repiratory tract	(ii)	Cellular barriers
C.	Polymorphonuclear leucocytes and natural killer cells	(iii)	Physiological barriers
D.	Interferons	(iv)	Physical barriers

	A	B	C	D
(a)	(iii)	(iv)	(ii)	(i)
(b)	(ii)	(iii)	(i)	(iv)
(c)	(iv)	(iii)	(ii)	(i)
(d)	(iii)	(ii)	(i)	(iv)

7. Match the column I (Disease) with column II (vaccine) and choose the correct option:

	Column I		Column II
A.	Tuberculosis	(i)	Harmless virus
B.	Whooping cough	(ii)	Inactivated toxin
C.	Diphtheria	(iii)	Killed bacteria
D.	Polio	(iv)	Harmless Bacteria

(a) A-(iv), B-(iii), C-(ii), D-(i)
(b) A-(i), B-(ii), C-(iv), D-(iii)
(c) A-(ii), B-(i), C-(iii), D-(iv)
(d) A-(iii), B-(ii), C-(iv), D-(i)

8. Which one of the following options gives the correct matching of a disease with its causative organism and mode of infection?

	Disease	Causative organisms	Mode of Infection
(a)	Elephantiasis	Wuchereria bancrofti	With infected water and food
(b)	Malaria	Plasmodium vivax	Bite of male Anopheles mosquito
(c)	Typhoid	Salmonella typhi	With inspired air
(d)	Pneumonia	Streptococcus pneumoniae	Droplet infection

9. Match the column I with column II and chose the correct option:

	Column I		Column II
A.	Pneumonia	1.	Rhino viruses
B.	Common cold	2.	Haemophillus influenza
C.	Filariasis	3.	Microsporum
D.	Ringworms	4.	Wuchereria bancrofti

	A	B	C	D
(a)	1	2	3	4
(b)	3	1	4	2
(c)	2	1	4	3
(d)	1	2	4	3

10. Match each item in Column I with one item in Column II and choose your answer from the codes given below:

	Column I (Type of secondary metabolite)		Column II (example)
I.	Alkaloid	1.	Abrin
II.	Toxin	2.	Morphine

III. Lectin 3. Vinblastin
IV. Drug 4. Concanavaline A

Codes

	I	II	III	IV
(a)	1	2	3	4
(b)	2	1	4	3
(c)	2	1	3	4
(d)	1	2	4	3

11. Match each item in Column I with one item in Column II and choose your answer from the codes given below:

Column I	Column II
I. Malaria	1. Sporozoan
II. Dysentary	2. Amoeboid
III. Sleeping sickness	3. Cilliate
IV. Balantidiasis	4. Flagellate

Codes

	I	II	III	IV
(a)	1	2	3	4
(b)	2	1	4	3
(c)	2	1	3	4
(d)	1	2	4	3

12. Match the following columns

Column I	Column II
A. Psychotropic drug	1. Cocaine
B. Sedative	2. LSD
C. Opiates	3. Barbiturates
D. Stimulants	4. Morphine
E. Hallucinogens	5. Pimozide

Codes

	A	B	C	D	E
(a)	5	3	4	1	2
(b)	5	2	1	4	3
(c)	2	5	4	1	2
(d)	4	3	4	2	1

13. Match the names of disease listed under column I with meanings given under column II, choose the answer which gives the correct combination of the alphabets of the columns.

Column I (Name of disease)	Column II (Meanings)
A. Jaundice	p. Allergic inflammation of nose
B. Stenosis	q. Loss of motor functions
C. Rhinitis	r. Heart vaive defect
D. Paralysis	s. Increase in bile pigments in the blood
	t. Septal defect of heart

(a) A-q; B-t; C-r; D-p
(b) A- s; B-p; C-q; D-r
(c) A-s; B-r; C-p; D-q
(d) A-s; B-t; c-p; D-q

14. Match the disease in Column I with the appropriate items (pathogen/prevention/treatment) in Column II.

Column I	Column II
1. Amoebiasis	(i) *Treponema pallidum*
2. Diphtheria	(ii) Use only sterilized food and water
3. Cholera	(iii) DPT Vaccine
4. Syphilis	(iv) Use oral rehydration therapy

(a) (1) - (i), (2) - (ii), (3) - (iii), (4) - (iv)
(b) (1) - (ii), (2) - (iv), (3) - (i), (4) - (iii)
(c) (1) - (ii), (2) - (i), (3) - (iii), (4) - (iv)
(d) (1) - (ii), (2) - (iii), (3) - (iv), (4) - (i)

15. Which one of the following sets of items in the options 1 - 4 are correctly categorized with one exception in it?

	Items	Category	Exception
(a)	UAA, UAG,UGA	Stop codons	UAG
(b)	Kangaroo, Koala, Wombat	Australian marsupials	Wombat
(c)	*Plasmodium*, Cuscuta, *Trypanosoma*	Protozoan parasites	Cuscuta
(d)	Typhoid, Pneumonia, Diphtheria	Bacterial diseases	Diphtheria

16. Identify the molecules (a) and (b) shown below and select the right option giving their source and use.

(a) 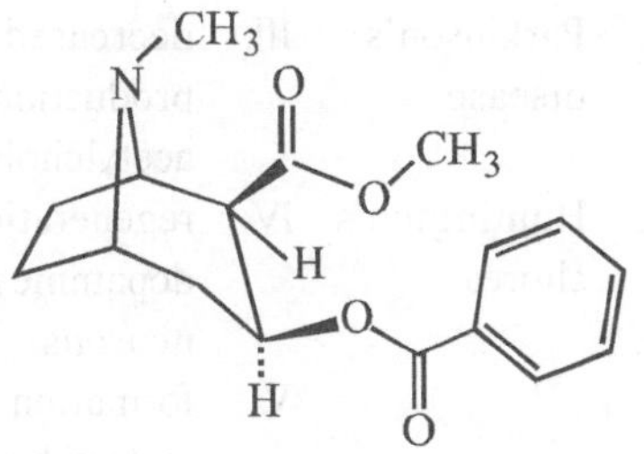 (b)

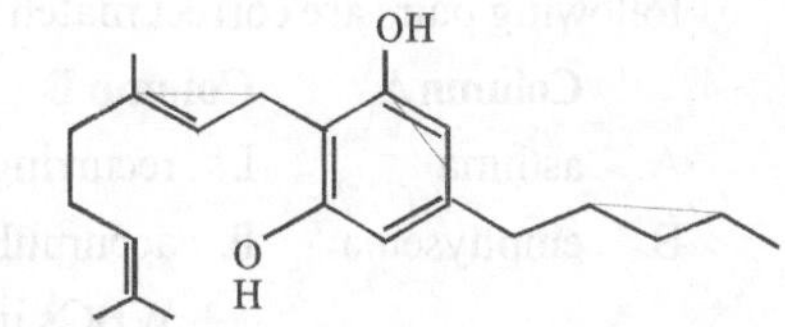

Options

	Molecule	Source	Use
(a)	Cocaine	*Erythroxylum coca*	Accelerates the transport of dopamine
(b)	Heroin	*Cannabis sativa*	"Depressant and slows down body functions"
(c)	Cannabinoid	*Atropabella dona*	Produces hallucinations
(d)	Morphine	*Papaver somniferum*	Sedative and pain killer

17. Match the following sexually transmitted diseases (Column –I) with their causative agents (Column- II) and select the correct option?

	Column- I		Column -II
A.	Gonorrhoea	I.	HIV
B.	Syphilis	II.	Neisseria
C.	Genital warts	III.	Treponema
D.	AIDS	IV.	Human papilloma virus

(a) A–II; B–III; C–IV; D–I
(b) A–III; B–IV; C–I; D–II
(c) A–IV; B–II; C–III; D–I
(d) A–IV; B–III; C–II; D–I

18. Match the following bacteria with the diseases

	Column-I		Column-II
A.	*Treponema pallidum*	I.	Plague
B.	*Yersinia pestis*	II.	Anthrax
C.	*Bacillus anthracis*	III.	Syphilis
D.	*Vibrio*	IV.	Cholera

(a) A – III; B – I; C – II; D – IV
(b) A – IV; B – I; C – II; D – III
(c) A – III; B – II; C – I; D – IV
(d) A – I; B – III; C – II; D – IV

19. Which one of the following is a correct match?

(1) Bhang – Analgesic
(2) Cocaine – Opiate narcotics
(3) Morphine – Hallucinogen
(4) Barbiturate – Tranquiliser

20. Match the following

	Set I		Set II
A.	LSD	I.	Euphorian effect
B.	Disulfiram	II.	Parasympathetic
C.	Cocaine	III.	*Cannabis*
D.	Scopolamine	IV.	Ergot alkaloid
E.	Hashish	V.	Antabuse

(a) A – IV; B – V; C – I; D – II; E – III
(b) A – IV; B – I; C – V; D – II; E – III
(c) A – IV; B – V; C – II; D – I; E – III
(d) A – V; B – IV; C– I; D – II; E – III

21. Column A represent diseases and column B represent their symptoms, which of the following pairs are correct match for them?

	Column A		Column B
A.	asthma	I.	recurring of bronchitis
B.	emphysema	II.	accumulation of WBCs in alveolus
C.	pneumonia	III.	allergy

(a) A – III; B – I; C – II
(b) A – II; B – I; C – III
(c) A – III; B – II; C – I
(d) A – II; B – III; C – I

22. Column I lists the components of body defence and column II lists the corresponding descriptions. Match the two columns. Choose the correct option from those given.

	Column I		Column II
A.	active natural immunity	I.	injection of gamma globulins
B.	first line of defence	II.	complement proteins and interferons
C.	Passive natural immunity	III.	direct contact with the pathogens that have entered inside
D.	second line of defence	IV.	surface barriers
		V.	antibodies transferred through the placenta

(a) A – IV; B – III; C – V; D – II
(b) A – III; B – IV; C – II; D – V
(c) A – III; B – IV; C – V; D – II
(d) A – V; B – III; C – II; D – I

23. Column I lists some disorders associated with brain. Column II lists the causes for these disorders. Match the two columns and identify the correct option from those given.

	Column I		Column II
A.	Epilepsy	I.	degeneration of neurons in the cerebral cortex
B.	Alzheimer's disease	II.	irregular electrical discharge in the neurons
C.	Parkinson's disease	III.	decreased production of acetylcholine
D.	Huntington's chorea	IV.	regeneration of dopamine releasing neurons
		V.	formation of blood clots in brain

(a) A – V; B – IV; C – III; D – I
(b) A – II; B – III; C – I; D – IV
(c) A – II; B – III; C – IV; D – I
(d) A – II; B – IV; C – III; D – I

24. Match the disease given in column I with the appropriate items (pathogen/ prevention/ treatment) given in column II.

	Column-I (Diseases)		Column-II (Pathogen/prevention/ treatment)
A.	Amoebiasis	I.	*Lassa virus*
B.	Diphtheria	II.	Use only sterilized food and water
C.	Cholera	III.	DPT vaccine
D.	Rabies	IV.	Use oral rehydration therapy

(a) A – II; B – III; C – IV; D – I
(b) A – I; B – II; C – III; D – IV
(c) A – II; B – IV; C – I; D – III
(d) A – II; B – I; C – III; D – IV

25. Which one of the following options gives the correct matching of a disease with its causative organism and mode of infection?

	Disease	Causative organisms	Mode of Infection
(a)	Elephantiasis	*Wuchereria bancrofti*	With infected water and food
(b)	Malaria	*Plasmodium vivax*	Bite of male *Anopheles* mosquito
(c)	Typhoid	*Salmonella typhi*	With inspired air
(d)	Pneumonia	*Streptococcus pneumoniae*	Droplet infection

26. Select the correct match of the symptoms of diseases given in column I with their respective pathogen of the diseases given in column II.

Column I	Column II
A. Appearance of dry, scaly lesions on various parts of the body such as skin nails and scalp.	I. *Entamoeba histolytica*
B. Chronic inflammation of the lymphatic vessel of lower limbs.	II. *Ascaris lumbricoides*
C. Fever, chills, cough, headache and in severe cases the lips and finger nails may turn gray to bluish in colour.	III. *Haemophilus influenzae*
D. Constipation, abdominal pain and cramps, stool with excess mucous and blood clots.	IV. *Wuchereria bancrofti*
E. Internal bleeding, muscular pain, fever, anaemia and blockage of intestinal passage.	V. *Microsporum*

(a) A – I; B – II; C – III; D – IV; E – V
(b) A – III; B – V; C – II; D – IV; E – I
(c) A – III; B – I; C – V; D – II; E – IV
(d) A – V; B – IV; C – III; D – I; E – II

27. Given figure shows the human lymphatic system with some part marked as A, B, C and D identify the correct part

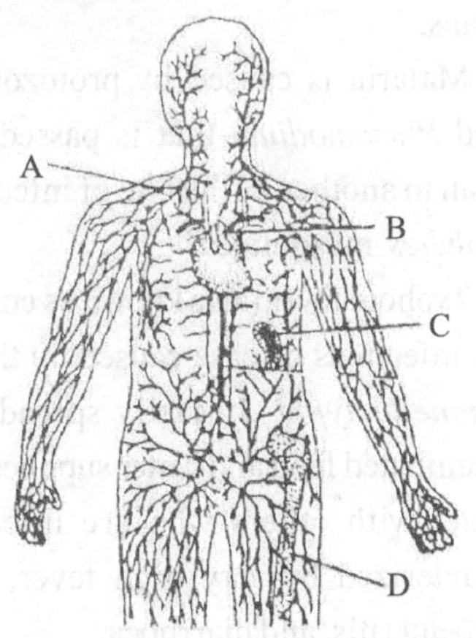

(a) A - lymph nodes (primary lymphoid organ), B - thymus (primary lymphoid organ), C - spleen (secondary lymphoid organ), D - bone marrow (secondary lymphoid organ)
(b) A - lymph nodes (primary lymphoid organ), B - thymus (secondary lymphoid organ), C - spleen (primary lymphoid organ), D - bone marrow (primary lymphoid organ)
(c) A - lymph nodes (secondary lymphoid organ), B - thymus (primary lymphoid organ), C-spleen (secondary lymphoid organ), D - bone marrow (primary. lymphoid organ)
(d) A- lymph nodes (primary lymphoid organ), B - thymus (secondary lymphoid organ), C - spleen (secondary lymphoid organ), D - bone marrow (secondary lymphoid organ)

28. The diagram given below shows an antibody molecule with their parts labelled as A, B, C, D, E & F. Identify the part marked as A, B, C, D, E and F.

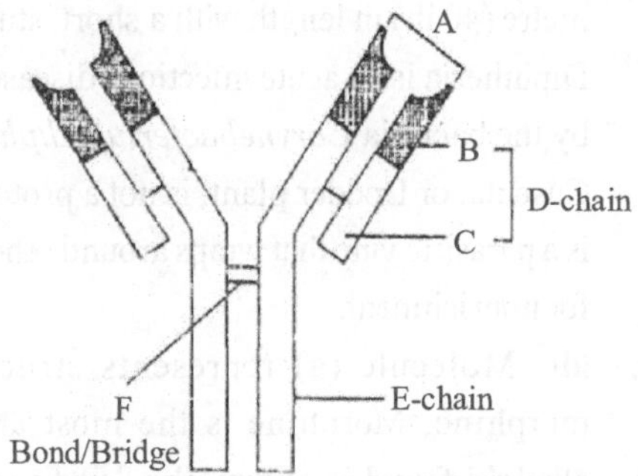

(a) A-Antigen binding site; B-Variable region (of L-Chain); C - Constant region (of L-Chain); D - Light polypeptide chain (L-Chain); E-Heavy polypeptide chain (H-Chain); F - Disulfide bond.
(b) A - Antigen binding site; B-Constant region (of L-Chain); C - Variable region (of L-Chain); D - Light polypeptide chain (L-Chain); E-Heavy polypeptide chain (H-Chain); F - Disulfide bond.

(c) A-Antigen binding site; B-Variable region (of L-Chain); C - Constant region (of L-Chain); D - Heavy polypeptide chain (L-Chain); E - Light polypeptide chain (H-Chain); F - Hydrogen bond

(d) A-Antigen binding site; B-Variable region (of L-Chain); C - Constant region (of L-Chain); D - Light polypeptide chain (L-Chain); E - Heavy polypeptide chain (H-Chain); F - Hydrogen bond

Solutions

1. **(a)** **2.** **(b)** **3.** **(c)** **4.** **(a)** **5.** **(b)**
6. **(a)** **7.** **(a)** **8.** **(d)** **9.** **(c)** **10.** **(b)**
11. **(d)** **12.** **(a)** **13.** **(c)**

14. **(d)**

Amoebiasis	:	Use only sterilized food and water
Diphtheria	:	DPT Vaccine
Cholera	:	Use oral rehydration therapy
Syphilis	:	*Treponema pallidum*

15. **(c)** UAG is also a stop codon. Wombats are also Australian marsupials. They are short-legged, muscular quadrupeds, approximately 1 metre (40 in) in length with a short, stubby tail. Diphtheria is an acute infectious disease caused by the bacteria *Corynebacterium diphtheriae*. Cuscuta, or Dodder plant, is not a protozoan. It is a parasitic vine that wraps around other plants for nourishment.

16. **(d)** Molecule (a) represents structure of morphine. Morphine is the most abundant alkaloid found in opium, the dried sap (latex) derived from shallowly slicing the unripe seedpods of the opium, or common and/or edible, poppy-*Papaver somniferum*. Morphine is a potent opiate analgesic drug that is used to relieve severe pain.

17. **(a)** **18.** **(a)** **19.** **(d)** **20.** **(a)** **21.** **(a)**
22. **(c)** **23.** **(c)**

24. **(a)** A : Amoebiasis refers to infection caused by *Entamoeba histolytica*. It may cause dysentery and invasive extra-intestinal disease.

B : Diphtheria is a bacterial (*Corynebacterium diphtheria*) infection and spreads through respiratory droplets (such as from a cough or sneeze) of an infected person or someone who carries the bacteria but has no symptoms.

C : Cholera is an infectious disease that causes severe watery diarrhea, which can lead to dehydration and even death if untreated. It is caused by eating food or drinking water contaminated with a bacterium called *Vibrio cholerae*.

D : Rabies is a viral illness spread via the saliva of an infected animal. It is caused by the rabies (lassa) virus which infects the brain and ultimately leads to death.

25. **(d)** (a) Elephantiasis is caused by *Wuchereria bancrofti* which is transmitted from human to human via the female mosquito when it takes a blood meal. The parasite grows into an adult worm that lives in the lymphatic system of humans.

(b) Malaria is caused by protozoan species called *Plasomodium* that is passed from one human to another by the bite of infected female *Anopheles* mosquitoes.

(c) Typhoid fever (also known as enteric fever) is an infectious disease caused by the bacteria *Salmonella typhi*. It easily spreads through contaminated food and water supplies and close contact with others who are infected. It is characterized by very high fever, sweating, gastroenteritis, and diarrhoea.

26. **(d)** A : Appearance of dry, scaly lesions on various parts of the body such as skin nails and scalp is the symptoms of ringworm disease caused by *Microsporum*. Ringworm is a fungal disorder.

B : Chronic inflammation of the lymphatic vessel of lower limbs is the symptoms of elephantiasis disorder which is caused by *Wuchereria bancrofti*.

C : Fever, chills, cough, headache and in severe cases the lips and finger nails may turn gray to bluish in colour are the symptoms of pneumonia. Pneumonia is caused by *Haemophilus influenzae* and *Streptococcus pneumonia*.

D : Constipation, abdominal pain and cramps, stool with excess mucous and blood clots are the symptoms of amoebiasis. Amoebiasis is caused by *Entamoeba histolytica*.

E : Internal bleeding, muscular pain, fever, anaemia and blockage of intestinal passage are the symptoms of ascariasis which is caused by common roundworm, *Ascaris lumbricoides*.

27. **(c)** Lymphatic system is the network of vessels through which lymph drains from the tissues into the blood. In the given figure of human lymphatic system, the parts marked as A, B, C and D are respectively lymph nodes (secondary lymphoid organ), thymus (primary lymphoid organ), spleen (secondary lymphoid organ), and bone marrow (primary lymphoid organ).

28. **(a)** In the given diagram of an antibody molecule, the part marked as A, B, C, D, E and F are respectively antigen binding site, variable regions (of L chain), constant region (of L chain), light polypeptide chain (L chain), heavy polypeptide chain (H chain) and disulfide bond.

CHAPTER

Strategies for Enhancement in Food Production

1. Match the column I with the column II and choose the correct option.

	Column I		Column II
A.	Sericulture	I.	Bee keeping
B.	Pisciculture	II.	Rearing of silkworm
C.	Apiculture	III.	Micropropagation
D.	Tissue culture	IV.	Rearing of fishes
E.	Green Revolution	V.	Fish production
F.	White Revolution	VI.	Crop production
G.	Blue Revolution	VII.	Milk production

(a) A - IV, B - III, C - II, D - I, E - VI, F - VII, G - V
(b) A - IV, B - I, C - II, D - III, E - VII, F - VI, G - V
(c) A - I, B - II, C - III, D - IV, E - VI, F - VII, G - V
(d) A - II, B - IV, C - I, D - III, E - VI, F - VII, G - V

2. Match the column I with column II and choose the correction option.

	Column I		Column II
A.	Many people have deficiencies as they cannot buy fruits & vegetables	I.	Single cell proteins
B.	Crops with higher vitamins, proteins and fats	II.	Micropropagation
C.	Growing microbes as the alternative source of proteins	III.	Somaclones
D.	Capacity to generate plant from a single cell or explant	IV.	Hidden hunger
E.	Production of thousand plants through tissue culture	V.	Biofortification
F.	Genetically identical plants	VI.	Totipotency

(a) A - IV; B - V; C - VI; D - I; E - II; F - III
(b) A - IV; B - V; C - VI; D - I; E - III; F - II
(c) A - IV; B - V; C - I; D - VI; E - II; F - III
(d) A - VI; B - V; C - I; D - IV; E - II; F - III

3. Which is correctly matched ?

(a) apiculture – honey bee
(b) pisciculture – silk moth
(c) sericulture – fish
(d) aquaculture – mosquito

4. Match the following columns and choose the correct option :

	Column-I		Column-II
A.	Mutation breeding	I.	Laborious and expensive process to obtain gene variation
B.	Selection	II.	Hybrid vigour can be maintained for several generations
C.	Hybridisation	III.	Simplest and easiest method of plant improvement
D.	Introduction	IV.	Oldest breeding method
		V.	Quick method to obtain gene variation

(a) A - V; B - IV; C - I; D - II

(b) A - V; B - IV; C - I; D - III

(c) A - IV; B - II; C - III; D - I

(d) A - I; B - II; C - IV; D - V

5. Consider the following two statements:

I. An effective germplasm collection is the prerequisite of any successful plant breeding program.

II. enetic variability is the root of any breeding program.

(a) Both I and II are true and II explains I

(b) Both I and II are true and II dose not explains I

(c) I is true but II is false

(d) I is false but II is true

6. Identify the option where all columns are not correctly matched:

	Crop	Variety	Resistant to diseases
(a)	Wheat	Himgiri	Leaf rust
(b)	*Brassica*	Pusa swarnim	White rust
(c)	Cowpea	Pusa komal	Black rot
(d)	Chilli	Pusa sadabahar	Leaf curl

7. Match each item in column I with one item in column II and chose your answer from the codes given below:

Column I	Column II
A. Pusa Swarnim	I. Cauliflower
B. Pusa Shubhra	II. Brassica
C. Pusa Koma	III. Okra
D. Pusa Sawami	IV. Cow pea

	A	B	C	D
(a)	I	II	III	IV
(b)	II	I	IV	III
(c)	II	I	III	IV
(d)	I	II	IV	III

8. Which one is the wrong pairing for the disease and its causal organism?

(a) Late blight of potato-Alternaria solani

(b) Black rust of wheat-Puccinia graminis

(c) Loose smut of wheat-Ustilago nuda

(d) Root-knot of vegetables-Meloidogyne sp.

9. In the following table identify the correct matching of the crop, its disease and the corresponding pathogen.

	Crop	Disease	Pathogen
(a)	Citrus	Canker	*Pseudomonas rubrilineans*
(b)	Potato	Late blight	*Fusarium udum*
(c)	Brinjal	Root-knot	*Meloidogyne incognita*
(d)	Pigeon pea	Seed gall	*Phytophthora infestans*

10. Which one of the following pairs is mismatched?

(a) Bombyx mori – silk

(b) Pila globosa – pearl

(c) Apis indica – honey

(d) Kenia lacca – lac

11. Which one of the following pairs is mismatched?

(a) Apis indica – honey

(b) Kenia lacca – lac

(c) Bombyx mori – silk

(d) Pila globosa – pearl

12. Match Column-I with Column-II.

Column-I	Column-II
(A) Saprophyte	(i) Symbiotic association of fungi with plant roots
(B) Parasite	(ii) Decomposition of dead organic materials
(C) Lichens	(iii) Living on living plants or animals

(D) Mycorrhiza	(iv)	Symbiotic association of algae and fungi

Choose the correct answer from the options given below:

	A	B	C	D
(a)	(i)	(ii)	(iii)	(iv)
(b)	(iii)	(ii)	(i)	(iv)
(c)	(ii)	(i)	(iii)	(iv)
(d)	(ii)	(iii)	(iv)	(i)

13. Which of the following is a correct match between crop, variety and resistance to diseases?

	Crop	Variety	Resistant to diseases
(a)	Wheat	Himgiri	White rust
(b)	*Brassica*	*Pusa sadabahar*	Black rot
(c)	Cowpea	*Pusa komal*	Bacterial blight
(d)	Chilli	*Pusa swarnim*	Chilly mosaic virus

14. Match column I with column II and select the correct option from given codes.

Column I	Column II
A. Brassica	I. Himgiri
B. Okra	II. Pusa Komal
C. Wheat	III. Pusa Gaurav
D. Cowpea	IV. Pusa Sawani

(a) A-III, B-IV, C-I, D-II
(b) A-I, B-III, C-II, D-IV
(c) A-IV, B-III, C-I, D-II
(d) A-II, B-IV, C-I, D-III

15. The process of protoplast isolation was primarily carried out by _________

(a) Henshel
(b) Bergman
(c) Klercher
(d) None of the above

16. Which statement is correct?

A. Somaclonal variations are the variations observed in plants generated from somatic cultures.

B. A transgenic crop is one that contains and expresses a transgene.

C. Chloromycetin is obtained from *Penicillium*.

D. Bioprospecting is the process of discovery and commercialization of new products basesd on biological resources.

(a) A, B, D
(b) B, C
(c) C, D
(d) A, B, C, D

17. Given flow chart represents different steps of MOET. Study the flow chart carefully and select the correct answer for (1), (2) and (3).

Cow is administered with (1) hormone

(2)

6-8 eggs per cycle are derived

Acritificially inseminated

Fertilised eggs at 8-32 cell stages are recovered

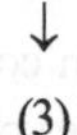

(3)

(a) 1-FSH, 2-Super ovulation due to induced follicular maturation, 3-Transfer to surrogate mother.
(b) 1-LH, 2-Super ovulation due to induced follicular maturation, 3-Transfer to surrogate mother.
(c) 1-Progesterone, 2-Super ovulation due to induced follicular maturation, 3-Transfer to surrogate mother.
(d) 1-FSH, 2-Transfer to surrogate mother, 3-Super ovulation due to induced follicular maturation.

18. Study the flow chart and answer the following given questions respectively:

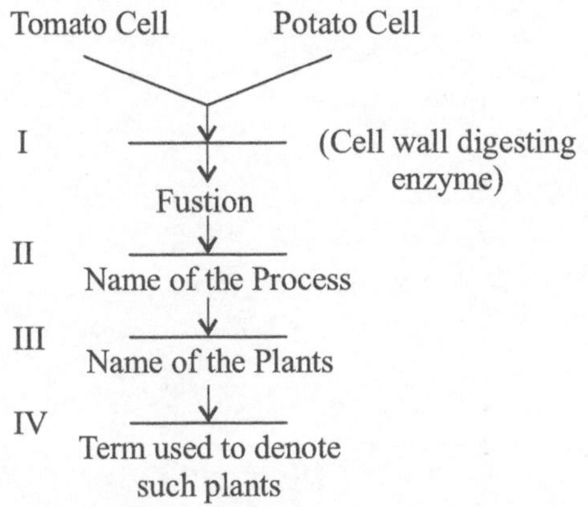

(a) I-Amylase, II-Protoplast fusion, III-Potato, IV-Somaclones

(b) I-Cellulase, II-Somatic hybridisation, III-Pomato, IV-Somatic hybrids.

(c) I-Amylase, II-Mristem culture, III-Pomato, IV-Somaclones.

(d) I-Polyethylene glycol, II-Somatic hybridisation, III-Pomato, IV-Somatic hybrids.

19. Find the wrong match.

(a) Wheat – Pusa Shubra

(b) Cauliflower – Pusa Snowball K-1

(c) Chilli – Pusa Sadabahar

(d) Brassica – Pusa Swarnim

20. Find the mis-match:

(a) Explant – Plant part used for tissue culture

(b) Somaclones – Variations produced during micropropagation

(c) Callus – Undifferentiated mass of cells

(d) Totipotency – Capacity to generate a whole plant from any cell

21. ______ is an instrument that helps to achieve specific temperature and pressure for scientific/ medical and industrial applications.

(a) Sterilizers (b) Autoclave

(c) Electrosurgical unit (d) None of the above

22. ______ is the result of an artificial hybridization between radishand cabbage

(a) Brassicaceae (b) Raphanobrassica

(c) Hirschfeldia incana (d) None of the above

Solutions

1. (a) 2. (c) 3. (a) 4. (b) 5. (a)
6. (c) 7. (b) 8. (a) 9. (c) 10. (b)
11. (d) 12. (d) 13. (c) 14. (a)
15. (c) 16. (a) 17. (a)
18. (b)

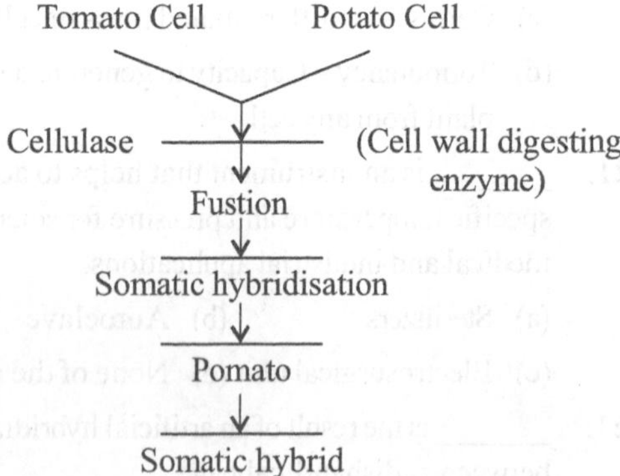

19. (a) 20. (b) 21. (b) 22. (b)

CHAPTER

Microbes in Human Welfare

1. Match different organisms in column I with their uses in coulmn II and select the correct answer from the given codes.

	Column-I		Column-II
A.	*Lactobacillus acidophilus*	(i)	Formation of dough
B.	*Saccharomyces cerevisiae*	(ii)	Single cell proteins
C.	*Propionibacterium sharmanii*	(iii)	Conversion of milk into curd
D.	*Spirulina*	(iv)	Formtion of Swiss cheese

(a) A-(iii), B-(i), C-(ii), D-(iv)
(b) A-(iii), B-(i), C-(iv), D-(ii)
(c) A-(i), B-(iii), C-(iv), D-(ii)
(d) A-(i), B-(iii), C-(ii), D-(iv)

2. Which of the following antibiotics is not correctly matched with the source from which it is obtained?

	Antibiotic	Source
(a)	Penicillin	*Penicillium chrysogenum*
(b)	Bacitracin	*Bacillus licheniformis*
(c)	Griseofulvin	*Penicullium griseofulvum*
(d)	Streptomycin	*Bacillus griseus*

3. Identify the blank spaces A, B, C and D in the following table and select the correct answer.

Type of microbe	Scientific name	Commercial product
Bacteium	A	Streptokinase
B	*Aspergillus niger*	Citric acid
Fungus	*Trichoderma polysporum*	C
Bacterium	D	Butyric acid

(a) A-*Streptococcus* B-Fungus C-Cyclosporin A D-*Clostridium butylicum*
(b) A-*Clostridium butylicum* B-*Streptococcus* C-Fungus D-Cyclosporin A
(c) A-*Streptococcus* B-Yeast C-Cyclosporin A D-*Lactobacillus*
(d) A-*Streptococcus* B-Cyclosporin A C-Statins D-*Clostridium butylicum*

4. A drug used for patient A is obtained from the organism B. Identify A and B in the above statement and select the correct answer.

	A	B
(a)	Swine flu	*Monascus purpureus*
(b)	AIDS	*Pseudomonas denitrificans*
(c)	Heart	*Penicillium chrysogenum*
(d)	Organ transplant	*Trichoderma polysporum*

5. Identify the blak spaces A, B, C and D in the table given below and select the correct answer.

Type of micorbe	Scientific name	Product	Medical application
Fungus	A	Cyclosporin A	B
C	*Monascus purpureus*	Stain	D

(a) A-*Trichoderma polysporum*, B-As an immunosuppressive agent, C-Yeast (Fungus), D-Lowering of blood cholesterol
(b) A-*Trichoderma polysporum*, B-Lowering of blood cholesterol, C-Yeast (Fungus), D-As and immunosuppressive agent
(c) A-Yeast (Fungus), B-Lowering of blood cholesterol, C-*Trichoderma polysporum*, D-As an immunosuppressive agent
(d) A-*Streptococcus*, B-As an immunosuppressive agent, C-Barterium, D-Lowering of blood cholesterol

6. Identify the blank spaces A, B, C and D in the following table and select the correct answer.

Type of microbe	Scientific name	Commercial product
Bacterium	A	Lactic acid
Fungus	B	Cyclosporin A
C	*Monascus purpureus*	Statins
Fungs	*Penicillium notalum*	D

(a) A-*Lactobacillus* B-*Trichoderma polysporum* C-Yeast D-Penicillin
(b) A-*Acetobacter* B-*Trichoderma polysporum* C-Yeast D-Streptomycin
(c) A-*Lactobacillus* B-*Aspergillus niger* C-Alge D-Penicillin
(d) A-*Lactobacillus* B-*Trichoderma polysporum* C-Agaricus D-Penicillin

7. Match column I with column II and select the correct answer from the given codes

Column-I	Column-II
A. The stage in which of physical tretment of sewage is done	(i) Anaerobic digestion activated sludge and production of biogas
B. The stage in which biological treatment of sewage is done	(ii) Activated sludge
C. Name of the sediment in primary treatment	(iii) Aeration tanks
D. It is carried ot aeration tanks from primary settling	(iv) Primary effluent
E. Name of the sediment in secondary treatment	(v) Primary sludge
F. Site of flocs growth	(vi) Secondary teatment
G Function of sludge digester	(vii) Primary treatment

(a) A-(vii), B-(vi), C-(v), D-(iv), E-(ii), F-(iii), G-(i)
(b) A-(i), B-(iii), C-(v), D-(vii), E-(ii), F-(iv), G-(vi)
(c) A-(i), B-(ii), C-(iii), D-(iv), E-(v), F-(vi), G-(vii)
(d) A-(vii), B-(vi), C-(i), D-(ii), E-(iii), F-(iv), G-(v)

8. Match column I with column II and select the correct answer from the given codes.

Column-I	Column-II
A. Methanogens	(i) BOD
B. Fermentors	(ii) Methane rich fuel gas
C. Organic waste in water	(iii) Production of methane
D. Biogas	(iv) Large vessels for growing microbes

(a) A-(ii), B-(iv), C-(iii), D-(i)
(b) A-(iv), B-(iii), C-(iv), D-(i)
(c) A-(ii), B-(i), C-(iv), D-(iii)
(d) A-(iii), B-(iv), C-(i), D-(ii)

9. Match column I with column II and select the correct option from the codes given below.

Column-I	Column-II
A. Statins	(i) Biogas
B. Dung	(ii) *Saccharomyces cerevisae*
C. Ethanol production	(iii) *Monascus purpureus*
D. Cyclosporin A	(iv) *Trichoderma polysporum*

(a) A-(iii), B-(i), C-(iv), D-(ii)
(b) A-(i), B-(iii), C-(iv), D-(ii)
(c) A-(iii), B-(ii), C-(iv), D-(i)
(d) A-(iii), B-(i), C-(ii), D-(iv)

10. Match clumn I with column II and select the correct answer from the given codes.

Column-I	Column-II
A. *Trichoderma*	(i) Free living nitorgen fixing bacteria
B. *Streptomyces*	(ii) Biocontroal agent
C. *Azospirillum*	(iii) Lactic acid
D. *Lactobacillus*	(iv) Source of antibiotic

(a) A-(ii), B-(iii), C-(iv), D-(i)
(b) A-(ii), B-(iv), C-(i), D-(iii)
(c) A-(iii), B-(i), C-(ii), D-(iv)
(d) A-(iv), B-(ii), C-(i), D-(iii)

11. Match column I with column II and select the correct answer form the given codes.

Column-I	**Column-II**
A. Mycrrhizae	(i) Azadirachtin
B. *Bacillus thuringiensis*	(ii) Phosphorus nutrition
C. Root nodules	(iii) Leghaemoglobin
D. Biopesticide	(iv) Bioinsecticide

(a) A-(iii), B-(i), C-(ii), D-(iv)
(b) A-(ii), B-(iii), C-(iv), D-(i)
(c) A-(ii), B-(iv), C-(iii), D-(i)
(d) A-(iii), B-(iv), C-(ii), D-(i)

12. Match column I with column II and select the correct answer from the given codes.

Column-I	**Column-II**
A. Ganga action plan	(i) N_2fixing cyanobacterium
B. Bt cotton	(ii) Ministry of environment and forests
C. *Rhizobium*	(iii) Insect resistant plant
D. *Nostoc*	(iv) N_2 fixing bacterium

(a) A-(ii), B-(iii), C-(iv), D-(i)
(b) A-(iii), B-(ii), C-(iv), D-(i)
(c) A-(ii), B-(iv), C-(iii), D-(i)
(d) A-(i), B-(iii), C-(ii), D-(iv)

13. Match column I with coulmn II and select the correct answer from the given codes.

Column-I	**Column-II**
A. *Azolla*	(i) Symbiotic N_2-fixer
B. Rotenone	(ii) Symbiotic association with N_2-fixing cyanobacteria
C. *Crotolaria*	(iii) Natural *juncea* insecticide
D. *Frankia*	(iv) Green manure

(a) A-(ii), B-(iii), C-(iv), D-(i)
(b) A-(ii), B-(iv), C-(iii), D-(i)
(c) A-(ii), B-(i), C-(iv), D-(iii)
(d) A-(i), B-(iii), C-(iv), D-(ii)

14. Match column I with column II and setect the correct option from the given codes.

Column-I	**Column-II**
A. Streptokinase	(i) *Trichoderma Polysporum*
B. Statins	(ii) *Streptococcus*
C. Cyclosporin A	(iii) *Monasus purpureus*
D. Penicillin	(iv) *Penicillium*

(a) A-(ii), B-(iii), C-(i), D-(iv)
(b) A-(i), B-(ii), C-(iii), D-(iv)
(c) A-(iv), B-(i), C-(iii), D-(ii)
(d) A-(iii), B-(ii), C-(i), D-(iv)

15. Match column I with column II and select the correct option using the codes given below.

Column-I	**Cloumn-II**
A. Citric acid	(i) *Trichoderma*
B. Cyclosporin A	(ii) *Clostridium*
C. Statins	(iii) *Aspergillus*
D. Butyric acid	(iv) *Monascus*

(a) A-(iii), B-(i), C-(ii), D-(iv)
(b) A-(iii), B-(i), C-(iv), D-(ii)
(c) A-(i), B-(iv), C-(ii), D-(iii)
(d) A-(iii), B-(iv), C-(i), D-(ii)

16. Match the following:

List-I	**List-II**
(i) Statins	A. *Propionibacterium shermanii*
(ii) Swiss cheese	B. *Steptococcus*
(iii) Cyclosporin A	C. *Aspergillus niger*
(iv) Citric acid	D. *Trichoderma polysporum*
(v) Clot buster	E. *Monascus purpureus*

(a) (i)-E, (ii)-A, (iii)-D, (iv)-C, (v)-B
(b) (i)-B, (ii)-A, (iii)-D, (iv)-E, (v)-C
(c) (i)-E, (ii)-A, (iii)-B, (iv)-C, (v)-D
(d) (i)-C, (ii)-E, (iii)-A, (iv)-D, (v)-B
(e) (i)-E, (ii)-C, (iii)-A, (iv)-D, (v)-B

17. Match the microbes in column I with their commercial/industrial products in column II and choose the correct answer.

	Column-I	Column-II
A.	*Aspergillus niger*	1. Ethanol
B.	*Clostridium butylicum*	2. Statins
C.	*Saccharomyces cerevisiae*	3. Citric acid
D.	*Trichoderma polysporum*	4. Butyric acid
E.	*Monascus purpuerus*	5. Cyclosporin A

18. Match the items in column I with those in column II and choose the correct answer.

	Column-I	Column-II
P.	Blue green algae as biofertilsers	i. Ectomycorrhiza
Q.	Fungi as biofertilsers	ii. *Thiobacillus* sp.
R.	Free living nitrogen fixing bacteria	iii. *Anabaena* sp.
S.	Phosphate solubilising bacteria	iv. *Clostridium* sp.
		v. *Azospirillum* sp.

(a) P-iii, Q-i, R-v, S-ii
(b) P-v, Q-i, R-ii, S-iv
(c) P-v, Q-iv, R-i, S-ii
(d) P-iv, Q-ii, R-v, S-i

19. Match the following columns.

	Column-I	Column-II
A.	*Plasmodium ovale*	1. Benign tertiary malaria
B.	*Plasmodium malariae*	2. Wild teriary malaria
C.	*Plasmodium vivax*	3. Malignant tertiary malaria
D.	*Plasmodium falciparum*	4. Quartan malaria

Codes:

	A	B	C	D		A	B	C	D
(a)	1	2	3	4	(b)	3	1	2	4
(c)	2	1	3	4	(d)	2	4	1	3

20. Match the following columus.

Column-I	Column-II
A. African sleeping sickness	1. *Sacculina*
B. Dumdum fever	2. *Haemophilus influenzae*
C. Pneumonia	3. *Leishmania donovani*
D. Parasitic castration	4. *Trypanosoma gambiense*
	5. *Leishmania tropica*

Codes:

	A	B	C	D		A	B	C	D
(a)	4	3	2	1	(b)	3	4	1	2
(c)	3	1	2	4	(d)	4	3	1	5

21. Match the following columns.

Column-I	Column-II
A. Filariasis	1. Amoebic dysentery
B. Amoebiasis	2. Whooping cough
C. Trypanosomiasis	3. Sleeping sickness
D. Pertusis	4. Elephantiasis

Codes:

	A	B	C	D		A	B	C	D
(a)	4	3	2	1	(b)	2	1	3	4
(c)	4	1	3	2	(d)	2	3	1	4

22. Match the following columns.

Column-I	Column-II
A. HIV infection	1. Widal test
B. Typhoid	2. Biopsy
C. Cancer	3. Tuberculin analysis
D. Tuberculosis	4. ELISA

Codes:

	A	B	C	D		A	B	C	D
(a)	1	3	4	2	(b)	3	2	4	1
(c)	4	1	2	3	(d)	2	4	3	1

23. Match the following columns.

Column-I	Column-II
A. *Glossina sp.*	1. Tse-tse fly
B. *Panstrangylus sp.*	2. Chagas disease
C. *Coxiella*	3. Q-fever
D. *Closteidum sp.*	4. Tetanospasmin

Codes:

	A	B	C	D		A	B	C	D
(a)	2	3	1	4	(b)	4	3	2	1
(c)	3	4	1	2	(d)	1	2	3	4

24. Watch each disease with its correct type of vaccine.

Column-I	Column-II
A. Tuberculosis	1. Harmless virus
B. Whooping cough	2. Inactivated toxin
C. Diphtheria	3. Killed bacteria
D. Pilio	4. Harmless bacteria

Codes:

	A	B	C	D		A	B	C	D
(a)	2	1	3	4	(b)	3	2	4	1
(c)	4	3	2	1	(d)	1	2	3	4

19. Match the microbes in column I with their commercial/industrial products in column II and choose the correct answer.

Column I	Column II
A. *Aspergillus niger*	I. Ethanol
B. *Clostridium butylicum*	II. Statins
C. *Saccharomyces cerevisiae*	III. Citric acid
D. *Trichoderma polysporum*	IV. Butyric acid
E. *Monascus purpureus*	V. Cyclosporin A

(a) A – IV; B – V; C – II; D – I; E – III
(b) A – V; B – IV; C – I; D – II; E – III
(c) A – III; B – IV; C – I; D – V; E – II
(d) A – III; B – IV; C – V; D – I; E – II

20. Match the following list of microbes and their importance:

A. *Sacharomyces* immunosuppressive agents	I. Production of *cerevisiae*
B. *Monascus Purpureus*	II. Ripening of Swiss cheese
C. *Trichoderma* ethanol	III. Commercial production of *polysporum*
D. *Propionibacterium sharmanii*	IV. Production of blood cholesterol lowering agents

(a) A – IV; B – III; C – II; D – I
(b) A – IV; B – II; C – I; D – III
(c) A – III; B – I; C – IV; D – II
(d) A – III; B – IV; C – I; D – II

21. Choose the right combination

Column-I	Column-II
A. *Escherichia coli*	I. Nif gene
B. *Rhizobium melilotae*	II. Digestive hydrocarbon of crude oil
C. *Bacillus thuringiensis*	III. Production of human insulin
D. *Pseudomonas putida*	IV. Biological control of fungal disease
	V. Bio-decomposed insectiside

(a) A – III; B – I; C – V; D – IV
(b) A – I; B – II; C – III; D – IV
(c) A – II; B – I; C – III; D – IV
(d) A – III; B – I; C – V; D – II

22. Match the items in Column 'I' and Column 'II' and choose correct answer.

Column-I	Column-II
A. Lady bird	I. *Methanobacterium*
B. Mycorrhiza	II. *Trichoderma*
C. Biological control	III. Aphids
D. Biogas	IV. *Glomus*

The correct answer is:
(a) A-II, B-IV, C-III, D-I
(b) A-III, B-IV, C-II, D-I
(c) A-IV, B-I, C-II, D-III
(d) A-III, B-II, C-I, D-IV

23. Match the column I and column II and choose the correct combination of alphabets of the two columns

Column-I Types of Bacteria	Column-II Activity
A. *Streptomyces*	I. Food poisoning
B. *Rhizobium*	II. Source antibiotics
C. *Nitrosomonas*	III. Nitrogen fixation
D. *Acetobacter*	IV. Nitrification
	V. Vinegar synthesis

(a) A-IV, B-V, C-I, D-III
(b) A-V, B-I, C-III, D-IV
(c) A-II, B-III, C-I, D-V
(d) A-II, B-III, C-IV, D-V

24. Match the following and choose the correct combination.

Column-I	Column-II
A. *Escherichia coli*	I. 'nif' gene
B. *Rhizobium meliloti*	II. Digests hydrocarbons of crude oil
C. *Bacillus thuringiensis*	III. Human insulin production
D. *Pseudomonas putida*	IV. Biocontrol of fungal disease
	V. Biodegradable insecticide.

(a) A-III, B-I, C-V, D-II
(b) A-III, B-I, C-V, D-IV
(c) A-I, B-II, C-III, D-IV
(d) A-II, B-I, C-III, D-IV

25. Match the column I and column II and find the correct option.

Column I	Column II
A. Dextran	I. Clarification of juices
B. Invertase	II. Used as clot buster
C. Streptokinase	III. Hydrolysis of sucrose
D. Protease	IV. Polymerization of simple sugar

(a) A – IV; B– III; C – II; D – I
(b) A– III; B– II; C– I; D– IV
(c) A– I; B– IV; C– III; D– II
(d) A– II; B– I; C – IV; D – III

Solutions

1. **(b)**
2. **(d)** Streptomycin is obtained from *Streptomyces griseus*. It is found useful in meningitis, pneumonia, tuberculosis and local infections.
3. **(a)**
4. **(d)** Cycolsporin A is a cyclic oligopeptide obtained through fermentative activity of fungs *Trichoderma polysporum*. It has anti-fungal, anti-inflammatory and immunosuppressive propeties. It inhibits activation of T-cells and therefore, prevents rejection reactions in organ transplantation.

5. **(a)** **6.** **(a)** **7.** **(a)** **8.** **(b)** **9.** **(d)**
10. **(b)** **11.** **(c)** **12.** **(a)** **13.** **(a)** **14.** **(a)**
15. **(b)** **16.** **(a)** **17.** **(c)** **18.** **(a)** **19.** **(c)**
20. **(d)** **21.** **(d)** **22.** **(b)** **23.** **(d)** **24.** **(c)**
19. **(c)** **20.** **(d)** **21.** **(d)** **22.** **(b)** **23.** **(d)**
24. **(a)** **25.** **(a)**

CHAPTER 33

Biotechnology: Principles and Processes

1. Select the correctly matched pair.
   (a) Cosmid – Cannot be used in human genome project
   (b) BAC – 300-350 kb of foreign DNA
   (c) YAC – Can clone fragments upto 45kb in length only
   (d) Phagemid – An RNA based cloning vector carrying an origin of relication derived from adenovirus.

2. Which of the following is correctly matched?
   (a) *Agrobacterium tumefaciens* – Tumour
   (b) *Thermus aquaticus* – Bt-gene
   (c) pBR322 – Enzyme
   (d) Ligase – Molecular scissors
   (e) *Hind* II – Plasmid vector

3. Match the tissue/molecules mentioned in column I with those of their degrading enzymes mentioned in column II and select the correct option from the given codes.

	Column I		Column II
A.	Cell wall	(i)	Proteases
B.	RNA	(ii)	Pectinases
C.	Histone	(iii)	Ribonucleases
D.	Pectin	(iv)	Cellulase

   (a) A-(iv), B-(iii), C-(i), D-(ii)
   (b) A-(ii), B-(i), C-(iv), D-(iii)
   (c) A-(i), B-(ii), C-(iii), D-(iv)
   (d) A-(iii), B-(iv), C-(ii), D-(i)

4. Match the items in column I with their uses in column II and choose the right option.

	Column I		Column II
A.	ELISA	(i)	Antigen-antibody interaction
B.	PCR	(ii)	Gene amplification
C.	Biolistics	(iii)	Direct introduction of recombinant DNA
D.	Micro-injection	(iv)	Gold coated DNA

   (a) A-(iii), B-(iv), C-(i), D-(ii)
   (b) A-(ii), B-(i), C-(iv), D-(iii)
   (c) A-(iv), B-(i), C-(ii), D-(iii)
   (d) A-(i), B-(iv), C-(ii), D-(iii)
   (e) A-(i), B-(ii), C-(iv), D-(iii)

5. Match the items in column I with their uses in column II and choose the right option.

	Column I		Column II
A.	*Bacillus thuringiensis*	(i)	Restriction endonuclease
B.	*Agrobacterium tumefaciens*	(ii)	Thermostable DNA polymerase
C.	*Thermus aquaticus*	(iii)	Insecticidal protein
D.	*Escherichia coli*	(iv)	Ti plasmid

   (a) A-(iii), B-(iv), C-(i), D-(ii)
   (b) A-(ii), B-(i), C-(iv), D-(iii)
   (c) A-(iv), B-(i), C-(ii), D-(iii)
   (d) A-(i), B-(iv), C-(ii), D-(iii)
   (e) A-(iii), B-(iv), C-(ii), D-(i)

6. Which of the following is not correctly matched for the organisms and its cell wall degrading enzyme?
   (a) Algae – Methylase
   (b) Fungi – Chitinase
   (c) Bacteria – Lysozyme
   (d) Plant cells – Cellulase

7. Match the entries in column I with those of column II and choose the correct answer.

	Column I		Column II
A.	Restriction endo-nucleases	(p)	Kohler and Milstein
B.	Polymerase chain reaction	(q)	Alec Jeffreys
C.	DNA fingerprinting	(r)	Arber
D.	Monoclonal antibodies	(s)	Karry Mullis

(a) A - (r), B - (s), C - (q), D - (p)
(b) A - (r), B - (q), C - (s), D - (p)
(c) A - (q), B - (r), C - (s), D - (p)
(d) A - (q), B - (s), C - (r), D - (q)

8. Match column I with column II with respect to the nomeclature of restiction enzyme *Eco*RI and select the correct answer from the given codes.

	Column I		Column II
A.	E	(i)	I^{st} in order of identification
B.	co	(ii)	Name of genus
C.	R	(iii)	Name of species
D.	I	(iv)	Name of strain

(a) A – (iii), B – (i), C – (ii), D – (iv)
(b) A – (ii), B – (i), C – (iii), D – (iv)
(c) A – (i), B – (ii), C – (iii), D – (iv)
(d) A – (ii), B – (iii), C – (iv), D – (i)

9. Match column I with column II and select the correct answer form the given codes.

	Column I		Column II
A.	amp^R gene	(i)	Artificial plasmid
B.	Separation of DNA	(ii)	Selectable marker fragments
C.	*Hind*III	(iii)	Electrophoresis
D.	pBR322	(iv)	***Haemophilus influenzae***

(a) A – (iii), B – (ii), C – (i), D – (iv)
(b) A – (iv), B – (i), C – (iii), D – (ii)
(c) A – (ii), B – (iii), C – (iv), D – (i)
(d) A – (ii), B – (iv), C – (i), D – (iii)

10. Match the terms given in column I with their definitions in column II and select the correct answer from codes given below.

	Column II		Ciolmn II
A.	Transformation	(i)	Sequences cut by restriction enzymes
B.	Recognition site	(ii)	process by which DNA fragments are separated based on their size
C.	Gel electrophoresis	(iii)	Plasmid DNA that has incorporated human DNA
D.	Recombinant DNA	(iv)	Process by which bacteria take up pieces of DNA from the envirment

(a) A – (iii), B – (i), C – (ii), D – (iv)
(b) A – (iv), B – (i), C – (ii), D – (iii)
(c) A – (i), B – (ii), C – (iii), D – (iv)
(d) A – (ii), B – (iii), C – (iv), D – (i)

11. Match column I with column II and select the correct answer from the given codes.

	Column II		Ciolmn II
A.	Recombinant DNA techonology	(i)	Chilled ethanol
B.	Precipitation of DNA	(ii)	DNA staining
C.	Trajnsposons	(iii)	Jumping genes
D.	Ethidium bromide	(iv)	Genetic engineering

(a) A – (iv), B – (i), C – (iii), D – (ii)
(b) A – (i), B – (iii), C – (ii), D – (iv)
(c) A – (ii), B – (i), C – (iii), D – (iv)
(d) A – (iv), B – (ii), C – (i), D – (iii)

12. Match column I (enzyme) with column II (characteristic/activity) and select the correct answer from the given codes.

	Column II		Ciolmn II
A.	Taq DNA polymerase	(i)	Cleaves the ends of linear DNA
B.	Exonuclease	(ii)	Breakdown of fungal cell wall
C.	Protease	(iii)	Stable above 90°C
D.	Chitinase	(iv)	Made only by eukaryotic cells
		(v)	Degradation of proteins

(a) A – (iii), B – (iv), C – (i), D – (ii)
(b) A – (iv), B – (iii), C – (i), D – (ii)
(c) A – (ii), B – (i), C – (v), D – (iii)
(d) A – (iii), B – (i), C – (v), D – (ii)

13. Given table given an account of differences between PCR and gene cloning. Which of the following points shows the incorrect difference?

	Parameter	PCR	Gene cloning
1.	Efficient	More	Less
2.	Apparatus Requirement	DNA	Restriction enzyme, ligase, vector, bacterial cell
3.	Manipulation	*in vitro*	*in vitro* and *in vivo*
4.	Cost	More	Less
5.	Automation	Yes	No
6.	Error probability	Less	More
7.	Time for a typical experiment	2-4 days	4 hours
8.	Application	More	Less

(a) 1 and 3 (b) 4, 5 and 6
(c) 4 and 7 (d) 4, 7 and 8

14. Match the scientists in column I with their related discoverise in column II and select the correct option from the given codes.

	Column II		Ciolmn II
A.	Kary Mullis	(i)	Father of genetic engineering
B.	Paul Berg	(ii)	Nobel prize for the discovery of restriction endonucleases
C.	Stanley Cohen and Herbert Boyer	(iii)	Developed polymerase chain reaction
D.	Arber, Smitjh and Nathan	(iv)	Isolated an antibiotic resistant gene from a plasmid of the bacterium *Salmonella typhimurium*

(a) A – (iii), B – (i), C – (iv), D – (ii)
(b) A – (iii), B – (iv), C – (i), D – (ii)
(c) A – (iv), B – (ii), C – (iii), D – (i)
(d) A – (i), B – (iii), C – (iv), D – (ii)

15. Which of the following is correctly matched?

(a) *Agrobacterium tumefaciens* – Tumour
(b) *Thermus aquaticus* – *Bt* gene
(c) pBR322 – Enzyme
(d) Ligase – Molecular scissors
(e) *Hind* II – Plasmid vector

16. Match the following Columns.

	Column I		Column II
A.	Bacterial enzymes used to cut DNA at defined sequences	1.	Recognition sequences
B.	Sequences cut by restriction enzymes	2.	Plasmids
C.	Ends left on DNA segments cut by DNA restriction enzymes	3.	Sticky ends
D.	Circular pieces of DNA found in bacteria	4.	Restriction enzymes

Codes

	A	B	C	D
(a)	1	4	3	2
(b)	4	1	3	2
(c)	1	4	2	3
(d)	4	3	2	1

17. Match the following Columns.

	Column I		Column II
A.	Bacterial viruses	1.	Transformation
B.	Process by which bacteria take up pieces of DNA from the environment	2.	Cloning vector
C.	*Hind* II	3.	*Haemophyllus influenzae*
D.	vehicle that move DNA from one organism to another	4.	Bacteriophges

Codes

	A	B	C	D
(a)	2	3	4	1
(b)	1	3	4	2
(c)	4	1	3	2
(d)	1	4	3	2

18. Match the following Columns.

	Column I		Column II
A.	A molecule used to carry foreign into bacteria	1.	Restriction enzymes
B.	A rapid way to amplify DNA in the laboratory	2.	Recombinant DNA
C.	A way to separate DNA fragments based on their size	3.	PCR
D.	Molecular scissors	4.	Vector
E.	A gene sequence from more than one origin	5.	Gel electrophoresis

Codes

	A	B	C	D	E
(a)	4	3	5	1	2
(b)	2	4	3	1	5
(c)	5	4	3	2	1
(d)	1	5	4	2	3

19. Identify the correct match for the given apparatus.

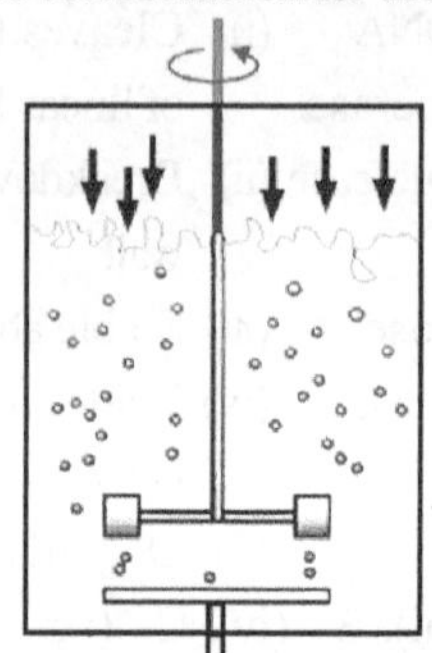

	Apparatus	Function
(a)	Gene gun	Vectorless direct gene transfer
(b)	Column chromatography	Separation of chlorophyll pigments
(c)	Sparged tank bioreactor	Carry out fermentation process
(d)	Respirometer	Finding out rate of respiration

20. Choose the correct option.

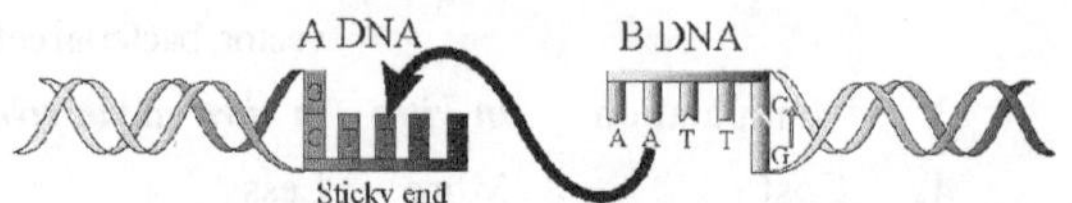

	A DNA	B DNA	Enzyme recognizing palindrome	Enzyme joining the sticky ends
(a)	Vector	Foreign	DNA ligase	EcoRI
(b)	Vector	Foreign	EcoRI	DNA ligase
(c)	Vector	Foreign	Exonuclease	DNA ligase
(d)	Vector	Foreign	DNA ligase	Exonuclease

21. Identify the correct match for the given figure.

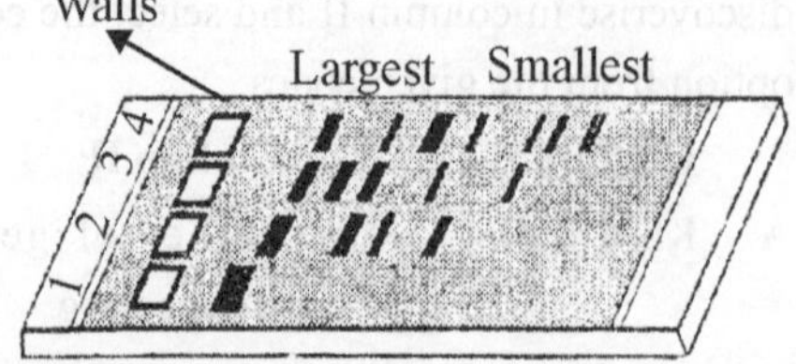

(a)	Electrophoresis	Differential migration of DNA fragments.
(b)	Column chromatography	Separation of chlorophyll pigments.
(c)	Gene cloning	Technique of obtaining identical copies of a particular DNA segment or a gene.
(d)	Microinjection	Technique of introducing foreign genes into a host cell.

22. Identify the correct option.

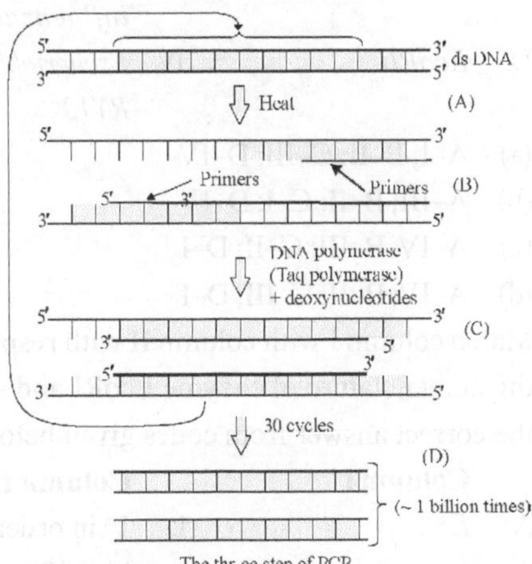

The thr ee step of PCR

(a) A-Denaturation, B-Annealing, C-Extension, D-Amplified
(b) A-Annealing, B-Denaturation, C-Extension, D-Amplified
(c) A-Denaturation, B-Annealing, C-Amplified, D-Extension
(d) A-Annealing, B-Denaturation, C-Amplified, D-Extension

23. Match the following columns.

	Column I		Column II
A.	Plasmids	I.	Virus infecting bacteria
B.	Bacteriophages	II.	Natural polymer of D-galactose
C.	Cosmids	III.	Hybrid vector derived from plasmids
D.	Agarose	IV.	Circular extrachromosomal DNA

(a) A–II; B–I; C–III; D–IV
(b) A–IV; B–I; C–III; D–II
(c) A–III; B–II; C–I; D–IV
(d) A–I; B–IV; C–III; D–II

24. Match the following columns.

	Column I		Column II
A.	Arber, Nathan and Hamilton Smith	I.	Isolated first restriction endonuclease from bacteria
B.	Paul Berg	II.	Term biotechnology
C.	Herbert Boyer and Stanley Cohen	III.	Father of genetic engineering
D.	Karl Erkey	IV.	First recombinant DNA

(a) A–I; B–IV; C–III; D–II
(b) A–III; B–II; C–I; D–IV
(c) A–I; B–III; C–IV; D–II
(d) A–IV; B–III; C–I; D–II

25. Which of the following is correctly matched?

(a) *Agrobacterium tumefaciens* - tumour
(b) *Thermus aquaticus* - Bt-gene
(c) pBR322 - enzyme
(d) Ligase - molecular scissors

26. Which one of the following option is correct for A, B, C and D?

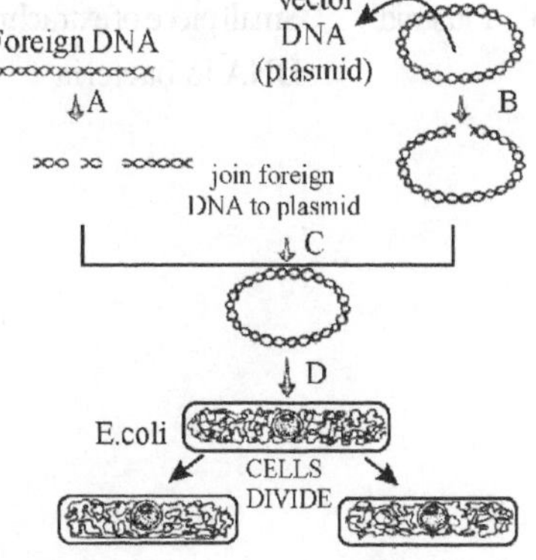

	A	B	C	D
(a)	Exonuclease	Endonuclease	DNA	Transformation ligase
(b)	Exonuclease	Exonuclease	DNA	Transformation ligase
(c)	Exonuclease	Endonuclease	Hydro- lase	Transduction
(d)	Restriction endonuclease	Restriction endonuclease	DNA ligase	Transformation

27. Which of the following pairs are correctly matched?
(a) Central dogma — Codon
(b) Okazaki fragments — Splicing
(c) RNA polymerase — RNA primer
(d) Restriction enzyme — Genetic engineering

28. Match List I with List II and select the correct option

List I	List II
A. *Bacillus thuringiensis*	I. Production of chitinases
B. *Rhizobium meliloti*	II. Scavenging of oil spills
C. *Escherichia coli*	III. Incorporation of '*nif*' gene
D. *Pseudomonas putida*	IV. Production of *Bt* toxin
E. *Trichoderma*	V. Production of human insulin

(a) A – II; B – IV; C – I; D – V; E – III
(b) A – II; B – IV; C – V; D – I; E – III
(c) A – IV; B – III; C – V; D – II; E – I
(d) A – III; B – IV; C – V; D – I; E – II

29. Which one of the following pairs is not correctly matched?

(a)	Plasmid	Small piece of extrachromosomal DNA in bacteria
(b)	Interferon	An enzyme that interferes with DNA replication
(c)	Cosmid	A vector for carrying large DNA fragments into host cells
(d)	Myeloma	Antibody-producing tumour cells

30. Match the following columns.

Column I	Column II
A. *Eco RI*	I. *E. Coli R 245*
B. *Hind III*	II. *Bacillus amyloliquefaciens*
C. *BamHi*	III. *Haemophilus influenzae*
D. *EcoRII*	IV. *Escherichia coli RY13*

(a) A–I; B–II; C–III; D–IV
(b) A–III; B–II; C–I; D–IV
(c) A–IV; B–III; C–II; D–I
(d) A–IV; B–II; C–III; D–I

31. Match column I with column II with respect to the nomenclature of enzyme EcoRI and select the correct answer from codes given below.

Column I	Column II
A. *E*	I. 1st in order of identification
B. *co*	II. Name of genus
C. R	III. Name of species
D. I	IV. Name of strain

(a) A–III; B–IV; C–I; D–II
(b) A–II; B–III; C–IV; D–I
(c) A–II; B–I; C–IV; D–III
(d) A–II; B–III; C–I; D–IV

Solutions

1. **(b)** Bacterial artificial chromosome (BAC) vectors are based on natural, extra-chromosomal plasmid of *E.coli*. These vectors can accommodate upto 300-350 kb of foreign DNA and are also being used in genome sequencing project.
2. **(a)** Ti plasmid (tumour inducing) from the soil bacterium *Agrobacterium tumefaciens* is effectively used as vector for gene transfer to plant cells. The part of Ti plasmid transferred into plant cell DNA, is called the T-DNA. This T-DNA with desired DNA spliced into it, is inserted into the chromosome of the host plant where it produces copies of itself, by migrating from one chromosomal position to another at random.
3. **(a)** 4. **(e)** 5. **(e)**
6. **(a)** Cell wall of algae is made up of cellulaose, pectin and mucilage. These substances cannot be degraded by methylase. Methylase is a type of transferase enzyme that transfers a methyl group from a donor to a acceptor.
7. **(a)** 8. **(d)** 9. **(c)** 10. **(b)** 11. **(a)**
12. **(d)**
13. **(c)** The cost of gene cloning is far more than PCR because gene cloning requires many intricate steps. PCR takes less than 4 hours while gene cloning can take days.
14. **(a)**
15. **(a)** *Agrobacterium tumefaciens* (updated scientific name: *Rhizobium radiobacter*) is the causal agent of crown gall desease (the formation of tumour) in over 140 species of dicot. It is a rod-shaped, Gram negative soil bacterium (Smith, *et. al*, 1907). Symptoms are caused by the insertion of a small segment of DNA, knwon as T-DNA (transfer DNA) into the plant cell, which is incorporated at a semi-random location into the plant genome.
16. **(b)** 17. **(c)** 18. **(a)** 19. **(c)** 20. **(b)**
21. **(a)** 22. **(a)**
23. **(b)** Plasmid Circular - extrachromosomal DNA
Bacteriophages - Virus infecting bacteria
Cosmids - Hybrid vector derived from plasmids
Agarose - Natural polymer of D - galactose
24. **(c)** Arber, Nathan and Hamilton Smith - Isolated first restriction endonuclease from bacteria
Paul berg - Father of genetic engineering
Herbert Boyer and Stanley Cohen - First recombinant DNA
Karl Erkey - Term biotechnology
25. **(a)** 26. **(d)** 27. **(d)** 28. **(c)**
29. **(b)** Interferons are antiviral proteins which were produced by "Charles Weismann" (1980) by recombinant DNA technology in *E. coli*.
30. **(c)** *EcoRI* - *Escherichia coli RY13*
HindII - *Haemophilus infulenzae*
BamHI - *Bacillus amyloliquefaciens*
EcoRII - *E. coli R 245*
31. **(b)** E - Name of genus
co - Name of species
R - Name of strain
I - 1st in order of identification

CHAPTER

Biotechnology and Its Applications

1. Select the correct set of the names for A, B, C and D.

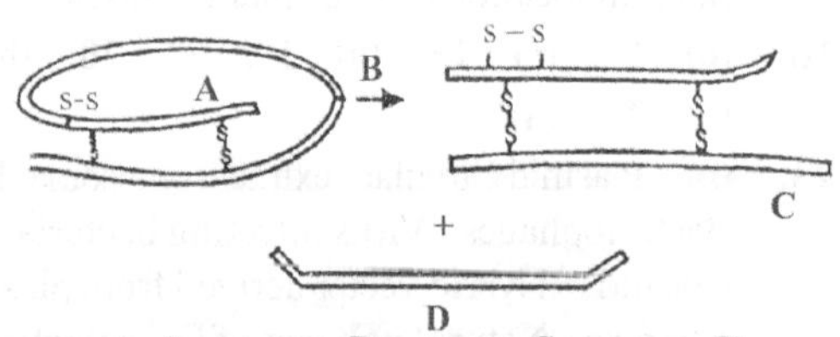

	A	B	C	D
(a)	Proinsulin	Peptide	Free C-Peptide	Insulin
(b)	Proinsulin	Peptidase	Insulin	Free C-Peptide
(c)	Proinsulin	Peptide	Insulin	Free C-Peptide
(d)	Insulin	Peptidase	Proinsulin	Free C-Peptide

2. Match the following and choose the correct option.

Column I	Column II
A. Golden Rice	I. Cry protein
B. Bt toxin	II. Rich in vitamin A
C. RNAi	III. First trangenic cow
D. Rosie	IV. Gene silencing

(a) A–II; B–I; C–IV; D–III
(b) A–II; B–I; C–III; D–IV
(c) A–II; B–III; C–I; D–IV
(d) A–IV; B–I; C–II; D–III

3. Match the following and choose the correct option.

Column I	Column II
A. Biopiracy	I. Search for unknown compounds
B. Bioprospecting	II. Hybridoma technology
C. Monoclonal antibodies.	III. Mobile genetic element
D. Transposon	IV. Bioresources

(a) A–II; B–I; C–IV; D–III
(b) A–II; B–I; C–III; D–IV
(c) A–II; B–III; C–I; D–IV
(d) A–IV; B–I; C–II; D–III

4. Match the following and choose the correct option.

Column I	Column II
A. Forensic science	I. AIDS
B. ELISA	II. First man made hormone
C. Humulin	III. Emphysema
D. α-1-antitrypsin	IV. DNA fingerprinting

(a) A–II; B–I; C–IV; D–III
(b) A–II; B–I; C–III; D–IV
(c) A–II; B–III; C–I; D–IV
(d) A–IV; B–I; C–II; D–III

5. Match the following columns.

Column I	Column II
A. Gene therapy	I. Effort to fix functional gene
B. Humulin	II. A single-stranded DNA of RNA tagged with a radioactive molecule
C. Probe	III. Diabetes
D. ELISA	IV. Diagnostic test

(a) A–I; B–III; C–II; D–IV
(b) A–IV; B–II; C–III; D–I
(c) A–II; B–III; C–I; D–IV
(d) A–III; B–I; C–IV; D–II

6. Which of the following is/are true ?

I. Biowar – Biowar is the use of biological weapons against humans and or their crops and animals.

II. Bioethics – Bioethics is the unauthorised use of bioresources and traditional knowledge related to bioresources for commercial benefits.

III. Biopatent – Exploitation of bioresources of other nations without proper authorization.

(a) II only (b) I only
(c) I and II only (d) I and III only

7. Which one of the following is the correctly matched pair of a product and the microorganism responsible for it ?
(a) Ethyl alcohol – Yeast
(b) Acetic acid – *Lactobacillus*
(c) Cheese – *Nitrobacter*
(d) Curd – *Azotobacter*

8. There are set of healthcare products. Match them with organisms which are genetically engineered for respective product

A. Insulin	I. *Escherichia coli / Saccharomyces*
B. Somatotropin	II. *Escherichia coli / yeast*
C. Interferon	III. GM *Escherichia coli*
D. Interleukins	IV. hGR in *Escheri chia coli*
	V. Humulin through *Escherichia coli*

(a) A–V; B–IV; C–I; D–II
(b) A–V; B–I; C–II; D–IV
(c) A–V; B–III; C–IV; D–I
(d) A–V; B–IV; C–III; D–II

9. Match the column I with column II and choose the correct option:

Column I	Column II
A. *Cry IAc*	1. *Escherichia coli*
B. *Cry I Ab*	2. *Agrobacterium*
C. Hirudin	3. Control cotton boll worms
D. Ti-plasmid	4. Control corn borer
	5. Introduced in *Brassica napus*

	A	B	C	D
(a)	2	3	1	5
(b)	3	2	4	1
(c)	1	2	3	4
(d)	3	4	5	2

10. Match the column I with column II and choose the correct option:

Column I	Column II
A. Bt- cotton	1. Insecticide
B. Flavr-Savr tomato	2. Delayed Ripening
C. Hirudin	3. Prevents blood clotting
D. Golden rice	4. Prevent Blindness
	5. Vitamin B-rich

(a) A-2, B-3, C-1, D-5
(b) A-3, B-2, C-4, D-1
(c) A-1, B-2, C-3, D-4
(d) A-5, B-3, C-1, D-2

11. GM plants, whose genes have been altered by manipulation, are useful in many ways. Match the column I with column II and choose the correct option:

Column I	Column II
A. Reduce reliance on chemical pesticides	I. Salt tolerant transgenic tomato
B. Enhanced nutritional value of food	II. Flavr-savr tomato
C. Reduce post harvest losses	III. Nematode resistant tobacco
D. Tolerant to abiotic stresses	IV. Golden rice

(a) A-III, B-IV, C-I, D-II
(b) A-II, B-IV, C-III, D-I
(c) A-II, B-IV, C-I, D-III
(d) A-III, B-IV, C-II, D-I

Solutions

1.	**(b)**	**2.**	**(a)**	**3.**	**(d)**	**4.**	**(d)**	**5.**	**(a)**
6.	**(b)**	**7.**	**(a)**	**8.**	**(a)**	**9.**	**(d)**	**10.**	**(d)**
11.	**(d)**								

CHAPTER

Organisms and Populations

1. Match the association in Column I with the type of interaction given in Column II and mark the correct option:

	Column I		Column II
A.	Barnacles on whale	I.	Predation
B.	Butterfly and birds	II.	Parasitism
C.	Goats and tortoise	III.	Competition
D.	Copepods on marine fish	IV.	Commensalism

(a) A- (I), B- (IV), C- (III), D- (II)
(b) A- (IV), B- (I), C- (II), D- (III)
(c) A- (III), B- (I), C- (IV), D- (II)
(d) A- (IV), B- (I), C- (III), D- (II)

2. What is the sequence of phases in the growth curve?

	(a)	(b)	(c)
(a)	Lag	Log	Inflexion phase
(b)	Lag	Stationary	Log
(c)	Log	Lag	Stationary
(d)	Lag	Log	Stationary

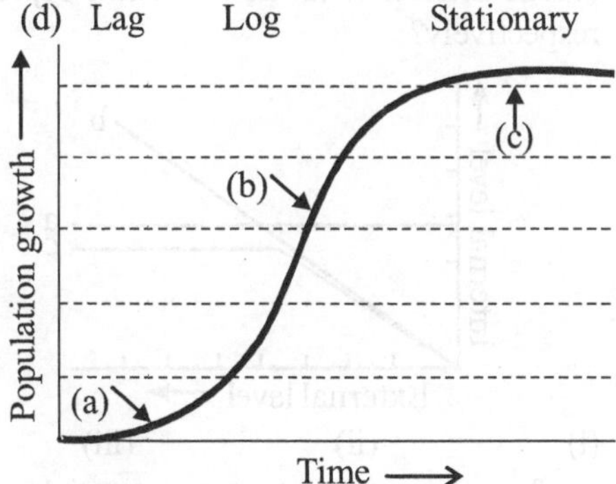

3. Match the columns and find out the correct combination:

A.	Bamboo	1.	Breeds many times in its lifetime
B.	Fish	2.	Produce a large number of small sized organization
C.	Mammal	3.	Breeds only once in its life time
D.	Bird	4.	Produce a small number of large sized organisms

(a) A-3, B-2, C-4, D-1
(b) A-1, B-2, C-3, D-4
(c) A-2, B-4, C-1, D-3
(d) A-4, B-1, C-3, D-2

4. Match the columns and find out the correct combination:

A.	Stable population	1.	Triangular
B.	Declining population	2.	Urn Shaped
C.	Growing population	3.	Bell shaped
D.	Migration	4.	Inward & outward movement

(a) A-3, B-2, C-1, D-4
(b) A-3, B-2, C-4, D-1
(c) A-3, B-1, C-2, D-4
(d) A-2, B-3, C-1, D-4

5. Match the column I with II and choose the correct option:

A.	Mutualism	1.	Ticks & lice
B.	Commensalism	2.	Liver fluke
C.	Ectoparasite	3.	Lichens
D.	Endoparasite	4.	Sea-anemone and clown fish

(a) A-4, B-3, C-1, D-2
(b) A-3, B-4, C-1, D-2
(c) A-3, B-4, C-2, D-1
(d) A-1, B-3, C-2, D-4

6. Identify the correct match from the column I, II and III regarding lake stratification:

Column I	Column II	Column III
1. Littoral zone	A. Maximum Phytoplankton	(i) Maximum Diversity
2. Limnetic zone	B. Aphotic zone	(ii) P/R = 1
3. Profundal zone	C. Ecotone	(iii) Euphotic zone
4. Compensation zone	D. Disphotic zone	(iv) Mainly occupied by heterotrophs

(a) 2-A-(ii), 1-C-(i), 3-B-(iv), 4-D-(iii)
(b) 1-C-(i), 2-A-(iv), 3-B-(iv), 4-D-(ii)
(c) 2-D-(iii), 2-B-(iv), 3-B-(i), 4-D-(ii)
(d) 2-B-(iii), 1-B-(iv), 3-A-(ii), 4-D-(iv)

7.

	A	B	C
	Mutualism	**Parasitism**	**Commensalism**
(a)	Barnacle & Whale	Loranthus & Mango	Yucca plant & pronuba moth
(b)	Leech on cattle	Orchid & Bee	Pilot fish & shark
(c)	Fig tree & wasp	Viscum & Oak	Orchid & mango
(d)	Sucker fish & shark	Lichen	Ticks on dog

8. Which one is correct?

(a) Cold area animals	Small in size	Large surface area	Low volume
(b) Warm area animals	Small in size	Low surface area	Large volume
(c) Warm area animals	Small in size	Large surface area	Low volume
(d) Cold area animals	Large in size	Small surface area	Small volume

9. Match Column-I with Column-II.

Column-I	Column-II
(A) Saprophyte	(i) Symbiotic association of fungi with plant roots
(B) Parasite	(ii) Decomposition of dead organic materials
(C) Lichens	(iii) Living on living plants or animals
(D) Mycorrhiza	(iv) Symbiotic association of algae and fungi

Choose the correct answer from the options given below:

	(A)	(B)	(C)	(D)
(a)	(i)	(ii)	(iii)	(iv)
(b)	(iii)	(ii)	(i)	(iv)
(c)	(ii)	(i)	(iii)	(iv)
(d)	(ii)	(iii)	(iv)	(i)

10. The figure given below is a diagrammatic representation of response of organisms to abiotic factors. What do a, b and c represent respectively?

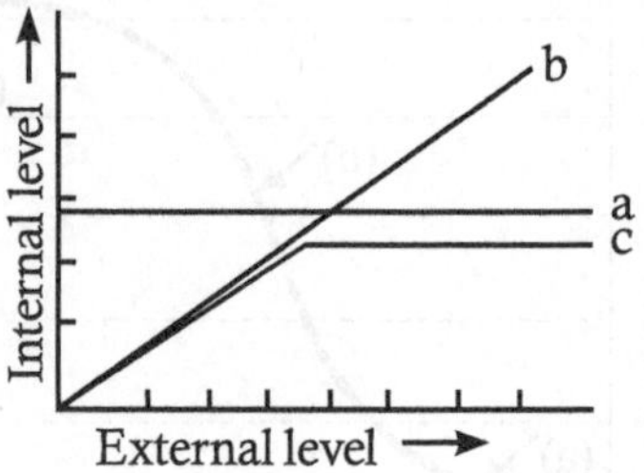

Internal level →
External level →
b
a
c

	(i)	(ii)	(iii)
(a)	conformer	regulator	partial regulator
(b)	regulator	partial regulator	conformer
(c)	partial regulator	regulator	conformer
(d)	regulator	conformer	partial regulator

11. Which one of the following pairs is mismatched?

(a) Tundra - Permafrost
(b) Savanna - Acacia trees
(c) Prairie - Epiphytes
(d) Coniferous forest - Evergreen trees

12. Which of the following is a correct pair?

(a) Cuscuta – parasite
(b) Dischidia – insectivorous
(c) Opuntia – predator
(d) Capsella – hydrophyte

13. Match column-I with column-II and choose the correct answer.

Column-I	Column-II
A. Pacific Salmon fish	I. Produces a small number of large sized offspring
B. Mammals	II. Produces a large number of small sized offspring
C. Oysters	III. Breed only once in their lifetime
D. Birds	IV. Breed many times during their lifetime

(a) A – III, B – IV, C – II, D – I
(b) A – I, B – IV, C – II, D – III
(c) A – IV, B – II, C – I, D – III
(d) A – II, B – IV, C – III, D – I

14. Match Column - I with Column - II and choose the correct option.

Column I	Column II
A. Pacific salmon fish	I. Verhulst - pearl logistic growth
B. $Nt = N_0 e^{rt}$	II. Breed only once in life time
C. Oyster	III. Exponential growth
D. $dN/dt = rN \frac{[K-N]}{K}$	IV. A large number of small sized offsprings

(a) A – IV; B – III; C – I; D – II
(b) A – III; B – IV; C – I; D – II
(c) A – III; B – I; C – IV; D – II
(d) A – II; B – III; C – IV; D – I

15. The density of a population in a given habitat during a given period, fluctuates due to changes in four basic processes. On this basis choose the correct option to fill up A and B boxes in the given diagram.

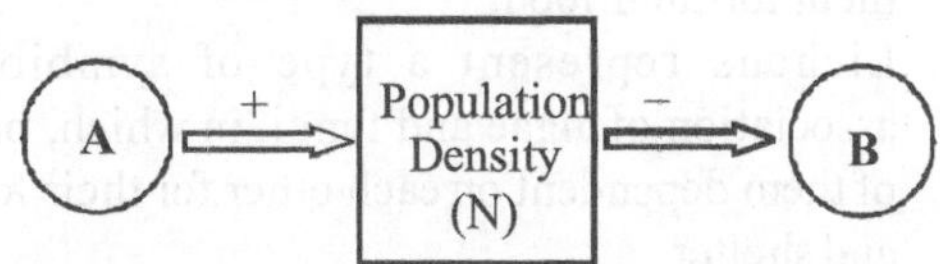

(a) A = Natality + Immigration, B = Mortality + Emigration
(b) A = Natality + Mortality, B = Immigration + Emigration
(c) A = Birth rate + Death rate, B = Mortality + Emigration
(d) A = Natality + Emigration, B = Mortality + Immigration

16. Identify I to IV which affect the population density.

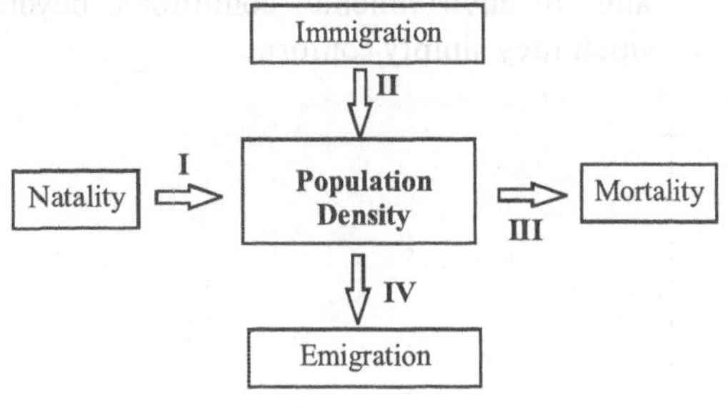

	I	II	III	IV
(a)	Increase	Decrease	Increase	Decrease
(b)	Decrease	Increase	Decrease	Increase
(c)	Increase	Increase	Decrease	Decrease
(d)	Decrease	Decrease	Increase	Increase

Solutions

1. (d) 2. (d) 3. (a) 4. (a) 5. (b)
6. (b) 7. (c) 8. (c)

9. **(d)** Saprophytes are organisms which live on dead organic matter and help in their decomposition.

Parasites is an organisms that live in or on other living plants and animals and dependent on them for their food.

Lichens represent a type of symbiotic association of algae and fungi, in which, both of them dependent on each other for their food and shelter.

Mycorrhiza is also a type of symbiotic association of fungi and plant roots, e.g., *Cycas* coralloid root.

10. **(d)** In the graph, the line 'a' represents regulator, line 'b' represents conformer and line 'c' represents partial regulator. Organism that are able to maintain homeostasis by physiological means that ensures constant body temperature are called regulators. Organism that are not able to maintain a constant internal temperature are called conformers.

Partial regulators are organisms that have the ability to regulate, but only over a limited range of environmental conditions, beyond which they simply conform.

11. **(c)** Prairie is a grass land, and epiphytes and ephemerals are found in desert. In Tundra, much of the ground stays frozen round the year, this condition is called permafrost. The *Acacia* trees are common in African savannas. In coniferous forest, all plants do not shed their leaves at the same time hence forest remain evergreen.

12. **(a)** *Opuntia* is a xerophyte. *Cuscuta* is a parasite. *Capsella* is not a hydrophyte.

13. **(a)** 14. **(d)**

15. **(a)** Population density due to changes in the following basic process - A: Natality + Immigration; B: Mortality + Emigration

Natality is the proportion of births to the total population in a place in a given time. Immigration is the number of individuals of the same species that have come into the habitat from elsewhere during the time period under consideration. Mortality is the number of deaths in the population during a given period of time. Emigration is the number of individuals of the population who left the habitat and have gone elsewhere during a given period of time.

16. **(c)** According to the given figure, I, II, III and IV (which affects the basic process of population density) are respectively increase, increase, decrease and decrease.

CHAPTER

Ecosystem

1. Identified A, B, C and D.

	Trophic levels	Examples
Tertiary consumer	Fourth trophic level (Top carnivore)	(D)
↑ (A)	Third trophic level (Carnivore)	Birds, fishes, and wolf
↑ Primary consumer	Second trophic level (Herbivore)	Zooplankton, grasshopper and cow
↑ (B)	First trophic level (C)	Phytoplankton, grass and trees

(a) A – Primary producer; B – Second consumer; C – Man / Lion; D – Plants

(b) A – Secondary consumer; B – Primary producer; C – Man / lion; D – Plants

(c) A – Primary producer; B – Secondary consumer; C – Plants; D – Man / lion

(d) A – Secondary consumer; B – Primary producer; C – Plants; D – Man / lion

2. Identified A, B, C and D of a nutrient cycle.

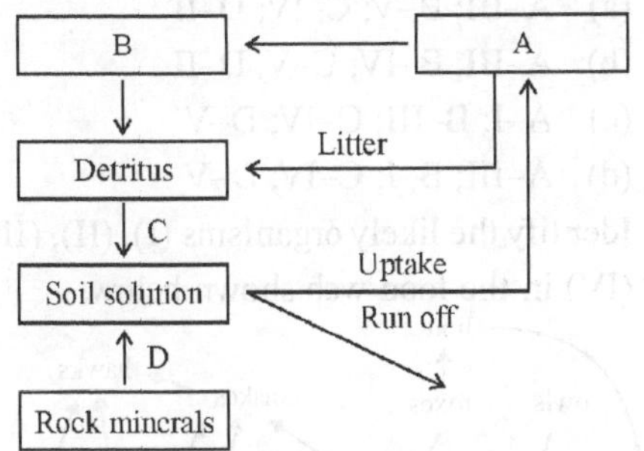

(a) A – Consumers; B – Decomposition; C – Producers; D – Weathering

(b) A – Consumers; B – Weathering; C – Producers; D – Decomposition

(c) A – Producers; B – Consumers; C – Decomposition; D – Weathering

(d) A – Consumers; B – Producers; C – Decomposition; D – Weathering

3. Match the following and choose the correct option

A.	Primary succession	I.	Autotrophs
B.	Climax community	II.	Community that has com pleted succession
C.	Consumer	III.	Colonization of a new environment
D.	Producer	IV.	Animals

(a) A – III; B – II; C – IV; D – I

(b) A – III; B – I; C – IV; D – II

(c) A – I; B – III; C – II; D – IV

(d) A – II; B – III; C – IV; D – I

4. Match the following columns.

	Column I		Column II
A.	Scavengers	I.	Autotrophs
B.	Parasites	II.	Heterotrophs
C.	Producers	III.	Consumers of dead bodies
D.	Phagotrophs	IV.	Consumers that feed on a small part of a living being

(a) A–III; B–V; C–I; D–II

(b) A–III; B–I; C–II; D–IV

(c) A–I; B–II; C–IV; D–III

(d) A–IV; B–III; C–II; D–I

5. Identify A, B and C from the given flow chart.

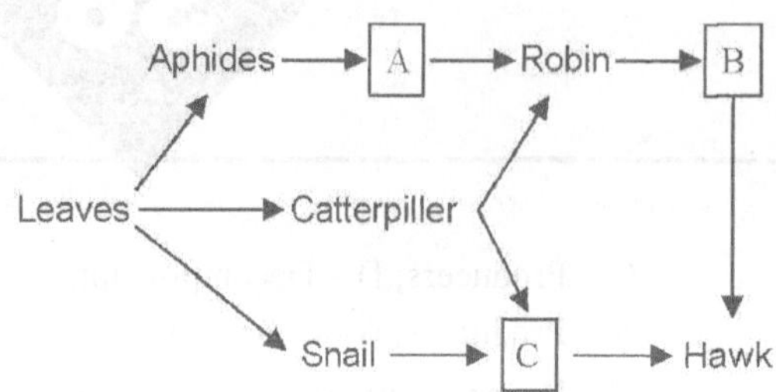

(a) A-Bulbul, B-Snake, C-Monkey
(b) A-Beetle, B-Lizard, C-Praying mantis
(c) A-Ladybird, B-Snake, C-Pigeon
(d) A-Lizard, B-Bird, C-Snake

6. Match the two sets

	Column I		Column II
A.	Pioneers	I.	Vegetation which modifies its own environment and thus causing its own replacement
B.	Autogenic	II.	Replacement of existing community by external conditions.
C.	Allogenic	III.	Establishment succession
D.	Ecesis	IV.	Primary colonisers

(a) A – IV; B – I, C – II; D – III
(b) A – I; B – II, C – III; D – IV
(c) A – II; B – I, C – IV; D – III
(d) A – I; B – IV, C – III; D – II

7. Match the following columns.

	Column I		Column II
A.	Inorganic substances	I.	Light, temperature and humidity
B.	Organic compounds	II.	Soil, pH and minerals.
C.	Climatic factors	III.	Proteins, carbohydrates and lipids, nucleic acid
D.	Edaphic factors	IV.	Carbon, nitrogen, oxygen and water.

(a) A–III; B–I; C–II; D–IV
(b) A–IV; B–III; C–I; D–II
(c) A–I; B–II; C–III; D–IV
(d) A–IV; B–II; C–I; D–III

8. Match the names of organisms given under column I with the ecological names given under column II. Choose the answer which gives the correct combinations of the two columns.

	Column I (Organisms)		Column II (Ecological names)
A.	Grass	I.	Decomposer
B.	Grasshopper	II.	Secondary carnivore
C.	Frog	III.	Producer
D.	Hawk	IV.	Primary consumer
		V.	Primary carnivore

(a) A–III; B–V; C–IV; D–II
(b) A–III; B–IV; C–V; D–II
(c) A–I; B–III; C–IV; D–V
(d) A–III; B–I; C–IV; D–V

9. Identify the likely organisms (I), (II), (III) and (IV) in the food web shown below.

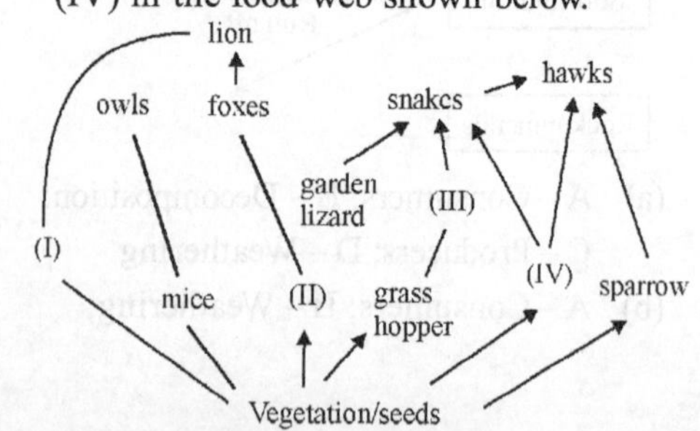

	(I)	(II)	(III)	(IV)
(a)	Deer	Rabbit	Frog	Rat
(b)	Dog	Squirrel	Bat	Deer
(c)	Rat	Dog	Tortoise	Crow
(d)	Squirrel	Cat	Rat	Pigeon

10. Match the following and select the correct option

(A) Earthworm	(I) Pioneer species
(B) Succession	(II) Detritivore
(C) Ecosystem service	(III) Natality
(D) Population growth	(IV) Pollination

	(A)	(B)	(C)	(D)
(a)	(I)	(II)	(III)	(IV)
(b)	(IV)	(I)	(III)	(II)
(c)	(III)	(II)	(IV)	(I)
(d)	(II)	(I)	(IV)	(III)

11. Given below is a simplified model of phosphorus cycling in a terrestrial ecosystem with four blanks (A-D). Identify the blanks:-

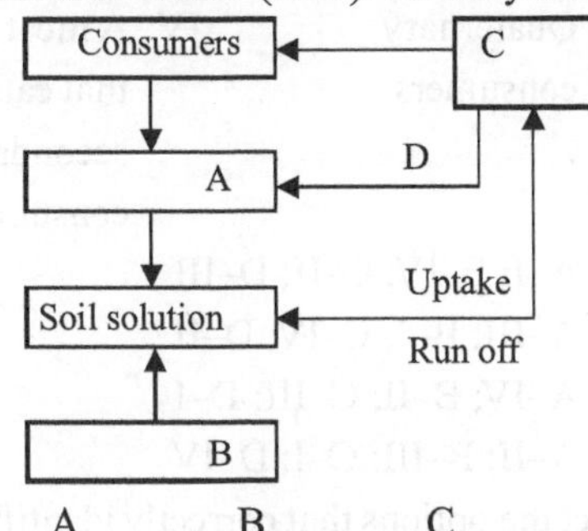

	A	B	C	D
(a)	Rock	Detritus minerals	Litter fall	Producers
(b)	Litter fall	Producers	Rock	Detritus minerals
(c)	Detritus minerals	Rock	Producer	Litter fall
(d)	Producers	Litter fall	Rock	Detritus minerals

12. In which of the following both pairs have correct combination ?

(a)	Gaseous nutrient cycle	Carbon and sulphur
	Sedimentary nutrient cycle	Nitrogen and Phosphorus
(b)	Gaseous nutrient cycle	Nitrogen and sulphur
	Sedimentary nutrient cycle	Carbon and Phosphorus
(c)	Gaseous nutrient cycle	Sulphur and Phosphorus
	Sedimentary nutrient cycle	Carbon and Nitrogen
(d)	Gaseous nutrient cycle	Carbon and Nitrogen
	Sedimentary nutrient cycle	Sulphur and Phosphorus

13. Match the following and choose the correct option –

Column I	**Column II**
A. Standing state	I. Perfect
B. Gaseous cycles	II. Amount of nutrients
C. Standing crop	III. Imperfect
D. Sedimentary cycles	IV. Living matter at different trophic levels

(a) A – II, B – I, C – IV, D – III
(b) A – I, B – II, C – III, D – IV
(c) A – III, B – II, C – IV, D – I
(d) A – I, B – IV, C – III, D – II

14. Answer the correct set

Column I	**Column II**
A. Gross primary	I. Total assimilation productivity
B. Secondary productivity	II. Remains mobile and does not remain in-situ
C. Transducers	III. Green plants
D. Food web	IV. Interlocking pattern

(a) A–I; B–II; C–III; D–IV
(b) A–II; B–III; C–IV; D–I

(c) A–III; B–IV; C–I; D–II
(d) A–I; B–III; C–II; D–IV

15. Study the following columns and choose the correct option.

Column I	Column II
A. Population	I. Parts of the earth consisting of all the ecosystems of the world.
B. Community	II. Assemblage of all the individuals belonging to different species occurring in an area
C. Ecosystem	III. Group of similar individuals belonging to the same species found in an area.
D. Ecosphere	IV. Interaction between the living organisms and their physical environment components.
	V. Classification of organisms based on the type of environment.

(a) A–III; B–II; C–I; D–IV
(b) A–V; B–II; C–III; D–IV
(c) A–II; B–III; C–V; D–I
(d) A–III; B–II; C–IV; D–I

16. Choose the correct combination of labelling of the zones in water in a lake

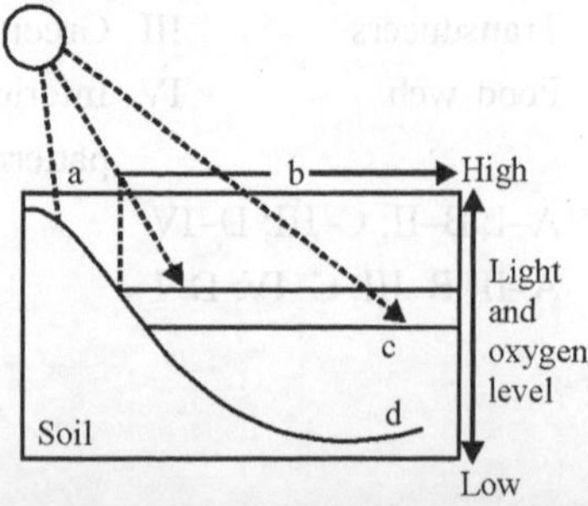

(a) a-Limnetic zone, b-Profundal zone, c-Littoral zone, d-Benthic zone
(b) a-Littoral zone, b-Benthic zone, c-Profundal zone, d-Limnetic zone
(c) a-Littoral zone, b-Limnetic zone, c-Profundal zone, d-Benthic zone
(d) a-Limnetic zone, b-Littoral zone, c-Benthic zone, d-Profundal zone

17. Match the following columns.

Column I	Column II
A. Primary consumers	I. A meat eater that eats primary consumers.
B. Secondary consumers	II. A meat eater that eats tertiary consumers.
C. Tertiary consumers	III. A organism eater that eats producers.
D. Quaternary consumers	IV. A meat eater that eats secondary consumers.

(a) A–I; B–IV; C–II; D–III
(b) A–III; B–I; C–IV; D–II
(c) A–IV; B–II; C–III; D–I
(d) A–II; B–III; C–I; D–IV

18. Select the options that correctly identifies A, B and C in the given table.

Organisms	Trophic Level	Type of Food Chain
Eagle	*A*	Grazing
Earthworm	Primary consumer	*B*
C	Secondary consumer	Grazing

(a) A-Secondary consumer, B-Grazing, C-Algae
(b) A-Top carnivore, B-Detritus, C-Frog
(c) A-Scavenger, B-Grazing, C-Hawk
(d) A-Decomposer, B-Detritus, C-Perch

19. Match the following columns.

	Column I		Column II
A.	Primary succession	I.	Colonisation of a new environment
B.	Climax community	II.	Ecosystem development
C.	Pioneer community on	III.	Crustose lichens lithosphere
D.	Ecological succession	IV.	Community that has completed succession

(a) A–III; B–II; C–I; D–IV
(b) A–IV; B–III; C–II; D–I
(c) A–I; B–II; C–III; D–IV
(d) A–IV; B–III; C–I; D–II

20. Match the following columns.

	Column I		Column II
A.	First trophic level	I.	Producer
B.	Decomposer	II.	Consumer
C.	Primary productivity	III.	Phytoplankton
D.	Secondary productivity	IV.	Stratification
		V.	Bacteria

(a) A–I; B–V; C–III; D–IV
(b) A–II; B–III; C–IV; D–V
(c) A–III; B–V; C–I; D–II
(d) A–III; B–V; C–II; D–I

21. Match the sets

	Column I		Column II
A.	*Artemisia tridentata*	I.	Grow better in over grazed area
B.	*Capparis spinosa*	II.	Dominate in areas destructed by fires
C.	*Pteridium aquilina* and *Pyronema*	III.	Indicates intense soil erosion
D.	*Amaranthus* and *Chenopodium*	IV.	Saline soils

(a) A–I; B–II; C–III; D–IV
(b) A–II; B–III; C–IV; D–I
(c) A–III; B–I; C–II; D–IV
(d) A–IV; B–III; C–II; D–I

22. Match column A with column B and select the correct option.

	Column I		Column II
A.	Pyramid of energy	I.	Xerosere
B.	First group of	II.	Always plant in bare area inverted
C.	Pyramid of biomass	III.	Hydrosere in aquatic habitat
D.	Succession in	IV.	Pioneers desert area
		V.	Always upright

(a) A – II; B – I; C – V; D – III
(b) A – V; B – IV; C – II; D – I
(c) A– V; B – III; C – II; D – IV
(d) A – II; B – III; C – V; D – I

23. Given food web contains some missing organisms A, B, C and D. Identify these organisms and select the correct answer.

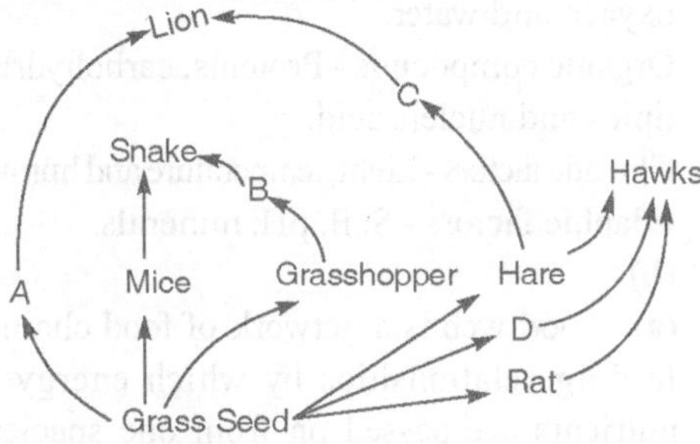

(a) A-Deer, B-Frog, C-Foxes, D-Sparrow
(b) A-Dog, B-Squirrel, C-Deer, D-Hawks
(c) A-Cat, B-Eagle, C-Cow, D-Rat
(d) A-Eagle, B-Sparrow, C-Dog, D-Cat

24. Match the following columns.

	Column I		Column II
A.	Xeroseres	I.	Ecological succession starts on terrestrial habitat.

B.	Hydroseres	II.	Succession begins from open water
C.	Lithoseres	III.	Successions begin on sand
D.	Psammoseres	IV.	Succession start on a bare rock

(a) A – III; B – I, C – II; D – IV
(b) A – IV; B – III, C – I; D – II
(c) A – I; B – II, C – IV; D – III
(d) A – II; B – IV, C – III; D – I

Solutions

1. **(d)** 2. **(c)** 3. **(a)**
4. **(a)** Scavengers - Consumers of dead bodes
Parasites - Consumers that feed on a small part of a living being
Producers - Autotrophs
Phagotrophs - Heterotrophs
5. **(c)** *Leaves → Aphids → Ladybird → Robin → Snake → Hawk Leaves → Snail → Pigeon → Hawk*
6. **(a)**
7. **(b)** Inorganic substances - Carbon, nitrogen, oxygen and water.
Organic compounds - Proteins, carbohydrates, lipids and nucleic acid.
Climatic factors - Light, temperature and humidity.
Edaphic factors - Soil, pH, minerals.
8. **(b)**
9. **(a)** Food web is a network of food chains or feeding relationships by which energy and nutrients are passed on from one species of living organisms to another.
10. **(d)**
11. **(c)** Phosphorus is an important element for living beings. Consumers obtain phosphorus directly or indirectly from plants. Phosphorus is also present in phosphatic rocks. It is released during the decomposition of plant and animal remains. The released phosphorus may reach the deeper layers of soil and gets deposited as phosphate rocks. All plants and animals eventually die and in due time, their organic remains or debris decay through the action of micro-organism and the phosphates are released into the water for recycling.
12. **(d)** Carbon and Nitrogen are gaseous nutrient cycle. Sulphur and phosphorus are sedimentary nutrient cycle.
13. **(a)** 14. **(a)**
15. **(d)** Population consists of organisms of same species, community have organisms of different species and ecosystem include biotic and abiotic components. Ecosphere is part of the earth consisting of all the ecosystems of the world.
16. **(c)**
17. **(b)** Primary consumer : That eats autotrophs.
Secondary consumer : A meat eater that eats primary consumers.
Tertiary consumer : A meat eater that eats secondary consumers.
Quaternary consumer : A meat eater that eats tertiary consumers.
18. **(b)** A-Top carnivore, B-Detritus, C-Frog.
19. **(c)** Primary – Colonisation of a new succession environment
Climas community – Community that has completed succession
Pioneer community – Crustose lichen on lithosphere
Ecological – Ecosystem development succession
20. **(c)** First trophic level - Phytoplankton
Decomposer – Bacteria
Primary productivity – Producer
Secondary productivity – Consumer
21. **(c)** 22. **(b)**
23. **(a)** A-Deer, B-Frog, C-Foxes, D-Sparrow
24. **(c)** Xeroseres: Ecological succession start on terrestrial habitat
Hydroseres: Succession begins from open water
Lithoseres: Succession starts on a bare rock.
Psammoseres: Succession begins on sand.

CHAPTER

Biodiversity and Conservation

1. Match items given in column I with those given in column II.

	Column I		Column II
A.	Rhinoceros	I.	Bharatpur
B.	Tiger project in Karnataka	II.	Tropical evergreen forest
C.	Assemblage protection	III.	Kaziranga
D.	Silent valley	IV.	National park
		V.	Bandipur

(a) A–V; B–III; C–I; D–IV
(b) A–II; B–IV; C–III; D–II
(c) A–IV; B–III; C–II; D–V
(d) A–III; B–V; C–I; D–II

2. Which one of the following is the correct matched pair of an endangered animal and National Park?

(a) Rhinoceros - Kaziranga National Park
(b) Wild ass - Dudhwa National Park
(c) Great Indian bustard - Keoladeo National Park
(d) Lion - Corbett National Park

3. Given below is the representation of the extent of global diversity of invertebrates. What groups the four portions (A-D) represent respectively?

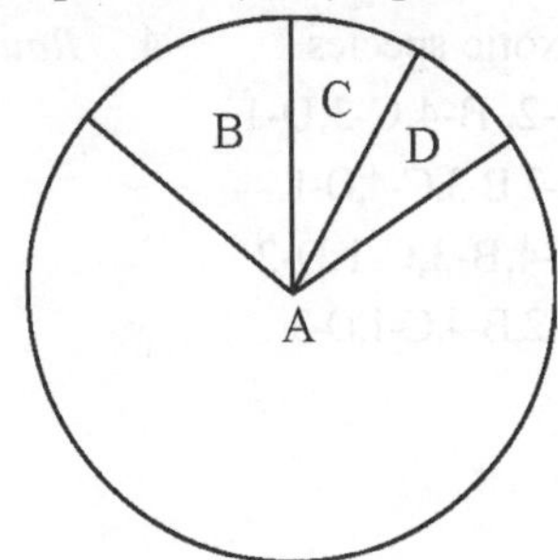

	A	B	C	D
(a)	Insects	Crustaceans	Other animal groups	Molluscs
(b)	Crustaceans	Insects	Molluscs	Other animal groups
(c)	Molluscs	Other animal groups	Crustaceans	Insects
(d)	Insects	Molluscs	Crustaceans	Other animal groups

4. Find the wrongly matched pair:

(a) Endemism- Species confined to a region and not found anywhere else
(b) Hot spots- Western Ghats
(c) Sacred groves- Jaintia Hills of Rajasthan
(d) *Ex-situ* conservation- Zoological park

5. Match the column -I with column -II

	Column I		Column II
A.	Bihar	I.	Indian elephant
B.	Rajasthan	II.	Gazello
C.	Madhya Pradesh	III.	Leopard
D.	Uttar Pradesh	IV.	Barasingha
E.	Gujarat	V.	Sloth Bear
		VI.	Asiatic Lion

(a) A–I; B–III; C–V; D–II; E–IV
(b) A–V; B–II; C–IV; D–III; E–VI
(c) A–III; B–V; C–II; D–IV; E–I
(d) A–VI; B–V; C–IV D–III; E–II

6. Which one of the following pairs is not correctly matched :
   (a) Manas Sanctuary – Assam
   (b) Kanha National Park – Madhya Pradesh
   (c) Dachigam Sanctuary – West Bengal
   (d) Bandipur Sanctuary – Karnataka

7. Identify the correctly matched pair :
   (a) Rann of Kutch – Wild ass
   (b) Corbett Park – Bustard
   (c) Kaziranga – Elephant
   (d) Gir Forest – Rhino

8. Given below is the representation of the extent of global diversity of *invertebrates*. What groups the four portions (A-D) represent respectively?

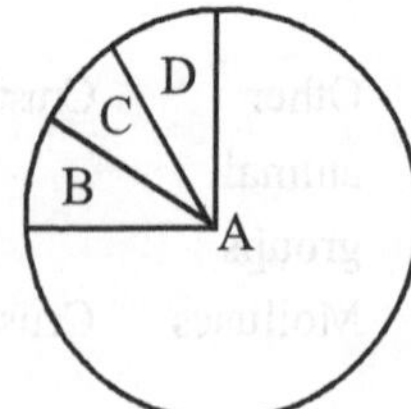

	A	B	C	D
(a)	Insects	Crustaceans	Other animal groups	Molluscs
(b)	Crustaceans	Insects	Molluscs	Other animal groups
(c)	Molluscs	Other animal groups	Crustaceans	Insects
(d)	Insects	Molluscs	Crustaceans	Other animal groups

9.

Column-I	Column-II
1. Silent valley	(A) Kaziranga
2. Rhinoceros	(B) Bandipur
3. Tiger project in Karnataka	(C) In situ
4. National Park	(D) Tropical evergreen forest

(a) I-B, II-A, III-D, IV-C
(b) I-D, II-A, III-B, IV-C
(c) I-A, II-C, III-B, IV-D
(d) I-B, II-A, III-C, IV-D

10. Match the following columns and select the correct option:

A. Alpha diversity	1. Richness of different species in a habitat
B. Beta diversity	2. Richness of different species along with a gradient from one habitat to another habitat within the community.
C. Gamma diversity	3. Richness of different species in different habitat.

(a) A-1,B-2, C-3
(b) A-1,B-3, C-2
(c) A-2, B-1, C-3
(d) A-3,B-2,C-1

11. Match the following columns:

Column I	Column II
A. Lungs of planet	1. *Lantana camara*
B. Reserpine	2. Amazon rain forest
C. Anti-cancer drug	3. Yew Tree
D. Exotic species	4. *Rauwolfia*

(a) A-2, B-4,C-3,D-1
(b) A-2,B-3,C-4,D-1
(c) A-4,B-3,C-1,D-2
(d) A-2,B-4,C-1,D-3

12. Given below are pie diagrams A, B and C related to proportionate number of species of major taxa of invertebrates, vertebrates and plants respectively. Critically study and fill in the blanks I, II, III and IV.

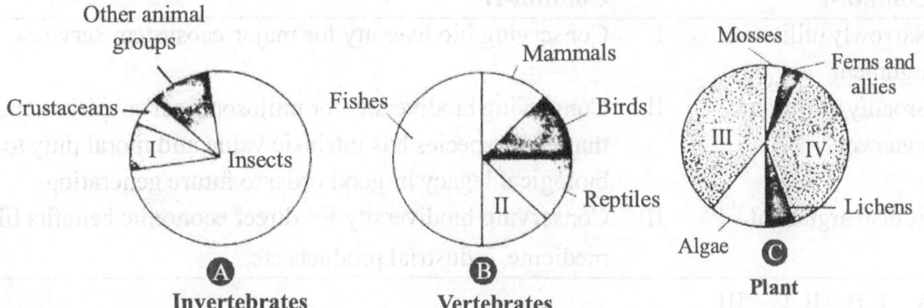

(a) I- Molluscs, II-Amphibians, III-Fungi, IV-Angiosperms
(b) I- Molluscs, II-Amphibians, III-Angiosperms, IV-Fungi
(c) I- Hexapoda, II-Amphibians, III-Fungi, IV-Angiosperms
(d) I- Turtles, II-Amphibians, III-Fungi, IV-Angiosperms

13. Given below is the representation of the extent of global diversity of invertebrates. What groups the four portions (A-D) represent respectively?

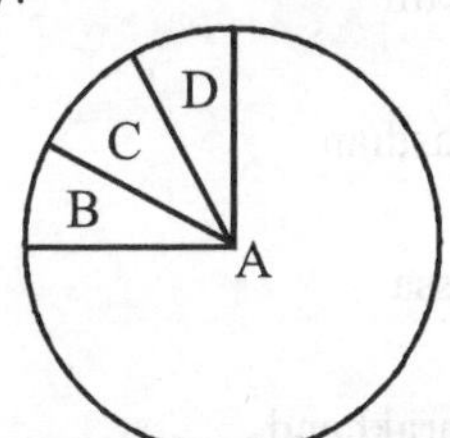

	A	B	C	D
(a)	Insects	Crustaceans	Other animal groups	Molluscs
(b)	Crustaceans	Insects	Molluscs	Other animal groups
(c)	Molluscs	Other animal groups	Crustaceans	Insects
(d)	Insects	Molluscs	Crustaceans	Other animal groups

14. Which of the following boxes show maximum, greater and minimum diversity ?

A

Animals	Species	Members
Bird	I	1
Bird	II	1
Bird	III	4

B

Animals	Species	Members
Bird	I	2
Bird	II	2
Mammal	III	2

C

Animals	Species	Members
Bird	I	2
Mammal	II	2
Insect	III	2

(a) A- Minimum diversity, B - Greater diversity, C - Maximum diversity
(b) A - Maximum diversity, B - Greater diversity, C - Minimum diversity
(c) A - Maximum diversity, B - Minimum diversity, C - Greater diversity
(d) A - Minimum diversity, B - Maximum diversity, C - Greater diversity.

15. Match the following and choose the correct option.

	Column-I		Column-II
A.	Narrowly utilitarian argument	I.	Conserving biodiversity for major ecosystem services
B.	Broadly utilitarian argument	II.	Conserving biodiversity for philosophical or spiritual need to realise that every species has intrinsic value and moral duty to pass our biological legacy in good order to future generation.
C.	Ethical argument	III.	Conserving biodiversity for direct economic benefits like food, medicine, industrial products etc.

(a) A – I, B – II, C – III
(b) A – III, B – I, C – II
(c) A – II, B – I, C – III
(d) A – I, B – III, C – II

16. Match the following.

	Column-I		Column-II
(A)	Ranthambore National Park	(i)	Assam
(B)	Kaziranga National Park	(ii)	Rajasthan
(C)	Jim corbett National Park	(iii)	Orissa
(D)	Nandan kanan zoological Park	(iv)	Uttarakhand

(a) (A) - (i), (B) - (ii), (C) - (iii), (D) - (iv)
(b) (A) - (ii), (B) - (iii), (C) - (iv), (D) - (i)
(c) (A) - (ii), (B) - (i), (C) - (iv), (D) - (iii)
(d) (A) - (iii), (B) - (ii), (C) - (i), (D) - (iv)

Solutions

1. **(d)** 2. **(a)** 3. **(d)** 4. **(c)** 5. **(b)**
6. **(c)** 7. **(a)**
8. **(d)** Arthropoda is the largest phylum of Animalia which includes insects. Over two-thirds of all named species on earth are arthropods. They have organ system level of organisation. Mollusca is the second largest animal phylum. They are terrestrial or aquatic (marine or fresh).
9. **(b)** 10. **(a)** 11. **(a)**
12. **(a)** In the given pie diagrams (A, B and C), the proportionate number of species of major taxa of invertebrates, vertebrates and plants respectively marked as I (mollusca), II (amphibians), III (Fungi), IV (Angiosperms)
13. **(d)** Arthropoda is the largest phylum of Animalia which includes insects. Over two-thirds of all named species on earth are arthropods. They have organ system level of organisation. Mollusca is the second largest animal phylum. They are terrestrial or aquatic (marine or fresh).
14. **(a)** A, B and C respectively show minimum, greater and maximum diversity. Since the number of individuals in all the three boxes are same but the variety of animals in all the boxes are different, like box A shows diversity of single animal - bird, box B shows diversity of birds and mammals whereas box C shows diversity of three animals - birds, mammals and insects.
15. **(b)** A - III, B - I, C - II
16. **(c)** Ranthambore National Park is a vast wildlife reserve near the town of Sawai Madhopur in Rajasthan, northern India. It is a former royal hunting ground and home to tigers, leopards and marsh crocodiles. Kaziranga National Park is a protected area in the northeast Indian state of Assam. It is a home to tigers, elephants and the world's largest population of Indian one-horned rhinoceroses. Jim Corbett National Park is a forested wildlife sanctuary in northern India's Uttarakhand State. Rich in flora and fauna, it is known for its Bengal tigers. Nandankanan Zoological Park is a 437-hectare zoo and botanical garden in Bhubaneswar, Orissa, India. It serves the first captive gharial breeding center of India.

CHAPTER

Environmental Issues

39. Match the following columns.

	Column I		Column II
A.	Suspended solids	I.	Nitrates ammonia, phosphate sodium calcium
B.	Colloidal matterials	II.	Faecal matter, bacteria, paper and cloth fibres
C.	Dissolved materials	III.	Sand, silt and clay

(a) A–I; B–II; C–III
(b) A–II; B–III; C–I
(c) A–III; B–I; C–II
(d) A–III; B–II; C–I

35. Match the sources of solid waste in Column A with the type of solid waste in column B.

	Column I		Column II
A.	Old newspapers	I.	Municipal solid wastes
B.	Construction site	II.	Industrial solid wastes
C.	Discarded medicines	III.	Hospital solid wastes and syringes

(a) A–II; B–III; C–I
(b) A–I; B–III; C–II
(c) A–I; B–II; C–III
(d) A–II; B–III; C–I

5. Identify the correctly matched pair.

(a) Basal Convention - Biodiversity Conservation
(b) Kyoto Protocol - Climatic change
(c) Montreal Protocol - Global warming
(d) Ramsar Convention - Ground water pollution

13. The below diagram shows a scrubber. Identify A, B, C and D.

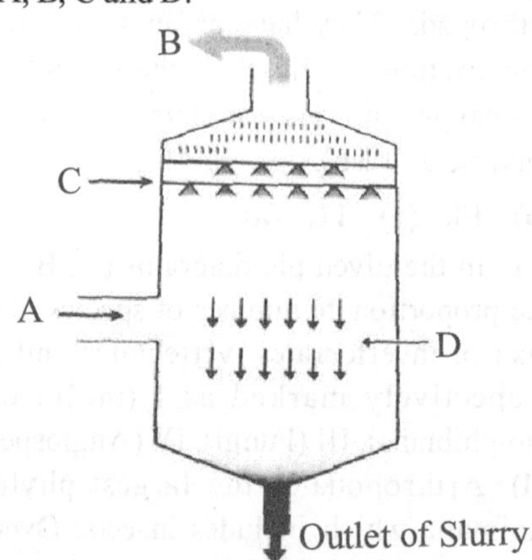

(a) A-Particulate matter, B-Clean air, C-Dirty air, D-Dust particle
(b) A-Dirty air, B-Clean air, C-Water lime spray, D-Slurry outlet
(c) A-Slurry outlet, B-Dirty airm, C-Particulate matter, D-Clean air
(d) A-Dust particle, B-Clean air, C-Particulate matter, D-water spray

27. Match the following items in column I with column II and choose the correct answer.

	Calumn I		Column II
A.	Arsenic	I.	Minamata disease
B.	Nitrate	II.	Itai-itai
C.	Mercury	III.	Blue-baby syndrome
D.	Cadmium	IV.	Skeletal fluorosis
E.	Fluoride	V.	Black-fool disease

(a) A–II; B–III; C–V; D–I; E–IV
(b) A–V; B–III; C–I; D–II; E–IV
(c) A–III; B–IV; C–V; D–I; E–II
(d) A–V; B–IV; C–III; D–II; E–I

41. Match the following columns.

	Column I		Column II
A.	Particulate pollutants	I.	Hydrogen sulphide
B.	Gaseous pollutants	II.	Carbon monoxide
		III.	Metallic particles
		IV.	Dust particles
		V.	Soot
		VI.	Aerosol
		VII.	Smoke
		VIII.	Nitrogen dioxide
		IX.	Sulphus dioxide

(a) A–III, IV, V, VI, VII; B–I, II, VIII, IX
(b) A–III, IV, V, B–I, II, VI, VII, VIII, IX
(c) A–III, IV, V, VI; B–I, II, VII, VIII, IX
(d) A–I, II, III, IV; B–V, VI, VII, VIII, IX

7. Match the following and select the correct option.

	Column I		Column II
A.	Emphysema	(i)	Increase in the concentration of non-biodegrable substances in food chains
B.	ADA deficiency	(ii)	a-1 antitrypsin
C.	Eutrophication	(iii)	Bone marrow transplantation
D.	Biomagnification	(iv)	Nutrient enrichment of water body

(a) A-(iii), B-(ii), C-(iv), D-(i)
(b) A-(ii), B-(iii), C-(iv), D-(i)
(c) A-(i), B-(iii), C-(ii), D-(iv)
(d) A-(iv), B-(ii), C-(iii), D-(i)

8. Match the column I with column II and choose the correct option:

	Column I		Column II
A.	Environment Protection Act	1.	1947
B.	Air Pollution and Control of Pollution Act	2.	1987
C.	Water Act	3.	1986
D.	Amendment of Air Act to include noise	4.	1981

(a) A-3, B-4, C-1, D-2
(b) A-1, B-3, C-2, D-4
(c) A-4, B-1, C-2, D-3
(d) A-3, B-4, C-2, D-1

9. Match the columns I with column II and choose the correct option:

	Column I		Column II
A.	UV rays	1.	Biomagnification
B.	Biodegradable organic matter	2.	Eutrophication
C.	DDT	3.	Snow blindness
D.	Phosphates	4.	BOD

(a) A-2, B-1, C-4, D-3
(b) A-3, B-2, C-4, D-1
(c) A-3, B-4, C-1, D-2
(d) A-3, B-1, C-4, D-2

10. Match the column I with column II and find out the correct combination:

	Column I		Column II
A.	Ozone depletion	1.	Thickness of ozone
B.	Greenhouse gas	2.	CFCs
C.	Decibels	3.	Units of sound
D.	Dobson units	4.	Methane

(a) A-2, B-3, C-4, D-1
(b) A-2, B-4, C-3, D-1
(c) A-3, B-2, C-4, D-1
(d) A-4, B-2, C-3, D-1

11. Match the items given in Column I with those in Column II and select the correct option given below

	Column-I		Column-II
A.	Eutrophication	i.	UV-B radiation
B.	Sanitary landfill	ii.	Deforestation
C.	Snow blindness	iii.	Nutrient enrichment
D.	Jhum cultivation	iv.	Waste disposal

	A	B	C	D
(a)	ii	i	iii	iv
(b)	i	iii	iv	ii
(c)	i	ii	iv	iii
(d)	iii	iv	i	ii

12. Identify the correctly matched pair.
(a) Basal Convention - Biodiversity Conservation
(b) Kyoto Protocol - Climatic change
(c) Montreal Protocol - Global warming
(d) Ramsar Convention - Ground water pollution

13. Which one of the following pairs is mismatched?
(a) Fossil fuel burning - release of CO_2
(b) Nuclear power - radioactive wastes
(c) Solar energy - green house effect
(d) Biomass burning - release of CO_2

Solutions

1. (d) Suspended Solid - Sand, silt and clay Colloidal Materials -Faecal matter, bacteria, paper and cloth fibres Dissolved Materials-Nitrates. ammonia phosphates, sodium and calcium
2. (c)
3. (b) Kyoto Protocol (1997) : International conference held in Kyoto, Japan obtained commitments from different countries for reducing overall greenhouse gas emissions at a level 9% below 1990 level by 2008-2012.
Montreal Protocol (1987) : Industrialized countries agreed to limit production of chloroflourocarbons to half the level of 1986.
4. (b) 5. (b)
6. (a) Particulate pollutants, metallic particles, soot aerosol, smoke and dust particles. Gasesous pollutants Hydrogen sulphide, carbon monoxide, nitrogen dioxide and sulphur dioxide.
7. (b) 8. (a) 9. (c) 10. (b)
11. (d) Snow blindness, also called arc eye or photokeratitis, is a painful eye condition caused by overexposure to ultraviolet (UV) light. When too much UV light hits the transparent outer layer of your eyes, called the cornea, it essentially gives your cornea a sunburn. Snow blindness symptoms can be disorienting.
12. (b) Kyoto Protocol (1997) : International conference held in Kyoto, Japan obtained commitments from different countries for reducing overall greenhouse gas emissions at a level 9% below 1990 level by 2008-2012.
Montreal Protocol (1987) : Industrialized countries agreed to limit production of chloroflourocarbons to half the level of 1986.
13. (c) Solar energy coming to the earth is not responsible for green house effect. It is the increase in green house gases in atmosphere like CO_2 which is released by complete combustion of fossil fuels or biomass in industries or transportation vehicles that prevent the reradiation of infrared radiation from the earth and result in increase in temperature of the earth.

Assertion Reason
Question Bank

INDEX

Chapter

1

The Living World

Directions: In the following questions, a statement of assertion is followed by a statement of reason. Mark the correct choice as:

(a) If both Assertion and Reason are true and Reason is the correct explanation of Assertion.

(b) If both Assertion and Reason are true but Reason is not the correct explanation of Assertion.

(c) If Assertion is true but Reason is false.

(d) If both Assertion and Reason are false.

1. **Assertion :** Botany deals with the study of plants and zoology deals with the study of animals.
   Reason : Biology is the study of living beings.
2. **Assertion :** Study of internal structure is called anatomy.
   Reason : It is useful for phylogentic study.
3. **Assertion :** The science of classifiying organisms is called taxonomy.
   Reason : Systematics and taxonomy have same meaning.
4. **Assertion :** Chemotaxonomy is classifying organisms at molecular level.
   Reason : Cytotaxonomy is classifying organisms at cellular level.
5. **Assertion:** Living organisms are regarded as closed systems.
   Reason: Energy of living organisms can not be lost or gained from external environment.
6. **Assertion:** Both internal as well as external growth is show by living organisms.
   Reason: Living organisms undergo the process known as accretion.
7. **Assertion:** Metabolism refers to the sum of chemical reactions that occur within living organisms.
   Reason: Metabolic reactions occur simultaneously inside living organisms.
   [AIIMS 2002]
8. **Assertion:** One of the defining property of living organisms is consciousness.
   Reason: Human being is the only organism that has self consciousness.
9. **Assertion:** Living organisms are self replicating, evolving and self regulating unit.
   Reason: These are capable of responding to external stimuli.
10. **Assertion:** All organisms reproduce for perpetuation of a population.
    Reason: Reproduction is an all inclusive characteristic of living organisms.
11. **Assertion:** Living organisms possess specific individuality with the definite shape and size.
    Reason: Both living and non living entities resemble each other at the lower level of organization.
12. **Assertion:** The growth in living organisms is from inside.
    Reason : Plants grow only upto certain age.
13. **Assertion:** Growth in living organism occurs by division of cells and increase in biomass.
    Reason: Growth in living organism occurs by accumulation of material by external agency.
14. **Assertion:** Consciousness and response to stimuli can be considered as defining property of living organism.
    Reason: The external environmental stimuli can be physical, chemical or biological.
15. **Assertion:** Reproduction cannot be refered as defining property of living organism.
    Reason: There are some living organism that do not reproduce e.g. mules, worker bees, infertile human, etc.
16. **Assertion:** A living organism is unexceptionally differentiated from a non living structure in the basis of responsiveness.
    Reason: Response to stimuli is a defining property of living organism.

17. **Assertion:** In fungi, vegetative reproduction occurs by fragmentation and budding.
Reason: Asexual reproduction in fungi, occurs through formation of asexual spores.

18. **Assertion :** Whittaker's classification for algae is not acceptable.
Reason : Whittaker grouped algae in different kingdoms.

19. **Assertion :** Systematics is the branch of biology that deals with classification of living organisms.
Reason : The aim of classification is to group the organisms.

20. **Assertion :** To give scientific name to plant, there is ICBN.
Reason : It uses articles, photographs and recommendations to name a plant.

21. **Assertion:** Systematics is defined as the science of diversity of organisms in evolutionary context.
Reason: It includes inter-relationship between organisms.

22. **Assertion:** New names in binomial nomenclature are derived from Latin or are latinised.
Reason: Latin is a technical language.

23. **Assertion:** Both words are separately underlined in binomial nomenclature.
Reason: Underlining indicates their Latin origin.

24. **Assertion:** Classification is necessary to study all living organisms.
Reason: Individuals are grouped into categories in classification.

25. **Assertion:** Binomial nomenclature is system of providing name with two.
Reason: Each name consists first of a specific name and second of a generic name.

26. **Assertion:** Unicellular green algae were not included in protista by Whitttaker.
Reason: Distinction between unicellular and multicellular organisms is not possible in case of algae.

27. **Assertion:** ICBN is responsible for giving scientific name to plant.
Reason: It uses articles, photographs and recommendations to name a plant.

28. **Assertion :** Formation of new species is called speciation.
Reason : The deme has a common gene pool.

29. **Assertion :** Phylogeny is the developmental history of a species.
Reason : Species is the basic unit of taxonomy.

30. **Assertion :** Taxon and category are different things.
Reason : Category shows hierarchical classification.

31. **Assertion :** The hierarchy includes seven obligate categories.
Reason : Intermediate categories are used to make taxonomic positions more informative.

32. **Assertion :**The species is reproductively isolated natural population.
Reason : Prokaryotes cannot be kept under different species on the basis of reproductive isolation.

33. **Assertion:** There are some similarities between cats and dogs.
Reason: Cats and dogs belong to the same family Canidae.

34. **Assertion:** Order is a taxonomic category that includes one or more genera.
Reason: All the genera in an order have some similar features and correlated characters.

35. **Assertion:** Whittaker's classification for algae is not accepable.
Reason: Whittaker grouped algae in different kingdoms.

36. **Assertion:** The hierachy includes seven obligate categories.
Reason: Intermediate categories are used to make taxonomic positions more informative.

37. **Assertion:** Bacteria, Protista do not have circulatory system.
Reason: These organisms live in moist and watery environment.

38. **Assertion:** The scientific terms for the categories like dogs, cats, mammals, plants, animals etc. is taxa.
Reason: The taxa can indicate categories at very different level.

39. **Assertion:** The family Solanaceae includes a number of genera like *Solanum, Petunia, Atropa,* etc.
Reason: Family contains one or more related genera.

40. **Assertion:** Species constitute a group of individuals with fundamental similarities.

Reason: *Indica, leo, tuberosum* represent such group of individuals.

41. **Assertion:** Flora contains the actual account of habitat and distribution of plants of a given area.

Reason: Monographs contain detailed information on any taxon.

42. **Assertion:** Botanical gardens are grown for educational and scientific purposes.

Reason: Zoological parks are the places where wild animals are kept in protected environments.

43. **Assertion:** Herbarium sheets carry a label.

Reason: Label provides information about data and place of collection.

44. **Assertion:** Herbarium is also known as "Dry garden"

Reason: It is a collection of plant parts that have been dried, pressed, preserved on sheets.

45. **Assertion:** Keys are analytical in nature.

Reason: These are based on couplet.

46. **Assertion:** Information for identification of names of species is provided by monographs.

Reason: Monographs contain information on more than one taxon.

Solutions

1. (a) Biology (Bio-living, logy-science). The study of living beings is called biology. Living beings on earth are mainly classified into two forms-plants and animals. Botany and zoology are the fundamental branches of biology. Word botany has been derived from greek word *botane* which means pasture or plants and zoology has been derived from word zoo-animals, logos-study. Theophrastus and Aristotle is called the father of botany and father of zoology respectively.
2. (b) Anatomy is the study of internal structure which can be observed with unaided eye after dissection. By studying anatomy of large number of organisms, it is useful for knowing phylogenetic similarity (homology) and phylogenetic dissimilarity (analogy).
3. (c) Taxonomy is the science of identification, nomenclature and classification of organisms. But taxonomy and systematics are different terms. Systematics is the branch of biology that deals with diversity of organisms at every level of classification.
4. (b) All the members of a species have similar karyotype (cytotaxonomy) - there is similarity in the number, size, shape and behaviour of chromosomes. At the molecular level, there is similarity in the types of proteins, enzymes, hormones and other biochemicals.
5. (d) Living organisms are regarded as open system as energy flow is the key function of an ecosystem.
6. (d) Living organisms show internal growth due to addition of materials and formation of cells inside the body. Such a method is called intussusception. While, non-living things grow due to addition of similar materials to their outer surface. The process is called accretion.
7. (b) All living organisms are made of chemicals. These chemicals, small and big, belonging to various classes, sizes, functions, etc., are constantly being made and changed into some other biomolecules. These conversions are chemical reactions or metabolic reactions. There are thousands of metabolic reactions occurring simultaneously inside all living organisms, be they unicellular or multicellular.
8. (b) All living organisms have an inherent ability to sense their surroundings or environment and respond to their environmental stimuli. Plants and animals both respond to the external stimuli. Responses of animals are rapid and can easily be observed because they escape by moving away from the site or environmental stress. The plants, on the other hand, cannot move. They face the stresses and adapt themselves by their slow physiological responses. Human beings are slightly different. They are the only organisms who are aware of themselves, i. e., have self -consciousness.
9. (b) Living beings are objects exhibiting growth, development, responsiveness and other characteristics of life. They have their own specific form and structure. Living organisms exhibit properties such as metabolism, growth, reproduction, consciousness, etc. Thus, living organisms are considered as self replicating, evolving and self regulatory interactive systems capable of responding to external stimuli, sharing a common genetic material to varying degree both horizontally and vertically.
10. (d) Reproduction is the formation of new individuals of the similar kind. Reproduction is not essential for survival of the individuals. It is required for perpetuation of a population. Many organisms do not reproduce, e.g., mules, sterile worker bees, infertile human couples. Therefore, reproduction is not an all inclusive characteristic of living organism.

11. (b) Both living and non-living entities resemble each other at the lower level of organization.

12. (c) Growth is the act or process, or a manner of growing; development; gradual increase. It is an exclusive event in majority of the higher animals and plants. In plants, growth occurs continuously throughout their life span and in animal, growth is seen only up to a certain age. In living organisms, growth is from inside. Therefore, it cannot be taken as a defining property of living organisms.

13. (d) Accumulation of material by external agency cause extrinsic growth which can not be the feature of living organism.

14. (b) All organisms, from primitive prokaryotes to most advanced and complex eukaryotes, are able to sense and respond to environmental factors. The stimuli are perceived by sense organs in higher animals through sensory receptors e.g. eyes, ears, nose. Plants do not possess such sense organs. However, they do respond to external factors such as light, water, temperature, pollutants, other organism, etc. Human beings have an additional facility of self conciousness (awareness of self). Consciousness and response to stimuli are said to be the defining properties of living organisms.

15. (d) A mule is a hybrid of male donkey and female horse. It inherited size and intelligence from the horse and firm footedness, great tolerance and ability to live on rough food from the donkey. However, with all its hybrid vigour, the mule is sexually sterile (i.e. unable to reproduce) and have to be produced every time anew. Honey bees are colonial, social and polymorphic insects. Three types of individuals (castes) are found in the colony of honey bees: (i) Queen which is fertile female. (ii) Drones which are males. (iii) Workers are sterile females and perform various duties of the colony.
A large number of couples are infertile. It means they are unable to produce children inspite of unprotected sexual activities. Thus, inability to conceive or produce children even after unprotected sexual cohabitation is called as infertility.

16. (a) All organisms from primitive prokaryotes to most advanced and complex eukryotes are able to sense and respond to environmental factors. The stimuli are perceived by sense organs in higher animals through sensory receptors. Consciousness and response to stimuli are said to be the defining properties of living organism.

17. (b) In fungi, vegetative reproduction occurs by fragmentation, budding (yeast), sclerotia, rhizomorphs, etc. Asexual reproduction occurs through formation of asexual spores such as zoospores, sporangiospores, chlamydospores, oidia, coidia, etc.

18. (a) In Whittaker's classification, algae are grouped in three kingdoms - Monera (blue-green algae), Protista (dinoflagellates, diatoms, euglenoids) and Plantae (red algae, brown algae and green algae). Though plant kingdom of Whittaker is often called metaphyta or multicellular plants, the algae included in this kingdom also contain a number of unicellular and colonial forms. The most accepted classification of algae is given by Fritsch. He classified all algae into 11 classes.

19. (b) Systematics is related with classification, of organisms. In classification, the organisms are grouped on the basis of their characters or phylogeny, etc.

20. (a) Anyone can study, describe, identify and give a name to an organism provided certain rules are followed. These rules are formed and standardised by International Code of Botanical Nomenclature (ICBN). It uses articles, photographs and recommendations.

21. (b) Simpson (1961) has defined systematics as the branch of biology that deals with the diversity of organism at every level of classification. It deals with cataloging plants, animals and other organisms into categories that can be named, remembered, compared and studied. Study of only one organism of a group provides sufficient

information about the remaining members of that group. It also helps in developing evolutionary relationships with or without the help of taxonomic studies of fossils.

22. (c) Binomial nomenclature is the system of providing organisms with appropriate and distinct names consisting of two were taken from Latin and Greek languages. New names are now derived either from Latin language or are latinised. This is because Latin language is dead and, therefore, it will not change in form or spelling with passage of time.

23. (a) Both the words in binomial nomenclature when handwritten, are separately underlined, or printed in italics to indicate their latin origin.

24. (a) It is nearly impossible to study all the living organisms. Classification refers to the process by which individuals are grouped into categories. So, classification makes it possible to study all the living organisms by studying the categorywise characteristics

25. (c) Binomial nomenclature is the system of providing organisms with appropriate and distinct names consisting of two words, first generic and second specific.

26. (a) Unicellular green algae were not included in protista by Whittaker. Distinction between unicellular and multicellular organism is not possible in case of algae.

27. (a) International Code of Botanical Nomenclature (ICBN) is responsible for giving scientific name to plants. It uses articles, photos and recommendations to plant.

28. (b) All new species develop from the pre-existing species. The phenomenon of development of a new species from pre-existing one is called speciation. A species is a collections of demes. The deme is a groups of populations with a common gene pool.

29. (b) Phylogeny is the developmental history of a species or a group of species. Species is the basic unit of taxonomy. It is a natural population of individuals or group of population which resemble one another in all essential morphological and reproductive characters so that they are able to interbreed freely and produce fertile offspring.

30. (a) A category is a rank or level in the hierarchial classification of organisms. Taxon is a unit in classification which may represent any level of grouping of organisms based on certain common characteristics. There is some confusion in the use of taxon and category, for example Bryophyta is a taxon while division is a category.

31. (b) The hierarchy includes seven obligate categories - kingdom, division or phylum, class, order, family, genus and species. In order to make taxonomic position of species more precise, certain categories have been added to this list. They are called intermediate categories, *e.g.*, subkingdom, superphylum or superdivision, superclass, subclass, superorder, suborder, superfamily, subfamily, tribe, subspecies, variety etc.

32. (b) The species is genetically distinct and reproductively isolated natural population. Sexual reproduction is absent in prokaryotes and some protists. In such cases, morphological differences, cytotaxonomy and chemo-taxonomy are resorted to.

33. (c) Family is a group of related genera with still less number of similarities as compared to genus and species e.g., a cat and a dog, have some similarities and some differences as well. They are separated into two different families - Felidae and Canidae, respectively.

34. (d) Family is a taxonomic category which contains one or more related genera. All the genera of a family have some common features or co-related characters. Whereas, order includes one or more related families.

35. (a) R.H. Whittaker (1969), an American Taxonomist, classified all organisms into five kingdoms: Monera, Protista, Fungi, Plantae and Animal. Plantae includes green algae, brown algae, red algae, bryophytes, pteridophytes, gymnosperms and angiosperms.

36. (b) Taxonomy is based on a hierarchy of classification; the lower you go in the hierarchy, the more closely related the living things are. These groups, from largest to smallest are Kingdom, Phylum, Class, Order, Family, Genus, and Species. Intermediate categories are used to make taxonomic positions more informative.

37. (b) In animals that do not contain a circulatory system, the transport of substances occurs by cell to cell diffusion. Bacteria, Protista do not have circulatory system. These organisms live in moist and watery environment.

38. (a) To study the organism dogs, cats, mammals, wheat, rice, plants, animals, etc. are convenient categories. Plants, animals, mammals, dogs, etc. all are taxa, which represent taxa at different levels.

39. (a) Family is a taxonomic category which contains one or more related genera. All the genera of a family have some common features and they are seperable from genera of a related family by important characteristics. The family Solanaceae includes a number of genera like *Solanum, Petunia, Atropa,* etc. due to certain similarities.

40. (b) Species refer to a group of organisms with fundamental similarities. A species is distinguished from the other closely related species based on distinct morphological differences. e.g., *Mangifera indica* (Mango), *Solanum tuberosum* (potato) and *Panthera leo* (lion). Therefore, all the three names, *indica*, *tuberosum* and *leo*, represent the specific epithets, while the first words *Mangifera*, *Solanum* and *Panthera* are genera.

41. (b) Floras, manuals, monographs, etc. are some important taxonomic aids that help in the correct identification. Flora provide the index to the plant species found in a particular area. Manuals are useful in providing information for identification of names of species found in an area. Monographs have information of any taxon.

42. (b) Botanical gardens are sufficiently large sized tracts where plants of various types and areas are grown for scientific and educational purposes. Zoological parks are the places where wild animals are kept in protected environments under human care and which enable us to learn about their food habits and behavior.

43. (a) A herbarium is a collection of preserved plant specimens and associated data used for scientific study. It carries a label. It provides information about data and place of collection.

44. (a) Herbarium is also known as "Dry garden". It is a collection of plant parts that have been dried, pressed and preserved on sheets. The procedure of pressing and drying specimens for storage has been an amazingly successful one in terms of preservation of detail and specimen longevity, and the plants so preserved provide a concrete basis for past, present and future studies.

45. (b) Key is a taxonomical aid used for identification of plants and animals based on the similarities and dissimilarities. The keys are based on contrasting characters generally in a pair called couplet. Keys are generally analytical in nature.

46. (d) Manuals are useful in providing information for identification of names of species found in an area. Monographs contain information on any one taxon.

Chapter 2

Biological Classification

Directions: In the following questions, a statement of assertion is followed by a statement of reason. Mark the correct choice as:

(a) If both Assertion and Reason are true and Reason is the correct explanation of Assertion.

(b) If both Assertion and Reason are true but Reason is not the correct explanation of Assertion.

(c) If Assertion is true but Reason is false.

(d) If both Assertion and Reason are false.

1. **Assertion :** Bacteria are prokaryotic.
Reason : Bacteria do not possess true nucleus and membrane bound cell organelles.

2. **Assertion :** Bacterial photosynthesis occurs by utilizing wavelength longer than 700 nm.
Reason : Here reaction centre is P-890.

3. **Assertion :** Sandfly transmits Kala-azar.
Reason : In Kala-azar, the parasite damages the brain.

4. **Assertion :** *Escherichia coli*, *Shigella* sp. and *Salmonella* sp. are all responsible for diarrhoeal diseases.
Reason : Dehydration is common to all types of diarrhoeal diseases and adequate supply of fluids and electrolytes should be ensured.

5. **Assertion :** Gram-negative bacteria do not retain the stain when washed with alcohol.
Reason : The outer face of the outer membrane of gram-negative bacteria contains lipopolysaccharides, a part of which is integrated into the membrane lipids.

6. **Assertion:** Two kingdom classification was insufficient.
Reason: Majority of organisms failed to fall into either of the categories in two kingdom classification.

7. **Assertion:** Archaebacteria are able to survive in harsh habitats.
Reason: Archaebacteria survive in extreme conditions due to the presence of peptidoglycan in their cell wall.

8. **Assertion:** Several ruminant animals contain methanogens within their gut.
Reason: Methanogens help in the production of methane from dung of ruminants.

9. **Assertion:** The nitrogen-fixing bacteria in leguminous plant nodules live as symbionts.
Reason: Leg-haemoglobin synthesized by leguminous plants protect bacteria.

10. **Assertion:** Bacteria are classified among plants.
Reason: They have cell walls.

11. **Assertion:** Bacteria do not always move with the help of flagella.
Reason: Rotary motion of flagellum is employed by flagellated bacteria for movement.

12. **Assertion:** Some bacteria have the capacity to retain Gram stain after treatment with acid alcohol.
Reason: They are known as gram positive as they are attracted towards positive pole under influence of electric current.

13. **Assertion:** Chemosynthesis is not carried out by autotrophic bacteria.
Reason: Chemosynthetic bacteria trap the small amount of energy released from inorganic compound's oxidation to use in the reactions that synthesize carbohydrates.

14. **Assertion :** Exotoxins are released by Gram +ve bacteria causing diseases to animals.
Reason: Exotoxins are proteins that react with WBC of animals.

15. **Assertion:** All food chains will come to stand still if bacteria disappear from earth.
Reason: Bacteria are only associated with the soil fertility and hardly any role for food chains.

16. **Assertion:** Broad spectrum antibiotics are produced by *Streptomyces*.
Reason: Antibiotics can destroy microorganisms by inhibiting DNA replication or protein synthesis.

17. **Assertion:** Bacterial cell wall is characterised by having mucopolysaccharides.
Reason: Acetyl muramic acid is an example of mucopolysaccharide.

18. **Assertion:** *Anabaena* inhabits root nodules of leguminous plants .
Reason: Leguminous plants are an example of symbiotic nitrogen fixation.

19. **Assertion:** *Bacillus butschli* is true bacterium.
Reason: Its cell wall is composed of acetyl muramic acid.

20. **Assertion:** Pili are motile appendages found in some bacteria.
Reason: These participate in conjugation.

21. **Assertion:** Cell secretion does not occur in bacteria.
Reason: Golgi complex is absent in bacteria.

22. **Assertion:** Methanogens are obligate anaerobes.
Reason: Halophiles are salt loving bacteria.

23. **Assertion:** Cyanobacteria are unicellular and colonial.
Reason: Blue green algae are chemosynthetic.

24. **Assertion:** Cyanobacteria are photosynthetic autotrophs.
Reason: Cyanobacteria have chlorophyll a and b similar to green plants.

25. **Assertion :** Plasmids are double-stranded extra chromosomal DNA.
Reason: Plasmids are possessed by eukaryotic cells.

26. **Assertion :** *Euglena* is studied as an animal as well as a plant.
Reason :*Euglena* is more an animal than a plant.

27. **Assertion :** *Amoeba* contains a contractile vacuole.
Reason : It helps in both digestion and osmoregulation.

28. **Assertion :** Chemosynthesis is an autotrophic nutrition.
Reason : Chemoautotrophs contain chlorophyll pigments.

29. **Assertion:** Cell wall of chrysophytes are indestructible.
Reason: Cell walls of chrysophytes have layer of magnesium pectate embedded in it.

30. **Assertion:** The protoplasm of plasmodial slime mould is considered purest in the world.
Reason: Protoplasm of plasmodium is differentiated into an outer enucleated and central nucleated portions.

31. **Assertion:** Sporozoans may have silica shells on their surface.
Reason: Shells of sporozoans render protection from acidic environment of the host.

32. **Assertion:** *Euglena* is called as plant animal.
Reason: Pellicle of *Euglena* is made up of cellulose and not protein.

33. **Assertion:** Chemosynthetic autotrophic bacteria oxidise various inorganic substances.
Reason: Energy released during oxidation is used in ATP production.

34. **Assertion:** Slime moulds show alternation of generation.
Reason: The sporangia bearing slime moulds represent haplophase.

35. **Assertion:** *Trichomonas vaginalis* causes infection only in women.
Reason: *Trichomonas buccalis* lives in the buccal cavity.

36. **Assertion:** Erythrocytic merozoites form gametocytes.
Reason: Gametocytes are of two types - male and female.

37. **Assertion:** *Plasmodium* causes disease in female *Anopheles* mosquitoes.
Reason: Female *Anopheles* mosquitoes feed on plasmodial blood.

38. **Assertion:** Malarial fever appear at merozoite stage of *Plasmodium.*
Reason: The infective stage of *Plasmodium* is sporozoite.

39. **Assertion:** Schizogony is an asexual reproduction of female *Anopheles* mosquito.
Reason: It takes place only in human liver cells.

40. **Assertion:** Kingdom-Protista forms a link between monerans and and the other organism like plants, animal and fungi.
Reason: Protist reproduce sexually and asexually by a process involving cell fusion and zygote formation.

41. **Assertion:** *Euglena* cannot be classified on the basis of two kingdom system.
Reason: *Euglena* is a plant due to presence of chlorophyll.

42. **Assertion:** The protist feeds on red blood corpuscles.
Reason: Amoebiasis is caused by *Amoeba*.

43. **Assertion :** Aflatoxins are produced by *Aspergillus flavus.*
Reason : These toxins are useful to mankind.

44. **Assertion :** *Saccharomyces ellipsoidens* is Wine yeast and *Saccharomyces cerevisiae* is Baker's yeast.
Reason : Yeast is used to make dry ice.

45. **Assertion :** *Neurospora* is commonly called water mould.
Reason : It belongs to basidomycetes fungi.

46. **Assertion:** Phycomycetes are commonly known as sac fungi.
Reason: In phycomycetes, ascospore (sexual spores) are produced endogenously in sac like asci.

47. **Assertion:** Deuteromycetes is known as fungi imperfecti.
Reason: In Deuteromycetes, only the asexual phase is known.

48. **Assertion:** "Fungi imperfecti" does not show alternation of generation.
Reason: The diploid phase is present in only zygote.

49. **Assertion:** *Rhizopus* and *Mucor* are used in liquor industry.
Reason: These cause fermentation.

50. **Assertion:** Morels and Truffles are edible fungi.
Reason: Ascocarps are edible.

51. **Assertion:** Yeast are the best source of vitamin B complex.
Reason: *Ashbya gossypii* is a filamentous yeast.

52. **Assertion:** *Claviceps* produces lysergic acid.
Reason: It is carcinogenic.

53. **Assertion:** Mushrooms are called fairy rings.
Reason: Mushroom consists of two parts-stipe and pileus.

54. **Assertion:** Actinomycetes are mycelial bacteria.
Reason: They are called ray fungi.

55. **Assertion :** Symbiosis is furnished by mycorrhiza.
Reason : In mycorrhiza, symbiosis is established between fungus and alga.

56. **Assertion:** Viruses are nucleoproteins and lack cell organelle, *etc.*
Reason: Viruses are not considered organism.
[AIIMS 1998]

57. **Assertion :** TMV is a virus which causes mosaic disease.
Reason : TMV has RNA as genetic material.
[AIIMS 2001]

58. **Assertion:** Mycoplasmas are pathogenic in animals and plants.
Reason: Mycoplasmas lack cell wall and can survive without oxygen.

59. **Assertion:** "Contagium Vivum Pasteur Fluidum" was coined by Pasteur.
Reason: Pasteur found that virus infected plant of tobacco can cause infection in healthy plant.

60. **Assertion:** Virus is an obligate parasite.
Reason: Virus is host specific.

61. **Assertion:** In lichens, mycobiont and phycobiont are symbiotically associated in algae which is predominant and fungi is a subordinate partner.
Reason: In this symbiotic association, the fungus provides food while the alga protects fungus from unfavourable conditions.

62. **Assertion:** These lichens are upright and have pendulous organisation and are attached to substratum by a discoid structure.
Reason: Fruticose are well branched leafy lichens.

Solutions

1. **(a)** Bacterial cell is prokaryotic. It lacks true nucleus and membrane bound organelles.
2. **(b)** Bacteria utilize the wavelengths longer than 700 nm for photosynthesis and the reaction centre is P-890 the reductant is NADH + H^+. In bacteria, donor may be H_2S or malate or succinate.
3. **(c)** *Leishmania donovani* causes kala-azar. The parasite is transmitted by sandfly. The parasite lives inside the cells of liver, spleen, lymph glands, white blood corpuscles and inner wall cells of blood capillaries. In sleeping sickness disease, the parasite damages the brain.
4. **(b)** *E. coli*, *Shigella sp.* and *Salmonella sp.* causes diarrhoea. It is due to intake of contaminated water.
5. **(a)** Gram negative bacteria contain lipopolysaccharide in its membrane.
6. **(a)** Two kingdom classification (founded by Linnaeus) worked well for a long time. However, this system failed to distinguish between the eukaryotes and prokaryotes, unicellular and multicellular organisms, photosynthetic and non-photosynthetic organisms. Although, classification of organisms (into plants and animals) was easily done and was easy to understand, but a large number of organisms did not fall into either category. Hence, the two kingdom classification used for a long time was found inadequate.
7. **(c)** Archaebacteria are special since they live in some of the most harsh habitats such as extreme salty areas (halophiles), hot springs (thermoacidophiles) and marshy areas (methanogens). Archaebacteria differ from other bacteria in having a different cell wall structure and this feature is responsible for their survival in extreme conditions. Archaebacteria are characterised by absence of peptidoglycan in their cell wall. Instead cell wall contains protein and non cellulosic polysaccharide.
8. **(b)** Methanogens occur in marshy areas where they convert formic acid and carbon dioxide into methane with the help of hydrogen. Some of the methanogen archaebacteria live as symbionts (e.g., *Methanobacterium*) inside rumen or first chamber in the stomach of herbivorous animals that chew their cud (ruminants, e.g., cow, buffalo) and thus, helps in production of methane from dung of these animals. These archaebacteria are helpful to the ruminants in fermentation of cellulose.
9. **(a)** *Rhizobium* form a symbiotic association with roots of leguminous plants producing root nodules. These bacteria reside inside the nodules and reduce atmospheric nitrogen (N_2) to ammonia. The fixed nitrogen is taken up by plant. In return, the plant provides both nutrients and protection to bacteria.
10. **(a)** Plant cells are characterized by the presence of a rigid cell wall on the basis of which they can be differentiated from animal cells. Hence, in two kingdom classification, bacteria were classified among plants. However, according to the five-kingdom classification, bacteria are grouped under kingdom Monera.
11. **(b)** Myxobacteria do not have flagella and move by gliding movement.
12. **(c)** The cell wall of Gram-negative bacteria contains alcohol-soluble lipid, while the cell wall of Gram-positive bacteria lacks the lipids and therefore resist decolourisation and retain the primary stain, appearing violet. Gram-negative bacteria are decolorized by organic solvents and therefore, take the counter stain, appearing red. Gram + ve bacteria are not attracted towards positive pole under influence of electric current.
13. **(d)** Chemosynthetic bacteria are without photosynthetic pigments. For the synthesis of their own organic food (carbohydrates), they obtain carbon from

CO_2 of the atmosphere and necessary energy from oxidation of inorganic or organic compounds, such as hydrogen sulphide (H_2S), ferrous compounds (Fe^{2+}), molecular hydrogen (H_2), ammonia (NH_3) and nitrites (NO_2^-).

14. (a) Mostly pathogenic gram +ve bacteria releases exotoxins outside the cell thus, killing the W.B.C. and causing disease.

15. (c) Bacteria play an important and dual role by disposing off the dead bodies and wastes of organism and by increasing the fertility of soil.

16. (a) *Streptomyces* is used for production of broad spectrum antibiotics where living microorganism is capable of inhibiting or destroying other many types of microbes.

17. (d) Chemically bacteria consists of acetylglycosamine, acetyl muramic acid and a peptide chain of four or five amino acids. All these chemicals together form a polymer called peptidoglycan (= murein or mucopeptide). Some other chemical substances deposited on the cell wall are - teichoic acid, protein, polysaccharides, lipoproteins and lipopolysaccharides.

18. (a) *Anabaena* found symbiotically in the root nodules of many leguminous plants helps in N_2 fixation.

19. (a) *Bacillus butschli* is the Gram positive bacterium and its cell wall consist of acetyl muramic acid.

20. (a) In some bacteria, nonmotile appendages called pili or fimbriae are also present. They take part in sexual reproduction, i.e., conjugation.

21. (a) Cell secretion occurs even in the prokaryotic cells (bacteria) in relation to the production of a variety of enzyme in the medium. While, golgi complex and other membrane bound organelles are absent in prokaryotes.

22. (b) Methanogens are obligate anaerobes and used in biogas fermenters to produce methane. e.g. *Methanobacterium*, *Methanococcus*, etc. Halophiles are salt loving bacteria as they are found in to live in environments with a very high salt concentration.

23. (c) Cyanobacteria or Blue green algae are photosynthetic prokaryotes with chlorophyll a, carotenoids and phycobillins. They may be unicellular, colonial or filamentous and marine or terrestrial.

24. (c) Cyanobacteria (also referred to as blue-green algae) are photosynthetic autotrophs. They have chlorophyll a similar to green plants.

25. (c) In addition of bacterial chromosomes, many bacteria have accessory rings of DNA called plasmids. Plasmids are absent in eukaryotic chromosome.

26. (b) *Euglena* is a typical example of mastigophora. It is phytoflagellate as it possesses both chloroplast and flagella. It is autotrophic in sunlight, but becomes heterotrophic in dark. Because of its two fold nutritional abilities, it is usually studied as a plant as well as an animal. But it is more an animal than plant because of

(a) The absence of cellulose cell wall overlying the plasma membrane.

(b) Presence of centriole.

(c) Reserve food is paramylon which is not a true starch.

(d) Response to various stimuli like an animal.

27. (c) Contractile vacuole in *Amoeba* is a single, clear, rounded, pulsating structure which is filled with a watery fluid and enclosed by a unit membrane. It helps in the osmoregulation and excretory activities. Digestion in *Amoeba* occurs in the food vacuoles. These are spherical species small and large, contain water and food in various phases of digestion. As soon as the egestion of non digestible food occurs through body, these disappear.

28. (b) Chemoautotrophs developed the ability to synthesize organic molecules from inorganic raw materials. Chlorophyll pigments are present in photoautotrophs. The photo-autotrophs utilize the solar energy absorbed by them in synthesizing organic compounds. Certain chemo-autotrophs include green sulphur bacteria.

29. (c) Chrysophytes include diatoms and golden algae (desmids). They are found in fresh water as well as in marine environments. The cell walls are embedded with silica and thus, the walls are indestructible.

30. (a) Vegetative part of slime moulds does not possess cell wall they either occur as free living amoeboid mass of protoplasm (plasmodium) or aggregation of amoebae (pseudoplasmodium). The protoplasm of plasmodial slime mould is considered as purest in the living world. It is differentiated into outer enucleated (hyaloplasm) and central nucleated portions. At maturity, it may contain several hundred to many thousand nuclei. The protoplasm is vacuolated.

31. (d) Sporozoans are endoparasites. Their body is covered with an elastic pellicle or cuticle. Thus, these do not have silica shells on their surface.

32. (c) *Euglena* is studied as plant as well as animal. It is called plant animal. Plant characters of *Euglena* are presence of chloroplasts with chlorophyll and holophytic (photosynthetic) nutrition in presence of light while, animal characters of *Euglena* are presence of pellicle which is made up of proteins and not of cellulose, presence of stigma and paraflagellar body (photosensitive structures), presence of contractile vacuole (not found in plants) and presence of longitudinal binary fission.

33. (b) Chemoautotrophic bacteria are able to manufacture their organic food from inorganic raw materials with the help of energy derived from exergonic chemical reactions involving oxidation of an inorganic substance present in the external medium. The chemical energy obtained from oxidation reaction is trapped in ATP molecules.

34. (a) Slime moulds exhibit alternation of generation. The diploid plasmodium is a sporophyte. Under certain conditions, it bears sporangia. These sporangia bearing plasmodium and spore producing sporangia constitute the sporophyte generation. It is a diplophase reduction division which takes place at the time of differentiation of resting spore. The resting spores germinate to produce the haploid, uninucleate swarm cells or myxamoebae. The latter meet and fuse in pairs to form a zygote. The haploid resting spores and the swarm cells or myxamoebae represent the haploid or gametophyte generation.

35. (b) *Trichomonas vaginalis* infects vagina of women and causes the disease known as leucorrhoea. In males, the parasite produces irritation in urethra. *Trichomonas buccalis* resides in the buccal cavity, which is nearly harmless.

36. (b) Some erythrocytic merozoites enter fresh RBCs and form rounded gametocytes (gamonts). The gametocytes are of two types – (i) Smaller male gametocytes or microgamete and (ii) Larger female gametocytes or macrogamete.

37. (d) The sexual phase of the malarial parasite occurs in the *Anopheles* mosquito. As the female *Anopheles* mosquitoes feed on blood, only they can serve as vector hosts of malarial parasites. The parasite does not harm the mosquito.

38. (b) When the mosquito bites man, sporozoites present in the salivary gland of female *Anopheles* mosquito are injected into the blood of the man. The erythrocytic schizont gives rise to merozoites. Malaria fever occurs when schizonts in red blood corpuscles burst and set free their contained merozoites and malarial pigment (haemozoin) in the blood plasma.

39. (c) Schizogony is an asexual reproduction in which schizont is formed. From the human blood, sporozoites enter the liver cells. The sporozoite grows in size to become a rounded schizont called cryptozoite. The latter divides to form cryptomerozoites. The cryptomerozoites formed during pre-erythrocytic schizogony may enter the human RBCs to start the erythrocytic schizogony, while some of them enter new liver cells to repeat hepatic (liver) schizogony.

40. (b) Phylogenetically the Kingdom-Protista acts as a connecting link between the prokaryotic Kingdom- Monera and the complex multicellular kingdom- Fungi, Plantae and Animalia. They reproduce asexually and sexually.

41. (c) *Euglena* is a green coloured, single celled organism, which moves like animals. Some taxonomists considered it as a plant and included it in the plant kingdom on the basis of chlorophyll, while other included it in the animal kingdom along with the flagellated protozoans because of the locomotion by flagella.

42. (c) Person suffering from amoebic dysentery has repeated blood mixed with slimy and foul smelling motions. The protist feeds on red blood corpuscles by damaging the wall of large intestine and reaching the blood capillaries.

43. (c) Aflatoxins, are produced by *Aspergillus flavus*. Contaminated food is the main source of infection. This toxin causes aflatoxicosis which may lead to haemorrhage and diseases of liver.

44. (b) The two common yeasts used by brewing industry are *Saccharomyces cerevisiae* (Beer or Baker's yeast) and *S. ellipsoidens* (Wine yeast). In the baking or brewing industry, CO_2 is the useful product. It is collected, solidified and sold as "dry ice".

45. (d) *Neurospora* belongs to class ascomycetes in which ascospores are produced in sac like asci . *Neurospora* is commonly called as pink or red bread mould. It can be grown easily in laboratory conditions so, used in genetics experiments.

46. (d) Ascomycetes is commonly known as sac-fungi. Sexual spores of Ascomycetes are produced endogenously in sac like asci. Members of Phycomycetes are found in aquatic habitats and on decaying wood in moist and damp places or as obligate parasites on plants.

47. (a) Deuteromycetes are commonly known as imperfect fungi because only the asexual or vegetative phases of these fungi are known and perfect or sexual stage is either absent or not known.

48. (c) Fungi imperfecti is that group of fungi where only the imperfect stage (asexual stages) is present. The only known method of reproduction is by conidia (asexual reproduction). As sexual reproduction is absent in this group therefore, diplophase is also absent.

49. (a) Both *Rhizopus* and *Mucor* species are used in alcoholic fermentation. Both of these produce a number of organic acids like citric acid, lactic acid and fumaric acid.

50. (a) The frutifications of some ascomycetes, i.e., ascocarps are edible, e.g., morels, truffles.

51. (b) Yeasts are the best sources of vitamin B complex. Riboflavin (B_6) is obtained from a filamentaous yeast, *Ashbya gossypii*.

52. (c) A derivative of ergot known by name of lysergic acid (LSD) is used in experimental psychiatry, as it is a hallucinogen.

53. (b) The basidiocarps or mushrooms often lie in rings. Therefore, these are also known as fairy rings. Each basidiocarp consists of two parts-stipe and pileus. The stipe or stalk is fleshy while, pileus is umbrella-like cap of the mushroom.

54. (a) Actinomycetes are mycelial (aseptate, branched filamentous) bacteria which form radiating colonies in culture hence, formerly called ray fungi. e.g. *Streptomyces*.

55. (c) Mycorrhiza represents mutualistic symbiosis between fungus and roots of higher plants. Fungus helps in absorption of minerals and water more efficiently and protect plant roots from infection. Fungus also gets food from plant.

56. (a) Virus is a small infectious agent that can only replicate inside the cells of another organism. Viruses are not considered as organisms as they have no independent machinery.

57. (b) In TMV, the chromosome consists of single stranded, linear RNA molecule coiled into a regular spiral. TMV causes mosaic disease in tobacco and some other plants.

58. (b) Mycoplasmas or mollicutes are the simplest and the smallest of free living prokaryotes, they can survive without oxygen. Mycoplasmas are heterotrophic in

their nutrition. Some of them live as saprophytes but majority parasitise plants and animals. The parasitic habit is due to the inability of the most mycoplasmas to synthesise the required growth factors.

59. (d) M.W. Beijerinek (1898) demonstrated that the extract of the infected plants of tobacco could cause infection in healthy plants and called the fluid as Contagium Vivum Fluidum (infectious living fluid).

60. (b) Virus is an obligate parasite. It is inert outside the host cell. A virus does not grow, divide or reproduce like typical organisms. Instead it multiplies by independent formation of its parts using host cell's machinery and then assembly of parts to produce virus particles. Viruses are host specific.

61. (d) Lichens are symbiotic associations i.e., mutually useful associations between algae and fungi. The algal component is known as phycobiont and fungal component as mycobiont, which are autotrophic and heterotrophic, respectively. Algae prepare food for fungi and fungi provide shelter and absorb mineral nutrients and water for its partner. Fungi dominate the relationship.

62. (c) Fruticose are well branched shruby lichens with upright and pendulous organization. These are attached to substratum by a discoid structure. Plant body can be divided into prostrate, leafy and lobed thallus.

Chapter 3

Plant Kingdom

Directions: In the following questions, a statement of assertion is followed by a statement of reason. Mark the correct choice as:

(a) If both Assertion and Reason are true and Reason is the correct explanation of Assertion.
(b) If both Assertion and Reason are true but Reason is not the correct explanation of Assertion.
(c) If Assertion is true but Reason is false.
(d) If both Assertion and Reason are false.

1. **Assertion :** Algae and fungi are grouped in thallophyta.
   Reason : Algae and fungi show no differentiation in thallus.
2. **Assertion :** *Chlorella* could be utilised to keep the air pure in space vehicles.
   Reason : The space travelers feed on *Chlorella* soup.
3. **Assertion :** Members of phaeophyceae vary in colour from olive green to various shades of brown
   Reason : Phaeophyceae possess chlorophyll a, c, carotenoids and xanthophylls. **[AIIMS 2006]**
4. **Assertion:** Rhodophyta is red in colour of due to abundant formation of r-phycoerythrin.
   Reason: r-phycoerythrin is able to absorb blue green wavelength of light and reflect red colour.
5. **Assertion:** The colour of brown algae varies from olive green to brown.
   Reason: In brown algae, fucoxanthin is responsible for colour variation.
6. **Assertion:** Plant body is usually grass green in colour in Chlorophyceae.
   Reason: Members of Chlorophyceae possess chlorophyll a, c, carotenoids and xanthophyll.
7. **Assertion:** *Chlorella* and *Spirulina* are used as a food supplement by space travellers.
   Reason: These are unicellular algae.
8. **Assertion:** Each group of algae show predominance of one pigment.
   Reason: The algae are classified on this basis.
9. **Assertion:** Only red algae are able to flourish at the great depths of sea.
   Reason: Red algae has the pigments r-phycoerythrin and r-phycocyanin.
10. **Assertion:** Carpogonium of red algae bears trichogyne.
    Reason: Trichogyne helps in reproduction.
11. **Assertion:** *Spirogyra* is slippery to touch.
    Reason: *Spirogyra* consists of a gelatinous sheath.
12. **Assertion:** Isogamy is a primitive type of sexual reproduction.
    Reason: The gametes are of different sizes.
13. **Assertion:** *Chlorella* could serve as a potential source of food and energy.
    Reason: *Chlorella,* when dried, has 15% protein, 45% fat, 10% carbohydrate, 20% fibre, and 10% minerals and vitamins.
14. **Assertion:** *Spirogyra* shows haplontic life cycle.
    Reason: Zygotic meiosis ocurs in *Spirogyra*.
15. **Assertion:** Red algae contributes in producing coral reef.
    Reason: Some red algae secrete and deposit calcium carbonate on their walls. **[AIIMS 2004, 2011]**
16. **Assertion:** In rhodophyceae, the cell wall is made of cellulose.
    Reason: The flagella number is two in class Rhodophyceae.
17. **Assertion :** Red algae contributes in producing coral reefs.
    Reason : Some red algae secrete and deposit calcium carbonate over their walls.
18. **Assertion:** Only anisogamous type of reproduction is seen in algae.
    Reason: Gametes can never be non-flagellated in algae.

19. **Assertion:** The peristome is a fringe of teeth-like projections found at the mouth of the capsule.
Reason: It may be of two types nematodontous and orthodontus.
20. **Assertion:** Mosses are of great ecological importance.
Reason: They prevent soil erosion by forming dense mat on the soil.
21. **Assertion :** Mosses are evolved from algae.
Reason : Protonema of mosses is similar to some green algae.
22. **Assertion:** In mosses, spores are contained within the capsule.
Reason: The spores are formed by mitotic division in mosses.
23. **Assertion:** Bryophytes are claimed to be terrestrial amphibians.
Reason: They require an external layer of water on the soil surface for their existence.
24. **Assertion:** Bryophytes and tracheophytes have an embryo stage in their life cycle.
Reason: Embryophyta are terrestrial plants.
25. **Assertion:** The sex organs in bryophytes are jacketed.
Reason: Bryophytes are land plants.
26. **Assertion:** Bryophytes are mostly land dwellers.
Reason: Water is necessary to complete their life-cycle.
27. **Assertion:** The bryophytes exist in two phases gametophyte and sporophyte.
Reason: The sporophyte is nutritionally independent.
28. **Assertion:** Bryophytes, unlike thallophytes, show formation of embryo.
Reason: The embryo gives rise to gametophyte of bryophytes.
29. **Assertion:** Archegonium is the female sex organ in bryophytes.
Reason: Algae also possess the archegonium.
30. **Assertion:** Bryophyte has an independent embryo.
Reason: The zygote of thallophyte is dependent.
31. **Assertion:** Liverworts fail to spread to a new locality through fragmentation.
Reason: Gemmae are helpful in propagating liverworts in different locality.
32. **Assertion:** Sperms of *Riccia* are biflagellate.
Reason: The sperms can swim.
33. **Assertion:** Among the liverworts, the sporogonium of *Riccia* is the simplest.
Reason: Sporophyte consists of capsule only.
34. **Assertion:** In *Funaria,* the young stem is photosynthetic.
Reason: It contain hydroids.
35. **Assertion:** *Funaria* multiplies vegetatively by means of bulbils.
Reason: Bulbils and tubers are two distinct structures.
36. **Assertion:** In *Funaria,* gemmae formation occurs in unfavourable condition.
Reason: The gemmae form on the stem and leaves.
37. **Assertion:** In *Funaria* is monoecious.
Reason: Cross fertilization occurs in *Funaria.*
38. **Assertion:** In *Funaria*, the antheridia are projected from surface.
Reason: Its antheridial cluster is surrounded by perigonial leaves.
39. **Assertion:** Mosses are used as indicators of pollution.
Reason: They absorb metals.
40. **Assertion:** Bryophytes and pteridophytes contain well-developed antheridia.
Reason: Biflagellate sperms are formed by their antheridia.
41. **Assertion:** In Liverworts, both male and female sex organs may be present on same thalli or different thalli.
Reason: A sporophyte is formed from the zygote which is differentiated into foot, seta and capsule.
42. **Assertion:** Bryophytes are known as the amphibians of plant kingdom.
Reason: They are found in swamps and the areas where land and water meet.
43. **Assertion:** Zygote produces a multicellular sporophyte in pteridophytes.
Reason: The dominant phase in life cycle of pteridophytes is sporophyte.
44. **Assertion:** *Selaginella* and *Salvinia* are homosporous.
Reason: In *Selaginella* and *Salvinia,* similar kind of spores are produced .
45. **Assertion:** The sorus of *Pteridium* is of coenosorus type.
Reason: *Pteridium* lacks sori.

46. **Assertion:** Coenosorus lacks true indusium.
Reason: Indusium covers sori.

47. **Assertion:** The scales which cover young rhizome and leaves of *Dryopteris* are called ramenta.
Reason: *Pteridium* lacks ramenta.

48. **Assertion:** The scale leaves present on the long shoots are called cataphylls.
Reason: Cataphylls lack mid rib.

49. **Assertion:** Water is required for fertilization process in ferns.
Reason: Malic acid of archegonial neck attracts antherozoids.

50. **Assertion:** Sporophytes of pteridophyta are dominant individuals.
Reason: They do not show the formation of true root.

51. **Assertion:** *Adiantum caudatum* is called walking fern.
Reason: It can reproduce by its leaf tips.

52. **Assertion :** *Pinus* displays the alternation of generations.
Reason : The gametophyte is dependent upon the sporophyte phase.

53. **Assertion :** Conifer trees produce a large quantity of wind borne pollen grains.
Reason : The pollen grains have wings.
[AIIMS 2007]

54. **Assertion:** Gymnosperms do not produce fruit.
Reason: Ovules of gymosperms are enclosed within the ovaries.

55. **Assertion:** Gametophyte is dominant in diplontic life cycle.
Reason: In diplontic life cycle, free living sporophyte is absent.

56. **Assertion:** In gymnosperms, stomata are found on the surface of leaves.
Reason: Cuticle of leaves is thin in gymnosperms.

57. **Assertion:** *Pinus* shows the alternation of generations.
Reason: The gametophyte is dependent upon the sporophyte phase.

58. **Assertion:** *Pinus* embryo has many cotyledons.
Reason: It shows polyembryony.

59. **Assertion:** The female cones take a long time to mature.
Reason: The seeds are shed when the cone is 22 months old.

60. **Assertion:** The female cones are same in number as the male cones.
Reason: Male and female cones appear alternately on the same branch of the *Pinus*.

61. **Assertion:** *Pinus* is monoecious.
Reason: Each sporophyll bears only one microsporangia.

62. **Assertion:** The mesophyll of *Pinus* shows no distinction as mesophyll and palisade.
Reason: Parenchymatous cells are present in mesophyll of *Pinus*.

63. **Assertion:** *Pinus* shows formation of annual rings.
Reason: It grows in areas of environmental fluctuation.

64. **Assertion:** In gymnosperms, plants lack well-developed vessels and fibres.
Reason: Companion cells are absent in gymnosperm.

65. **Assertion:** Gymnosperms seeds are naked.
Reason: They lack ovary wall.

66. **Assertion:** *Pinus* has a pyramidal appearance.
Reason: The older parts of long shoot have scars of fallen dwarf shoots.

67. **Assertion:** The female cone of *Cycas* is not a true cone.
Reason: Its formation checks the growth of the stem.

68. **Assertion:** All living species of *Cycas* are dioecious.
Reason: *Cycas* contains male and female cones on the separate plant.

69. **Assertion:** The male of *Cycas* changes in size when the microspores became mature.
Reason: The microspores are dispersed by wind.

70. **Assertion:** The leaves in gymnosperm are well adapted to withstand extremes of temperature, humidity and wind.
Reason: Unlike bryophytes and pteridophytes, in gymnosperms, the male and female gametophytes do not have an independent free living existence.

71. **Assertion:** The male and female gametophytes do not have independent existence in gymnosperms.
Reason: They remain within the sporangia retained on the sporophyte.

72. **Assertion :** Angiosperm and Gymnosperms both form spermatophyta.
Reason : Angiosperm and Gymnosperms both form triploid endosperm.

73. **Assertion:** Stamens are comparable to microsporophylls.
Reason: Ovules are comparable to megasporophylls.

74. **Assertion:** Biennial plants flower in two years.
Reason: Biennial plants live for two years.

75. **Assertion:** Flagellate male gametes are absent in angiosperms.
Reason: For fertilization, sperms are not dependent on water.

76. **Assertion:** Ovules form seeds upon fertilization.
Reason: Ripened ovary forms fruit.

77. **Assertion:** Pyrenoids are utilised during starvation.
Reason: Pyrenoids are proteinaceous bodies.

78. **Assertion:** The eye-spot is present in the cell in green algae.
Reason: Eye-spot is meant for respiration.

79. **Assertion:** Flower is an aggregation of sporophylls.
Reason: In angiosperms, sporophylls are modified.

80. **Assertion:** Plants show alternation of generation [between haploid gametophytic (n) phase and diploid sporophytic (2n) phase].
Reason: Plantae includes eukaryotic, heterotrophic, chlorophyll containing organism.

81. **Assertion:** Each cell of the embryo sac is haploid in angiosperms.
Reason: In angiosperms, meiosis preceeds embryo sac formation.

Solutions

1. (a) On the basis of
(i) Thallus like non-vascular plant body.
(ii) Simple, unicellular non-jacketed sex organs and
(iii) No embryo development after gametic union, the algae and fungi have long been grouped together in thallophyta. The algae and fungi are the result of parallel development and do not indicate any phylogenetic relationship.

2. (b) *Chlorella* could be utilised to keep the air in space vehicles pure and supply food in space stations and prolonged space flight trips. The space travellers could feed on *Chlorella* soup. It is nourishing but not appetizing food.

3. (a) Phaeophyceae possesses chlorophyll a, c, carotenoids and xanthophylls. Members of phaeophyceae show variations in colour from olive green to different shades of brown depending upon the amount of xanthophyll pigments.

4. (a) The red colour of Rhodophyta is due to abundan of the pigment r-phycoerythrin. Phycoerythrin absorbs blue green wavelengths of light and reflects red light where a imparts red colour to algae.

5. (b) Brown algae show a range of colour from olive green to various shades of brown depending upon the amount of fucoxanthin the xanthophyll pigment, present in them.

6. (c) Chlorophyceae are commonly called green algae. The plant body may be unicellular, colonial or filamentous. They are usually grass green in colour due to the dominance of pigments, chlorophyll a and b.

7. (b) Unicellular algae *Chlorella* and *Spirullina* are rich source of proteins and hence are used as food supplement by space travellers.

8. (a) The colour of the algal thallus is due to the presence of definite chemical compounds in their cells and varies in different classes of algae. These are called pigments. Each pigment has its own characteristic colour. The particular colour of an alga is due to the predominance of one pigment in a combination of several others. Each group of algae has its own particular combination of pigments and a characteristic colour which is not found in other algal groups.

9. (a) The red algae flourish and occur in abundance at great depths of sea where other plants do not. The sunlight, as it penetrates water, portions of spectrum such as red, orange, yellow and green light rays which are of short wavelengths are filtered out. Only the blue and violet rays of greater wavelengths remain and penetrate to great depths. The green pigment chlorophyll cannot trap these light rays of great wavelength and the green plants are thus, unable to carry on photosynthesis at these depths. The red pigment r-phycoerythrin and a blue pigment γ-phycocyanin which are characteristic pigments of all the red algae, can utilize wavelengths of light (blue and violet rays) not absorbed by chlorophyll.

10. (a) The carpogonium (female sex organ) in one of the simplest red alga *Nemalion*, consists of a swollen base containing the female nucleus and an elongated terminal hair-like structure called the trichogyne. During fertilization, the spermatium (male gamete) discharges its contents into the latter. The spermatium nucleus migrates downwards to fuse with the egg nucleus in the basal swollen part of the carpogonium. Soon after fertilization, the trichogyne disintegrates.

11. (a) The outermost portion of pectose changes into pectin in *Spirogyra*. The latter dissolves in water to form a gelatinous sheath which is slimy. It envelopes the entire filament. This makes filament slippery to touch.

12. (c) The fusing gametes in the lower forms of algae are similar in size, structure and behaviour. They are indistinguishable with respect to sex. Such gametes are called isogametes. Sexual reproduction involving the fusion of isogametes is termed isogamous. It is a primitive type of sexual reproduction.

13. (c) *Chlorella* could serve as a potential source of food and energy because of its photosynthetic efficiency. When dried, it has about 45% protein, 20%, fat, 20% carbohydrate, 5% fibre and 10% minerals and vitamins.

14. (a) Haplontic life cycle is characterized by a haploid thallus and zygotic meiosis. It is also called as haplobiontic because only a single type of free living individual is involved in the life cycle. *Spirogyra* shows haplontic life cycle and therefore, it shows zygotic nucleus as well.

15. (a) In some species of red algae, the cell walls become hardened with calcium carbonate. These algae are hence, important for the formation of coral reefs. Coral reefs are formed through the accumulation of calcareous exoskeletons of coral animals, calcareous red algae and molluscs. They form the foundation of reefs by secreting a calcium carbonate skeleton and provide protection for the coral polyps. Calcium carbonate is continuously secreted by the coral colony.

16. (c) Flagella is absent in class Rhodophyceae.

17. (a) Red algae generally grow attached to rocky stones. Some deep water red algae are calcareous and build up hard stony thalii responsible for the production of lime stones and coral reefs.

18. (a) In algae, sexual reproduction takes place by fusion of two gametes. These gametes can be flagellated and similar in size (*Chlamydomonas*) or non-flagellated (non-motile) but similar in size (*Spirogyra*). Such reproduction is called isogamous. Fusion of two gametes that are dissimilar in size, as in some species of *chlamydomonas* is termed as anisogamous. Fusion between one large, non-motile female gamete and a smaller, motile male gamete is termed oogamous.

19. (b) The peristome teeth are present at the mouth of capsule. The teeth may be solid cellular tissue or composed only of the thickened portions of the cell walls of adjacent cells. When the teeth of peristome are solid structures composed of bundles of dead cells, it is termed *nematodontous* peristome. It is found in *Polytrichum*, *Pogonatum* and *Tetraphis*. If peristome composed of thin, membranous, transversely barred teeth, each tooth is made up of the thickened portions of the cell walls of adjacent cells. Such a peristome is called orthodontous.

20. (b) Mosses and lichens are the first organisms to colonise rocks and hence, are of great ecological importance. They cause decomposition of rocks making the substrate suitable for the growth of higher plants. Mosses form dense mats on the soil, and reduce the impact of falling rain and prevent soil erosion.

21. (a) According to some botanists, mosses originated from algae. Protonema of mosses is similar to certain algae.

22. (c) In mosses, vegetative reproduction takes place by fragmentation and budding in the secondary protonema. The zygote develops into a sporophyte after fertilisation and consists of a foot, seta and capsule. The sporophyte in mosses is more elaborate as compared to that in liverworts. The capsule contains spores. Spores are formed after meiosis and develop into new gametophyte.

23. (a) Bryophytes require an external layer of water on the soil surface for their existence and thus are called terrestrial amphibians. The external supply of water is required for

(a) dehiscence of antheridia and archegonia

(b) swimming of male gametes to reach archegonia

(c) protection from transpiration and desiccation as the plant body is not covered by cuticle

(d) supply of water to all plants through capillarity in the absence of vascular tissues.

24. (b) Bryophytes and tracheophytes possess an embryo stage and are collectively called embryophyta. They are terrestrial plants. Bryophytes are nonvascular while tracheophytes possess vascular tissue.

25. (a) Bryophytes are a group of non-vascular land plants. The sex organs in the bryophytes are multicellular and jacketed. The jacket of sterile cells around the sperms and eggs is an adaptation to a land habitat. It protects the sex cells against the drying effects of air.

26. (b) Majority of the bryophytes are land dwellers and inhabit damp, shaded and humid localities. A few of them live in or float on water. The bryophytes cannot carry on their reproductive activities without sufficient moisture. Presence of water is necessary.

27. (c) The bryophytes have evolved a life which comprises of two phases-gametophyte and sporophytes. The gametophyte (haploid) is concerned with sexual reproduction and constitutes the most conspicuous, nutritionally independent phase in the life cycle. The sporophyte is partly or wholly dependent on the gametophyte for nutritional purpose.

28. (c) In thallophytes (algae and fungi), the formation of embryo is absent. In bryophytes, the zygote, on germination, does not produce the gametophyte plant. It undergoes segmentation to form an embryo. The embryo (diploid) by further segmentation and differentiation gives rise to sporophyte. The sporophyll obtains its nourishment directly from the parent gaemtophyte to which it is organically attached.

29. (c) Archegonium is the female sex organ of the bryophytes. It appears for the first time in the liverworts and mosses and continues in the pteridophytes. Archegonium is absent in thallophtes (algae and fungi). Sex organs in them are male gametes and female gametes.

30. (d) In bryophytes, the zygote, on germination, does not produce the gametophytic plant. It undergoes segmentation to form an embryo. But the embryo formation and its development to sporogonium and sporophyte are dependent on gametophyte plant as the sporophyte is dependent on the gametophyte for nutrition. They organically remain attached to the gametophytic plant. In algae, the zygote is independent and it does not form the sporophyte.

31. (b) Fragmentation leads to an increase in the number of plants in a locality but it does not permit the spread of the plant to an entirely new locality. Gemmae are easily carried as they are small and sufficiently buoyant. They spread by water and wind currents to new habitats when detached, where each grows into a new individual immediately.

32. (a) Each sperm of *Riccia* is a minute, slender and curved structure. It bears a pair of whiplash flagella at its anterior end. The sperms do not leave the antheridium until enough moisture is present that allow them to swim about.

33. (a) The sporogonium (capsule) of *Riccia* is the simplest among the liverworts. It lacks the foot and the seta. Elaters are absent. Unlike other liverworts, in *Riccia*, the embryo, sporogonium and spore mother cells develop no chloroplasts. Thus, no photosynthesis occurs there. The sporophyte is totally dependent upon the gametophytic thallus.

34. (b) The cortical cells in young stems of *Funaria,* contain chloroplasts, and thus, they are photosynthetic. The central cylinder forms the core of the stem. It consists of vertically elongated, thin-walled, narrow, compactly arranged cells lacking protoplasm. These thin walled, elongate, dead cells with non-lignified walls are commonly called as hydroids.

35. (c) In some mosses, the formation of small, underground resting, bud-like structures called the tubers has also been reported. Formerly, these underground bud-like structures were called the bulbils. The tubers develop singly on stem, leaves and rhizoids as small, spherical storage organs containing starch. These serve as means of perennation and enable the plant to survive over periods unfavourable for vegetative growth.

36. (b) In *Funaria*, the gemmae develop on the stem and leaves of the gametophore at the onset of conditions unfavourable for growth or during injury. These detached gemmae directly develop into new leafy gametophores under conditions favourable for vegetative growth.

37. (b) *Funaria* is monoecious. The antheridia (male sex organ) are formed at the summit of a relatively small, main leafy shoot which develops first from the parent plant.
The female branch arises later as a lateral outgrowth from the base of the parent male shoot. When the two kinds of the sex organs are borne in separate clusters on two distinct branches of the same plant, the arrangement is called monoecious.

38. (b) In *Funaria,* the antheridia project from the surface of the receptacle and are aggregated to form a cluster. The leaves surrounding the antheridial cluster are known as the perigonial leaves. The antheridial cluster with the surrounding perigonial leaves is called the perigonium.

39. (a) Rubling and Tyler (1979) showed that air dried mosses can absorb metals. The accumulation of heavy metal cations in mosses enables them to be used as pollution indicators.

40. (d) In bryophytes, antheridia are well developed and often possess a stalk. In pteridophytes, antheridia are less developed and are generally devoid of a stalk. Pteridophytes have multiflagellate sperm formed from androcyte cell of antheridium. Bryophytes have biflagellate sperm.

41. (b) In Liverworts, antheridia(male) are produced on antheridiophore and archegonia(female) are borne on special stalked structure called archegoniophore. Both male and female sex organs may be present on same thalli or different thalli. Sporophyte is formed from the zygote which is differentiated into foot, seta and capsule.

42. (b) Bryophytes are the dwellers of transitional habitat between the aquatic and terrestrial habitats. It is represented by the swamps and the areas where water and land meet. Bryophytes usually grow in amphibious situation and cannot complete their life cycle without external water.

43. (b) Gametophytes bear male and female sex organs called antheridia and archegonia, respectively in pteridophytes. Water is required for transfer of the male gametes released from the antheridia, to the mouth of archegonium. Fusion of male gamete with the egg present in the archegonium results in the formation of zygote. Zygote thereafter produces a multicellular well-differentiated sporophyte, the dominant phase of the pteridophtyes.

44. (d) All the spores are of similar kinds in majority of the pteridophytes; such plants are called homosporous. Genera like *Selaginella* and *Salvinia* produce two kinds of spores i.e. macro (large) spores and micro (small) spores, hence, are known as heterosporous.

45. (c) The sporangia of *Pteridium* are not grouped together in small seprate sori, but the sorus is continuous along the under margin of the pinnules, often for considerable distances. This type of sorus is known as continuous linear sorus (coenosorus).

46. (b) Indusium is an membranous epidermal outgrowth covering the sori in some ferns. The coenosorus is surrounded by two well formed indusial lips, between which the receptacle lies. The outer indusial lip is well-developed and is formed by the reflexed margin of the pinnule, which overlaps the coenosorus and its sporangia. This is commonly called the false indusium.

47. (b) In *Dryopteris,* young rhizome and leaves are covered with dry, brown, chaffy scales known as ramenta. In *Pteridium,* the rhizome and the leaves especially while young, are covered by a felt of simple hairs, and the scales are conspicuously absent.

48. (d) The scale leaves are present both on the long and dwarf branches. They fall off as the branches mature. The scale leaves on the dwarf shoots are called the cataphylls and possess a distinct midrib.

49. (c) In ferns, fertilization usually takes place if the prothalli are watered from above as they would be by rain in the ordinary course of nature. They possess flagella for swimming towards archegonia through water. The discharged matter at the mouth of the opened archegonial neck probably contains some chemical substance, e.g. malic acid, which by positive chemotaxis attracts the free swimming antherozoids, that penetrate the neck and reach the ovum which is deeply seated.

50. (c) In the pteridophytes, the sporophyte gains physiological independence and develops into the dominant, typically photosynthetic phase of the life cycle. It is organized into stem, leaves and roots. *Psilophyta* (a pteridophyte division) lack true roots.

51. (c) Leaf tips of *Adiantum caudatum*, develop adventitious buds for vegetative propagation. Leaf tip when reaches the ground, develops into new plant, therefore, it appears that the plant is walking.

52. (b) *Pinus* show alternation of generations. The sporophyte phase is of long duration and is represented by the huge pine tree, which bears the staminate and ovulate cones since meiotic divisions occur at the same time of the differentiation of the pollen grains and megaspores.

53. (a) In pinus, a conifer tree, the microspores are produced by microsporogenesis in microsporangium. Each microsporangium has an inner nourishing layer known as tapetum. A large number of dusty and two winged microspores are present. On maturity, the microsporangium wall bursts and microspores are released in the air which is called "shower of sulphur."They are dispersed by wind due to presence of wings.

54. (c) The gymnosperms are plants in which the ovules are not enclosed by any ovary wall and remain exposed, before and after fertilisation as well. The seeds that develop post-fertilisation, are not covered or are naked. After fertilization, zygote develops into an embryo and ovules into naked seeds.

55. (d) The diploid sporophyte is the dominant, photosynthetic and independent phase of the plant gametophyte in diplontic lifecycle. It is highly reduced and is retained within sporangia.

56. (d) In gymnosperms, the leaves are well-adapted to withstand extreme conditions of temperature, humidity and wind. The needle -like leaves reduce the surface area. Their thick cuticle and sunken stomata help in reducing water loss.

57. (b) *Pinus* shows alternation of generations. The sporophyte phase is long and represented by the huge pine tree bearing the staminate and ovulate cones. Meiotic divisions occur at the same time as the differentiation of the pollen grains and megaspores.

58. (b) The embryo in *Pinus* is straight and consists of a short axis bearing a ring of about ten slender, yellow cotyledons at the end that is away from the micropylar end. In *Pinus,* more than one embryo is developed from a single egg by the splitting of the product of a single fertilization termed as cleavage polyembrony.

59. (b) The ovulate or female cones take about three years to mature. The mature cones are hard, woody and very large in size. Many important changes take place in the female cone during the interval of about thirteen months between pollination and the actual act of fertilization.

60. (d) Female cones or ovulate cones are less in number and arise as single or in a small clusters of two to four, each as a bud in the axial of a scale leaf towards the end of the new shoots of unlimited growth (long shoots) which do not bear the male cones.

61. (c) *Pinus* is monoecious for it bears both types of cones on the same tree on separate branches. The male cone comprises of a number of small spirally arranged microsporophylls. Each microsporophyll bears two microsporangia or pollen sacs on the lower surface of its horizontal position.

62. (c) The parenchymatous mesophyll is present within the hypodermis of *Pinus* leaf. It is compact and shows no differentiation into palisade and spongy tissues. It consists of thin walled cells which contain numerous chloroplasts and abundant starch. The mesophyll thus function as the chlorophyll bearing tissue which manufactures food for plants.

63. (a) The secondary wood shows well marked growth rings which are formed annually due to environmental fluctuations. Each annual ring possesses a zone of spring and an autumn wood. Spring wood is formed during spring season under availability of enough water and minerals. It possess large polygonal, thin walled and wide tracheids with large bordered pits. Autumn wood is formed during autumn season. It possesses smaller, thick walled and narrow tracheids with small bordered pits. It is evident that the size of tracheids shows a marked variation with regards to amount of moisture available in the respective season.

64. (c) In gymnosperms, xylem lacks true vessels and wood fibres. It consists of tracheids that are arranged in uniform radial rows and xylem parenchyma only. The phloem contains sieve tubes and parenchyma cells. There are no companion cells.

65. (a) The gymnosperms have their ovules freely exposed before and after fertilization. They are not enclosed by any ovary wall. The seeds formed by them lack seed coat. Hence, due to absence of ovary wall and seed coat, their seeds are naked.

66. (b) Long branches of *Pinus* gradually become shorter towards the apex. Hence, the pine tree has a conical or pyramidal appearance. Long branches bear short branches and older portion of long branches display the scars of fallen short branches.

67. (c) There is no true and compact or properly organised female cone in *Cycas*. Megasporophylls are loosely arranged and thus, form a loose female strobilus. The growing point of the stem is unaffected by their development and continues its growth through the loose strobilus.

68. (a) All living species of *Cycas* are dioecious as the male and female structures occur on separate plants. The microsporophylls are aggregated into large compact male strobili or cones. The megasporophylls are loosely arranged. They do not form a true cone.

69. (a) When the microspores mature, the male cone elongates considerably and rapidly. The scales separate from one another so that sporangia are exposed. The sporangia lose water and with the loss of water from its cells, the exothecium shrinks. The sporangia thus, opens by a slit on its outer face. The spores fall out and the liberated spores are dispersed by wind.

70. (b) The leaves in gymnosperm are well adapted to withstand extremes of temperature, humidity and wind. In conifers, the needle like leaf reduce the surface area. Their thick cuticle and sunken stomata also help to reduce the water loss. Unlike bryophytes and pteridophytes, in gymnosperms, the

male and female gametophytes do not have an independent free living existence. They remain within the sporangia retained on the sporophytes.

71. (a) Gametophytes are retained within sporangia in gymnosperms.

72. (c) In angiosperms, endosperm is formed through triple fusion (fusion of sperms with two polar nuclei of the central cell) and is triploid. In gymnosperms, endosperm is formed before fertilization and therefore, it is haploid.

73. (b) Stamens are specialized microsporophylls. Each stamen has a narrow stalk or filament and a broader tip called anther. Anther develops four microsporangia or pollen grains. Carpels are specialized megasporophylls. Each carpel has a swollen base named ovary. The interior of ovary contains one or more placentae for bearing ovules.

74. (b) Biennial plants survive for two favourable seasons. During the first season, the plants grow in size and store food. In the second season, they bear flowers that form fruits.

75. (a) Angiosperms is the most highly evolved group of plant kingdom. It is adapted for terrestrial habitats. Swimming habit of sperms is completely absent in angiosperm. The pollen grains reach the stigma by an external agency and deliver the male gamete in the ovule through pollen tube.

76. (b) Fertilized ovules ripen to form seeds. The seeds are covered by fruits. Technically, a fruit is a ripened ovary. Gymnosperms contain ovules but they lack ovary, therefore, seeds are formed but are not fruits. Angiosperms contain both ovule and ovary and therefore, are seed bearing and fruit forming plants.

77. (b) The chloroplasts of green algae contain one or more distinct, rounded, proteinaceous bodies called the pyrenoids. These diminish in size and ultimately disappear if the plant is under conditions of starvation. They reappear when the conditions become favourable.

78. (c) The eye spot is usually associated with the chloroplast in green algae. It is considered as a photoreceptive organ.

79. (b) Sporophylls are organised into flowers in angiosperm. Both microsporophylls and megasporophylls are specialised. A microsporophyll or stamen consists of a filament and an anther. A megasporophyll or carpel is rolled and partly sterilised to produce a stigma, style and ovary containing ovules.

80. (c) The plant cell wall have eukaryotic structure with prominent chloroplast. Life cycle consists of alternating haploid gametophyte and diploid sporophyte generations. Plantae includes eukaryotic, autotrophic, chlorophyll containing organisms.

81. (a) Pistil consists of an ovary enclosing one to many ovules in angiosperms. Highly reduced female gametophytes termed embryo sacs are present within ovules. The embryo-sac formation is preceded by meiosis and thus, each of the cells of an embryo-sac is haploid.

Chapter

4

Animal Kingdom

Directions: In the following questions, a statement of assertion is followed by a statement of reason. Mark the correct choice as:
(a) If both Assertion and Reason are true and Reason is the correct explanation of Assertion.
(b) If both Assertion and Reason are true but Reason is not the correct explanation of Assertion.
(c) If Assertion is true but Reason is false.
(d) If both Assertion and Reason are false.

1. **Assertion:** Radial symmetry in animal helps in detecting food and danger.
   Reason: It enables the animal to respond to stimuli from any direction.
2. **Assertion:** Animals that have an exoskeleton, lacks an endoskeleton.
   Reason: Skeleton cells in the embryonic stage migrate to either stage and produce exoskeleton or endoskeleton but never both.
3. **Assertion :** Cold blooded animals do not have fat layer.
   Reason : Cold blooded animals use their fat for metabolic process during hibernation.
   [AIIMS 1997]
4. **Assertion :** The skeleton of sponges is made up of spicules.
   Reason : Composition of spicules help in classification of sponges.
5. **Assertion :** Sponges belong to Porifera.
   Reason : Sponges have canal system.
6. **Assertion :** Sponges have body organization of "cellular level".
   Reason : There is some physiological division of labour.
7. **Assertion:** Sponges exhibit cellular level of organization.
   Reason: In sponges, cells are arranged as loose cell aggregates.
8. **Assertion:** *Leucosolenia* shows ascon type of canal system.
   Reason: Water passes through ostia $\rightarrow$ spongocoel $\rightarrow$ osculum in *Leucosolenia*.
9. **Assertion:** Sponges do not show any animal nature.
   Reason: Sponges are sessile having specialized structures for capturing food or eliminating wastes.
10. **Assertion:** In ctenophores, digestion is chiefly extracellular.
    Reason: Digestive tract is incomplete in ctenophores.
11. **Assertion:** Cnidoblasts are present on the tentacles and the body in cnidarians.
    Reason: Cnidoblasts are used for anchorage, defence and capture of the prey.
12. **Assertion:** Coelenterates are known as Radiata.
    Reason: These are bilaterally symmetrical organism.
13. **Assertion:** *Hydra* is green in colour.
    Reason: Green colour is due to the presence of chlorophyll in their body wall.
14. **Assertion:** Nerve cells in coelenterata have complete co-ordination in their body.
    Reason: True nerve cells occur for the first time in coelenterate.
15. **Assertion:** *Obelia* is dimorphic in nature.
    Reason: Polyp and gonangia form are exhibited by *Obelia*.
16. **Assertion:** Coelenterates show alternation of generation.
    Reason: Asexual generation is followed by sexual generation in coelenterates.
17. **Assertion:** Coelenterata are diploblastic animals.
    Reason: They have cellular level of organization.
18. **Assertion:** Platyhelminthes are generally hermaphrodites.
    Reason: Fertilization is internal in Platyhelminthes.
19. **Assertion:** *F. hepatica* undergoes both aerobic and anaerobic respiration.
    Reason: *Fasciola* respires only in absence of oxygen.

20. **Assertion:** There is no chance of malaria to a man by the bite of male *Anopheles* mosquito.
Reason: It carries a virulant strain of *Plasmodium*.
21. **Assertion:** Cephalization is advantageous to an animal.
Reason: It improves the appearance of the animal.
22. **Assertion :** Tapeworm, roundworm and pinworm are endoparasites of human intestine.
Reason : Improperly cooked food is the source of intestinal infections.
23. **Assertion:** Aschelminthes are called as pseudocoelomates.
Reason: In aschelminthes, mesoderm is present as scattered pouches in between ectoderm and endoderm.
24. **Assertion:** Both digested and semi-digested food is absorbed by body surface in tapeworms.
Reason: Tapeworms lack digestive organs.
25. **Assertion:** *Plasmodium vivax* is responsible for malaria.
Reason: Malaria is caused by polluted water.
26. **Assertion:** Cutaneous glands help in regulation of body temperature.
Reason: Cutaneous glands are produced from stratum germinativum.
27. **Assertion :** Annelids are ureotelic.
Reason : Only excretory product of annelids is uric acid.
28. **Assertion:** Metamerism is the characteristic of phylum annelida.
Reason: Metamerism is one type of body segmentation.
29. **Assertion:** Blood is red in annelida.
Reason: RBCs are absent in them.
30. **Assertion:** Spermathecae are the main part of reproductive system of annelida.
Reason: These help in sperm transfer.
31. **Assertion :** Blood is colourless in insects.
Reason : Insect blood has no role in O_2 transport.
32. **Assertion :** Typhlosole increases the effective area of absorption in the intestine.
Reason : Typhlosole, present in the intestine, is the characteristic feature of cockroach.
33. **Assertion:** Lateral line system is found in fishes and aquatic larval amphibians.
Reason: Lateral line system has receptor of sensory cells derived from ectoderm.
34. **Assertion:** Open circulatory system is found in most arthropods.
Reason: Arthropods contain haemolymph which directly bathes internal tissues and organ.
35. **Assertion:** Moulting or ecdysis occurs only in invertebrates.
Reason: Moulting usually takes an average time of five weeks in birds.
36. **Assertion:** Phylum arthropoda is the largest phylum of Kingdom animalia.
Reason: It includes the largest number of animals with approx. 900,000 species.
37. **Assertion:** Arthropods are able to survive in adverse conditions.
Reason: Arthropods have developed sense organs, compound eyes and taste receptors.
38. **Assertion:** Feather-like gills are present in mantle cavity in molluscs.
Reason: These gills have both respiratory and excretory functions.
39. **Assertion:** Circulatory system is of closed type in mollusca.
Reason: The blood of mollusca contains haemoglobin.
40. **Assertion:** 'Calabar swelling' is caused by 'eye worm'.
Reason: *Loa loa* is called the 'eye worm'.
41. **Assertion:** Detorsion is the characteristic of mollusca.
Reason: Detorison is an arrested stage of torsion.
42. **Assertion** : Torsion can be seen in ctendium.
Reason : Ctenidium acts as the respiratory organ.
43. **Assertion :** Ambulacral system plays a major role in locomotion of echinoderm.
Reason : Hydraulic pressure of fluid and contraction of muscle of tube feet make possible movement of echinoderm.
44. **Assertion:** Tube feet are characteristic organs of echinodermata.
Reason: Tube feet have an important role in respiration.
45. **Assertion:** Water vascular system is the characteristic of echinoderms.
Reason: Main function of water vascular system is locomotion.

46. Assertion : Acraniata is a group of organisms which do not have distinct cranium.
Reason : It includes small marine forms without head. **[AIIMS 1997, 2012]**

47. Assertion: The body of hemichordates is divisible into proboscis, collar and trunk.
Reason: Proboscis gland helps in digestion.

48. Assertion: Acraniata is a group of organisms which do not have distinct cranium.
Reason: Acraniata constitutes small marine forms without head.

49. Assertion: Characters of cyclostomes show an advance over *Amphioxus*.
Reason: Cyclostomes have some degenerated characters.

50. Assertion: *Amphioxus* has a simple organization compared to vertebrates.
Reason: *Amphioxus* lacks many important craniate structures.

51. Assertion: Glochindium larva rapidly disperse to a great distance.
Reason: Glochindium is parasitic on fish.

52. Assertion: Respiration in *Amphioxus* is done by both water and blood.
Reason: *Amphioxus* is aquatic and possesses blood.

53. Assertion: *Herdmania* has digestion mechanism like higher group of animals.
Reason: Liver of *Herdmania* possess several enzymes required for digestion.

54. Assertion: In *Balanoglossus,* notochord is replaced by pygochord.
Reason: Pygochord supports adbominal region.

55. Assertion: *Balanoglossus* are also known as "acorn worms".
Reason: The word 'acorn worm' has no meaning.

56. Assertion: *Wuchereria* are triploblastic with the presence of an excretory pore.
Reason: They have muscular pharynx.

57. Assertion: Claspers are a distinguishing feature of males in class Chondrichthyes.
Reason: Claspers help in copulation.

58. Assertion: Osteichthyes fish swim constantly to avoid sinking.
Reason: In fishes of class Osteichthyes, air bladder is absent.

59. Assertion: A shark can stay at a desired level in water without swimming.
Reason: It has a buoyancy-regulating organ called as the swim bladder.

60. Assertion: In fishes, heart is venous.
Reason: Only veins are present in the heart of fishes.

61. Assertion: Ampullae of lorenzini are found beneath the skin of head region in fishes.
Reason: Ampullae of lorenzini acts as receptors.

62. Assertion: Lateral line canal is one of the main characteristics of fishes.
Reason: Lateral line canal is a system of sense organ concerned with life in water.

63. Assertion: Lateral line system is found in fishes and aquatic larval amphibians.
Reason: Lateral line system has receptor of sensory cells derived from ectoderm.

64. Assertion: Amphibian males and females produce lot of gametes.
Reason: Males lack copulatory organ in amphibians.

65. Assertion: Parental care is seen in amphibians.
Reason: Amphibians have taken several method to protect their eggs and offspring.

66. Assertion: In frogs, the entire skin serves as tangoreceptors.
Reason: Tactile organs and patches are present throughout the skin of frog.

67. Assertion: "Lymph heart" is present in frog.
Reason: Lymph in frog is circulated by lymph heart.

68. Assertion: In frog, most of the absorption takes place in intestine.
Reason: The intestine in frog is the coiled structure.

69. Assertion: Amphibians are poikilothermal.
Reason: Amphibians often undergoes summer sleep.

70. Assertion: *Calotes*, *Crocodilus* and *Chelone* are members of class Reptilia.
Reason: Heart is three chambered in *Calotes*, *Crocodilus* and *Chelone*.

71. Assertion: King cobra is adaptive to oriental realm.
Reason: Interaction of king cobra and kangaroo is prevented by wallace line.

72. Assertion: The fangs of snake is the maxillary teeth.
Reason: The poison apparatus in snake consists of poison gland, ducts and fangs.

73. Assertion: In reptiles, hemipenes is present.
Reason: Hemipenes is the combination of both ovary and penis.

74. **Assertion :** Birds have one ovary.
Reason : This reduces the body weight for flight.

75. **Assertion :** All birds, except the ones like koel (cuckoo) build nests for retiring and taking rest during night time (day time for nocturnal).
Reason : Koel lays its eggs in the nests of tailor bird.

76. **Assertion:** Skin is moist in birds.
Reason: This reduces effects of friction due to flying in air.

77. **Assertion:** Air sacs are connected to lungs in class Aves.
Reason: These help in the process of respiration.

78. **Assertion:** The birds can maintain a constant body temperature.
Reason: Birds possess feathers covering their body.

79. **Assertion:** There are no mammary gland in birds.
Reason: Pigeons secrete 'pigeon's milk'.

80. **Assertion :** Bats and whales are classified as mammals.
Reason : Bats and whales have four-chambered heart.

81. **Assertion :** The duck-billed *Platypus* and the spiny anteater, both are egg-laying animals yet they are grouped under mammals.
Reason : Both of them have 7 cervical vertebrae and 12 pairs of cranial nerves.

82. **Assertion :** Holoblastic cleavage with almost equal sized blastomeres is a characteristic of placental animals.
Reason : Eggs of most mammals, including humans, are of centrolecithal type.

83. **Assertion:** In mammals, teeth are heterodont.
Reason: Mammalian teeth are embedded in a socket of jaw.

84. **Assertion:** Lophodont dentition is also found in the mammals.
Reason: Lophodont type of dentition is specially for herbivore mammals.

85. **Assertion:** Baleen is an example of aquatic adapation.
Reason: Baleen is a balloon like structure present beneath the skin of mammals.

86. **Assertion:** Coprophagy is the characteristic of mammal.
Reason: Coprophagy is found in all mammals.

87. **Assertion:** Both true ribs and floating ribs are present in mammals.
Reason: By nature, sternal ribs are true ribs as, they possess all the characters of ribs.

Solutions

1. **(a)** Radial symmetry is advantageous for an animal in responding to stimuli from any direction thereby allowing it to detect food and danger easily.
2. **(d)** Many animals have an endoskeleton and exoskeleton such as Chelon-turtle or Testudo-tortoise. Exoskeleton of other animals include chitinous plate, calcareous shell, horny scales, feathers, hair, claws, nails, hoofs, horns and antlers.
3. **(c)** Cold blooded animals do not need to stay warm and can let their body temperatures get closer to that of their surroundings. Thus, they do not need to have extra insulation.
4. **(b)** Spicules help in making skeleton of sponges. These are made up of silica, calcium or spongin substances. The structure of spicules also help in classification of sponges.
5. **(b)** Sponges belong to Porifera and they have characteristic canal system.
6. **(b)** Sponges are multicellular but they have cellular level of body organization *i.e.*, true tissue, movable parts, or appendages are not formed. Although, there is some physiological division of labour, accompanied with structural differentiation amongst body cells. But here, similar cells are arranged neither in permanent layer nor masses to form tissues.
7. **(a)** All members of animalia are multicellular, but all of them do not exhibit the same pattern of organization of cells. In sponges, the cells are arranged as loose cell aggregates, *i.e.*, they exhibit cellular level of organisation while, higher animals have tissue or further organ system level of organization.
8. **(a)** *Leucosolenia* shows simplest type of canal system. In this, surrounding water enters the canal system through ostia. This water of sea enters into the spongocoel and is pushed out readily through osculum. Course taken by the water current in the body of sponge may be shown as under.

$$\text{Ingressing} \xrightarrow[\text{Ostia}]{\text{Through}} \text{Spongocoel} \xrightarrow[\text{Osculum}]{\text{Through}} \text{To outside}$$

9. **(d)** Robert Grant (1857) was the first to recognise and prove the true animal nature of sponges. The animal nature of sponges was well established on the following grounds-
   (i) Sponges feed on in water solid particles. Their mode of nutrition is truly holozoic.
   (ii) Sponge cells are devoid of cellulose cell walls.
   (iii) Life cycle of sponges include swimming ciliated larval stages resembling those of other marine animals. Sponges are sessile and digestion is very simple without any apparent way of capturing food or eliminating wastes.
10. **(d)** Digestive tract in ctenophores consists of mouth, pharynx or stomodaeum, stomach or infundibulum, anal canals and two anal pores. Since there are mouth and anal pores present, the digestive tract is complete. Thus, digestion is both extracellular and intracellular.
11. **(b)** Cnidoblast cells are present on the tentacles and the body of cnidarians. A cnidoblast (also called nematoblast) has nematocyst known as 'stinging organ' (consisting of capsule, shaft and thread tube) used for anchorage, defence and offence.
12. **(c)** Coelenterata is the phylum of acoelomate and radially symmetrical lower invertebrates. Due to their radial body symmetry, they are also known as radiata. Bilateral symmetry starts from the phylum platyhelminthes.

13. (c) *H. viridis* is green in colour. Its bright green colour is not because of chlorophyll containing chloroplasts, but due to the presence of symbiotic zoochlorallae, *Chlorella vulgaris*, a unicellular green alga, that lives in its gastrodermal cells.

14. (a) Coelenterates possess a very primitive type of nervous system. This system is composed of many nerve cells. In coelenterates, separate mechanisms for digestion, respiration, excretion and reproduction etc. have evolved for the first time. Thus, there is a constant need to maintain coordination between these systems. Nerve cells are developed for this purpose, for the first time in coelenterates.

15. (a) Hydroid colony of Obelia is dimorphic, exhibiting two types of individuals or zooids which differ both morphologically as well as physiologically. These two zooids are-

(i) Polyps – the nutritive zooid of the colony

(ii) Gonangium – the reproductive zooid.

16. (a) Alternation of generations may be defined as a phenomenon whereby, during the life history of an organism, a diploid asexual phase and a haploid sexual phase regularly alternates with each other. This type of true alternation of generations is also called metagenesis. In coelenterates, an asexual polypoid generation appears to alternate regularly with a sexual medusoid generation.

17. (c) Tissue level of organization is observed in Phylum - Coelenterata or Cnidaria. Cellular level of organization is only present in Cnidarians.

18. (b) Platyhelminthes are generally hermaphrodites, i.e., both the sexes are present in one organism. These show internal as well as cross fertilization where male gametes of one organism fertilize female gametes of another organism.

19. (c) *F. hepatica* undergoes both aerobic and anaerobic respiration depending on the availability of oxygen. Oxygen content in bile being extremely low, respiration in *F. hepatica* is anaerobic or anoxybiotic. This is an exothermic reaction involving release of energy. While, if free oxygen is available, aerobic respiration takes place.

20. (c) Malaria can not be transmitted by the bite of male *Anopheles* mosquito as it does not carry active stage of *Plasmodium*.

21. (c) Cephalization is the differentiation of head at anterior end. This does not play any role in improving the appearance of an animal but it results in accumulation of nervous tissue and sense organs in head so as to integrate the activities of the nervous system.

22. (b) Tapeworm, roundworm & pinworm are all endoparasites. The main cause of the intestinal infection is improperly cooked food. However, tapeworm infection occur by eating improperly cooked food, roundworm is transmitted by contaminated food & water and pinworm or ringworm is transmitted through food or improper sanitary condition.

23. (a) In aschelminthes, the body cavity is not lined by mesoderm, instead, the mesoderm is present as scattered pouches in between the ectoderm and endoderm. Hence, they are called pseudocoelomates.

24. (a) As tapeworm is an endoparasite, it does not have alimentary canal therefore, digested food of the host is diffused directly through the general body surface.

25. (c) *Plasmodium vivax* is responsible for malaria. It is spread by the bite of female *Anopheles* mosquito. Thus, malaria is not caused by polluted water.

26. (b) Sweat glands produced from stratum germinativum plays an important role in the regulation of body temperature. When the body temperature rises too much, the sweat glands are stimulated to take up water from blood vessels and to pour out their secretion on the general surface of the skin. Evaporation of sweat from the body surface uses up latent heat of vaporization from the skin, thus the extra heat of the body is used up and the body cools down reducing the temperature.

27. (c) Aquatic annelids excrete ammonia, and terrestrial species (earthworm) excrete urea.

However, earthworms are less ureotelic than other terrestrial animals. Excretory fluid contains 40% urea, 20% ammonia and 40% amino acids and other nitrogenous compounds, but no uric acid or urate.

28. (b) The body of annelids is divided into segments called metameres, externally ring like grooves (annuli) and internally by vertical partitions called septa. The external segmentation corresponds to internal segmentation. This phenomenon is called metamere or metameric segmentation. Phylum annelida represents the first group of metazoan animals developing a true coelom with metameric segmentation.

29. (b) In annelida, blood is red due to the presence of haemoglobin or erythrocruorin dissolved in plasma. RBCs are absent in them. Blood corpuscles are colourless. Instead of blood, leeches posses reddish haemocoelomic fluid that flows in haemocoelomic channels.

30. (a) In annelida, four pairs of flask shaped sacs, each with a diverticulum for storage of sperms and large ampulla for their nourishment is present. Spermathecae occur in 6-9 segments. These receive sperm during copulation. As cross fertilization occurs in earthworm, the sperms of one worm is transferred to spermathecae of the other.

31. (b) Insect blood is colourless and does not play any role in transport of oxygen. Insects have tracheal respiration.

32. (d) Typhlosole is the characteristic feature of earthworm. It can be defined as an extra flap of tissue or an infolding along the inner wall of intestine. The typhlosole in earthworm increases the surface area of the intestine for efficient secretion and absorption during digestion.

33. (a) Lateral line system of fishes and aquatic larval amphibians whose receptors are group of sensory cells derived from ectoderm.

34. (a) Most arthropods, certain molluscs and tunicates contain open circulatory system. In them, a fluid composed of blood mixes with tissue fluid bathing internal tissues and organs directly. It oozes through spaces or cavities that surround the organs, this mixture of fluid is usually referred to as haemolymph.

35. (d) Moulting or ecdysis occurs not only in invertebrates, but in birds also. In birds, shedding and replacement of feathers is moulting or ecdysis which takes place gradually, that is, about six weeks on an average. At the base of each feather follicle, a dermal papilla persists from which new feathers will form. Thus, there is a continuous replacement of feather throughout life.

36. (a) Among all the phylum of Kingdom animali, arthropoda is the largest whereas the second largest phylum is phylum mollusca that includes 60, 000 species.

37. (b) Arthropods survive adverse conditions because of its unique cuticle, segmentation and jointed appendages. These provide arthropods an advantage of protection on land and the ability to move quickly.

38. (b) In molluscs, the space between the mantle and the hump is called mantle cavity in which feather-like gills are present. They have both respiratory as well as excretory functions.

39. (d) In mollusca, circulatory system is of open type with a heart made up of two auricles and a ventricle. Haemoglobin is found to be present in blood.

40. (b) One of the important human filaria is the African eye-worm *Loa loa,* transmitted by mangofly chiefly found in Africa. They commonly invade subcutaneous tissue and during their migration may pass across the eye-ball, hence the name eyeworm.

Loa microfilariae could be very injurious and fatal when they penetrate brain and spinal cord as these carry neurotropic viruses. During their migration, these cause itense itching and swelling. These also cause swelling and pain in eyes which are known as "calabar swellings".

41. (b) Torsion or twisting is a process during larval development of gastropods, which rotates the viscero- pallium anti clockwise brought 180° from its initial position, so that mantle cavity, with its pallial complex, is through in front of the body in adult. Changes occuring in torsion are to a certain extent reversible. This reversion is known as detorsion and it is a very characteristic of the whole group of the euthyneura. Formerly, this condition was looked upon as an arrested stage in the torsion, but there is the same reduction of the paired parts of the pallial complex as in the specialized streptoneura. Total detorsion, as shown by the typical opisthobranchia is accompained by the reduction of disappearance of the shell.

42. (b) Ctenidium is a gill situated on the right side of the branchial chamber. It helps in respiration by beating cilia. During development, ctenidium shifts from left side to right side which is called "torison". It is characteristic feature of gastropods.

43. (a) The water vascular system is a unique organ system that functions in locomotion, feeding, respiration and excretion. Ambulacral canal is connected to outside through external tube feet. Hydraulic pressure of fluid and contraction of muscle of tube feet make possible movement of Echinoderm.

44. (c) Each ambulacral groove of echinoderms contain two double rows of short, tubular retractile projections, called as podia or tube feet, that end in suckers. Tube feet are characteristic organs of echinoderms serving variously for locomotion, capturing of food, respiration etc.

45. (b) Water vascular system of ambulacral system is a unique system of echinoderms which helps mainly in locomotion. It is in fact a modified part of coelom consisting of a system of canals containing sea water and amoeboid corpuscles. It helps in locomotion by providing a hydraulic pressure mechanism of tube feet may serve for respiratory exchange of gases. Tube feet also help in anchoring the body to substratum and in capturing and handling the food.

46. (b) Cephalochordates and urochordates are acraniates. These are marine animals without cranium, jaws, vertebral column and paired appendages. Notochord is present and they are less developed than craniates.

47. (c) Hemichordates are worm-like marine animals. Their body is composed of an anterior probosics, a collar and a long trunk. Proboscis gland is excretory in function.

48. (b) Acraniata includes marine forms without head or cranium. These lack jaws, vertebral column and paired appendages.

49. (b) Following are the characters of cyclostomes showing an advance over *Amphioxus*. A distinct head, however may be secondary, a so-called cranium, a more advanced brain, pro and mesonephric kidneys, secondary notochord, vertebrae introduced (lampreys) etc. Cyclostomes also have some particular specialization like tongue apparatus, sucking mouth with horny teeth, sac-like gill pouches, separate branchial sac with branchial basket etc.

The degenerated characters of cyclostomes are –

(i) tongue apparatus (ii) rudimentary paired eyes in hagfishes (iii) lack of exoskeleton (iv) reduced liver and lack of gall bladder and bile duct in adult lamperey.

50. (a) *Amphioxus* is devoid of heart, head, kidneys and paired limbs. Paired sense organs are absent also receptors are of primitive type. A complete notochord is persistant with no vertebral column. These show that it is has a simple organization compared to vertebrates because many important craniate structures are lacking in it. But it is definitely a simple chordate having a large number of primitive characters such as a notochord, dorsal hollow nerve cord, and gill clefts.

51. (a) The life cycle of fresh water mussel, including a parasitic glochidium larva on a fish host has many advantages. Besides affording protection and a means of nourishment, it ensures a far wide and more rapid dispersal of the species. A fish may carry these tiny parasites to great distances before they drop off. Considering the sluggish habits and poor

locomotory ability of the mussels, this is probably the only way to ensure their proper distribution.

52. **(a)** In *Amphioxus*, some exchange of O_2 and CO_2 occurs between the water current and blood through the gill-clefts, but this appears doubtful since the blood contains no respiratory pigment. The pharyngeal wall of *Branchiostoma* is richly vascular and the water current entering the pharyngeal cavity brings O_2. The blood flows so close to the surface that some exchange between blood and water can easily occur. It appears more probable that an exchange of gases occurs over the whole surface of the body and particularly in the walls of atrium.

53. **(a)** Digestion mechanism of *Herdmania* is similar to that of higher group of animals due to possessing several enzymes used in digestion. In *Herdmania,* the liver secretes a yellowish-brown digestive fluid into the stomach, it has many enzymes, an amylase which splits carbohydrates into maltose, a protease which breaks down proteins and a weak lipase which probably acts on fats. And also secretion of pyloric gland probably has an accessory digestive function similar to that of pancreas.

54. **(d)** Pygochord is longitudinal rod like structures extending from the ventral side of the intestine to the body wall, in the post hepatic region of the trunk. Its cells are vacuolated. It supports the post hepatic region of the body but probably also performs some other functions not yet understood.

55. **(c)** Balanoglossus belongs to class enteropneusta. In certain cases, the proboscis pore does not communicate with the proboscis coelom, but terminates blindly, and may send off a narrow tubular diverticulum which opens into the neurocoel. The proboscis sits in the collar somewhat like an acorn in its cup, a character that has given the name "acorn worm" to the group.

56. **(b)** *Wuchereria bancrofti* belonging to phylum Aschelminthes is a dreaded human endoparasite of human blood and lymph. It consists of muscular pharynx and an excretory pore.

57. **(b)** In Chondrichthyes, males can be distinguished from a female, as the former has a pair of hard elongated claspers attached to the pelvic fins. Claspers are an external appendage designed to deliver sperm inside a female. These claspers help in copulation.

58. **(d)** Members of class Chondrichthyes are marine with streamlined body having cartilaginous endoskeleton. Due to the absence of air bladder, these have to swim constantly to avoid sinking, air bladder is present in Osteichthyes thus, helping in regulation of buoyancy.

59. **(d)** Shark is a cartilagenous fish and lack buoyancy regulating organ called swim bladder. These fishes need to swim constantly or will sink to the bottom. Thus, these cannot stay at a desired level in water without swimming.

60. **(c)** In fishes, the heart is mainly two chambered containing one auricle and one ventricle. Heart of *Scoliodon* receives only deoxygenated or venous blood, hence named as venous heart. The auricle opens to the ventricle through atrioventricular aperture. Mainly the impure blood passes from the heart to the gills only once. Therefore, they have single circulation only.

61. **(b)** The ampullae of Lorenzini are found in clusters on the dorsal and ventral surfaces of the head embedded below the skin but opening externally on the surface of the skin. These were formerly regarded as neuromast organs but Sand (1938) has proved that these are thermoreceptor organs. Thus, these are responsible for sending signals to the brain in response to change in temperature of water.

62. **(a)** A faint line runs on either side of the body extending from the head to the posterior end of the tail, this is called lateral line (also called neuromast system). It marks the position of an underlying canal which runs along side of the body and contains special receptor organs. The lateral line canal extends anteriorly into the head, where it branches into several canals; at intervals these canals open to the exterior through the pores. These canals contain neuromast organs like rheoreceptors or current receptors. The latter can perceive vibration of very low frequency and detect disturbances in water.

63. (b) Lateral line system is made up of sensory cells of ectodermal origin. It is meant for balancing the body while swimming. So, is found in fishes and larval forms of amphibians.

64. (b) In amphibians, fertilization is external, hence, males and females produce a lot of gametes and release in water to maximize the chances of fertilization. Males of class Amphibia generally lack copulatory organs. The reproductive tracts open outside through cloacal aperture.

65. (a) Parental care is clearly seen in amphibians. They protect their eggs by keeping them – (i) In enclosures in the water, (ii) In holes near water, (iii) In nests, on trees or on rocks, overhanging water, (iv) In transparent gelatinous bag in the water, (v) On trees or in moss, away from water. They also show direct nursing by the parent.

66. (a) The entire skin of frog serves as organs of touch as it is abundantly supplied with sensory nerve endings situated in the spaces between the cells. Thus, the skin is called tangoreceptor. At places, groups of epidermal cells-tactile organs and patches are present. The tactile organs make the skin of frog sensitive to touch, heat, cold and the effects of the chemicals.

67. (d) From the diffused lymphatic system, lymph is pumped back into veins by two pairs of lymph hearts. One of which is situated just behind the transverse processes of the third vertebra opening into the sub scapular veins, the second pair of lymph hearts is found on either side at the end of the urostyle. They open into the femoral vein.

68. (b) In frog, most of the absorption takes place in intestine. The intestine of frog is so formed, that it gives the greater surface area. The intestine is the longest part of the alimentary canal where the absorption of the digested food materials take place. To increase the absorptive surface of the intestine, the internal lining of the intestine forms transverse folds in the duodenum and longitudinal folds in the region of the ileum and rectum.

69. (a) Amphibia is cold blooded or ectothermal animal as its body temperature does not remain constant but fluctuates with that of environment. Thus, it is called poikilothermal animal. In winter, the temperature of the body activities ceases down. In this condition, it can not live more on the land, so it takes winter sleep or hibernation in underground. Similarly, during the summer it once again goes underground to sleep as its all body activities are slowed down due to high temperature. This is known as summer sleep.

70. (c) *Calotes, Crocodilus* and *Chelone* are members of class Reptilia. Heart is four chambered in *Crocodilus* while three chambered in *Calotes* and *Chelone.*

71. (b) Realm is a large landscape (generally subcontinental) having its unique biodiversity. South Asia (including India) occurs in oriental realm; king cobra is endemic here and kangaroo is found in Australian realm. Wallace line is the imaginary line seperating oriental and Australian realms.

72. (b) The poison apparatus of snake consists of a pair of poison glands, their ducts and a pair of fangs. The poison glands are situated one on either side of the upper jaw. These glands are possibly the superior labial glands or parotid glands. The fangs are sharply pointed and are enlarged maxillary teeth.

73. (c) Hemipenes are the copulatory organs found in *Uromastix* and some other reptiles. These are two eversible hollow sacs lying under the skin behind the cloacal aperture at the base of the tail. Proximally, the hemipenes communicate with the urodaeum of the cloaca. During

copulation, only one hemipenes, is inserted into the cloaca of the female. Erection of the hemipenes is due to the muscular action and filling with blood, then they are everted and become cylindrical and project beyond the cloaca.

74. (a) Birds have many adaptations for flight. They have pneumatic bones and only one ovary which reduces their body weight.

75. (c) Koel (*Eudynemis*) lays eggs in crow's nest for incubation and rearing.

76. (d) The characteristic features of Aves (birds) are the presence of feathers. Most of them can fly except flightless birds (*e.g.*, Ostrich). Skin of birds is dry as it is without glands except the presence of oil glands at the base of the tail.

77. (a) Respiration is by lungs in class Aves (birds). However, the lungs are spongy and inelastic. Air sacs are connected to lungs to supplement respiration.

78. (a) Birds have a constant body temperature which commonly remains in between 104° to 112°F even in subzero weather. Thus, they are called homeothermal. The feathers serve the most important function of retention of heat as the plumage forms an efficient, non-conduction covering with its innumerable dead air spaces, useful in insulation. In cold weather, the heat loss is reduced to minimum by fluffing out the feathers, which increases the depth of insulating material by adding to the air spaces within the feathery layers. In warm weather, the feathers are often held close to the body to allow some escape of body heat.

79. (b) Pigeon is a bird species known to produce milk even though they lack mammary glands. Milk starts to be produced in the crop of the parent birds two days before the egg hatch. During lactation, a curd-like substance is created from fat filled cells that line the crop and regurgitated to feed the squab.

80. (b) Bats and whales are the members of class Mammalia. The bats are the only mammals which have wings and can really fly while whales are the largest animals in existence. Both bats and whales have four chambered heart but birds and crocodiles also have four chambered heart.

81. (a) The duck billed *Platypus* and the spiny anteater are primitive oviparous, reptile-like mammals and are included in class mammalia. Both of them have 12 pairs of cranial nerves and 7 cervical vertebrae.

82. (c) Cleavage in placental mammals is holoblastic because of microlecithal eggs.

83. (b) In class Mammalia, teeth are of different types (heterodont) and are embedded in the socket of jaw (thecodont). These are developed twice during the life time of the animal (diphyodont) *i.e.*, milk and permanent teeth.

84. (b) In lophodont condition, found in elephants, there is an intricate folding of enamel and dentine. Cresentic enamel cusps are connected by several transverse ridges called lophos. A single large lophodont molar, 30 cm by 10 cm is present at one time in each half of each jaw. These are adapted to grind all sorts of plants, including grasses.

85. (c) Whale lack teeth. Instead, the upper jaw carries two transverse rows of numerous triangular fringed horny plates of baleen or whale bone. This serves as the effective sieve for straining plankton (mostly krill) which forms their chief food.

86. (c) Coprophagy is found in certain mammals (e.g. rabbits). This is the process by which many rodents form a special kind of faeces from the contents of the caecum and these are reingested, so that the food passes through the digestive system second time. Rabbit is coprophagus in habit, eating its own faeces in order to get maximum amount of nutrient from its food.

87. (b) All the sternal parts of the thoracic ribs except the last five are attached to the sternum below by hyaline cartilage. Therefore, they are called as true ribs. While, last two pairs of ribs (11th and 12th pair) provided with the sternal parts but they are not connected with the sternum and hence known as floating ribs. Floating ribs are responsible for protecting the kidney.

Chapter

5

Morphology of Flowering Plants

Directions: In the following questions, a statement of assertion is followed by a statement of reason. Mark the correct choice as:

(a) If both Assertion and Reason are true and Reason is the correct explanation of Assertion.

(b) If both Assertion and Reason are true but Reason is not the correct explanation of Assertion.

(c) If Assertion is true but Reason is false.

(d) If both Assertion and Reason are false.

1. **Assertion :** Apical meristem of root is subterminal.
   Reason : At the terminal end of root, root cap is present.
2. **Assertion:** Fibrous root stem.
   Reason: Fibrous root system is found in dicots only.
3. **Assertion :** Ginger has a prostrate-growing rhizome.
   Reason : Shoot growth is not effected by gravity.
4. **Assertion:** *Avicennia* has pneumatophores.
   Reason: Pneumatophores help the plant to get oxygen for respiration.
5. **Assertion:** Roots do not possess nodes but no leaves or buds.
   Reason: Root branches arise endogenously.
6. **Assertion:** Root caps are absent in floating aquatic plants.
   Reason: Root pockets are present in aquatic plants.
7. **Assertion:** Root pockets are very similar to root caps.
   Reason: Root caps and root pockets have the ability to regenerate.
8. **Assertion:** Root hairs are not present on whole of root surface.
   Reason: Root hairs absorb water.
9. **Assertion:** Deep feeder tap root system is called racemose tap root system.
   Reason: It is found in trees.
10. **Assertion:** *Orchis* root resembles human hand.
    Reason: It is an example of fasciculated fleshy roots.
11. **Assertion:** *Momordica* roots look like necklace.
    Reason: *Momordica* possess moniliform roots.
12. **Assertion:** Assimilatory roots can photosynthesize.
    Reason: Assimilatory roots possess chlorophyll.
13. **Assertion:** Epiphytes are called space parasites.
    Reason: Their roots possess velamen.
14. **Assertion:** Pneumataphores are seen in *Rhizophora*.
    Reason: From the region of elongation, some of the epidermal cells form root hairs.
15. **Assertion :** Bud may form leaves and flowers.
    Reason : Bud is a condensed shoot.
16. **Assertion:** Stems of some plants protect them from browsing animals.
    Reason: Axillary buds of stems of these plants are modified into thorns.
17. **Assertion:** Stem develops from the hypocotyl of embryo.
    Reason: Internodes bear axillary buds.
18. **Assertion:** Thorns of *Artabotrys* are modified floral stalks.
    Reason: The upper floral buds develop thorns in *Antigonon*.
19. **Assertion:** Prickles lack vascular cylinder.
    Reason: Prickles show deposition of silica or calcium carbonate.
20. **Assertion:** Small leaflets are present on the phyllode of *Parkinsonia aculeata*.
    Reason: Phyllode does not bear leaves and flowers.
21. **Assertion :** A simple leaf has undivided lamina.
    Reason : Leaves showing pinnate and palmate venations have various type of incisions.
22. **Assertion :** Whole compound leaf of *Clematis* converts into tendril.
    Reason : *Gloriosa superba* shows whole leaf tendril.

23. **Assertion :** Leaves of *Bryophyllum, Begonia* help in vegetative multiplication.
Reason : Leaves of these plants possess adventitious buds.
24. **Assertion:** The leaf base is swollen in some leguminous plants.
Reason: The swollen leaf base is called pulvinus.
25. **Assertion:** Leaves of monocot plants generally possess reticulate venation.
Reason: Leaves of dicot plants generally possess parallel venation.
26. **Assertion:** In alternate type of phyllotaxy, the arrangement of leaves is such that a single leaf arises at each node in alternate manner.
Reason: The alternate type of phyllotaxy is seen in china rose and mustard plant.
27. **Assertion:** Phyllotaxy deals with arrangement of leaves.
Reason: Foliage denotes all leaves of a plant.
28. **Assertion:** In spiral phyllotaxy, only leaf is present on each node.
Reason: In opposite phyllotaxy, two leaves are borne on a node.
29. **Assertion:** Prickles of plant have multiple roles along with protection of plant.
Reason: They are superficial in origin.
30. **Assertion:** Leaves are formed in caducous plants.
Reason: In deciduous plants, all leaves fall together.
31. **Assertion:** Onion leaves are centric and green.
Reason: Aerial leaves of onion store food.
32. **Assertion:** Both china rose and rose bear stipules.
Reason: They are of adnate types.
33. **Assertion:** Leaves of *Bryophyllum, Begonia* help in vegetative multiplication.
Reason: Leaves of these plants possess adventitious buds.
34. **Assertion:** Spathe, a bract of spadix attracts pollinators.
Reason: It is often brightly cloloured.
35. **Assertion:** Food is stored in leaf bases.
Reason: Buds develop from the leaf bases.
36. **Assertion:** In leguminous plants, leaf base becomes swollen, called pulvinus.
Reason: In *Alstonia,* leaves show alternate phyllotaxy.
37. **Assertion :** In corymb, all the flowers lie at the same level.
Reason : Pedicels of all the flowers are of same length.
38. **Assertion :** An incomplete flower can be perfect.
Reason : Perfect flowers (incomplete) are called neuter.
39. **Assertion :** A plant having unisexual flowers are called dioecious.
Reason : Mango is a polygamous plant.
40. **Assertion:** The cymose type of inflorescence has limited growth.
Reason: In cymose inflorescence, the main axis terminates in a flower.
41. **Assertion:** In some flowers like lily, perianth is a term used when calyx and corolla are not distinct.
Reason: Calyx and corolla are the reproductive organs.
42. **Assertion:** In imbricate aestivation, out of five petals, one is completely internal, one is completely external and in each of the remaining three petals, one margin is internal and the other is external.
Reason: Ascending imbricate aestivation is found in *Cassia* and gulmohur.
43. **Assertion:** In cymose branching, growth of terminal bud stops after some time.
Reason: The growth of the main stem is definite.
44. **Assertion:** Persistent sepals of *Physalis* are called accrescent.
Reason: In Guava, the sepals are marcescent.
45. **Assertion:** The flowers of hypanthodium are never exposed.
Reason: Hypanthodium flowers are bisexual.
46. **Assertion:** Verticillaster is a cymose inflorescence.
Reason: The main axis and lateral branches of inflorescence end in flowers.
47. **Assertion:** Flower of racemose inflorescence are pollinated by insects.
Reason: In racemose head infloresence, the florets are arranged in a centripetal fashion.
48. **Assertion:** In cymose inflorescence, the main and the lateral axis end in a flower.
Reason: The arrangement of flower in this inflorescence is centrifugal.
49. **Assertion:** Compound umbel is branched.
Reason: In compound umbel, both involucre and involucels are present.
50. **Assertion:** In cyathium, several male flowers surround a single female flower.
Reason: The involucre is nectariferous.

51. **Assertion:** In china rose, the flowers are actinomorphic.
Reason: They are hypogynous with twisted aestivation.

52. **Assertion:** Monoadelphous stamens are found in pea.
Reason: Diadelphous stamens are found in china rose.

53. **Assertion :** In hemianatropous ovule, the funicle lies perpendicular to body of ovule.
Reason : Here, body of ovule is rotated by 90°.

54. **Assertion:** The symbol for inferior ovary is $\underline{G}$.
Reason: Adhesion is indicated by enclosing the figure within bracket.

55. **Assertion:** The floral formula of family Solanaceae is

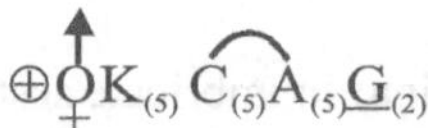

Reason: This floral formula tells that flower is bisexual, sepals five, petals five, stamens five and gynoecium tricarpellary, trilocular with many ovules.

56. **Assertion:** The filaments are free and the anthers are fused in syngenesious stamens.
Reason: In synandrous stamens, both filaments and anthers are fused.

57. **Assertion:** Parietal placentation is the placentation in which the placenta forms a ridge along the ventral suture of ovary and ovules are borne on this ridge forming two rows.
Reason: The marginal placentation has ovules developed on the inner wall of the ovary or on peripheral part.

58. **Assertion :** Coconut tree is distributed in coastal areas over a large part of the world.
Reason : Coconut fruit can float and get dispersed over thousands of kilometers before losing viability. **[AIIMS 2004]**

59. **Assertion:** Fruit is the mature or ripened ovary developed after fertilisation.
Reason: Parthenocarpic fruit is formed without fertilisation of the ovary.

60. **Assertion:** Seed coat is the outermost covering of a dicotyledonous seed.
Reason: The seed coat has two layers-outer testa and inner hilum.

61. **Assertion:** In syconous type of fruit, the achenes formed are fewer than the total number of flowers in the inflorescence from which it is formed.
Reason: Upper and middle flowers cannot develop into fruits.

62. **Assertion:** Some fruits are furnished with hooks, spines, barbs or other devices for sticking to the body of animals unwillingly.
Reason: Such fruits are dispersed by animals unwillingly.

63. **Assertion:** The mesocarp of drupe is not edible in all cases.
Reason: Coconut is a fibrous drupe.

64. **Assertion:** Fruit of wheat is a caryopsis.
Reason: Its pericarp is well differentiated.

65. **Assertion:** Achenial fruits are single seeded fruits.
Reason: Capsular fruits are multiseeded fruits.

66. **Assertion:** Samara is a winged achenial fruit.
Reason: Wings may or may not develop from its pericarp.

67. **Assertion :** Many plants are propagated vegetatively even though they bear seeds.
Reason : Potatoes multiply by tubers, apple by cutting etc.

68. **Assertion:** Maize is an albuminous seed.
Reason: Endosperm is completely absorbed by its growing embryo.

69. **Assertion:** Human travellers also disperse seeds and fruits.
Reason: Generally seeds of economically important crops are introduced to new areas.

70. **Assertion:** In dicotyledonous seeds, cotyledons are often fleshy and full of reserve food.
Reason: Generally monocotyledonous seeds are endospermic.

71. **Assertion:** Heterophylly is observed in many aquatic plants.
Reason: Aquatic plants survive in two different conditions of the environment.

72. **Assertion :** Citrus is a palmate compound leaf.
Reason : Citrus has single functional leaflet.

73. **Assertion :** In fabaceae family, monocarpellary, unilocular ovary is present.
Reason : In fabaceae, placentation is parietal. **[AIIMS 2010]**

74. **Assertion:** An ascending taxonomic sequence of *Gossypium herbaceum* indicates its placement in progressively higher groups.
Reason: Ascending taxonomic hierarchy indicates that a taxon is treated as belonging to a number of taxa.

Solutions

1. (a) Root cap is the terminal part of root.
2. (c) A number of thin, thread-like branched roots develop from the base of the stem in fibrous root system. The roots are of nearly equal size. They form a bunch which helps in holding the soil firmly. It provides good anchorage to the plant, helps in proper absorption of water and minerals. This root system is found in many monocots. Examples of plants having fibrous root system are wheat and barley.
3. (b) Ginger is horizontal in position and generally branched and producing aerial leaves or shoots above ground and adventitious roots on lower side in favourable season. Thus, shoot growth is not effected by gravity.
4. (a) In plants such as *Avicennia,* growing in swampy areas, many roots come out of the ground and grow vertically upwards. Such roots are called pneumatophores which help to get oxygen for respiration. These roots are also known as respiratory roots.
5. (b) Root is typically a non green underground cylindrical structure forming the descending axis of the plant which gives rise to endogenous branches and does not possess nodes, leaves or buds. Presence of nodes and internodes is the characteristic feature of stems.
6. (b) The root cap protects the root meristem from friction of the soil particles. In the process, its outer cells are continuously peeled off and replaced by new cells formed from root meristem. In floating aquatic plants, the root apices possess finger glove-like coverings called root pockets instead of root cap.
7. (d) Root pockets are present in floating aquatic plants. They act as balancers. They are structurally similar to root caps but differ from them, in the fact, that the damaged root pockets are not regenerated. *Pandanus*, possess multiple root caps with a number of sheaths found successfully one after the other because they are not peeled off in the absence of soil friction.
8. (b) Root hair zone is 1-6 cm in length. The root hairs increase the exposed surface of the root for absorption of water and minerals.
9. (a) Deep feeder tap root system has an elongated tap root which penetrates the deeper layers of the soil. It is mostly found in trees. Deep feeder tap root is also called racemose tap root system. In surface feeders, the tap root does not elongate very much. The secondary roots spread to a greater extent. Such a system is also named as cymose tap root system.
10. (c) The fleshy roots are thickened like the palm of human hand. They similarly possess finger like outgrowth, *e.g., Orchis*. They are palmate roots. Fasciculated fleshy roots are the swollen roots or root tubers occurring in clusters.
11. (b) Moniliform of beaded roots are swollen at regular intervals like beads of a necklace. Hence, the roots have the appearance of necklace. Such roots are found in *Discorealata, Momordica charauter* etc.
12. (a) Assimilatory roots are green roots (as they contain chlorophyll) which are capable of photosynthesis. *e.g., Taeniophyllum*, is a leafless epiphytic orchid with thick flattened photosynthetic roots.
13. (b) Epiphytes live on the surface of other plants for shelter and space only, hence are also called space parasites. Epiphytic roots possess a covering of dead spongy tissue known as velamen. They are able to absorb water from moist atmosphere, dew and rain with the help of velamen.
14. (c) The zone of elongation region of a root lies behind the growing point. The cells of this region are newly formed cells which lose the power of division. They elongate rapidly. This increases the length of the root. The root hair zone represents the zone of differentiation or maturation because of different types of primary tissues

differentiates or matures in this region. Some of the outer cells of this zone give rise to lateral tubular outgrowths called root hairs.

15. (a) A bud is a condensed immature or embryonic shoot having a growing point surrounded by closely placed immature leaves. The largest bud is cabbage. According to their nature, buds can be vegetative, reproductive and mixed.

16. (a) Stems are modified to perform different functions like storage, protection, mechanical support and photosynthesis etc. Axillary buds of stems may also get modified into woody, straight and pointed thorns. Thorns are found in many plants such as *Citrus, Bougainvillea,* etc. They protect plants from browsing animals and also reduce transpiraton .

17. (d) Stem is usually the above-ground erect ascending part of the plant body that develops from the plumule, grows by means of a terminal bud and shows distinction of nodes and internodes. The nodes bear leaves having auxillary buds.

18. (c) The pedicles or floral stacks of *Artabotrys* are modified into stiff curved thorns or hooks for climbing. In *Antigonon*, the flowers occur in bunches in the axils of scale leaves on the floral shoot. The upper floral buds develop into tendrils instead of forming flowers.

19. (c) Prickles are superficial outgrowths of stem or leaves which do not possess a vascular cylinder. They can be easily pulled off. Bristles are stiff hair which become thickened due to deposition of silica or calcium carbonate.

20. (b) Phyllodes do not bear leaves, branches, flowers, etc. In *Parkinsonia aculeata*, the rachis ends in a spine. Rachis are elongated, flattened and green to function as phyllodes. They bear small leaflets which fall off very easily.

21. (b) A leaf having a single or undivided lamina is called simple leaf. The lamina can have different types of incisions, which may reach upto half (-fid), more than half (-partite) or near the base or midrib (-sect). Depending upon the pinnate or palmate venation, the incisions are known as pinnatifid palmatifid, pinnatipartite, palmatipartite, pinnatisect and palmatisect etc.

22. (c) The petiole, rachis and the stalks of the leaflets in *Clematis* are sensitive to contact and can coil around the support to help the plant in climbing. In whole leaf tendril, the whole leaf is modified into a tendril for climbing. The leaf apices of *Gloriosa superba* are greatly elongated to function like the tendrils.

23. (a) Leaves of a number of plants develop or possess adventitious buds for vegetative propagation, *e.g., Bryophyllum. Begonia* leaf develops buds only when the leaf is injured or detached.

24. (b) Lowermost part of the leaf by which the leaf is joined to the node of the stem is the leaf base. It protects the young axillary bud. In many legumes, it is swollen. The swollen leaf base is known as pulvinus. It is responsible for sleep and shock movements of certain leaves, e.g., *Mimosa pudica* and *Cassia*.

25. (d) Venation is the arrangement of veins and the veinlets in the lamina of leaf. The venation is termed as reticulate when the veinlets form a network. When the veins run parallel to each other within a lamina, the venation is termed as parallel. Leaves of dicotyledonous plants generally possess reticulate venation, while parallel venation is the characteristic feature seen in most monocotyledons.

26. (b) Phyllotaxy is the arrangement of leaves on the stem or branch. The purpose or function of phyllotaxy is to arrange leaves in such a manner that all of them get proper exposure to sunlight. In alternate type of phyllotaxy, a single leaf arises at each node in an alternate manner. Only one leaf is borne on a node and the leaves of the adjacent nodes roughly lie towards the opposite sides. Alternate phyllotaxy is also known as spiral phyllotaxy. Alternate type of phyllotaxy is seen in China rose, mustard and sunflower plants.

27. (b) Leaf is a green, dissimilar exogenous lateral outgrowth which is borne on the node of a stem or its branch and is specialised to perform photosynthesis. All the green leaves of a plant are collectively called foliage. Phyllotaxy is the arrangement of leaves on the stem or its branches.

28. (b) In spiral arrangement, each node bears a leaf and the leaves of the adjacent nodes roughly lie towards the opposite sides. In opposite arrangement, two leaves are borne on the opposite sides of a single node. When three or more leaves develop on the nodes, they form whorled arrangement.

29. (b) Prickles are defensive organs of plants but prickles being usually curved are commonly used for climbing. They are superficial outgrowths of stem or leaves which do not possess a vascular cylinder.

30. (b) In caducous, leaves fall down soon after their appearance, *e.g.*, *Opuntia*. In deciduous plants, almost all leaves fall off almost simultaneously at the end of the growing season. The phenomenon is called leaf fall, *e.g.*, Mulberry, Poplar.

31. (c) A leaf is called centric leaf when the leaf is more or less cylindrical and directed upwards or downwards, as in onion. A centric leaf is equally illuminated on all sides and, therefore, it is evenly green. Centric leaves of onion is aerial. It is underground scale leaves of bulb which store food.

32. (c) China–rose has free lateral stipules and rose bears adnate stipules. Free lateral stipules are free stipules, usually small and green in colour, borne on the two sides of the leaf-base. Adnate stipules are two lateral stipules that grow along the petiole upto a certain height, adhering to it and making it somewhat winged in appearance.

33. (a) Leaves of a number of plants develop or possess adventitious buds for vegetative propagation, *e.g.*, *Bryophyllum*. *Begonia* leaf develops buds only when the leaf is injured or detached.

34. (a) The spadix contains a large green or coloured bract called spathe. For example, in banana and aroids, the brightly coloured spathe attracts insects to facilitate pollination.

35. (b) *Scilla* synthesise its food stored in the leaf bases. It is a photosynthethic plant. The bud also originates fom the leaf bases and this part contains the tunicated bulb.

36. (c) Leaf base is the lowermost part of the leaf by which the leaf is joined to the node of the stem. In leguminous plants, leaf base is swollen (pulvinus). *Alstonia* show whorled phyllotaxy. i.e. three or more than three leaves develop from a single node.

37. (c) In corymb, the main axis is shortened and lower flowers have much longer stalks or pedicels than the upper ones so that all the flowers are brought more or less to the same level. Corymb inflorescence is found in *Cassia sp.*

38. (c) A flower is regarded as complete if it has all the four floral whorls, *i.e.*, calyx, corolla, androecium and gynoecium. If any of these whorl in missing, the flower is described as incomplete. An incomplete flower can either be perfect, having male as well as female sex organs or imperfect with either of the sexes missing. When both the essential organs are absent, the flower is spoken as neuter.

39. (b) When a plant bears only one type of unisexual flowers, it is termed as dioecious. Some plants possess three types of flowers - perfect (intersexual), staminate and female or neuter. They are called polygamous. Polygamous plants as for example, mango and cashewnut bear perfect and imperfect flowers on the same individual.

40. (a) Inflorescence is the arrangement of flowers on the floral axis. Cymose inflorescence is the name of determinate or definite inflorescence in which the tip of the main axis terminates in a flower and further growth continues by one or more lateral branches which also behave like the main axis. The arrangement of flowers is either basipetal or centrifugal.

41. (c) Sepals or calyx constitute the outermost series of green foliaceous floral organs which are mainly meant for protecting other

floral parts in the bud condition. Petals or corolla constitute the upper or inner series of accessory floral organs which are leaf-like but brightly coloured to attract pollinating animals. Sepals and petals are nonessential or accessory floral organs or floral leaves which do not take any direct part in sexual reproduction. In plants, like lily there is no distinction of sepals and petals, the nonessential floral organs are collectively called perianth. The individual parts of the perianth are known as tepals.

42. (b) Aestivation is the arrangement of accessory floral organs (sepals or petals) in relation to one another in the floral bud. In imbricate aestivation, therc is an irregular overlapping of petals upon one another. Out of five petals, one is completely internal, one is completely external and in each of the remaining three petals, one margin is internal and the other is external. In ascending imbricate aestivation, posterior petal is internal *e.g., Cassia, Caesalpinia* and gulmohur.

43. (a) In cymose branching, the growth of the main stem is definite, that is the terminal bud does not continue to grow, but the main stem produces one or more lateral branches lower down, which grow more vigorously than the terminal one. In some plants, the terminal bud gets modified into a flower, tendril, thorn etc.

44. (b) Persistent sepals are called accrescent if they grow along with the fruit (*i.e., Physalis*). They (persistent sepals) are marcescent when they assume a dried up form before being shed, *i.e.,* Guava.

45. (c) Hypanthodium possesses a flask – shaped fleshy receptacle which possesses a narrow canal and a terminal pore at one end.

46. (a) Cymose inflorescence is determinate or definite inflorescence in which the tip of the main axis terminates in a flower and further growth continues by one or more lateral branches which also behave like the main axis.

Verticillaster is a special form of cymose inflorescence. The first axis ends in a flower, it bears two lateral branches, each ending in a flower, succeeding lateral branches are produced in an alternating manner.

47. (b) In racemose head, the main axis or receptacle is suppressed, becoming almost flat. It bears a mass of small sessile flowers (florets) on its surface, with one or more whorls of bracts at the base forming an involucre.

The florets are arranged in a centripetal fashion, *i.e.,* younger towards the centre and older towards the periphery. The advantages of this kind of inflorescence are that the head as a whole becomes more showy and attractive and the florets being close together, one or a few insects can pollinate most of them within a short time.

48. (a) In cymose inflorescence, the main axis ends in a flower and similarly the lateral axis also ends in a flower. Thus, the growth of each axis is checked. In cymose inflorescence, the terminal flower is always older and opens earlier than the lateral ones, *i.e.,* the order of opening of flowers is centrifugal.

49. (b) Compound umbel is branched umbel, where several small or daughter umbels arise from a common point in an umbellate fashion. A whorl of bracts, called involucre present at the base of the daughter umbels are called involucels.

50. (b) Cyathium is a special kind of inflorescence found in *Euphorbia, i.e., Poinsetia* and *Euphorbia.*

In cyathium, there is a cup – shaped involucre, often provided with nectar – secreting glands. The involucre encloses a single female flower in the centre, seated on a comparatively long stalk and a number of male flowers around this, seated on short slender stalks.

51. (b) In china rose (*Hibiscus rose-sinensis*) flowers are actinomorphic, hypogynous and twisted aestivation in corolla.

52. (d) Androecium is composed of stamens. A stamen or male reproductive organ of a flower is made up of two parts - a stalk -like filament and a knob like terminal anther. The free stamens are called polyandrous. The adelphous stamens are fused by their filaments only. The anthers are free. Fusion of filaments may produce one bunch or bundle and is called monodelphous *e.g.,* china rose. Fusion of filaments in two bundles is called diadelphous, *e.g.* pea.

53. (a) In hemianatropus ovule, the funicle lies at right angles to the body of the ovule. The body of the ovule is rotated by 90º.

54. (d) A flower is represented by a floral diagram and floral formula. The floral formula is represented by some symbols. $\underline{G}$ is the symbol for superior ovary. Fusion is indicated by enclosing the figure within bracket and adhesion by a line drawn above the symbols denoting the floral parts.

55. (c) The floral formula of family Solanaceae is

$$\oplus ⚥ K_{(5)} \overset{\frown}{C_{(5)} A_{(5)}} \underline{G}_{(2)}$$

Solanaceae is commonly called the potato family. This floral formula describes that the flower is bisexual, actinomorphic, sepals are five and united, petals are five and united, stamens are five, epipetalous and gynoecium is bicarpellary, and syncarpous, ovary is superior, bilocular and placenta is swollen with many ovules.

56. (b) In syngenesious condition, when the stamens are united by their anthers only, the filaments remaining free. In synandrous, stamens are fused by both their filaments as well as anthers.

57. (d) One or two alternate rows of the ovules occur longitudinally along the ridge in the wall of the ovary in the area of fusion of its two margins or ventral suture in marginal placentation. A true placenta is believed to be absent. Ovary is unilocular. Marginal placentation is found in monocarpellary pistils of Leguminosae (*e.g.,* Pea, *Cassia, Acacia*) and other plants (*e.g.,* Larkspur). In parietal placentation, two or more longitudinal placentae develop along the wall of a syncarpous or compound pistil. The ovary is usually unilocular or become falsely bi or tri locular due to ingrowth of placentae or formation of false septa. Parietal placentation is found in members of family Brassicaceae, *Capparis* and *Viola* etc.

58. (b) Coconut require the hot and wet climate hence it is grown in coastal areas. It is widely grown in coastal and deltic regions of tropical and subtropical countries. Coconut fruit show hydrochory *i.e.,* the dispersal takes place through water medium. Being the habitat of coastal area the fruit is so adapted that it can float and dispersed over thousand of kilometers before losing viability.

59. (b) True fruit (eucarp) is a ripened ovary which develops under the influence of ripening ovules and is meant for protecting them. It consists of a pericarp formed from the wall of ovary and seeds developed from ovules. False fruit is a fruit in which other floral parts like thalamus, base of sepals petals, etc. fuse with the pericarp, accessory fruit or pseudocarp. The examples of false fruit are apple, mulberry and strawberry etc. A fruit formed without fertilisation, *i.e.,* a seedless fruit is called parthenocarpic fruit *e.g.,* banana.

60. (c) Seed is the ripened ovule which contains an embryo or miniature plant which has adequate reserve food for future development of the embryo. A seed may have one or two coverings called seed coat. The outer or the only seed coat (if one is present) is called testa while the inner one is named as tegmen. The hilum is a scar on the seed coat through which developing seed attaches to fruit. It is the place where funiculus or stalk of the seed is borne.

61. (a) Syconous fruit develops from hypanthodium inflorescence in which 3 types of flowers are found i.e. male, female and sterile gall flowers. Male flowers and gall flowers cannot develop into fruits. So in syconous type of fruits, the achenes formed are fewer than the total number of flowers in the inflorescence.

62. (a) Many fruits are provided with hooks, barbs, spines, bristles, stiff hairs etc., on their surface by means of which they adhere to the body of woolly animals as well as to the clothing of mankind and are often carried by them to distant places. The animals are forced to carry such fruits and seeds.

63. (b) The pericarp of drupe is differentiated into epicarp, mesocarp and endocarp. Endocarp is stony. Hence, drupes are also called stone fruits. Coconut is called fibrous drupe due to fibrous mesocarp, possesses edible endosperm. Among drupes, the mango has edible mesocarp, cherry, peach, plum and *Zizyphus* have edible epicarp and mesocarp.

64. (c) Caryopsis is a superior achenial fruit where testa and pericarp are inseparably fused, *e.g.,* wheat, maize etc. Achenial fruits are single seeded indehiscent dry and simple fruits. The pericarp is dry and undifferentiated. The pericarp of wheat is thus, dry and it is fused with testa.

65. (b) Achenial fruits are single seeded dry indehiscent and simple fruits. The pericarp is dry and undifferentiated. Capsular fruits are many seeded dry and simple fruits in which the pericarp splits open to expose the seeds.

66. (c) Samara is an achenial fruit having winged pericarp, *e.g. Ulmus* (Elm). Achenial fruits are single seeded dry indehiscent and simple fruits. If the wings develop from places other than pericarp in achenial winged fruits then they are called samaroid *e.g.,* sepals in *Shorea*.

67. (c) Plants do propagate more by vegetative means since they multiply faster vegetatively.

68. (c) Albuminous seeds are those where endosperm is present, as in maize and castor bean. The endosperm persists in their seeds. In exalbuminous seeds, the endosperm is completely absorbed by the growing embryo and the food reserve gets stored in the cotyledons.

69. (b) Human travellers have always taken plants from one area to another. Potato was brought from New World by the Portuguese. Many economically important crops and plants such as maize, tobacoo, groundnut, chillies, tea, cabbage, cauliflower, rubber etc. are dispersed by man, as they have been introduced to new areas from their original home. However, many weeds are also dispersed alongwith useful plants.

70. (b) In both monocots and dicots, food reserves are stored in the endosperm; however, in non-endospermic dicots, the cotyledons act as the storage.

71. (a) Heterophylly is seen in many aquatic plants, particularly those growing in shallow running water. Here, the floating or aerial leaves and the submerged leaves are of different kinds; the former are generally broad, more or less fully expanded and undivided or merely lobed; while the latter are narrow, ribbon-shaped, linear or much dissected. Examples are *Sagittaria, Ranunculus aquatilis, Limnophila heterophylla*.

72. (b) The palmate compound leaf is one in which the petiole bears leaflets at the tip like the fingers of the palm. Citrus is actually a palmate compound leaf where the two lateral leaflets have been suppressed and only the central leaflet is functional. Such a palmate compound leaf, with one functional leaflet is called unifoliate compound leaf.

73. (c) In fabaceae, ovary is present. Placentation is marginal with many ovules.

74. (a) *Gossypium herbaceum* belongs to family-Malvaceae. Taxonomic hierarchy is the system by which various taxonomic categories are arranged in a proper descending order. The ascending taxonomic hierarchy shows that a taxon belongs to a number of taxa and its placement in progressively higher groups.

Chapter 6

Anatomy of Flowering Plants

Directions: In the following questions, a statement of assertion is followed by a statement of reason. Mark the correct choice as:

(a) If both Assertion and Reason are true and Reason is the correct explanation of Assertion.
(b) If both Assertion and Reason are true but Reason is not the correct explanation of Assertion.
(c) If Assertion is true but Reason is false.
(d) If both Assertion and Reason are false.

1. **Assertion :** Apical meristem of root is subterminal.
Reason: At the terminal end of root, root cap is present.
2. **Assertion :** Histogen theory is not applicable to shoot apex.
Reason : The shoot apex is not clearly divided into three layers.
3. **Assertion :** Higher plants have meristematic regions for indefinite growth.
Reason : Higher plants have root and shoot apices. **[AIIMS 1997]**
4. **Assertion:** Apical meristem and intercalary meristem both are primary meristems.
Reason: Both of these meristems appear early in life of a plant and help in the formation of the primary plant body.
5. **Assertion:** Lateral meristems include fascicular vascular cambium, interfascicular cambium and cork-cambium.
Reason: These are responsible for forming the secondary tissues.
6. **Assertion:** Higher plants have meristematic regions for indefinite growth.
Reason: Higher plants have root and shoot apices.
7. **Assertion:** Quiescent centre is found in the centre of the root apex.
Reason: It consists of actively dividing cells.
8. **Assertion:** Intercalary meristems increase length of plant like apical meristems.
Reason: It originates from the apical meristems.
9. **Assertion:** Apical and intercalary meristems contribute to the growth in length, while the lateral meristems cause increase in girth in maize.
Reason: Apical and intercalary meristems always increase the height of plants.
10. **Assertion:** In grasses and cereals, intercalary meristems are present.
Reason: Intercalary meristems form permanent tissues.
11. **Assertion:** Collenchyma forms the hypodermis of dicotyledon stems.
Reason : This is the reason for flexibility of dicotyledonous stems.
12. **Assertion :** Aerenchyma help in buoyancy to hydrophyte plants.
Reason : The large air chambers are present in aerenchyma.
13. **Assertion :** Collenchymatous cells show thickenings of pectin.
Reason : Collenchyma is thick walled dead tissue.
14. **Assertion:** A simple tissue is made of only one type of cells.
Reason: Various simple tissues in plants are parenchyma, collenchyma and sclerenchyma.
15. **Assertion:** Sclerenchyma cells do not possess plasmodesmata.
Reason: The cell walls of some permanent tissues are heavily lignified.
16. **Assertion:** Idioblasts are derived from parenchyma.
Reason: Secretory cells are modified parenchyma.
17. **Assertion:** Sclerenchyma consists of long narrow cells with thick lignified cell walls.
Reason: They are usually dead and without protoplasm.
18. **Assertion:** Many organs of aquatic plants float in water.
Reason: Large air gaps are present in the collenchyma tissues of lotus leaf.

19. **Assertion:** Sclereids are found in the fruit walls of nuts, pulp of fruits like guava, pear and sapota and seed coats of legumes.
Reason: Sclereids are spherical, oval or cylindrical, highly thickened dead cells with narrow lumen.

20. **Assertion :** In angiosperms, the conduction of water is more efficient because their xylem has vessels.
Reason : Conduction of water by vessel elements is an active process with energy supplied by xylem parenchyma rich in mitochondria.
[AIIMS 2006]

21. **Assertion :** Vessels are more efficient for water conduction as compared to tracheids.
Reason : Vessels are dead lignified.

22. **Assertion:** Xylem vessel is a long cylindrical tube like-structure made up of many cells each with lignified walls.
Reason: Presence of vessels is a characteristic feature of gymnosperms.

23. **Assertion:** Phloem fibres or bast fibres are made up of collenchymatous cells.
Reason: These are generally found in primary pholem.

24. **Assertion:** Cells are living and thin walled and their cell wall are made up of cellulose.
Reason: The radial conduction of water in plants takes place by the help of these tissues.

25. **Assertion:** Phloem transport the food materials usually from the leaves to other parts of the plant.
Reason: Phloem in the angiosperm is composed of sieve tube elements, companion cells, phloem parenchyma and phloem fibres.

26. **Assertion:** Thick cuticle is present in disease resistant plants mostly.
Reason: Disease causing agents cannot invade the cuticle and grow on cuticle.

27. **Assertion:** Xylem and phloem form conducting tissue of the plant.
Reason: Xylem and phloem are also called as hadrome and leptome respectively.

28. **Assertion:** Cuticle is also present in lower epidermal region of the leaf.
Reason: The lower epidermis contains a large number of stomata.

29. **Assertion :** Radial vascular bundles are found in roots.
Reason : Xylem & phloem occur in separate bundles and lie on different radii alternating with each other.

30. **Assertion :** Open vascular bundles are found in dicot stem & gymnosperm.
Reason : Cambium is absent in between xylem & phloem.

31. **Assertion :** Amphivasal vascular bundles are found in some monocots.
Reason : Xylem lie in centre surrounded by phloem.

32. **Assertion:** Cambium is a lateral meristem and cause growth in width.
Reason: Cambium is made up of fusiform and ray initials in stem. **[AIIMS 1998]**

33. **Assertion :** In collateral vascular bundles, phloem is situated towards inner side.
Reason : In monocot stem, cambium is present.
[AIIMS 1998]

34. **Assertion:** Each stoma is composed of two bean shaped cells known as guard cells.
Reason: Guard cells regulate the opening and closing of stomata.

35. **Assertion:** In a dicot stem, vascular bundles are conjoint, collateral and closed.
Reason: Vascular bundles are conjoint, collateral and open in monocot stem.

36. **Assertion:** All tissues lying inside vascular cambium are called as bark.
Reason: Bark is made up of phellogen, phellem and phelloderm lying inside secondary phloem.

37. **Assertion:** Stomata are absent in submerged hydrophytes.
Reason: Respiration occurs by means of air chambers in submerged plants.

38. **Assertion:** Vascular bundle of monocot stem is conjoint.
Reason: Vascular bundle of monocot stem are open and phloem parenchyma is absent.

39. **Assertion :** Petroplants produce large amount of latex.
Reason : The latex contains long chain hydrocarbons. **[AIIMS 2007]**

40. **Assertion:** Intercellular spaces are found in cortex region.
Reason: Intercellular spaces are absent in endodermis.

41. **Assertion:** Pith is large and well developed in monocots.
Reason: Monocot root do not undergo any secondary growth.

42. **Assertion :** In stem, pericycle take active part in secondary growth.
Reason : In root, pericycle take active part in secondary growth.

43. **Assertion:** The trichomes in the shoot system are usually multicellular.
Reason: These help in preventing water loss due to evaporation.

44. **Assertion:** Endodermis is also called as starch sheath in dicot stem.
Reason: The cells of the endodermis are rich in starch grains.

45. **Assertion:** The two cotyledons in seed are embryonic leaves.
Reason: The embryo contains radicle and plumule. **[AIIMS 2002]**

46. **Assertion:** Bulliform cells are useful in the unrolling of leaf.
Reason: Bulliform leaves store water. **[AIIMS 2011]**

47. **Assertion:** In dicot leaf, epidermis covers both the upper surface (adaxial epidermis) and lower surface (abaxial epidermis).
Reason: The adaxial epidermis bears more stomata than the abaxial epidermis.

48. **Assertion:** Xerophytic leaves may contain stomatal crypts or sunken stomata.
Reason: Spongy parenchyma is more in xerophytic leaves.

49. **Assertion:** The upper surface of the leaf is darker than the lower surface.
Reason: Spongy mesophyll contains less chloroplasts than palisade mesophyll cells.

50. **Assertion :** Annual rings do not occur in dicot trees growing on sea shore.
Reason : There is little climate variation.

51. **Assertion :** Tyloses are more abundant in duramen.
Reason: They provide rigidity & strength to heart wood.

52. **Assertion :** In woody stems, the amount of heart wood continues to increase year after year.
Reason : The cambial activity continues uninterrupted. **[AIIMS 2007]**

53. **Assertion:** Phellem or cork is impervious to water.
Reason: It is due to suberin deposition in the cell wall of cork.

54. **Assertion:** Heartwood the greater part of secondary xylem, is lighter in colour and consists of dead elements with highly lignified walls.
Reason: The peripheral region of the secondary xylem is dark brown in colour and is called sapwood.

55. **Assertion:** The wood is actually secondary xylem.
Reason: Secondary growth occurs in most of the monocot roots and stems.

56. **Assertion:** Cambium is a lateral meristem and cause growth in width.
Reason: It is made up of fusiform and ray initials in stem.

57. **Assertion:** Sapwood is less durable than the heartwood.
Reason: Hollow tree trunks are due to the disappearance of sapwood.

58. **Assertion:** Growth rings are also called as annual rings.
Reason: Generally growth ring is formed in each year.

59. **Assertion:** Secondary growth is usually seen in dicotyledonous stems.
Reason: The vascular cambium present between xylem and pholem possesses the ability to form secondary xylem and secondary pholem respectively.

60. **Assertion:** Epidermal cells have small amount of cytoplasm and a large vacuole.
Reason: Guard cells are dumb bell shaped in dicots and bean shaped in monocots.

61. **Assertion:** In dicot stem, vascular bundles are arranged in a ring.
Reason: In dicot roots, cambium develops in between xylem and phloem.

Solutions

1. (a) Root apical meristem is subterminal because of the presence of a protective terminal root cap over it.
2. (a) Histogen theory, which proposes that the three principal tissues of the root-vascular cylinder, cortex, and epidermis-originate from three groups of initial cells, or histogens, in the apical meristem-plerome, periblem, and dermatogen respectively. A fourth histogen, the calyptrogen, produces the root cap.
3. (a) The root apex and shoot apex are meristematic in nature. These meristematic tissues are embryonic in origin. They are primary in origin because it develops from embryonic tissues and primary in function because they form the primary structure of the plant cell, the root apex and shoot apex, that live till the death of the whole plant. Hence, plants have the feature of indefinite growth.
4. (a) Growth in plants is mostly restricted to specialised regions of active cell division called meristems. The meristems which occur at the tips of roots and shoots and produce primary tissues are called apical meristems. They cause growth in length. The meristem which occurs between mature tissues is known as intercalary meristem, commonly located at the bases of leaves, above the nodes (*e.g.*, grasses) or below the nodes (*e.g.*, mint). These help in elongation of the organs. Both apical meristems and intercalary meristems are primary meristems because they appear early in life of a plant and contribute to the formation of the primary plant body.
5. (b) Secondary meristem is the meristem that occurs in the mature regions of roots and shoots of many plants, particularly those that produce woody axis and appear later than primary meristem. These are cylindrical meristems. Fascicular vascular cambium, interfascicular cambium and cork cambium are examples of lateral meristems. These are responsible for producing the secondary tissues.
6. (a) Higher plants have root and shoot apices where the cells are in state of continuous division. Here, they can grow indefinitely. Such regions are not found in animals.
7. (c) Quiescent centre is found in the centre of the root apex. Cell divisions are very few in the quiescent centre as there is very little synthesis of new proteins, RNAs and DNA. Quiescent centre may function as reserve meristem.
8. (a) Intercalary meristems are intercalated in-between the permanent tissues. The activities of these meristems also add to the length of the plant or its organs. They originate from the apical meristems when their portions get detached due to the growth of the organs. For example, in the grasses when the internodes complete their elongation, some cells at the base retain their meristematic activity and function as intercalary meristems. They lie just above the node.
9. (d) Apical and intercalary meristems always increase the height of plants and lateral meristem is responsible for secondary growth and doesn't occur in monocots.
10. (b) Intercalary meristems are intercalated in between the permanent tissues. They may be present either at the base of the internode as in the stems of various grasses and wheat; or at the base of the leaf as in *Pinus*; or at the base of a node as in mint (*Mentha viridis*).
11. (a) Collenchyma cells are elongated cells with irregularly thick cell walls that provide support and structure. Their thick cell walls are composed of the compounds cellulose and pectin. These cells are often found under the epidermis, or the outer layer of cells in young stems and in leaf veins.
12. (c) Aerenchyma is a spongy tissue that forms spaces or air channels in the leaves, stems and roots of some plants, which allows exchange of gases between the shoot and the root.

13. (c) Collenchyma is made up of living cells with unevenly thickened cell wall. Their cell wall is made up of cellulose and pectin. Collenchyma are present beneath the epidermis of young stem, petioles and midrib of leaves, *etc*. These are absent in underground tissues and leaves and stems of monocots.

14. (b) The tissues in which the cells of which have lost the capacity to divide and have attained a permanent shape, size and function due to morphological, biochemical and physiological differentiation are permanent tissues. Permanent tissues can be classified as simple, complex and special on the basis of composition. A simple permanent tissue is that tissue which is made up of similar permanent cells that carry out the same function or have the same structure. Simple permanent tissues are of three types-parenchyma, collenchyma and sclerenchyma.

15. (a) Sclerenchyma is the supporting tissue in plants. Two types of sclerenchyma cells exist: fibers and sclereids. Their cell walls consist of cellulose, hemicellulose and lignin. Sclerenchyma provides the main structural support to a plant.

16. (b) Secretory cells are specialized parenchyma cells that produce nectar, oil, etc. Idioblasts are specialized non-green large-sized parenchyma cells which possess inclusions or ingredients like tannins, oils, crystals, etc.

17. (a) Sclerenchyma consists of long narrow cells with thick lignified cell walls having a few or numerous pits. They are usually dead and without protoplasm.

18. (c) Organs of aquatic plants are made of a special parenchyma tissue known as aerenchyma. It consists of a network of parenchyma cells which enclose very large air cavities. These air cavities store gases and make the aquatic plants light and buoyant. Collenchyma is simple permanent tissue with pectocellulose thickening in its wall and no intercellular gaps.

19. (b) Sclerenchyma is a simple supportive tissue with highly thick-walled cells with little or no protoplasm. Sclerenchyma is of two types: sclerenchymatous fibres and sclereids. Sclereids dead sclerenchymatous cells that are highly thickened with very narrow cavities. They are lignified and extremely thick walled. Sclereids are broader as compared to the fibres being isodiametric polyhedral, spherical, oval, short or cylindrical. They may also be branched. Sclereids may occur singly or in groups. The various types of sclereids are stone cells or Brachysclereids, Macroslereids, Osteosclereids. Astrosclereids, filiform sclereids and trichosclereids, etc. Sclereids are found in grit of guava, sapota, apple, pear, epidermal covering of some legume, seeds, etc.

20. (d) Xylem is the water conducting tissue. It consists of living cells like parenchyma and dead cells like tracheary elements.

21. (b) Vessels are more efficient for water conduction as compared to tracheids. Vessels resemble tracheids very much in structure and function. But unlike tracheids, these are like long tubes arranged in vertical row formed of cylindrical cells arranged to end with their end walls completely dissolved. These are also dead and lignified.

22. (c) Xylem is a complex tissue which performs the function of transport of water and minerals from roots to the stem and leaves. It also provides mechanical strength. Xylem consists of four types of cells namely tracheids, vessels, xylem fibres and xylem parenchyma.

23. (d) Phloem is a complex tissue meant for transport of food from leaves to the other body parts of the plant. Phloem is also called bast. It consists of four types of cells: sieve tubes, companion cells, phloem parenchyma and fibres. Sclerenchyma fibres found in the phloem are called phloem or *bast* fibres. Phloem fibres provide mechanical strength. the textile fibres of flax (*Linum usitatissimum*), hemp (*Cannabis*) and jute (*Corchorus* species) are phloem fibres which are used for making ropes and coarse textiles.

24. (b) Xylem parenchyma cells are living and thin walled and their cell walls are made up of cellulose. They store food materials in the form of starch or fat and other substances like tannins. The radial conduction of water takes place by the ray parenchymatous cells.

25. (b) Usually phloem transports food material from leaves to other parts of the plant. In angiosperm, phloem is composed of sieve tube elements, companion cells, phloem parenchyma and phloem fibres.

26. (a) Disease resistant plants possess thick cuticle so that infectious organisms can not grow or invade cuticle.

27. (a) Phloem transports organic food inside the body of the plant. Xylem performs the function of transport of water or sap inside the plant. Thus, they form the conducting elements in the plant. Haberlandt used the term leptome for phloem and hadrome for xylem.

28. (b) A distinct layer of cuticle is present in the lower epidermis. The cuticle is, however, less developed than at the upper epidermis. The lower epidermis contains a large number of pores called stomata. They lead internally into substomatal cavities.

29. (a) Radial vascular bundles occur in dicot & monocot roots. A vascular bundle, in which the primary xylem and primary phloem strands are separated from each other by non-vascular tissues and they are situated on alternate radii of an axis, is known as radial vascular bundle or radial bundle.

30. (c) Open vascular bundles are the feature of dicot stem and gymnosperm. The cambium present between xylem and phloem is called fascicular cambium. In closed vascular bundles, the cambium will be absent (fascicular cambium absent) and they do not show secondary growth (closed for secondary growth). In open vascular bundles, a layer of cambium will be present between the xylem and phloem and thus, they shows secondary growth.

31. (c) A vascular bundle in which xylem encircles the central strand of phloem is known as amphivasal bundle, also called leptocentric bundle. Ex. *Dracaena, Yucca.*

32. (b) Fusiform initials are vertically elongated cells that produce xylem and phloem elements. Ray initials are isodiametric and produce parenchymatous rays in secondary xylem and phloem.

33. (d) Collateral vascular bundles have the xylem pointing towards the inner side of the phloem. In the same way, in monocots, cambium is absent. Collateral vascular bundles are present in stems and leaves of angiosperms and gymnosperms.

34. (b) Stomata are structures present in the epidermis of leaves. Stomata regulate the process of transpiration and gaseous exchange. Each stoma is composed of two bean shaped cells known as guard cells. In grasses, the guard cells are dumb-bell shaped. The guard cells possess chloroplasts and regulate the opening and closing of stomata.

35. (d) In a dicot stem, each vascular bundle consists of phloem on the outer side, xylem towards the inner side and a strip of cambium in between the two. Phloem and xylem tissues lie on the same radius. Such vascular bundles are known as conjoint (with both phloem and xylem), collateral (phloem and xylem on the same radius) and open. In monocot stem, phloem lies towards the outside and the xylem on the inner side. Cambium is absent as the whole procambium is consumed in the formation of vascular tissues. The vascular bundles are, therefore, conjoint, collateral and closed.

36. (d) Bark consists of all tissues outside the vascular cambium. Phellem, phellogen and phelloderm constitute periderm.

37. (b) Stomata are absent in submerged hydrophytes. Air chambers help in gaseous exchange, O_2 liberated during photosynthesis is stored in these chambers and used in respiration. CO_2 released during respiration also remains in these chambers. CO_2 is used in photosynthesis.

38. (c) Vascular bundle of monocot stem are conjoint, collateral but closed. They lack cambium hence, seconday growth is absent. Phloem consists of sieve tubes, companion cells and a few phloem fibres. Phloem parenchyma is absent.

39. (a) Petroplants are plants having large amount of latex with long chain hydrocarbons. Latex of these plants are a good substitute for liquid fuels or petroleum. Cultivation of petroplants is a part of energy- cropping.

Dr. Calvin was the scientist who identified petrocrops. They have property of converting large amount of their photosynthates into latex along with hydrocarbons. Some important petrocrops are *Euphorbia antisyphilitica*, *E. lathyris*, *Calotropis procera etc*.

40. (b) In dicotyledonous root, the cortex consists of several layer thin walled parenchyma layer. These parenchyma cells have intercellular space. The inner most layer of the cortex is called endodermis. It surrounds the vascular tissue.

41. (b) Pith is well developed in the monocots and is small, inconspicuous in dicots. In monocot, there is no secondary growth due to absence of the vascular cambium between the xylem and phloem. But, secondary growth is the characteristic of dicot plants.

42. (d) The pericycle is located between the endodermis and phloem in plant roots. In dicot stems, it is situated around the ring of vascular bundles in the stele. In dicot roots, the pericycle strengthens the roots and provides protection for the vascular bundles. In plants, undergoing secondary growth, the pericycle contributes to the vascular cambium often diverging into a cork cambium.

43. (b) The epidermal hairs on the stem are called trichomes. The trichomes in the shoot system are usually multicellular. They may be branched or unbranched and soft or stiff. They may even be secretory. The trichomes help in preventing water loss due to transpiration.

44. (a) The innermost layer of the cortex is called endodermis. It is made up of closely packed living cells characterized by the presence of band like thickenings of lignin and suberin on their radial and tangential walls. These bands or strips are called casparian bands or strips. The cells of the endodermis are rich in starch grains and layer is also referred to as the starch sheath.

45. (b) During epigeal germination, cotyledons come out of the soil. The green cotyledons function as leaves of the seedling. They manufacture food and sustain the young seedling till the plumule gives rise to new leaves.

46. (b) In isobilateral leaves, the upper epidermis contains specialized cells, *i.e.*, bulliform or motor cells. They are highly vacuolate and can store water, if available. However, in case of water deficiency, the bulliform cells lose water and become flaccid. As a result, the leaf gets rolled up to reduce the exposed surface. The bulliform cells are also useful in the unrolling of leaf during its development.

47. (c) The upper surface of the leaf is called the adaxial or ventral surface, and the lower surface of the leaf is called outer, abaxial or dorsal surface. Most of the dicotyledonous leaves are dorsiventral. Epidermis covers both the upper and lower surfaces of the leaf. Both upper and lower epidermis consist of rectangular parenchymatous cells. The abaxial epidermis generally bears more stomata than adaxial epidermis. Sometimes adaxial epidermis may even lack stomata. A distinct layer of cuticle is present on the adaxial and abaxial epidermis. The cuticle prevents excessive transpiration.

48. (c) Spongy parenchyma is reduced in xerophytic leaves. Palisade parenchyma may occur on both the upper and lower sides with spongy parenchyma sandwiched between the two, *e.g., Nerium*.

49. (a) The palisade mesophyll cells lie below the upper epidermis. The spongy parenchyma or spongy mesophyll lies between the lower epidermis and the palisade parenchyma. The spongy mesophyll cells contain chloroplasts but fewer than present in the palisade parenchyma. As the chloroplasts are more abundant in the compact palisade mesophyll cells than the loosely arranged mesophyll cells, the upper surface of the leaf appears deeper green as compared to the lower surface.

50. (a) Annual rings do not occur in dicot tree growing on seashore because. Soil is sandy, there is little climatic variation and increased moisture.

51. (a) Tyloses are most abundant in heart wood (duramen), where wood parenchyma is scarce, in the xylem of woody plants as response to injury or as protection from decay in heartwood.

52. (a) In woody trees, the central portion of stem is dark in colour. It is hard and tough due to deposition of resins, tannins, gums and formation of tyloses. This central hard portion is called heart wood. It is formed by secondary growth. Due to cambial activity, secondary xylem becomes non-functional and forms heart wood or duramen. It is more durable and little susceptible to attack of pathogens. The cambial activity continues in this region.

53. (a) Phellogen produces cork or phellem on the outer side. It consists of dead and compactly arranged rectangular cells. Due to suberin deposition in the cell walls, these cells are impervious to water. The cork cells contain tannins. Hence, they appear brown or dark brown in colour. Cork prevents the loss of water by evaporation. Cork is light, compressible non-reactive and sufficiently resistant to fire. It is used as a stopper for bottles, shock absorption and insulation.

54. (d) The greater part of secondary xylem in old trees is dark brown due to deposition of organic compounds like tannins, resins, oils, gums, aromatic substances and essential oils in the central or innermost layers of the stem. These substances make it hard, durable and resistant to the attacks of microorganisms and insects. This region comprises dead elements with highly lignified walls called as heartwood. The heartwood does not conduct water but it gives mechanical support to the stem. The peripheral region of the secondary xylem, is lighter in colour and is known as the sapwood. It is involved in the conduction of water and minerals from the root to the leaf.

55. (c) Wood is the secondary xylem that forms the bulk of the stem. The secondary xylem consists of vessels, tracheids (both tracheary elements), wood fibres and wood parenchyma. Wood parenchyma may contain tannins and crystals besides storing food. Secondary xylem does not show distinction into protoxylem and metaxylem elements. Therefore, vessels and tracheids with annular and spiral thickenings are absent. Secondary growth occurs in most of the dicotyledonous roots and stems.

56. (b) Cambium is a lateral meristem. Its activity causes increase in width. It is composed of fusiform and ray initial.

57. (c) Various types of plant products like oils, resins, gums and tannins are deposited in the cells of the heartwood. They are antiseptic. The heartwood is, therefore, stronger and more durable than the sapwood. It is, however, liable to be attacked by wood rotting fungi. Hollow tree trunks are due to their activity. Sapwood (outer light coloured wood) is less durable because it is susceptible to attack by pathogens and insects.

58. (c) Trichomes are unicellular or multicellular outgrowths which are strictly epidermal in origin. Trichomes are of two kinds, hair and scales. Roots have unicellular root hair which arise as tubular unbranched out-growths of cells of piliferous layer or epiblema. They increase the absorptive surface of the root.

59. (a) Dicotyledonous stems usually display secondary growth in thickness, which is due to the activity of vascular cambium and cork cambium. Vascular cambium is present between phloem and xylem. Such vascular bundles because of the presence of cambium possess the ability to form secondary xylem and phloem tissues, and exhibit secondary growth.

60. (c) Epidermal cells are elongated compactly arranged and form continuous layer called epidermis. In monocotyledons (grasses), the guard cells are dumb bell shaped and in dicotyledonous the guard cells are bean or kidney shaped.

61. (b) Dicot stems show conjoint, collateral and open vascular bundle i.e. xylem and phloem are present at the same radii. The initiation of vascular cambium during secondary growth phase takes place in pericycle which is present in between xylem and phloem.

Chapter 7

Structural Organisation in Animals

Directions: In the following questions, a statement of assertion is followed by a statement of reason. Mark the correct choice as:

(a) If both Assertion and Reason are true and Reason is the correct explanation of Assertion.
(b) If both Assertion and Reason are true but Reason is not the correct explanation of Assertion.
(c) If Assertion is true but Reason is false.
(d) If both Assertion and Reason are false.

1. **Assertion :** Specialization of cells is advantageous for the organisms.
Reason : It increases the operational efficiency of an organism.
2. **Assertion :** The squamous epithelium is made of a single thin layer of flattened cells with irregular boundaries.
Reason : They are found in walls of blood vessels and air sacs of wings. **[AIIMS 2017]**
3. **Assertion :** Urinary bladder can considerably expand to accommodate urine.
Reason : It is lined by stretchable squamous epithelium.
4. **Assertion :** Columnar epithelium lining the intestinal mucosa appears to have a brush like appearance.
Reason : A large number of microvilli are present on brush bordered columnar epithelium.
5. **Assertion :** Surface of skin is impervious to water.
Reason : Surface of skin is covered by stratified cuboidal epithelium.
6. **Assertion:** Stomach and intestine of our body has columnar epithelium.
Reason: Columnar epithelium helps in secretion and absorption.
7. **Assertion:** Cell junctions are present in the epithelium and other tissues.
Reason: Among cell junctions, adhering junctions help to stop substances from leaking across a tissue.
8. **Assertion:** Simple epithelium covers surfaces exposed to mechanical or chemical abrasions.
Reason: Protection of underlying tissues is the major function of simple epithelium.
9. **Assertion:** Compound epithelium play important role in absorption, secretion and excretion.
Reason: Compound epithelium is found in the stomach lining.
10. **Assertion :** Cartilage (protein matrix) and bone (calcium matrix) are rigid connective tissue.
Reason : Blood is connective tissue in which plasma is the matrix.
11. **Assertion:** Connective tissues are most abundant and widely distributed in the body of complex animals.
Reason: Connective tissues link and support other tissues or organs of the body.
12. **Assertion:** Tendons attach one bone to another bone.
Reason: Ligaments attach skeletal muscles to bones.
13. **Assertion:** The cells of connective tissues except blood secrete fibres.
Reason: Fibres provide strength, elasticity and flexibility to the tissue.
14. **Assertion:** Presence of connective tissue inside the brain is essential for conduction of nerve impulse.
Reason: Connective tissue hold together the nerve cells of brain.
15. **Assertion:** Tendon is present in all bone joints.
Reason: Tendon connects the bones together and holds them in position.
16. **Assertion:** The cell secretes fibres of structural protein in all the connective tissues except blood.
Reason: Neuroglea is made up of more than one half the volume of neural tissue in our body.
17. **Assertion:** In skeletal muscles, a sheath of tough connective tissue encloses several bundles of muscle fibres.
Reason: These are involuntary in their action.

18. **Assertion :** WBCs accumulate at site of wounds by diapedesis.
Reason: It is squeezing of leucocytes from endothelium.
19. **Assertion :** Mast cells in the human body release excessive amounts of inflammatory chemicals which cause allergic reactions.
Reason : Allergens in the environment on reaching human body stimulate mast cells in certain individuals.
20. **Assertion :** Mast cells help in body defence.
Reason : Mast cells phagocytose & destroy microbes.
21. **Assertion:** Total count of RBC comes out to be very low in polycythemia.
Reason: Number of erythrocytes get reduced in the condition of polycythemia.
22. **Assertion:** Haemoglobin is said to be a conjugated protein.
Reason: It is composed of a protein called haem and a non protein iron porphyrin complex called globin.
23. **Assertion:** Histamine is involved in allergic and inflammatory reactions.
Reason: Histamine is a vasodilator.
24. **Assertion:** Chilling of blood decreases coagulation time.
Reason: Cold increases the action of coagulation promoting enzymes.
25. **Assertion:** Thrombin is necessary to initiate blood coagulation.
Reason: Thrombin helps in the formation of thromboplastins.
26. **Assertion:** The regulation of RBC production is accomplished by FSH.
Reason: Erythropoietin hormone circulates to kidney where it increases stem cell mitosis and speed up development of RBCs.
27. **Assertion:** Materials cannot be exchanged between epithelial cells.
Reason: Blood vessels are present in epithelial tissue.
28. **Assertion:** There is hepatic portal system in frogs.
Reason: It is venous connection between liver and intestine in frog.
29. **Assertion:** Mummies of Egypt still have their arteries preserved due to the presence of yellow elastic connective tissue.
Reason: Yellow elastic connective tissue have considerable strength and remarkable elasticity.
30. **Assertion:** Areolar tissue contains fibroblast, macrophages and mast cells.
Reason: Adhering junction helps to stop substances from leaking across tissue.
31. **Assertion:** Hardest tissue of the body is bone
Reason: Hardness of the bone is due to the calcification of its matrix.
32. **Assertion :** Intercalated discs are important regions of cardiac muscle cells.
Reason : Intercalated discs function as boosters for muscle contraction waves.
33. **Assertion:** Smooth muscles are known as involuntary muscles.
Reason: Smooth muscles are controlled by autonomic nervous system.
34. **Assertion:** Muscle cells are also called myofibrils..
Reason: Muscle cells are very thick and elongated.
35. **Assertion:** Thigh muscles can get tired but not the muscles of ventricle of heart.
Reason: Muscles of thigh are voluntary whereas that of heart are involuntary muscles.
36. **Assertion:** Non-striated muscles are said to be voluntary in nature.
Reason: Non-striated muscles can be moved according to will.
37. **Assertion:** Granulocytes are white blood cells.
Reason: They contain lobed nuclei and tiny granules.
38. **Assertion:** Osteocytes are present in spaces called lacunae.
Reason: Striated muscles fibres are bundles together in a parallel fashion.
39. **Assertion:** Neurons protect and support the neuroglial cells.
Reason: Neuroglial cells make up ninety per cent neural tissue in our body.
40. **Assertion:** Non-myelinated nerve fibres do not possess nodes of Ranvier.
Reason: This is due to the absence of nissl's bodies in node of Ranvier.
41. **Assertion:** Neuroglial cells protect and support the neurons.
Reason: When neuron is suitably stimulated, an electrical disturbance is generated which travels along its cytoplasm.

42. **Assertion:** Setae are absent in clitellum.
Reason: These help in locomotion.

43. **Assertion:** Blood glands are present in earthworm.
Reason: Earthworm has an open type of blood vascular system.

44. **Assertion:** Earthworms are known as friends of farmers.
Reason: Earthworms make burrows in the soil and make the soil porous, which helps in respiration and penetration of developing plant roots.

45. **Assertion:** In earthworm, setae are present in all segments except first, clitellum and last.
Reason: Earthworms are hermaphrodite and reproduce primarily by self-fertilization.

46. **Assertion:** Blood in cockroach is colourless haemolymph with no respiratory pigment.
Reason: Respiration in cockroach occurs through diffusion in haemolymph.

47. **Assertion:** Malpighian tubules is responsible for excretion in cockroach.
Reason: Each Malpighian tubule is lined by non-ciliated columnar cells.

48. **Assertion:** Eggs of cockroach are encased in capsules called oothecae.
Reason: Oothecae is a dark reddish to blackish brown capsule.

49. **Assertion:** Cockroach shows sexual dimorphism.
Reason: The female cockroach bears a pair of short thread like anal styles.

50. **Assertion:** Frog has short alimentary canal.
Reason: Frogs are carnivores.

Solutions

1. (a) Specialization of cells into tissue, organ and organ systems is advantageous for the organisms. It increases the operational efficiency through division of labour which avoids duplication of work.
2. (b) Squamous epithelium is a single layer of flattened cells in contact with basal lamina of the epithelium. This type of epithelium is often permeable and occurs where small molecules need to pass quickly through membranes.
3. (c) Urinary bladder is not lined by squamous epithelium but by transitional epithelium which is a stretchable compound epithelium. It has a single layer of cuboidal cells at the base, 2-3 middle layers of large polygonal cells and a superficial layer of large, broad rectangular cells. Stretching considerably flattens and broadens the cells of superficial and middle layers, hence causing expansion of the urinary bladder.
4. (a) Columnar epithelium is a type of simple epithelium characterised by the presence of tall column like cells. Its major function is absorption or secretion. It covers the inner surface of the intestine, stomach and gall bladder. In the intestine, it appears to have a brush like appearance on the free surface, which is due to the presence of large number of microvilli. Function of microvilli is to enhance absorption. Due to the presence of microvilli, the epithelium is also called as brush bordered columnar epithelium.
5. (c) Surface of skin is impervious to water because it is covered by stratified keratinised squamous epithelium. This epithelium has many superficial layers of horny, scale like remains of dead squamous cells and several deeper layer of living polygonal cells. Heavy deposits of the insoluble protein keratin are present in the dead superficial layers which makes this epithelium impervious to water. Stratified cuboidal epithelium, on the other hand, lines the inner surface of sweat gland, larger salivary and pancreatic ducts.
6. (a) The columnar epithelium is composed of a single layer of tall and slender cells. Their nuclei are located at the base. Free surface may have microvilli. They are found in the lining of stomach and intestine and help in secretion and absorption.
7. (c) All cells in epithelium are held together with little intercellular material. In nearly all animal tissues, specialized junctions provide both structural and functional links between its individual cells. Three types of cell junctions are found in the epithelium and other tissues. These are called as tight, adhering and gap junctions. Adhering junctions perform cementing function to keep neighbouring cells together.
8. (d) Simple epithelium does not cover surfaces exposed to mechanical or chemical abrasions because it is made up of a single layer of cells, hence it is not effective in protecting the underlying tissue. Simple epithelium occurs mainly on secretory and absorptive surfaces. There is another types of epithelial tissue called compound epithelium which being multilayered is effective in providing protection to underlying tissues, therefore, covers the surfaces exposed to mechanical and chemical abrasions.
9. (d) Compound epithelium performs the function of providing protection against chemical and mechanical stress. Thus, it has limited role in absorption, secretion and excretion. This epithelium is found in the moist surface of buccal cavity, pharynx, inner lining of duct of salivary gland but not in stomach lining.
10. (b) Cartilage comprises of mucopolysaccharide called chondroitin sulphate. Bone is a hard connective tissue while blood is a fluid connective tissue.
11. (b) Connective tissue is the most abundant and widely distributed tissue of the body. It connects different tissues or organs and

provides support to various structures of animal body. The connective tissue consists of living cells and extra-cellular matrix. It includes soft connective tissues and specialised tissues like cartilage, bone, adipose and blood.

12. (d) Tendon is made up of white fibrous tissue. Tendon connects a skeletal muscle to bone. It is tough and inelastic. Ligament is strong and elastic and made up of yellow elastic tissue with some collagen fibres. Ligament connects a bone to another bone.

13. (b) All cells of connective tissue except blood secrete fibres. Fibroblasts are the main cells of connective tissue, which secrete various types of fibres. There are three types of fibres secreted by connective tissue cells and each type is formed by proteins. These are collagen fibres (made up of collagen protein), elastic fibres (formed of elastin) and reticular fibres (made up of reticulin). All provide strength, elasticity and flexibility to the connective tissue.

14. (d) Ordinary connective tissue is absent inside the central nervous system. *i.e.* brain and spinal cord and has no function in the conduction of nerve impulse. The neurons of nerve tissue inside the brain and spinal cord are held together by supporting cells called neuroglia cells. Neuroglia cells resemble neurons and have long radiating processes but no nissl granules.

15. (d) It is not tendon but another type of connective tissue called ligament which is present in most of the bone joints and connect the bones together. Ligament also helps in holding the bones in position. Tendon, on the the other hand, is a dense, strong, fibrous connective tissue which forms strong inextensible attachment of a skeletal muscle to a bone.

16. (b) The cell secretes fibres of structural protein in all the connective tissues called collagen. Neuroglea is made up of more than one half the volume of neural tissue in human body

17. (c) Skeletal muscles action are voluntary i.e., they can be removed according to our will, walls of the blood vessels contain epithelial tissue not skeletal muscles.

18. (b) In wounds, germs are removed by WBCs accumulation at wound site by diapedesis. It is squeezing of leucocytes out from endothelium of capillaries to fight external agent.

19. (a) The symptoms of an allergic reaction develop in response to histamine. Mast cells release a large amount of histamine into the blood stream and it also act as initiator of the inflammatory response which aids the arrival of leucocytes at a site of infection. Histamine stimulates capillary dilation, increased capillary permeability, closure of bronchial tubes, mucus secretion, pain and swelling.

20. (c) Mast cells are large irregular cells with granular cytoplasm, present in the areolar connective tissue. These cells store inflammation producing substances such as histamine in dense granules. Mast cells defend themselves which in turn helps in body defence by attracting phagocytes to the injured tissue.

21. (d) Total count of RBC refers to the total number of red blood corpuscles (erythrocytes) present in one microlitre of the blood. It averages 5 million and 4.5 million in adult man and woman respectively. Total count of RBC comes out to be very low in condition of anaemia and after profuse bleeding. On the contrary, polycythemia is the condition which arises due to the abnormal rise in the total count of RBC.

22. (c) Conjugated proteins are the proteins which are formed by the binding of a simple protein with a non-protein prosthetic group. Conjugated chromoproteins are the pigment protein complexes. Hemoglobin is one such conjugated chromoprotein. It is composed of a simple protein called "globin" and non protein iron (Fe^{2+}) porphyrin complex called "heme". 100 ml of blood contains about 15g of hemoglobin. Four Fe^{2+} ions of heme can loosely bind to upto four molecules of oxygen, thus enabling hemoglobin to carry oxygen.

23. (a) Histamine is a derivative of the amino acid histidine produced by damaged cells of vertebrates. When released, it has the effect of dilating capillaries and lowering blood pressure. Histamine is involved in allergic and inflammatory reactions.

24. (d) Treating the blood to low temperatures (chilling) decreases the activity of coagulation promoting enzymes. So, at low temperatures it will take more time for the blood to clot i.e. the coagulation of blood gets delayed. Thus, chilling of blood increases the coagulation time (time taken for the blood to coagulate) and not decrease it.

25. (c) Blood coagulation is brought about by the hydrolysis of soluble protein fibrinogen to insoluble fibrin. This reaction is catalysed by the enzyme thrombin. Thrombin occurs in normal blood as an inactive globulin called prothrombin which is activated to thrombin by the action of another enzyme called prothrombinase before blood coagulation starts. Thromboplastins are the coagulation promoting substances released from clumped platelets and damaged tissue, which helps in the formation of the enzyme prothrombinase.

26. (d) Regulation of RBCs production is accomplished by hormone erythropoietin which is secreted by kidney. This hormone increases stem cell mitosis and speed up RBCs development in red bone marrow.

27. (d) Though blood vessels are absent in epithelial tissues, exchanges of materials takes place in them. Materials are exchanged between epithelial cells and vessels of the connective tissues by diffusion across the basement membrane. Also, epithelial tissues exchange materials through osmosis and filtration, (e.g. epithelial tissues of pulmonary vein, Bowman's capsule etc.).

28. (a) In frog, venous system has hepatic portal system. This system carries blood from the alimentary canal and its associated glands to the liver. It consists of a large hepatic portal vein that receives a number of tributaries from many organs.

29. (a) Yellow elastic connective tissue have considerable strength and remarkable elasticity. They are present in the wall of blood vessels, lungs, bronchioles, cartilage of larynx and trachea, etc. Many years old mummies still have their arteries intact due to well preserved elastic yellow fibres.

30. (c) Adhering junctions form a strengthening and interlocking belt encircling the exterior of adjacent cells and contribute to the stability and integrity of the cell layer.

31. (a) Hardest tissue of the body is bone. Its hardness is due to the calcification of its matrix. It has hard and non-pliable ground substances rich in calcium salts and collagen fibres which give strength to the bone.

32. (a) Cardiac muscle cells are short cylindrical cells joined end to end and by side branching to form a network. Intercalated discs are the dense junctions formed in between the cardiac muscle cells where they meet each other. Intercalated discs are the specialised regions of the cell membranes. As cardiac muscle possesses considerable rhythmicity and generates its own wave of excitation, these discs function as boosters for muscle contraction wave.

33. (a) Smooth muscles are found in the posterior part of oesophagus, stomach, intestine, blood vessels, iris of eye and dermis of skin. They are involuntary as their functioning cannot be directly controlled. Action of these muscles is controlled by autonomic nervous system.

34. (d) Since muscle cells are very thin and elongated, therefore, they are also called as muscle fibres and not myofibril. Myofibril is the unit of a striated muscle fibre. A striated muscle fibre is composed of many myofibrils arranged along the long axis of the fibre. A myofibril is made of two types of myofilaments : actin filaments and myosin filaments. Sliding of these myofilaments over one another cause the contraction and relaxation of the muscle fibre.

35. (b) The thigh muscles are the striated muscles which soon get fatigued due to overwork. These muscles show fast contractions and then get tired immediately due to accumulation of lactic acid. The muscles of heart wall are the cardiac muscles which are unfatiguable and show rhythmic and automatic contractions. They have specialised regions of the cell membranes which function as boosters for muscle contraction waves. Thigh muscles are called voluntary muscles because they can be moved at the will of organism whereas heart muscles cannot be moved at one's will and therefore are involuntary.

36. (d) Non striated or smooth muscles are said to be involuntary in nature because they do not contract or relax according to our will. Those muscles which can be moved according to will of the organism are called voluntary muscles. Striated or skeletal muscles are said to be voluntary in nature as they can be contracted or relaxed voluntarily.

37. (b) On the basis of presence of tiny granules and number of lobes in nucleus of their cytoplasm, white blood cells are divided into two groups
   (i) Granulocytes contain tiny granules and lobed nuclei in their cytoplasm.
   (ii) Agranulocytes have no cytoplasmic granules in their nuclei and are also undivided.

38. (c) The muscles of biceps are voluntary and striated are called flexor as they bend one part of limb on another at a joint.

39. (d) Neuroglia or neuroglial cells are specialized cells found in the brain and spinal cord supporting the neurons and their fibres. About 50 percent of all brain cells are neuroglial cells.

40. (c) Myelin sheath is a lipid rich insulating layer which covers some nerve fibres of nerve tissue. Such fibres are called myelinated or medullated nerve fibres. Each myelinated nerve fibre shows constrictions at regular intervals called nodes of Ranvier which results from interruption in the myelin sheath at those places. Non myelinated nerve fibres are not covered by any myelin sheath, consequently no nodes of Ranvier are present in them.

41. (c) If neuron is suitably stimulated, an electrical disturbance is generated which travels along its plasma membrane. Arrival of the disturbance at the neuron's ending, triggers the events that may lead to the stimulation of adjacent neurons and other cells.

42. (b) Except the first, last and clitellar segments of earthworm, each segment bears a ring of tiny curved, chitinous structures known as setae or chaetae. These are embedded in the skin. Each seta (singular of setae) lies in a setal sac, which is a small pit in the skin. The sac has special muscles to move the seta out or in and to bend it forward or backward. The setae hold the substratum firmly. Thus, it helps in locomotion.

43. (c) Earthworm has closed type of blood vascular system as the blood flows in the closed blood vessels. Due to closed circulatory system, blood is confined to the heart and blood vessels. Contractions keep blood circulating in one direction. Blood glands are present on the 4th, 5th and 6th segments. These produce blood cells and haemoglobin which is dissolved in blood plasma.

44. (a) Earthworms are known as 'friends of farmers' because they make the soil loose and porous by their burrowing habit. Thus, the soil provides quick aeration and absorption of water, thereby the roots of the plant get penetrated easily. Earthworms continuously bring the lower soil on the surface, and deposit it there. They plough the land and share the work of the farmers. The process of increasing fertility of soil by earthworm is called vermicomposting.

45. (c) Earthworm is hermaphrodite and reproduces primarily by cross-fertilization. The earthworm does not reproduce asexually. Except the first, the last and the clitellar segment, each segment bears a ring of tiny curved chitinous structure known as setae. Setae help in locomotion and copulation.

46. (c) The colourless blood or haemolymph of cockroach has a clear plasma and numerous white corpuscles called haemocytes. Being devoid of any respiratory pigment it does not serve for gaseous exchange. Its plasma contains about 70% water. In all terrestrial insects, like cockroach every tissue of body is in direct contact with atmospheric air for gaseous exchange.

47. (c) Excretion in cockroach is performed by Malpighian tubules. Each tubule is lined by glandular and ciliated cells. They absorb nitrogenous waste products and convert them into uric acid which is excreted out through the hindgut.

48. (b) The fertilized eggs of cockroach are encased in capsules called oothecae. Oothecae is a dark reddish to blackish brown capsule, about 3/8" (8 mm) long. They are dropped or glued to a suitable surface, usually in a crack or crevice with high relative humidity near a food source. On an average, females produce 9-10 oothecae, each containing 14-16 eggs.

49. (c) In cockroach, males and females have slightly different morphology, hence showing sexual dimorphism. One of the distinguishing features is presence of anal styles (paired thread - like structure) only in males. Females lack anal styles.

50. (a) The digestive system of frog consists of alimentary canal and digestive gland. Alimentary canal of frog is short because frogs are carnivores. Carnivores have shorter digestive tracts as meat is easier to digest than plant material.

Chapter 8

Cell: The Unit of Life

Directions: In the following questions, a statement of assertion is followed by a statement of reason. Mark the correct choice as:

(a) If both Assertion and Reason are true and Reason is the correct explanation of Assertion.

(b) If both Assertion and Reason are true but Reason is not the correct explanation of Assertion.

(c) If Assertion is true but Reason is false.

(d) If both Assertion and Reason are false.

1. **Assertion:** Organisms are made up of cells.
   Reason: Cells are structural unit of living organisms. A cell keeps its chemical composition steady within its boundary.
2. **Assertion:** Specialization of cells is useful for organism.
   Reason: It increases the operational efficiency of an organism.
3. **Assertion:** The number of cells in a multicellular organism is inversely proportional to size of body.
   Reason: All cells of biological world are alive.
4. **Assertion :** Living organisms possess specific individuality with the definite shape and size.
   Reason : Both living and non living entities resemble each other at the lower level of organisation.
5. **Assertion :** It is important that the organisms should have cell.
   Reason : A cell keeps its chemical composition steady within its boundary.
6. **Assertion:** The number of cells in a multicellular organism is inversely proportional to the size of body.
   Reason: All the cells in the biological world are of same size.
7. **Assertion:** Cell is an open system.
   Reason: Cell receives a number of materials including energy containing nutrients from outside.
8. **Assertion:** Smaller cells are usually metabolically active cells.
   Reason: Smaller cell nucleocytoplasmic ratio and surface volume ratio is higher.
9. **Assertion:** Rudolf Virchow modified the hypothesis of cell theory given by Schleiden and Schwann.
   Reason : Cell theory says that all cells arise from pre-existing cells.
10. **Assertion:** Schleiden and Schwann were the first to observe the cells and to put forward cell theory.
    Reason: The cells are always living unit.
11. **Assertion:** As per Schwann, cell wall is a unique character of the plant cell.
    Reason: Body of plants and animals are composed of cells and products of cells.
12. **Assertion:** Eukaryotic cells have membrane bound organelles.
    Reason: Prokaryotic cells lack membrane bound organelles.
13. **Assertion:** Ribosomes are non-membrane bound organelles found in the prokaryotic cells only.
    Reason: These are present only in the cytoplasm.
14. **Assertion:** Eukaryotic cells have more DNA than prokaryotic cells.
    Reason: Eukaryotes are genetically more complex than prokaryotes.
15. **Assertion:** Prokaryotes have a one envelop system.
    Reason: There is not even a single membrane that surrounds the prokaryotic cell.
16. **Assertion:** Lipids present in the outer and inner side of the bilayer membrane are commonly different.
    Reason : Oligosaccharides are attached to external surface as well as inner surface of a biomembrane. **[AIIMS 2009]**
17. **Assertion :** Cell membrane is semipermeable.
    Reason : The constituent molecules can freely move in the membrane.
18. **Assertion :** A cell membrane shows fluid behaviour.
    Reason : A membrane is a mosaic or composite of diverse lipids and proteins. **[AIIMS 2003, 2008]**

19. **Assertion :** Na^+-K^+ ATPase is an important membrane associated enzyme.
Reason : It helps in ion transfer across the membrane.
20. **Assertion:** Peripheral proteins are totally or partially buried in the membrane.
Reason: Integral proteins lie on the surface of membrane.
21. **Assertion:** Mesosomes are the infoldings of cell membrane. They helps in cell wall formation, DNA replication and respiration.
Reason: They increase the area of surface membrane.
22. **Assertion :** Cell wall is not found in animal cell.
Reason : Animal cells are covered by cell membrane. **[AIIMS 2001]**
23. **Assertion:** The endomembrane system comprises endoplasmic reticulum (ER), Golgi complex, lysosomes and vacuoles.
Reason: Mitochondria, chloroplast and peroxisomes are not the part of endomembrane system as their functions are not coordinated with the same.
24. **Assertion:** The endoplasmic reticulum which lacks ribosomes is called smooth endoplasmic reticulum (SER).
Reason: SER is mainly involved in protein synthesis.
25. **Assertion:** The Golgi apparatus mainly performs the function of packaging materials.
Reason: Materials to be packed in the form of vesicles from the ER fuse with trans face of the Golgi Apparatus.
26. **Assertion:** ER acts as a circulatory system.
Reason: ER functions as cytoskeleton
27. **Assertion :** Lysosomes help in photorespiration.
Reason : Lysosome have basic enzyme.
28. **Assertion:** Lysosomes are capable of digesting carbohydrates, proteins, lipids and nucleic acids.
Reason: Lysosomes are rich in hydrolytic enzymes like lipases, proteases and carbohydrases.
29. **Assertion:** Sphaerosome are single membrane bound and are associated with synthesis and storage lipids.
Reason: Lysosomes are double membrane vesicles budded off from Golgi apparatus and and contain digestive enzymes.
30. **Assertion :** Power house of cell is mitochondria.
Reason : ATP is produced in mitochondria. **[AIIMS 2001]**
31. **Assertion :** Mitochondria and chloroplasts are semi autonomous organelles.
Reason : They are formed by division of pre-existing organelles as well as contain DNA but lack protein synthesizing machinery **[AIIMS 2005, 2014]**
32. **Assertion:** The content of inner compartment of mitochondria is called matrix.
Reason: The outer membrane forms a number of infoldings called cristae.
33. **Assertion:** The number of mitochondria in a cell corresponds to the function of the cell.
Reason: Mitochondria are common to both plant and animal cells.
34. **Assertion:** The chromoplastin contains fat soluble carotenoid pigments like carotene and xanthophylls etc.
Reason: These pigments give yellow, orange or red colour to some part of the plant.
35. **Assertion:** Leucoplasts perform photoysnthesis.
Reason: Chloroplasts store fats, starch and proteins.
36. **Assertion:** Leucoplasts give rise to other types of plastids.
Reason: Chromoplasts do not get changed to other types of plastids.
37. **Assertion :** Centrosomes and centrioles are related to each other.
Reason : Centrosome usually contains two cylindrical structures called centrioles.
38. **Assertion:** The arrangement of axonemal microtubules in cilia or flagella is called 9 + 2 array.
Reason: The axoneme usually has nine pairs or doublets of radially arranged peripheral microtubules, and pair of centrally located microtubules.
39. **Assertion:** The fimbriae are elongated tubular structures made of special protein.
Reason: The pili are small bristle like fibres sprouting out of the cell.
40. **Assertion :** Plasmids are double-stranded extra chromosomal DNA.
Reason : Plasmids are possessed by eukaryotic cells.
41. **Assertion :** DNA is associated with proteins.
Reason : DNA binds around histone proteins that form a pool and the entire structure is called a nucleosome.

Solutions

1. (a) Cells are the basic structural and functional unit of organism.
2. (a) Specialization of the cell increases the efficiency of the cell for a particular function.
3. (d) The size and shape of the cell in multicellular organism depends upon the location and function performed by them.
4. (b) All living organisms have definite shape and size and all show specific individuality with an orderly mannered organisation whereas at the lower level of organisation, both the living and non living are made up of atoms.
5. (a) Metabolic reactions of a living organism can occur only in a delicately balanced environment in the non-living organisms. The cells are the life supporting chambers which have such a special environment. A living cell keeps its chemical composition steady within its boundary.
6. (d) Number of cells in a multicelluar organism are directly proportional to the size of the body. On the other hand, it is a fact that cell vary greatly in their size. *Mycoplasma* cells are the smallest, ranging from 0.1 to 0.3μm, whereas human cells, generally range from 20 to 30μm. Nerve cells are the longest.
7. (a) Cell is an isothermal open system as all the parts of the cell at any given time maintains the same temperature and pressure. Cell is an open system in which materials and energy are transferred between organisms and the exterior environment.
8. (a) Metabolically active cells are usually smaller due to higher nucleocytoplasmic ratio and higher surface volume ratio. The former will allow the nucleus to have better control of metabolic activities, while the latter will allow quicker exchange of materials between the cells and its outside environment.
9. (b) Schleiden and Schwann together formulated the cell theory. The theory however, did not explain as to how new cells were formed. Rudolf Virchow (1855) first explained that cells divided and new cells are formed from pre-existing cells (Omins cellua e cellua). He modified the hypothesis of Schleiden and Schwann to give the cell theory a final shape. The present cell theory states that: (i) all living organism are composed of cells and products of cells. (ii) all cells arise from pre-existing cells.
10. (d) They are credited with cell theory but the cells are not always the living unit. Cells die and still remain functional such as horny cells in animal and xylem vessels in plants.
11. (b) Based on his studies, Schwann proposed the hypothesis that the bodies of animal and plants are composed of cells and products of cells. Schleiden and Schwann together formulated the cell theory. Cell theory as understood is (i) All living organism are composed of cells and products of cells and (ii) all cells arise from pre-existing cells.
12. (b) Eukaryotic cells which have membrane bound distinct structures called organelles like nucleus, endoplasmic reticulum (ER), Golgi complex, lysosomes, mitochondria, microbodies and vacuoles. These are found in all protists, plants, animals and fungi. Prokaryotic cells lack such membrane bound organelles. Prokaryotic cells occur in bacteria, archaea, blue-green algae, mycoplasma and PPLO. Genetic material in these cells lies naked in the cytoplasm.
13. (d) Ribosomes are non-membrane bound organelles found in eukaryotic as well as prokaryotic cells. Within the cell, ribosomes are found not only in the cytoplasm but

also within the two organelles - chloroplasts (in plants) and mitochondria and on rough ER

14. (a) Eukaryotic cells have more DNA than prokaryotic cells because in eukaryotic cells complex chromosomes are composed of DNA and histone proteins. But in prokaryotic cells, histone protein is absent.

15. (c) Most prokaryotic cell particularly the bacterial cells have a chemically complex cell envelope. The cell envelope consists of a tightly bound three layered structure, i.e. the outermost glycocalyx followed by the cell wall and plasma membrane. Although each layer of the envelope performs distinct function, they act together as a single protective unit.

16. (c) Lipids present in the outer and inner side of the bilayer are commonly different, *e.g.*, lecithin on the outer side and cephalin on the inner side of erythrocyte membrane. Oligosaccoharides are attached to external surface of lipids and proteins of a bio-membrane. They are absent on the inner side.

17. (b) Cell membrane is semipermeable as it allows continuous flow of selected materials across it as required from time to time. On the other hand, constituent molecules of cell membrane are free to move inside membrane.

18. (a) With the help of freeze-fracture techniques in electron microscopy, the fluid mosaic model was put forward in 1970 by S.J. Singer and G.L. Nicolson. According to this model, plasma membrane is composed of phospholipids, extrinsic proteins. Selective permeability of plasma membrane can be explained with this model.

19. (a) Of all the membrane associated enzymes, Na^+–K^+ ATPase is one of the most important because of its role in ion transfer across the plasma membrane. This enzyme is dependent on the presence of lipids and is inactivated when all lipids are extracted.

20. (d) Membrane proteins are classified as integral or peripheral on the basis of ease of extraction. Peripheral proteins lie on the surface of membrane while the integral proteins are partially or totally buried in the membrane.

21. (b) A special membranous structure is the mesosome which is formed by the extension of plasma membrane into the cell. These extensions are in the form of vesicles, tubules and lamellae. They help in cell wall formation, DNA replication, respiration and distribution to daughter cell. They also help in secretion processes to increase the surface area of the plasma membrane and enzymatic content.

22. (a) Cell wall is characteristic feature of plant cells. Cell wall is absent in animals. Animals cells are covered by cell membrane.

23. (b) Endomembrane system refers to the grouping of some membrane organelles which function in close coordination with one another, viz., endoplasmic reticulum, Golgi complex, lysosomes and vacuoles. Functions of other organelles are not coordinated. They are not a part of endomembrane system, e.g., chloroplasts, mitochondria, peroxisomes and glyoxisomes etc.

24. (c) Smooth Endoplasmic Reticulum (SER) possesses smooth membranes which do not bear ribosomes. It is, therefore, also called agranular endoplasmic reticulum. SER is reponsible for synthesis of fats inside the cells of adipose tissue, formation of sphaerosomes, synthesis of glycogen as well as glycogenolysis (hydrolysis of glycogen) in liver cells, synthesis of sterols and steroid hormones as in the interstitial cells of testis and ovary and formation of visual pigments from vitamin A in retinal cells.

25. (c) The Golgi apparatus principally performs the function of packaging materials, to be delivered either to the intracellular targets or secreted outside the cell. Materials to be packaged in the form of vesicles from the ER fuse with the cis face of the Golgi apparatus and move towards the maturing face. That is, why the Golgi apparatus remains in close association with the endoplasmic reticulum.

26. (b) ER functions as cytoskeleton or intracellular and ultrastructural skeletal framework by providing mechanical support to colloidal cytoplasmic matrix. The ER may act as a circulatory system for intracellular circulation of various substances. Membrane flow may also be an important mechanism for carrying particles, molecules and ions into and out of the cells.

27. (d) Lysosomes have hydrolytic enzymes. These have no role in photorespiration.

28. (a) Lysosomes are single membrane bound small vesicles containing hydrolytic enzymes in the form of minute crystalline or semicrystalline granules of 0.5-0.8 μm. The important enzymes are acid phosphatases, sulphatases, proteases, peptidases, nucleases, lipases and carbohydrases. They are also called acid hydrolases because these digestive enzymes usually function in acidic medium with a pH of 4-5. These enzymes are capable of digesting carbohydrates, proteins, lipids and nucleic acids. Lysosomes are also called suicidal bags because of the presence of a large number of digestive enzymes or acid hydrolases in them which can cause cell lysis if a lysosome is burst.

29. (c) Double membrane are absent in lysosomes. They are enclosed by single lipoproteinaceous unit membrane.

30. (b) Mitochondria are called power house of a cell because they produce large amount of energy in the form of ATP.

31. (c) Mitochondria and chloroplasts both are double membrane organelles. They are semi autonomous as both their structure and functions are partially controlled by nucleus of the cell and partially themselves. Both possess their own DNA and arise from pre-existing cells. Synthesis of many amino acids occurs in mitochondria. The first formed amino acids are glutamic acid and aspartic acid.

Also, plastid manufactures some of its own proteins, enzymes and other chemicals because of the presence of 70S ribosomes which can help translate the coded information contained in mRNAs transcribed over chloroplast DNA.

DNA replication is the process of forming carbon copy of DNA. Whereas, transcription is the formation of RNA over DNA template.

32. (b) Each mitochondrion is a double membrane-bound structure with the outer membrane and the inner membrane dividing its lumen distinctly into two aqueous compartments, i.e., the outer compartment and the inner compartment. The inner compartment contains the matrix. The outer membrane forms the continuous limiting boundary of the organelle. The inner membrane forms a number of infoldings called the cristae towards the matrix. The cristae increase the surface area.

33. (d) Several functions of cell are carried out by mitochondria i.e. ATP synthesis, aerobic respiration, maternal inheritance etc.

34. (b) Chromoplasts are yellow or reddish in colour because of the presence of carotenoid pigments. Chlorophylls are absent. Chromoplasts are formed either from leucoplasts or chloroplasts. Change of colour from green to reddish during the ripening of tomato and chilli is due to transformation of chloroplasts to chromoplasts. The orange colour of carrot roots is due to chromoplasts.

35. (d) Chloroplasts perform photosynthesis while leucoplasts are storage plastids.

36. (b) Leucoplasts can change to other types of plastids, but chromoplasts cannot. Chromoplasts are formed either from leucoplasts or chloroplasts.

37. (a) The centrosome is the main place where cell microtubules get organized. Centrosome usually contains two cylindrical structure called centrioles. Centrioles are composed of grouping of microtubules arranged in 9 + 2 pattern. The pattern is so named because a ring of 9 microtubule "triplets" are arranged at right angles to one another. Centrioles found in

animal cells help to organize the assembly of microtubules during cell division. Centrioles replicate during the interphase stage of mitosis and meiosis.

38. (a) The study of a cilium or the flagella shows that they are covered with plasma membrane. Their core is called axoneme, it possesses a number of microtubules running parallel to the long axis. The axoneme usually has nine pairs or doublets of radially arranged peripheral microtubules, and a pair of centrally located microtubules. Such an arrangement of axonemal microtubules is referred to as the 9 + 2 array.

39. (d) Pili and fimbriae are surface structures of the bacteria but do not play a role in motility. The pili are elongated tubular structures made of a special protein (pilin). Pili develop in response to F^+ or fertility factor in Gram negative bacteria. The fimbriae are small bristle like fibres sprouting out of the cell. Fimbriae are involved in attaching bacteria to solid surfaces or host tissues. Some fimbriae cause agglutination of RBCs and help in mutual clinging of bacteria.

40. (c) Plasmid is extra-chromosomal DNA. It is also called fertility factor and is possessed by prokaryotic cells.

41. (a) A chain of DNA has 140 base pairs which makes $1\frac{3}{4}$ turns and twists around a histone octamer forming nucleosome. The core of nucleosome consists of 4 histones H_2A, H_2B, H_3 and H_4.

Chapter 9

Biomolecules

Directions: In the following questions, a statement of assertion is followed by a statement of reason. Mark the correct choice as:

(a) If both Assertion and Reason are true and Reason is the correct explanation of Assertion.

(b) If both Assertion and Reason are true but Reason is not the correct explanation of Assertion.

(c) If Assertion is true but Reason is false.

(d) If both Assertion and Reason are false.

1. **Assertion:** The living state is a equilibrium steady state to be able to perform work.
   Reason : Living process is a constant effort to prevent falling into non-equilibrium.
2. **Assertion:** Living organisms have more nitrogen and oxygen per unit mass than inanimate objects (e.g., earth crust).
   Reason: Living organisms have more Ca, Mg, Na in them than inanimate object.
3. **Assertion:** In living system, all the metabolic conversions are aided by catalyst.
   Reason: The catalyst which hasten the rate of a given metabolic conversion are not proteins.
4. **Assertion:** Secondary metabolites are produced in small quantities and their extraction from the plant is difficult and expensive.
   Reason: Secondary metabolites can be commercially produced by using tissue culture technique.
5. **Assertion :** Comparative biochemistry provides a strong evidence in favour of common ancestory of living beings.
   Reason : Genetic code is universal.
6. **Assertion :** Human diet should compulsorily contain glycine, serine and tyrosine.
   Reason : Essential amino acids can not be synthesized in the human body. **[AIIMS 2010]**
7. **Assertion :** The amino acid glycine comes under the category of nonessential amino acids.
   Reason : This is due to the fact that it can not be synthesised in the body. **[AIIMS 2011]**
8. **Assertion:** Amino acids are known as α-amino acids.
   Reason : Amino acids are organic compounds containing an amino group and carboxylic group as substituent on the α-carbon.
9. **Assertion:** Proteins are a heteropolymer.
   Reason : Dietary proteins are the source of non-essential amino acids.
10. **Assertion:** The long protein chain folds upon itself like a hollow ball giving rise to the tertiary structure.
    Reason : Tertiary structure gives a 3-dimensional view of a protein.
11. **Assertion:** Amino acids are amphoteric in their function.
    Reason: All amino acids are necessary for our body.
12. **Assertion:** Nine amino acids are essential amino acids for human.
    Reason: They are essential for human health.
13. **Assertion :** Vegetable oils are fats which are present in plant cells in soluble form.
    Reason : Vegetable oils occur only in cells of embryo.
14. **Assertion :** Unsaturated fats are more reactive compared with the saturated fats.
    Reason : Unsaturated fats have only single bonds in their structure. **[AIIMS 2010]**
15. **Assertion:** Palmitic acid has 20 carbon atoms including carboxyl carbon.
    Reason : Arachidonic acid has 16 carbon atoms including carboxyl carbon.
16. **Assertion :** Glycosidic bonds are formed by dehydration.
    Reason : In polysaccharides, individual monosaccharide is linked by glycosidic bond. **[AIIMS 2016]**
17. **Assertion:** The exoskeleton of arthropods is composed of complex polysaccharide called chitin.
    Reason : Plant cell walls are made of cellulose.
18. **Assertion :** In a DNA molecule, A–T rich parts melt before G–C rich parts.
    Reason: In between A and T, there are three H–bond, whereas in between G and C, there are two H-bonds. **[AIIMS 2017]**

19. **Assertion :** DNA molecules and RNA molecules are found in the nucleus of cell.
Reason : On heating, enzymes do not lose their specific activity.

20. **Assertion:** The heterocyclic compounds in nucleic acid are the nitrogenous bases.
Reason : Adenine and guanine are substituted pyrimidines while uracil, cytosine and thymine are substituted purines.

21. **Assertion:** The bonds attaching second and third phosphate in higher nucleotide are high energy bonds.
Reason: The bonds are attached against force of repulsion.

22. **Assertion :** Allosteric enzymes show feed back inhibition.
Reason : The inhibitor is competitive.
[AIIMS 2012]

23. **Assertion :** Enzymes have active sites and substrates reactive sites on their surfaces respectively.
Reason : Active and reactive sites push the enzyme and substrate molecules away from each other.

24. **Assertion :** Enzyme substrate complex does not remain throughout the reaction.
Reason : The greater the affinity of the enzyme for a substrate, the higher is the catalytic activity.

25. **Assertion :** Desmolysing enzymes are those which catalyse the reactions by hydrolysis.
Reason : Digestive enzymes are hydrolysing in nature.

26. **Assertion :** Coenzymes serve as co-factors in a number of different enzyme catalyzed reactions.
Reason : Coenzymes and prosthetic groups are cofactors.

27. **Assertion :** Enzymes are defined as biological proteins.
Reason : Chemically all enzymes are globular proteins.

28. **Assertion :** The higher the turn-over number the more efficient an enzyme is.
Reason : It is not dependent upon the number of active sites present over an enzyme.

29. **Assertion :** Enzyme becomes inactive below minimum temperature.
Reason : The inactivity of the enzymes is due to denaturation.

30. **Assertion :** Enzymes lower the activation energy.
Reason : A substrate molecule can be acted upon by a particular enzyme.

31. **Assertion:** All enzymes are not proteins.
Reason : RNA molecules that possess catalytic activity are called ribozymes.

32. **Assertion:** Inorganic catalysts work efficiently at high temperature.
Reason : Enzymes get damaged at high temperature.

33. **Assertion:** The inhibition of activity of succinic dehydrogenase by malonate is the example of competitive inhibition.
Reason : Competitive inhibition is the inhibition of enzyme activity when inhibitor closely resembles the substrate in its molecular structure.

34. **Assertion:** Each enzyme has a substrate binding site in its molecule which forms higly reactive enzyme-substrate complex.
Reason : The enzyme-substrate complex is long-lived and dissociates into its product and unchanged enzyme.

35. **Assertion:** Co-enzyme nicotinamide adenine dinucleotide (NAD) and NADP contain a vitamin.
Reason : The association of co-enzyme with apoenzyme is enduring.

36. **Assertion:** Most of the chemical reactions do not start automatically.
Reason : Reactant molecules have an energy barrier to become reactive.

37. **Assertion:** Hydrolases are the enzymes which catalyse the hydrolysis of ester, ether, peptide, glycosidic, C – C or P – N etc. bonds.
Reason : Lyases are the enzymes catalysing the linking together of 2 compounds like joining of C – O, C – N, P – O etc. bonds.

38. **Assertion:** The protein part of the enzyme is called apoenzyme and non-protein part of the enzyme is called co-factor.
Reason : Zinc is a co-factor for the proteolytic enzyme carboxypeptidase.

39. **Assertion:** Enzymes lower the activation energy.
Reason: A substrate molecule can be acted upon by a particular enzyme.

Solutions

1. **(d)** The living systems are in metabolic flux and thus, maintain the concentration of biomolecules, always remaining in non-equilibrium steady state where equilibrium is seldom achieved. No work can be carried out in equilibrium state. Living systems are therefore, regularly receiving an input of energy to prevent reaching an equilibrium and always remain in non-equilibrium steady state. Energy is obtained from metabolism. Metabolism and living state are thus, complementary and synonymous.
2. **(c)** After performing elemental analysis of a plant tissue, animal tissue, microbial paste (living matter) and of a piece of earth's crust (animate object), it was found that all living and non-living systems are made up of same chemical i.e., elements (e.g. carbon, hydrogen, oxygen and several others). Most living organisms have relatively high abundance of carbon and hydrogen than in earth's crust.
3. **(c)** All the catalysts including those which hasten the metabolic conversion rate are proteins.
4. **(b)** Secondary metabolites are biosynthetically derived from primary metabolites but more limited in distribution in plant kingdom being restricted to a particular taxonomic group. By culture media using tissue culture technique, secondary metabolites can be produced on a large scale.
5. **(b)** Comparative biochemistry provides a strong evidence for common ancestors of living beings (*e.g.* proteins lymph, enzymes, hormones, blood groups *etc.*)
6. **(d)** Essential amino acids are those which are taken from food and not synthesized in the body whereas non-essential amino acids need not be supplied in the diet and are synthesized in the body. Glycine, serine and tyrosine are non-essential amino acids.
7. **(c)** Non-essential amino acids are those amino acids which need not be supplied in the diet because they can be synthesised by the body, particularly from carbohydrate metabolites. Glycine is one such non essential amino acid. On the contrary, essential amino acids are those amino acids which can not be synthesised in the animal body and must be supplied with food in adequate amounts. Out of twenty amino acids, eight are considered essential in human diet.
8. **(a)** Amino acids are organic acids (with carboxylic group – COOH) having amino group ($-NH_2$) generally attached to α-carbon that also bears a variable hydrocarbon or alkyl group R and hydrogen. Amino acids are, therefore, substituted methanes where the four substituent groups occupy the four valency positions. These are hydrogen, carboxyl group and a variable group designated as R group.
9. **(c)** Each individual protein is a polymer of amino acids. As there are 20 types of amino acids, a protein is a heteropolymer and not a homopolymer. Amino acids can be essential or non-essential. Certain amino acids are essential for our health and they have to be supplied through our diet. Dietary proteins are thus, a source of essential amino acids. Non-essential amino acids are those amino acids which are synthesised in our body.
10. **(b)** The primary structure of protein depicts the sequence of amino acids in a chain or gives the positional information in a protein. Protein thread is folded in the form of a helix or in the sheet form in the secondary structure. The long protein chain is also folded upon itself like a hollow wollen ball, giving rise to the tertiary structure. This gives us a 3-dimensional view of a protein. Tertiary structure is absolutely necessary for many biological activities of proteins.
11. **(b)** Proteins and amino acids are amphoteric in nature, i.e., in aqueous they possess both

cationic and anionic groups. All the amino acids are necessary for the normal function of the body as they are building blocks of proteins and enzymes.

12. (a) Nine amino acids are referred to as the essential amino acids for human. They must be therefore, supplied through diet as our body cannot synthesize these.

13. (d) Vegetable oils and fats are present in plants in insoluble form. They are extracted mostly from seeds. In several cereals, they are obtained from embryo. Olive and palm oils are obtained from flesly pericarp of the fruit. Sometimes oils are also extracted from roots, stem and leaves.

14. (c) Compounds having double bond in their structure are more unstable compounds in comparison to single bond holders. Unsaturated fats those have double bonds in their structures are more reactive than saturated fats.

15. (d) Palmitic acids and arachidonic acids are simple fatty acids. A fatty acid has a carboxyl group attached to an R group. The R group could be a methyl ($-CH_3$), or ethyl ($-C_2H_5$) or higher number of $-CH_2$ groups (1 carbon to 19 carbons). For example, palmitic acid has 16 carbons including carboxyl carbon. Arachidonic acid has 20 carbon atoms including the carboxyl carbon.

16. (b) In polysaccharides, individual monosaccharide is linked by glycosidic bond. This bond is formed between two carbon atoms of two adjacent monosaccharides. A glycosidic bond is a type of covalent bond that joins a carbohydrate molecule to another group, which may or may not be another carbohydrate. Glycosidic bonds are formed by dehydration.

17. (b) Polysaccharides are complex carbohydrates which are formed by polymerisation of large number of monosaccharide monomers. Exoskeleton of arthropods, contains a complex polysaccharide called chitin. These complex polysaccharides are heteropolymers. Plant cell walls are made of cellulose. Paper made from plant pulp and cotton fibre is cellulosic. Cellulose is a homopolysaccharide.

18. (c) In a DNA molecule, A-T rich parts melt before G-C rich parts because there are two H-bond between A and T whereas in between G and C, there are three H-bond.

19. (d) We know that DNA molecules are found primarily in the nucleus of the cell but RNA molecules are found outside the nucleus. By heating, its special structural arrangement is changed irreversibly. This results in the conversion of enzyme into a fibrous or insoluble form. Due to this irreversible change, enzymes lose their specific activity when heated.

20. (c) Nucleic acids are polynucleotides. A nucleotide has three chemically distinct components. One is a heterocyclic compound, the second is a monosaccharide and the third a phosphoric acid or phosphate. The heterocyclic compounds in nucleic acids are the nitrogenous bases named adenine, guanine, uracil, cytosine and thymine. Adenine and guanine are substituted purines while the rest are substituted pyrimidines formed from the skeletal heterocyclic rings purine and pyrimidine respectively.

21. (a) Nucleotides which possess more than one phosphate group are called higher nucleotides. The second and third phosphates of higher nucleotides are attached against forces of repulsion between similarly charged phosphate radicals. Hence, the bonds attaching second and third phosphates are higher energy bonds.

22. (c) Feed back inhibition is a type of reversible inhibition found in allosteric enzymes. The inhibitor is non-competitive and is usually a low molecular intermediate or product of metabolic pathway having a chain of reactions involving a number of enzymes.

23. (c) Enzyme has specific site for substrates called as active sites and substrate has reactive sites. These active and reactive sites help in making of substrate enzyme complex.

24. (a) The enzymes substrate complex is short lived. The substrate is changed into products. These products remain

complexed with the active site of the enzyme for a brief period. They soon separate and the active site is free to perform another catalytic act. Enzyme activity depends upon their affinity of substrates. If turnover number of substrate is higher, then enzymes show high affinity towards substrate. The number of substrate molecules changed per minute by a molecule or enzyme is called turn over number.

25. (b) Desmolysing enzymes are those which catalyse reactions by the other methods other than hydrolysis, e.g., aldolases, dehydrogenases, oxidases, etc. Digestive enzymes function by catalysing hydrolysis. Larger molecules are broken into smaller ones. They are grouped into three types - proteolytic (breaks protein molecule), amylolytic (breaks sugar molecule) and lipolytic (breaks lipid molecule).

26. (b) Cofactor may be inorganic or organic in nature. Organic cofactors are of two types, coenzymes and prosthetic groups. Coenzymes are easily separable non-protein organic cofactors. Prosthetic groups are non-protein organic cofactors firmly attached to apoenzymes (protein part of enzyme).

27. (a) We know that all biological reactions are catalysed by special catalysts called enzyme, thus enzymes are defined as biological proteins. We also know that enzymes are small organic molecules which are weakly held to the protein and can be easily separated by dialysis. Therefore, chemically all enzymes are globular proteins.

28. (c) The number of substrate molecules changed per minute by a molecule or enzyme is called turn over number. The higher the turn-over number, the more efficient an enzyme is. It depends upon the number of active sites present over an enzyme.

29. (c) Enzyme becomes inactive below minimum temperature. Low temperature preserve the enzymes in the inactive state. High temperature destroys enzymes by causing their denaturation.

30. (b) Activation energy is an external supply of energy which is needed for the initiation of the chemical reaction. Activation energy required for such a large number of reactions cannot be provided by living systems. Enzymes lower the activation energy required for a reaction. Enzymes are generally specific for their substrates.

31. (a) Almost all enzymes are proteins. They may have additional inorganic or organic substances for their activity. Some RNA molecules behave like enzymes, which are called ribozymes.

32. (a) Inorganic catalysts work efficiently at high temperatures and high pressures, while enzymes get damaged at high temperatures (above 40°C). However, enzymes isolated from organisms who normally live under extremely high temperatures (e.g., hot vents and sulphur springs) are stable and retain their catalytic power even at high temperatures (upto 80°–90°C).

33. (a) The activity of an enzyme is highly specific to the presence of chemicals that bind to the enzyme. When the inhibitor closely resembles the substrate in its molecular structure and inhibits the activity of the enzyme, it is known as competitive inhibitor. Consequently, the substrate cannot bind and the enzyme action declines. The inhibition of succinic dehydrogenase by malonate which closely resembles the substrate succinate in structure is the example of competitive inhibition.

34. (c) A particular substrate molecule is acted upon by a particular enzyme. After coming in contact with the active site of the enzyme, the substrate molecules or reactants form a complex called enzyme-substrate complex. The enzyme substrate complex is short lived. In the complexed state, the molecules of the substrate undergo chemical change. The products remain attached to the enzyme for some time so that an enzyme product complex is also formed. However, the products are soon released and the freed enzyme is able to bind more substrate molecules.

35. (c) Co-enzymes are also organic compounds but their association with the apoenzyme is only transient, usually occurring during the course of catalysis. Co-enzymes serve as cofactors in a number of different enzyme catalyzed reactions. The essential chemical components of many co-enzymes are vitamins, e.g., co-enzyme nicotinamide adenine dinucleotide contain the vitamin niacin.

36. (a) The chemical or metabolic conversion refers to a reaction. Most of the chemical reactions do not start automatically because the reactant molecules have an energy barrier to become reactive. Therefore, an external supply of energy is needed for the start of the chemical reaction. It is called activation enegy. Enzymes lower the activation energy required for a reaction.

37. (c) Enzymes are of various types depending on their action. Hydrolases catalyse the hydrolysis of ester, ether, peptide, glycosidic, C – C, C – halide, P – N bonds etc. which are formed by dehydration and condensation. Hydrolases break up large molecules into smaller ones with the help of hydrogen and hydroxyl groups of water molecules. The phenomenon is called hydrolysis. Lyases are the enzymes which cause cleaveage, removal of groups without hydrolysis, addition of groups to double bonds or removal of a group producing double bond, e.g., histidine decarboxylase breaks histidine to histamine and CO_2.

38. (b) Cofactor is a small, heat stable and dialysable part of conjugate enzyme. It may be inorganic or organic in nature. Organic cofactors are of two types, coenzymes and prosthetic groups. Inorganic cofactors include ions of a variety of minerals e.g., calcium, iron, copper, zinc, magnesium, manganese, potassium, nickel, molybdenum, selenium, cobalt. They usually function as activators. Zinc is required for carboxypeptidase activity.

39. (b) The external supply of energy which is needed for the initiation of the chemical reaction is activation energy. Activation energy required for such a large number of reactions cannot be provided by living systems. Enzymes lower the activation energy required for a reaction. Enzymes are usually specific for their substrates.

Chapter 10
Cell Cycle and Cell Division

Directions: In the following questions, a statement of assertion is followed by a statement of reason. Mark the correct choice as:

(a) If both Assertion and Reason are true and Reason is the correct explanation of Assertion.
(b) If both Assertion and Reason are true but Reason is not the correct explanation of Assertion.
(c) If Assertion is true but Reason is false.
(d) If both Assertion and Reason are false.

1. **Assertion :** Interphase is resting stage.
   Reason : The interphase cell is metabolically inactive.
2. **Assertion :** Histones are basic proteins of major importance in packaging of eukaryotic DNA. DNA and histones comprise chromatin, forming the bulk of eukaryotic chromosome.
   Reason : Histones are 5 major types H_1, H_2A, H_2B, H_3 and H_4.
3. **Assertion :** DNA synthesis occurs in G_1 and G_2 periods of cell cycle.
   Reason : During G_1 and G_2 phase, the DNA content become double.
4. **Assertion:** Due to inactivation of the cell cycle, some cells undergo G_0 phase.
   Reason : G_0 phase occurs due to non-availability of mitogen and energy rich compounds.
5. **Assertion:** G_1 phase is the interval between mitosis and initiation of DNA replication.
   Reason : The cell is metabolically inactive during G_1 phase.
6. **Assertion:** Cell growth results in disturbing the ratio between the nucleus and cytoplasm.
   Reason : Mitosis helps the cell to restore the nucleocytoplasmic ratio.
7. **Assertion :** Cell growth is a continuous process in terms of cytoplasmic increase.
   Reason : DNA synthesis occurs only during two specific stages in the cell cycle.
8. **Assertion :** Every chromosome, during metaphase has two chromatids.
   Reason : Synthesis of DNA takes places in the S-phase of interphase.
9. **Assertion :** Mitosis maintains the genetic similarity of somatic cells.
   Reason : Chromosomes do not undergo crossing over.
10. **Assertion :** Karyokinesis occurs in M-phase.
    Reason : Cell division stops in M-phase.
11. **Assertion:** Prophase is the first stage of mitosis which follows S and G_1 phases of interphase.
    Reason : Prophase is marked by the initiation of clusters of chromosomes.
12. **Assertion:** During anaphase, centromere of each chromosomes splits and chromatids separate.
    Reason : Chromatids move to opposite poles.
13. **Assertion :** Mitosis is often called indirect division.
    Reason : Mitosis divides a parent cell into two daughter cells.
14. **Assertion :** Mitosis is important in the life of an organism, especially in the growth of a multicellular organism.
    Reason : Mitosis restores the nucleocytoplasmic ratio.
15. **Assertion :** In animal cells, the cytokinesis is marked by the appearance of a furrow in plasma membrane.
    Reason : In plant cells, the formation of the new cell wall starts with the formation of simple precursor called cell plate.
16. **Assertion:** Meiosis results in production of haploid cells.
    Reason: Synapsis occurs during leptotene. **[AIIMS 1998]**
17. **Assertion :** Meiosis II is known as equational or homotypic division.
    Reason : Meiosis II produces same number of chromosome in cell. **[AIIMS 2010]**

18. **Assertion :** The stage between two mitotic divisions is called interkinesis.
Reason : Interkinesis is generally long lived.
[AIIMS 2016]

19. **Assertion :** Diplotene is characterized by the presence of chiasmata.
Reason : Diplotene can last for months and years in oocytes of some vertebrates. **[AIIMS 2016]**

20. **Assertion :** Chiasmata is formed during diplotene.
Reason : Chiasmata are formed due to deposition of nucleoproteins.

21. **Assertion :** During zygotene, chromosomes show bivalent stage.
Reason : Bivalent is half the number of chromosomes.

22. **Assertion :** Meiosis takes place in pollen mother cells.
Reason : Each pollen mother cell produce 4 haploid pollen grains.

23. **Assertion :** Meiotic division results in the production of haploid cells.
Reason : Synapsis occurs during zygotene of meiosis.

24. **Assertion:** Crossing over leads to recombination of genetic material on the two chromosomes.
Reason : It is the exchange of genetic material between two homologous chromosomes.

25. **Assertion:** The process of pairing of the chromosomes is called synapsis.
Reason : Synapsis occurs during leptotene stage.

26. **Assertion:** Variations are critical for the process of evolution.
Reason : Meiosis increases the genetic variability in the population of organisms from one generation to the next.

27. **Assertion:** Reduction division occurs in anaphase-I. So there is no need of meiosis.
Reason: Meiosis-II occurs to separate homologous chormosomes.

28. **Assertion :** Meiotic division takes place in reproductive cells.
Reason : Synapsis occurs during zygotene of meiosis.

29. **Assertion :** Meiosis is known as reductional division.
Reason : During meiosis, the chromosome number get reduce by half of its total number.

Solutions

1. (c) Previously interphase was called resting stage because there is no apparent activity related to cell division. The interphase cell is metabolically quite active. Interphase consist of three subphases (G_1 , G_2 and S). Synthesis of DNA occurs in S phase. G_1 is the period between the end of mitosis and the start of S phase. G_2 is the interval between S phase and start of mitosis. As the synthesis of DNA occurs in S phase so, it is considered as metabolically active phase.

2. (b) Chromosome contains equal amounts of DNA and histone. The DNA and histone octamer forms a nucleosome. Histone is the protein found in eukaryotic chromosomes. There are 5 types of histone namely H_1, H_2A, H_2B, H_3 and H_4.

3. (d) The synthesis of DNA occurs only in a restricted portion of the interphase during S period, which is preceded and followed by two "gap" periods of interphase (G_1 and G_2) in which there is no DNA synthesis. G_1 is the period between the end of mitosis I and the start of DNA synthesis. S is the period of DNA synthesis and G_2 is the interval between the end of DNA synthesis and the start of mitosis. During G_1, a cell contains two times (4C) the amount of DNA present in the original diploid cell (2C). Following mitosis, the daughter cell again enter is the G_1 period and have a DNA content equivalent to 2C.

4. (a) The phase in which cells do not undergo S-phase after G_1-phase is known as G_0 phase or quiescent stage. It occurs due to non-availability of mitogen and energy rich compounds. The cells remain metabolically active, but no longer proliferate unless called on to do so depending on the requirement of the organisms.

5. (c) G_1 phase is also known as first growth phase or post mitotic gap phase. It is the phase between end of mitotic phase of previous cell and initiation of S-phase of next mitotic phase. During G_1 phase, the cell is metabolically active and continuously grows. In this phase, different types of RNA (*m*RNA, *t*RNA and *r*RNA) and proteins are synthesised.

6. (a) Mitosis causes the growth of multicellular organism. The nucleus controls the functions of cell. The size of nucleus does not change, but cytoplasm increases during cell growth. Increase in size disturbs the nucleo –cytoplasmic ratio. This ratio is restored to efficient level through cell division.

7. (c) DNA synthesis takes place only during one specific stage in cell cycle (interphase).

8. (a) In S phase or synthetic phase chromosomes replicates, DNA content doubles, i.e., 1C to 2C for haploid cells and 2C to 4C for diploid cells. Along with replication of DNA, new chromatin fibres are formed which remain attached in pairs and the number of chromosomes does not increase i.e. 1n to 1n and 2n to 2n. As the chromatin fibres are elongated chromosomes, each chromosomes comes to have two chromatin threads which are attached at centromere. During metaphase, every chromosome have two chromatids. The chromosomes separate from each other during anaphase.

9. (a) Mitosis keeps all the somatic cells of an organism genetically similar, resembling the fertilized egg. Mitosis involves replication and equitable distribution of all the chromosomes so that all the cells of a multicellular organism have the same number and type of chromosomes. This helps in proper co-ordination among different cells.

10. (d) M-phase represents the phase of actual division. It consists of karyokinesis (the division of nucleus) followed by cytokinesis (the division of cytoplasm). Cell divisions stop after M-phase.

11. (d) Prophase which is the first stage of mitosis follows the S and G_2 phases of interphase. In the S and G_2 phases, the new DNA molecules formed are not distinct but interwined. Prophase is marked by the initiation of condensation of chromosomal material. The chromosomal material becomes untangled during the process of chromatin condensation.

12. (b) In anaphase, centromeres of chromosomes start to divide into two, forming daughter chromatids with centromere in each. Daughter chromosomes are repulsive so, migrate towards opposite poles. Spindle fibres attached to the centromeres shorten and pull the chromosomes, the centromeres lead the path while the limbs trail behind. So, anaphasic chromosomes appear as V, L, J and L shaped.

13. (b) Mitosis is often said as an indirect division. It is the method of equal division of nuclei. It is an elaborate process which includes a series of important changes in the nucleus as well as in cytoplasm. Therefore, it is called indirect method of division. In direct division, the nucleus becomes constricted at the center, assuming an hour glass shape, and then divides into two. This is followed by cleavage or division of cytoplasm to form 2 daughter cells. It does not involve doubling of chromosomes. Also called amitosis.

14. (a) Mitosis results in the production of diploid daughter cells with identical genetic complement. In multicellular organism, growth is due to mitosis. Cell growth results in disturbing the ratio between the nucleus and the cytoplasm. It therefore, becomes essential for the cell to divide and to restore the nucleocytoplasmic ratio.

15. (b) In an animal cell, cytokinesis is marked by the appearance of a furrow in the plasma membrane. The furrow slowly deepens and ultimately joins in the centre dividing the cell cytoplasm into two. Plants cells however, are enclosed by a relatively inextensible cell wall, therefore they undergo cytokinesis by a different mechanism. In plant cells, wall formation starts in the centre of the cell and grows outward to meet the existing lateral walls. The formation of the new cell wall begins with the formation of a simple precursor called the cell-plate that represents the middle lamella between the walls of two adjacent cells.

16. (c) Synapsis occurs during zygotene stage. Synapsis is the pairing of homologous chromosomes which leads to the formation of bivalents.

17. (a) Meiosis II is known as equational or homotypic division like mitosis. It ensures the maintenance of constant number of chromosomes from generation to generation of a species.

18. (d) Interkinesis or interphase II is a period of rest that cells of some species enter during meiosis, between meiosis I and meiosis II. No DNA replication occurs during interkinesis however, it does occur during the interphase I stage of meiosis. Interkinesis is generally short lived.

19. (b) Diplotene is the longest and most active subphase of prophase I of meiosis. The beginning of diplotene is recognized by the dissolution of synaptonemal complex and the tendency of the recombined homologous chromosomes of the bivalents to separate from each other except at the sites of crossovers. These X-shaped structures are called chiasmata. Diplotene can last for months and years in oocytes of some vertebrate.

20. (c) The points of attachment between the homologous chromosomes after the partial dissolution of nucleoprotein complex are called chiasmata. It occurs during diplotene substage of prophase I.

21. (b) During zygotene, because of the pairing of the homologues, the nucleus contains half the number of chromosomes. Each unit is a bivalent composed of two homologous chromosomes.

22. (a) Meiosis occurs in pollen mother cells. All pollen mother cells are diploid and produce haploid pollen grains after meiosis.

23. (a) Diploid cell produce haploid cell by meiosis. It occurs due to synapsis. A chromosome has two chromatids, hence a bivalent has 4 chromatids.

24. (a) Crossing over occurs during pachytene. Recombination involves mutual exchange of the corresponding segments of non-sister chromatids of homologous chromosomes. It takes place by breakage and reunion of chromatid segments. Breakage, called nicking, is assisted by an enzyme endonuclease and reunion termed annealing, is aided by an enzyme ligase. Crossing over leads to recombination of genetic material on the two chromosomes.

25. (c) Synapsis occurs during zygotene stage of prophase. During this stage, chromosomes start pairing together and this process is called synapsis. Such paired chromosomes are called homologous chromosomes. Synapsis is accompanied by the formation of complex structure called synaptonemal complex. The compex formed by a pair of synapsed homologous chromosomes is called a bivalent or a tetrad.

26. (b) Meiosis involves the exchange of genes between homologous chromosomes. So, the gametes produced are genetically different from each other. Offsprings produced by the fusion of gametes also show recombinations or genetic variations. These variations in the offsprings make organisms more adaptable to the environment and these play a definite role in evolution.

27. (d) Anaphase-I involves separation of homologous chromosomes into different daughter cells. So, meiosis I is a reductional division. But each chromosome is still formed of two sister chromatids joined at the common centromere. Anaphase-I results in reduction in number of chromosomes but each chromosome has double the amount of DNA, so, meiosis-II occur, during which chromatids of each chromosome separate into different cells. Main aim of meiosis II is to separate genetically modified chromatids of each homologous chromosome formed during crossing over in meiosis-I.

28. (b) Meiotic division is a reductional division. It occurs in reproductive cells and maintains a fixed number of chromosomes in sexually reproducing organisms. Prophase-I of meiotic division is a long phase, which is divided into five sub-phases, i.e., leptotene, zygotene, pachytene, diplotene and diakinesis. In zygotene phase, homologous chromosomes pair up, this process is called synapsis. Each pair is called a bivalent.

29. (a) After meiosis, the chromosomes are reduced by half, producing haploid cells. The sperm and the egg are haploid cells and when they fuse during fertilisation, they produce original diploid cell.

Chapter 11

Transport in Plants

Directions: In the following questions, a statement of assertion is followed by a statement of reason. Mark the correct choice as:

(a) If both Assertion and Reason are true and Reason is the correct explanation of Assertion.

(b) If both Assertion and Reason are true but Reason is not the correct explanation of Assertion.

(c) If Assertion is true but Reason is false.

(d) If both Assertion and Reason are false.

1. **Assertion :** No energy expenditure is observed in the process of diffusion.
   Reason : Diffusion occurs along the concentration gradient, i.e., from a region of higher concentration to a region of lower concentration.
2. **Assertion :** β -cyanine does not diffuse to the outside of the cell through washed beet root slices when kept in cold water.
   Reason : Membrane is not permeable to pigment β -cyanine.
3. **Assertion:** A special type of diffusion of water through a semipermeable membrane is known as osmosis.

   Reason: The net direction and rate of osmosis only depends on the pressure gradient.
4. **Assertion:** In symport transport both molecules cross the membrane at the same time in the same direction.

   Reason: In antiport transport, both molecules move in opposite direction.
5. **Assertion:** In plant cells to counteract the increase in turgour pressure, the cell wall produces an equal and opposite pressure, *i.e.*, wall pressure.

   Reason: When plant cells undergo endosmosis, they swell but do not burst.
6. **Assertion:** If the process is in the order, limiting → incipient → evident, plasmolysis will be severe.

   Reason: Plasmolysis is exosmosis.
7. **Assertion:** In hypertonic solution, a plant cell shrinks.

   Reason: Due to plasmolysis in hypertonic solution, water moves out of the cells.
8. **Assertion:** Turgor pressure is the positive pressure that develops in the plant cell due to entry of water.

   Reason: During growth of cells, the turgor pressure is responsible for enlargement and extension.
9. **Assertion:** Osmotic pressure is equivalent numerically to the osmotic potential.

   Reason: Osmotic pressure is the negative pressure applied, while osmotic potential is positive.
10. **Assertion :** Pure water has maximum water potential.

    Reason : The osmotic potential is zero in purewater.
11. **Assertion :** Pure water is obtained by reverse osmosis from a solution through differentially permeable membrane.

    Reason : Water obtained from reverse osmosis is devoid of impurities and is extra pure.
12. **Assertion :** Water potential is new term for diffusion pressure deficit.

    Reason : Both diffusion pressure deficit and water potential have a negative value.
13. **Assertion:** By lowering O_2 tension, water absorption is reduced.

    Reason: Water absorption reduces due to the accumulation of CO_2.
14. **Assertion:** The more number of solute molecules, the lower (more negative) is Ψ_w.

    Reason: The free energy of water is reduced by the presence of solute particles and thus, decreases the water potential.

15. Assertion : When the ambient temperature is high and soil contains excess of water, the plants tend to lose water in the form of droplets from lenticels.

Reason : Root pressure regulates the rate of loss of water form lenticels. **[AIIMS 2006]**

16. Assertion : Light is very important factor in transpiration.

Reason : Light induces stomatal opening and darkness closing of stomata. Therefore, transpiration increases in light and decreases in dark. **[AIIMS 1999, 2015]**

17. Assertion : Wilting occurs due to loss in turgidity.

Reason : Turgor pressure checks the excessive entry of water into cells.

18. Assertion : Waxy and cutin coating on plant parts reduce the transpiration.

Reason : These adaptations are found in xerophytes.

19. Assertion : Guttation liquid is found on the margins of leaves.

Reason : Hydathodes are found on the margins.

20. Assertion : Plant parts become flaccid in wilting condition.

Reason : Temporary and permanent wilting result in plant death.

21. Assertion: For checking transpiration, film forming chemical should not be used.

Reason: Film forming chemicals interrupt photosynthesis and respiration.

22. Assertion: On the top of the water, oil will form a film affecting the amount of light entering the water.

Reason: Oil is a polar molecule, and forms hydrogen bonds.

23. Assertion: In transpiration process, water in liquid form reaches to plant surfaces.

Reason: At plant surface, water changes from liquid to vapour phase.

24. Assertion: Guttation is the loss of water in its liquified phases from the leaves.

Reason: Guttation takes place at night only.

25. Assertion : Cells of living plants do not burst on keeping in water, while an animal cell like RBCs bursts when kept in water.

Reason : The rigidity of cell wall is due of which plant cell maintains its shape and do not burst.

26. Assertion : To counteract the increase in turgor pressure in plant cells, the cell wall produces an equal and opposite pressure, i.e., wall pressure.

Reason : When plant cells undergo endosmosis, they swell but do not burst.

27. Assertion: For crops, arid areas are not suitable.

Reason : For planting crops in arid regions, antitranspirants are used.

28. Assertion : Long distance flow of photoassimilates in plants occurs through sieve tubes.

Reason : Mature sieve tubes have parietal cytoplasm and perforated sieve plates.

29. Assertion: For the lateral transport of water, the xylem ray parenchyma is responsible.

Reason: Through xylem and tracheids, only vertical movement of water is possible.

30. Assertion: During water apoplastic movement, water travels through the cells and their cytoplasm.

Reason: The symplastic movement of water takes place exclusively through the intercellular spaces and the walls of the cells.

31. Assertion: Ions are absorbed from the soil by active transport only.

Reason: The proteins present in the membranes of root hair cells passively pump ions from the soil into the cytoplasm of the epidermal cells.

32. Assertion : Cohesion force is also called as tensile strength.

Reason : Attraction of water molecule to polar surface or hydrophilic wall of the xylem tube causes adhesion force.

33. Assertion : Unidirectional flow of water, mineral and nitrogen occurs through xylem.

Reason : Direction of flow of organic and inorganic substances is unidirectional and occurs through phloem.

34. Assertion : Transpiration facilitate supply of water for photosynthesis, maintains shape and structure of plant and transport minerals from the soil to other parts of the plant.

Reason : Process of transpiration helps in translocation of inorganic and sugar molecules from the source to sink.

35. **Assertion:** Cohesion, adhesion and surface tension provides high tensile strength to water.
Reason: Capillarity is aided by small diameter of the tracheary elements.

36. **Assertion :** During rainy season wooden doors get stuck and do not open and shut properly.
Reason : Due to the process of imbibition, volume of wooden items increases, when they come in contact of water.

37. **Assertion :** Upward movement of water is called ascent of sap.
Reason : Upward movement of water occurs through xylem and phloem.

38. **Assertion :** Xylem is principal water conducting tissue.
Reason : It has been recognised by girdling or ringing experiment.

39. **Assertion:** Stomata are also known as "turgor operated valves"
Reason: Stomata show reversible turgor changes.

40. **Assertion:** On both surfaces the isobilateral leaf has equal number of stomata.
Reason: On upper surface the dorsiventral leaf has greater number of sotmata.

41. **Assertion:** Normally in the day stomata are open during day time and closed during the night.
Reason: The change in the turgidity of the guard cells causes the opening or closing of stomata.

42. **Assertion:** Bi-directional movement of organic solutes is present in the pholem.
Reason: The transportation depends on variability of source-sink relationship.

43. **Assertion:** The movement of substances in bulk from source to sink as a result of pressure differences is mass or bulk flow.
Reason: Water, minerals and food are generally moved by mass flow.

44. **Assertion:** To the plants, capillary water is not readily available as it lies below the level of roots.
Reason: The only water available to the plants is gravitational water.

45. **Assertion :** Sugars are translocated in non-reducing form in phloem.
Reason : Non-reducing sugars are most reactive sugars.

46. **Assertion :** In the ringing experiment, a narrow continuous band of issues external to the xylem is removed.
Reason : Ringing experiment proves the transport of solutes by phloem.

47. **Assertion :** The optimum amount of water soil can retain is known as its field capacity.
Reason : Water in excess of field capacity percolates to water table due to gravitation.

48. **Assertion:** In loam soil, field capacity is maximum.
Reason: The soil has maximum field capacity in water logging condition.

49. **Assertion:** Mostly by roots, plants absorb water.
Reason: In water absorption, root cap region participates actively.

50. **Assertion :** Water and mineral uptake by root hairs from the soil occurs through apoplast until it reaches endodermis.
Reason : Casparian strips in endodermis are suberized.

51. **Assertion :** Seeds and spores do not lose the viability in unfavourable periods.
Reason : Seeds and spores have high osmotic pressure.

Solutions

1. **(b)** Process diffusion can be defined more meaningfully as the net transport of solute or solvent from a region of higher chemical potential or higher concentration to lower chemical potential or lower concentration area where ion, atoms or molecules moves randomly without the involvement of energy.
2. **(b)** Process of diffusion can be summarised easily as the movement of uncharged ions, atoms or molecules through a biological membrane depends upon the permeability of biological membrane. Depending upon the permeability, the membrane may be semi permeable or differentially permeable, selectively permeable and impermeable. Here, the membrane is impermeable to pigment betacynin. That is why, pigment betacynin is unable to colourise the water.
3. **(c)** Osmosis is diffusion of water from its pure state (or dilute solution) into a solution (or stronger solution) when the two are separated by a semi-permeable membrane. The direction and rate of osmosis depend upon the sum of two forces, pressure gradient (gradient of Ψ_w) and concentration gradient (gradient of Ψ_s). The difference in the water potentials of solutions separated by a semipermeable membrane determine the net force or gradient.
4. **(b)** Some carrier proteins allow transport only if two types of molecules move together. This is known as co-transport. Symport and antiport are two types of co-transport. Symport allows both the molecules to move in same direction and antiport allows both the molecules to move in opposite direction.
5. **(a)** The pressure which develops in the confined part of an osmotic system due to osmotic entry of water into it is called turgor pressure. It is also called hydrostatic pressure or pressure potential. Wall pressure is the force exerted by the cell wall over the protoplast. Normally wall pressure is equal and opposite to turgor pressure except when the cell becomes flaccid.
6. **(b)** Under the influence of a hypertonic solution, shrinkage of the protoplast of a cell from its cell wall causes exosmosis or withdrawl of water from the central vacuole of cell. Simultaneously, the pressure on the wall is reduced and the elastic wall contracts causing a reduction in cell size. This first stage of plasmolysis is known as limiting plasmolysis. Initially the protoplast withdraws itself from the corners. This stage is known as incipient plasmolysis. Protoplast shrinks further and withdraws from the cell wall except at one or a few points due to continued exosmosis. It is known as evident plasmolysis. In such case, cells cannot survive.
7. **(a)** With regard to water movement the behaviour of the plant cells or tissues depends on the surrounding solution. In a hypertonic solution, when the cell or tissue is placed water moves out; it is first lost from the cytoplasm and then from the vacuole. When water is drawn out of the cell through diffusion into the extracellular (outside cell) fluid, it causes the protoplast to shrink away from the walls. The cell is said to be plasmolysed.
8. **(b)** Due to entry of water into it, a positive pressure develops in a plant cell or system. This positive hydrostatic pressure is also known as turgor pressure. Turgor pressure keeps the cells and their organelles stretched, this is essential for proper functioning of a cell. It gives support to non-woody tissues like parenchyma. During growth, turgor pressure is essential for cell enlargement.
9. **(c)** Osmotic pressure is defined as the pressure required to inhibit the entry of water into osmotically active solution across a semi permeable membrane. Thus, water will move from a region of lower osmotic pressure to a region of higher osmotic pressure. It is measured in atmospheres, bars or pascals. Osmotic pressure is numerically equal to osmotic potential (= solute, potential, Ψ_s) but osmotic potential has a negative value, whereas osmotic pressure (π, pi) has a positive value, ($\Psi_s = -\pi$).

10. (c) Water potential is the potential energy of water relative to pure water in reference conditions. Pure water has maximum water potential, whereas, addition of solutes to water lowers the water potential. Osmosis is a special type of diffusion in which water diffuses from its pure state i.e., higher water potential to concentrated solution i.e., lower chemical potential through a semipermeable membrane. Since pure water has no difference in chemical potential, it has zero osmotic potential.

11. (b) In pure water the impurities are negligible. Pure water is generally obtained by reverse osmosis but other sources like rain water, snow, etc., are also the souce of pure water.

12. (c) The reduction in the diffusion pressure of water in a solution over its pure state is called diffusion pressure deficit or DPD. It is a term coined by Meyer (1938). It has positive value. Water potential is a modern term coined by Slatyer and Taylor (1960) which is equivalent to DPD, but it has a negative value.

13. (b) In the soil, the accumulation of CO_2 appears to have a greater inhibitory effect on water absorption than do lowered oxygen tensions. An increase in CO_2 causes an increase in the viscosity of protoplasm and a decrease in the roots permeability to water thereby, bringing about a retardation in water absorption.

14. (a) Water molecules possess kinetic energy. Water molecules are in random motion in liquid and gaseous form. The greater the concentration of water in a system, greater is its kinetic energy or water potential. Pure water has greatest water potential i.e., zero. When a solute is added to pure water, it decreases the free energy of water and hence, decreases the water potential (Ψ_w).

15. (d) Root pressure is a pressure produced in the roots of plants, causing exudation of sap from cut stems and guttation of water from leaves. The pressure is generated by the concentration of solutes in the xylem of the root and stem which then causes water to move into the xylem by osmosis.

16. (a) Light is an important factor in transpiration. The stomata opens well on days when light is brighter. It is also evident on cloudy days that the stomata does not open well. Hence, light induces stomatal opening and darkness closing.

17. (b) Flowers, young stems and other softer organs are able to maintain their form due to turgidity or TP (turgor pressure). In case of loss of turgidity, the shoots droop down and the leaves show wilting. Turgor pressure (pressure potential or hydrostatic pressure) keeps a check on the excessive entry of water into cells.

18. (a) Waxy coating, thick cuticle, sunken stomata, hairy surface reduce transpiration and are characteristic of xerophytes which grow in places where water is not available in much quantity.

19. (a) Guttation drops are restricted to tips or margins of the leaves. Guttation takes place through special structures called hydathodes. They are usually found on the margins and tips of the leaves.

20. (c) In case of loss of turgidity, the shoots droop down and the leaves show wilting. In wilting, the individual cells of leaves and other softer parts become flaccid, due to loss of water from their interior. In temporary wilting, plants gain their turgidity when they are given water. If the soil does not obtain water periodically, the recovery may be only partial or it may not occur at all. The latter condition is known as permanent wilting.

21. (d) By forming a thin film on the transpiring surface, film forming chemicals check transpiration. To allow photosynthesis and respiration, they are sufficiently permeable to carbon dioxide and oxygen but prevent movement of water vapours through them. Such chemicals can be used as antitranspirants.

22. (c) Oil is a nonpolar molecule, that means it does not form hydrogen bonds with water and hence, does not dissolve.

23. (d) With water vapours, the intercellular spaces of the transpiring organ is almost saturated. When the stomata are open, the water vapours are drawn from the substomatal cavities to the outside air due to high DPD of the later. This increases the DPD of the substomatal air that draws more water vapours from the intercellular spaces. In turn, later get water vapours from the wet walls of mesophyll cells.

24. (c) Guttation is the loss or excretion of water in the form of liquid droplets from the leaves and other parts of an uninjured or intact plant. All plants do not show guttation. It is restricted to about 345 genera of herbaceous and some woody plants. Guttation occurs through special structures called hydathodes that are usually found on the margins and tips of the leaves. Common examples are found in garden nasturtium, oat and other cereals, balsam, tomato, cucurbits. Guttation usually occurs during periods of active growth when conditions favour more water absorption and less transpiration. It takes place either at night or early in the morning.

25. (a) The plant cell do not burst in hypotonic solution because of presence of cell wall but as animal cells are devoid of cell wall therefore, these get burst in hypotonic solution.

26. (a) Hydrostatic pressure develops in an osmotic system (plant cells) due to osmotic entry or exit of water from it. A positive hydrostatic pressure or turgor pressure develops in the confined part of an osmotic system due to osmotic energy of water into it. Due to turgor pressure the protoplast of a plant cell will press the cell wall to the outside. The cell wall, being elastic, presses the protoplast with an equal and opposite force. The force exerted by the cell wall over the protoplast is called wall pressure. If the cell wall is absent in the cell then it will not counteract hydrostatic pressure and will continue to absorb water till it bursts.

27. (b) In arid and unirrigated areas, crop plants cannot be grown due to excessive transpiration and reduced water availability. Antitranspirants are the substances that reduce the rate of transpiration. e.g., ABA. Antitranspirants will maintain a favourable internal water balance even in cases of very low water availability. It will allow farmers to grow crop profitably in unirrigated areas and help foresters to plant trees even in extreme arid or desert areas.

28. (a) Sieve tubes are the conducting elements of phloem (a permanent vascular tissue which conducts organic food in plant body) which are elongated tubular channels formed by end to end union of numerous cells. The septa between individual sieve tube cells or sieve elements are bulged out. They are called sieve plates possessing a number of perforations (sieve pores or sieve pits) and helps in conduction of food.

29. (c) In vertical direction, vessels and tracheids are oriented in the plant with respect to their long axis and water movement is predominantly in this direction, along with lateral water movement. Numerous pits through which water may pass perforate the side walls of vessel elements and tracheids. The xylem ray parenchyma greatly facilitates the lateral transport of water and nutrients.

30. (d) The apoplastic movement of water takes place exclusively through the walls of the cells and the intercellular spaces in-between the walls of the cells. Movement through the apoplast does not involve crossing the cell membrane. This movement is dependent on the gradient. The symplastic system is the system of interconnected protoplasts. Neighbouring cells are connected through cytoplasmic strands which extend through plasmodesmata. In symplastic movement, the water travels through the cells-their cytoplasm; intercellular movement is through the plasmodesmata. Symplastic movement may get aided by cytoplasmic streaming.

31. (d) In the soil, minerals are present in the form of ions. Ions cannot directly cross the cell membrane. Ions are absorbed from the soil by both passive and active (majorly) transport. In the membranes of root hair cells, specific proteins actively pump ions from the soil into the cytoplasm of the epidermal cells. Like all cells, the endodermal cells have many transport proteins that is embedded in their plasma membrane; they let some solute cross the membrane, but not others. Transport proteins of endodermal cells are control points, where a plant adjusts the quantity and types of solutes that reach the xylem.

32. (b) The force which is responsible to join water molecules to each other in water column is cohesion force. On the account of cohesion force, water column can bear a pull or tension up to 100 atm. Therefore, it is also known as tensile strength while the force between the wall of tracheary elements and water molecule is called as adhesion force which produces surface tension and which account for high capillarity through tracheids and vessels.

33. (c) Unidirectional flow of water, mineral and nitrogen occurs through xylem and direction of flow of organic and inorganic substances are multidirectional, which occurs through phloem.

34. (c) Transpiration plays an important role in the supply of water in photosynthesis and is regarded as a price paid for photosynthesis. A little amount of water (0.2%) is used in the process of photosynthesis. It also helps in maintaining the turgidity of cells and cause transpiration pull in the water column of xylem tissue. The later absorb water along with minerals from the soil. However, translocation of organic molecules like sugar takes place through phloem and another conductive tissue.

35. (b) Water molecules are held together by strong cohesion force which is because of hydrogen bonds amongst them. There is another force of adhesion that holds water to the walls of xylem vessels. Water molecules are attracted to one another more than the water molecules in the gaseous state. It produces surface tension that accounts for high capilarity through tracheids and vessels. In tracheary elements, water column is present. There is a continuous column of water from roots through the stem and into the leaves. These tracheary elements form continuous system through their unthickened areas. Since, a large number of tracheary elements are present together, no breakage in the continuity of water takes place even it there is a blockage of one or few of them.

36. (b) Wooden doors get stuck and become difficult to open and shut due to imbibition. Imbibition is a process in which water is absorbed by solids (colloids) causing them to enormously increase in volume.

37. (c) Sap is water with dissolved ingredients. The upward movement of water from roots towards the tips of stem branches and their leaves is called ascent of sap. It occurs through the tracheary elements of xylem.

38. (a) Harting performed ringing experiment to show path of water through xylem. Xylem is basic tissue for conduction of water in higher plants. It has vessels and tracheids which are well adapted for water translocation.

39. (a) Due to reversible turgor changes in the cells, many plant movements are produced. The opening and closing of stomata occurs by gain and loss of turgidity by their guard cells. Hence, they are often called "turgor operated valves".

40. (c) Tiny pore complexes found in epidermis of leaves and other soft aerial parts is known as stomata. The lower surface of a dorsiventral (often dicotyledonous) leaf has a greater number of stomata than the outer surface, whereas in an isobilateral (often monocotyledonous) leaf, stomata are about equal in number on both surfaces.

41. (a) Normally in the day time stomata are open and closed during the night. The immediate cause of the opening or closing of the stomata is a change in the turgidity of the guard cells. The inner wall of each guard cell, towards the pore or stomatal aperture, is thick and elastic. Within the two guard cells flanking each stomatal aperture or pore when turgidity increases, the thin outer walls bulge out and force the inner walls into a crescent shape, the opening of the stomata is also aided due to the orientation of the microfibrils in the cell walls of the guard cells. When the guard cells lose turgidity, due to water loss the elastic inner walls regain its original shape, the guard cells become flaccid and the stomata closes.

42. (a) The long distance movement of organic substances from the source or supply end (region of manufacture or storage) to the region of utilisation or sink is phloem transport. But depending on the season or need of the plants, the source and sink may be reversed. Sugar stored in roots may be mobilised to become a source of food in the early spring when the buds of trees act as sink and need energy for their growth and

development. Since the source-sink relationship is variable, the direction of movement of organic solutes in pholem can be upwards or downwards i.e., bidirectional.

43. (b) By means of diffusion, faciliated diffusion and active transport substances move through the plant. These methods cannot be used for long distance transport mass flow. Mass flow is the movement of substances in bulk from one point to another as a result of pressure differences between the two points. It is a characteristic of mass flow of that substance, whether in solution or in suspension, are swept along at the same pace, as in a flowing river. This is unlike diffusion where different substances move independently depending on their concentration gradients. Bulk flow can be achieved either through a positive hydrostatic pressure gradient (e.g., a garden hose) or a negative hydrostatic pressure gradient (e.g., suction through a start water and mineral, and food are generally moved chart a mass or bulk flow system). The bulk movement of substances through the conducting or vascular tissues of plants is known as translocation.

44. (d) After gravitational water has drained away, capillary water contains the bulk of water remaining in the soil. It is held in the soil by capillary forces. It is the readily available water to the plants and is the main source of all the water absorbed by plants. Gravitational water is not readily available to the plants and penetrates below the level of the roots.

45. (c) Sucrose is a non-reducing and most translocating sugar as phloem. Non-reducing sugars can be easily transported because they are less reactive.

46. (a) In ringing experiment, a continuous band of tissues, external to the xylem is removed. When such plant is placed in the light, after sometime, the tissue above the ring become swollen due to the accumulation of solutes. Due to swelling, ringing solutes are not transported towards the root side.

47. (b) Field capacity is the water retaining or holding capacity of soil which can be defined as the maximum amount of water retained per unit dry weight of the soil after stoppage of graviational flow of water, while excess water percolates to the fringe of water table.

48. (c) Field capacity is the optimum or maximum amount of water retained per unit dry weight of soil after the stoppage of gravitational flow. It is 25-35% common in loam soils. Soil moisture beyond field capacity produces water logging.

49. (c) Through their entire surface right from root, stem, leaves, flowers, etc. plants have the potentiality to absorb water. However, as water is available mostly in the soil, only the underground root system is specialized to absorb water. The most efficient region of water absorption in roots is the root hair zone.

50. (a) In plants, usually maximum water uptake is found in the root hair zone, as this part has the maximum surface area due to the presence of root hairs. These root hairs also withdraw from interspaces, which are not in contact with epiblema of the root. Whereas, the zone of mature cells cannot absorb water because of the presence of impermeable and suberised surface layer.

51. (a) A high osmotic pressure has been found to protect the plants against drought and frost injury. Seeds and spores are similarly able to pass through the unfavourable periods due to high osmotic pressure (or low solute potential).

Chapter 12

Mineral Nutrition

Directions: In the following questions, a statement of assertion is followed by a statement of reason. Mark the correct choice as:

(a) If both Assertion and Reason are true and Reason is the correct explanation of Assertion.

(b) If both Assertion and Reason are true but Reason is not the correct explanation of Assertion.

(c) If Assertion is true but Reason is false.

(d) If both Assertion and Reason are false.

1. **Assertion :** Hydroponics is used for solution culture.
   Reason : A balanced nutrient solution contains both essential and nonessential elements.
2. **Assertion :** In solution culture of plants, iron is added in the form of Fe-EDTA.
   Reason : Hydroponics setup is costly.
3. **Assertion :** Hydroponics requires purified water and mineral nutrient salts.
   Reason : Purified water and mineral salts are always not essential for the growth of hydroponics.
4. **Assertion :** Every plant can grow in a suitable mineral solution only (i.e., without soil).
   Reason : Hydroponics does not help in the identification of essential elements and deficiency symptoms of the plants.
5. **Assertion :** Manganese is an activator of enzyme nitrite reductase.
   Reason : Manganese deficient cells prefer ammonia over nitrate.
6. **Assertion :** Calcium is a constituent of cell wall.
   Reason : Calcium is required in mitotic division.
7. **Assertion :** Plants absorb sulphur in the form of sulphate ions.
   Reason : Sulphur bacteria are required for the formation of sulphate. **[AIIMS 2007]**
8. **Assertion:** Plants absorb calicum from soil in the form of calcium ions (Ca^{2+}).
   Reason: Calcium is required by meristematic and differentiating tissues.
9. **Assertion:** Certain essential elements are called structural elements of cells.
   Reason: These essential elements are the components of certain biomolecules.
10. **Assertion:** The main constituent of several coenzymes, vitamins and ferredoxin is sulphur.
    Reason: Sulphur is present in two amino acids - valine and cysteine.
11. **Assertion:** Plants obtain molybdenum in the form of molybdate ions (MoO_4^{2+}).
    Reason: Molybdenum is a component of pollen germination, cell elongation and cell differentation.
12. **Assertion :** Iron is a microelement.
    Reason : Microelements are required in traces only, less than 1mg/gm of dry matter.
13. **Assertion :** Magnesium is important in photosynthesis and carbohydrate metabolism.
    Reason : Mg^{++} is involved in the synthesis of nucleic acids.
14. **Assertion:** The technique of growing plants in a nutrient solution is known as hydroponics.
    Reason : Hydroponics is used for commercial production of vegetables such as tomato, seedless cucumber and lettuce.
15. **Assertion :** Some essential elements can alter the osmotic potential of a cell.
    Reason : Osmotic potential can be regulated by potassium.
16. **Assertion :** Activator of the enzyme reductase is manganese.
    Reason : Manganese deficient plants cells prefers ammonia over nitrate.
17. **Assertion :** Deficiency of sulphur causes chlorosis in plants.
    Reason : Sulphur is a constituent of chlorophyll, proteins and nucleic acids.
18. **Assertion:** The leaves of cauliflower become flaccid and brown in case of molybdenum deficiency.
    Reason: Cauliflower plant is affected by whiptail disease due to molybdenum deficiency.

19. **Assertion:** Deficiency of manganese causes exanthema disease.
Reason: Reclamation is a disease of legumes.
20. **Assertion:** When the availability of the essential nutrients falls below the cirtical concentration deficiency symptoms appear.
Reason: Critical concentration is that limited concentration of the essential element below which growth of the plant is reduced.
21. **Assertion:** Necrosis occurs due to deficiency of Ca, Mg, Cu and K.
Reason: Necrosis is the death of tissue, particularly leaf tissue.
22. **Assertion:** The most effective symptom of manganese toxicity is the appearance of brown spots surrounded by chlorotic veins.
Reason: Excess of manganese may induce deficiencies of iron, magnesium and calcium.
23. **Assertion:** The movement of ions into or out of the cells is usually called flux.
Reason: The entry or exit of ions to and from the symplast, is an active process.
24. **Assertion:** Nitrogen-fixing bacteria in root nodules of legumes survive in oxygen-depleted cells of nodules.
Reason: Leghaemoglobin completely removes oxygen from the nodule cells.
25. **Assertion:** Ammonia is converted into nitrate by soil bacteria like *Nitrosomonas* and *Nitrobacter*.
Reason: These nitrifying bacteria are photoautotrophs.
26. **Assertion:** Reduction of nitrogen to ammonia by living organisms is called nitrification.
Reason: Example of free-living nitrogen fixing anaerobic microbes are *Azotobacter* and *Beijerinckia*.
27. **Assertion:** The enzyme nitrogenase is a Mo-Fe protein and catalyses the conversion of atmospheric nitrogen to ammonia.
Reason: The enzyme nitrogenase is highly sensitive to the molecular oxygen.
28. **Assertion:** Reductive amination involves the transfer of amino group from one amino acid to the keto group of a keto acid.
Reason: In transmination reaction, ammonia reacts with α-ketoglutaric acid and forms glutamic acid.
29. **Assertion** : Leguminous plants are nitrogen fixers.
Reason : Leguminous plants have Rhizobium in their root nodules.
30. **Assertion:** Nitrate present in the soil is reduced to nitrogen by the process of denitrification.
Reason: Denitrification is carried by bacteria *Pseudomonas* and *Azotobacter.*
31. **Assertion:** As per carbonic acid exchange theory of mineral salt absorption, CO_2 released during respiration of roots forms H_2CO_3 when dissolved in soil water.
Reason: H_2CO_3 dissociates into H^+ and HCO_3^- ions, where H^+ ions exchange with anions adsorbed on clay particles.
32. **Assertion** : Active absorption of minerals is inhibited when the roots are deprived of oxygen.
Reason : Active absorption of minerals requires expenditure of metabolic energy, which comes from respiration in the presence of oxygen.
33. **Assertion:** In *Dionaea*, each lamina has marginal teeth.
Reason: Marginal teeth of *Dionaea* help in prey capturing.
34. **Assertion:** Use of fertilizers enhances crop productivity to a great extent.
Reason: Irrigation is very important in increasing crop productivity.
35. **Assertion:** Insectivorous habitat of plants is not meant to cope up with O_2 deficiency.
Reason: Insectivorous plants are partly autotrophic and partly heterotrophic.
36. **Assertion:** Leguminous plants are nitrogen fixers.
Reason: These plants have *Rhizobium* in their root nodules.
37. **Assertion:** Plants do not absorb nitrogen in the form of nitrate only.
Reason: Nitrogen is the most critical element.
38. **Assertion:** Plants do not possess excretory organs.
Reason: Plant usually absorb essential nutrients and lead a passive life.
39. **Assertion :** Plants lack excretory organs.
Reason : Plant usually absorb essential nutrients and lead a passive life. **[AIIMS 1997]**

Solutions

1. **(c)** Solution culture is being used for raising flowers and vegetables at home. This soilless production of plants is called hydroponics. A solution having all the essential elements in proper proportion is called normal or balanced nutrient solution.

2. **(b)** In solution culture, iron is added as Fe-EDTA. The agent which keeps metals in the soluble state is called chelating agent or ligand. Fe-EDTA complex is called chelate. The soilless production of plants is called solution culture or hydroponics. The cost of setting up a hydroponic system is very high.

3. **(c)** Due to exposure of the plant roots to a limited amount of the solution, there are chances that the concentrations of oxygen and other minerals in the plant roots would reduce. That's the reason that purification of water and nutrient salts are essential for hydroponics, so as to maintain an optimum growth of the plants.

4. **(c)** Hydroponics is a technique of growing plants in a nutrient solution. After that, a number of improvised methods have been employed to determine the mineral nutrients essential for plants. After a series of experiments in which the roots of the plants were immersed in nutrient solutions and an element was added/removed or given in varied concentration, a mineral solution suitable for the plant growth was obtained. By this method, essential elements were identified and their deficiency symptoms were discovered.

5. **(a)** Manganese plays an important role in nitrate reduction. Manganese acts as an activator for the enzymes nitrite reductase and hydroxylamine reductase. The preference of ammonia over nitrate as a nitrogen source by the manganese - deficient cells supports the above mentioned analysis of the role of manganese.

6. **(b)** Calcium is a constituent of cell walls in the form of calcium pectate. Calcium in small amounts is necessary for normal mitosis. Calcium may be involved in chromatin or mitotic spindle organization.

7. **(a)** Sulphur is a constituent of amino acids (cystein and cystine and methionine). Sulphur is present in the soil in the form of oxides. Sulphur bacteria convert them into sulphate ions.The plants absorb sulphur in the form of sulphate ions.

8. **(b)** Plants absorb calcium from the soil is absorbed by plants in the form of calcium ions (Ca^{2+}). Calcium is required by meristematic and differentiating tissues. During cell division it is used in the synthesis of cell wall, particularly as calcium pectate in the middle lamella. It is also needed during the formation of mitotic spindle. It activates certain enzymes and plays an important role in regulating metabolic activities.

9. **(a)** Some essential elements play a structural role in plants. These essential elements are carbon, hydrogen, oxygen and nitrogen. They are the building blocks of macromolecules that form the bulk of plant body. Carbon and hydrogen are components of all organic substances. Many of them also contain oxygen. Nitrogen is a constituent of amino acids, proteins, nucleic acids, chlorophyll, auxin, cytokinins and vitamins.

10. **(c)** Sulphur is an important macroelement of plants. Plants obtain sulphur in the form of sulphate (SO_4^{2-}). Sulphur is present in two amino acids –cysteine and methionine and is the main constituent of several coenzymes, vitamins (thiamine, biotin, coenzyme A) and ferredoxin.

11. **(d)** Plants obtain molybdenum in the form of molybdate ions $(MoO)_2^{2+}$. It is a component of several enzymes, including nitrogenase and nitrate reductase both of which participate in nitrogen metabolism.

12. **(a)** Micro elements are those essential elements which are required by plants in traces only, less than 1 mg/gm of dry matter. Iron occurs in the concentration of less than 1 mg/gm.

13. (b) Magnesium is a constituent of the chlorophyll molecule, without which photosynthesis would not occur. Many of the enzymes involved in carbohydrate metabolism require magnesium as an activator. Magnesium is also an activator for those enzymes involved in the synthesis of nucleic acids (DNA, RNA) from nucleotide polyphosphate.

14. (b) The production of plants without soil is called hydroponics. Solution culture is used for raising soilless flowers and vegetables. Plants are raised in small tanks of concrete or metal. The upper covering has supports for plants. The narrow tanks are provided with nutrient solution. A pump circulates air as well as nitrient solution. Roots of the plants are, therefore, regularly provided with aerated nutrient solution. Hydroponics is useful in areas having thin, infertile and dry soil.

15. (a) Some essential elements can alter the osmotic potential of a cell. Potassium plays an important role in the opening and closing of the stomata.

16. (a) Manganese plays in important role in nitrate reduction Manganese acts as activator of the enzymes nitrite reductase and hydroxylamine reductase.

17. (c) Due to deficiency of sulphur plant shows chlorosis (*i.e.*, yellowing due to degradation of chlorophyll) followed by anthocyanin development. The younger leaves show chlorosis before older ones. Sulphur is not the constituent of chlorophyll. The main constituent of chlorophyll is magnesium.

18. (a) In cauliflower plants whiptail disease is very common. The leaves first show an interveinal mottling and the leaf margins may become gray and flaccid and finally brown.

19. (d) Exanthema and reclamation are the most important disease due to copper deficiency. Exanthema is a disease of fruit tree. Reclamation is disease of cereals that occurs chiefly on newly reclaimed peat land.

20. (a) Critical concentration is that optimum concentration of an essential element below which growth of the plant is reduced. As each essential element has one or more specific structural and functional roles, its deficient supply results in appearance of abnormal signs called deficiency symptoms. Deficiency symptoms appear when the availability of the essential nutrients falls below the critical concentration. The symptoms disappear when the deficient element is supplied again.

21. (b) Necrosis is the premature death of cells in a living tissue. It is the symptom of a disease. This symptom can occur in any plant tissues such as leaves, petioles, stem etc. Necrosis may appear in small areas and goes up to large areas of plant tissues. The apical necrosis of young leaves extends toward the base along the margins. Necrosis occurs due to deficincy of Ca, Mg Cu and K.

22. (b) The necessity of micronutrients is always in low amounts while their moderate decrease causes deficiency symptoms and a moderate increase causes toxicity. Toxicity levels for any element also varies for different plants. Many times, excess of an element may inhibit the uptake of another element. For example, the prominent symptom of manganese toxicity is the appearance of brown spots surrounded by chlorotic veins. Manganese competes with iron and magnesium for uptake and with Magnesium for binding with enzymes. Manganese also inhibits calcium translocation in shoot apex. Therefore, excess of manganese may induce deficiencies of iron, magnesium and calcium.

23. (b) The movement of ions is usually called flux, the inward movement into the cells is influx and the outward movement is called as efflux. The entry or exit of ions to and from the symplast requires the expenditure of metabolic energy, which is an active process.

24. (c) *Rhizobium* species (e.g., *Leguminosarum*, *R. lupini* etc) live in symbiotic association in the root nodules of leguminous plants like, pea, gram etc. The bacteria cannot fix nitrogen in the soil. After entering the legume root, the bacterium induces a cell membrane. A pink-red pigment called leghaemoglobin lines the membrane and protects the bacteriods from the oxygen.

25. (c) Ammonia is first oxidised to nitrite by the bacteria *Nitrosomonas* and/or *Nitrosococcus*. The nitrite is further oxidised to nitrate with the help of the bacteria *Nitrobacter*, and/or *Nitrocystis*. These steps are called nitrification. These nitrifying bacteria are chemoautotrophs.

26. (d) Reduction of nitrogen to ammonia by living organism is called biological nitrogen fixation. Only certain prokaryotic species are capable of fixing nitrogen. The enzyme, nitrogenase which is capable of nitrogen reduction is present exclusively in prokarytoes. Such microbes are called N_2 fixers. *Azotobacter* and *Beijerinckia* are free living N_2-fixing aerobic bacteria.

27. (b) The enzyme nitrogenase is a Mo-Fe protein and catalyses the conversion of atmospheric nitrogen to ammonia, which is the first stable product of nitrogen fixation. The enzyme nitrogenase is highly sensitive to molecular oxygen; it requires anaerobic conditions. The nodules have adaptations that ensure that the enzyme is protected from oxygen.

28. (d) In reductive amination, in the presence of enzyme glutamate dehydrogenase and a reduced coenzyme (NADH or NADPH), ammonia can directly combine with α-ketoglutaric acid to form an amino acid. On the other hand, transamination is the transfer of amino group (> $CHNH_2$) of one amino acid with the keto group (> C - O) of keto acid. The enzyme required is transaminase or aminotransferase.

29. (a) Leguminous plants have nodules in their roots, in which *Rhizobium* is present. So, they are able to fix nitrogen.

30. (c) The nitrate formed by nitrification is absorbed by plants and is transported to the leaves. In leaves, it is reduced to form ammonia that finally forms the amine group of amino acids. Nitrate present in the soil is also reduced to nitrogen by the process of denitrification. Denitrification is carried by the bacteria *Pseudomonas* and *Thiobacillus*.

31. (c) According to carbonic acid exchange theory, CO_2 released during respiration of roots combines with soil water to produce carbonic acid (H_2CO_3). Carbonic acid dissociates into H^+ and HCO_3^- ions in soil solution. These H^+ ions may be exchanged for cations adsorbed on clay particles. The cations thus released into soil solution from the clay particles, may be adsorbed on root cells in exchange for H^+ ions.

32. (a) Active absorption requires energy for absorption of minerals. It comes from respiration that is aerobic resopiration. So, when roots are deprived of oxygen, active absorption of minerals is inhibited.

33. (a) The upper surface of each lamina lobe of *Dionaea* contains 3 sensitive spines. The leaf margin bears 12-20 curved spiny teeth. The marignal teeth get interlocked and the prey cannot escape.

34. (b) Phosphorus and potash are most common nutrients found deficient in Indian soil. Supply of these nutrients to soil artificially is necessary through fertilizers to keep the soil rich in plant nutrients for obtaining maximum yield. Irrigation practices also help in enhancing the crop yield. Thus, both fertilizers and irrigation are equally important for high crop yield.

35. (a) Insectivorous plants are partly autotrophic and partly heterotrophic as they capture insects to overcome their nitrogen deficiency.

36. (a) Leguminous plants have nodulated roots in which *Rhizobium* is present. So, these are able to fix nitrogen.

37. (a) Plants absorb nitrogen in the form of NO_3^- (nitrate) or NH_4^+ (ammonium) ion. They can absorb NH_2^- (nitrite) as well but nitrate does not accumulate in the soil. Only a small quantity of nitrate or ammonium is available in the lithosphere. Therefore, nitrogen is the nost critical element. Other critical elements are phosphorus and potassium.

38. (a) Plants absorb the essential nutrients from soil hence they lack excretory organs.

39. (b) Plants do lack excretory organs, but it is not due to absorption pattern or passive life. The carbon dioxide during respiration passes out through the stomata. The other waste materials come out in the form of alkaloids, gums and resins.

Chapter 13

Photosynthesis in Higher Plants

Directions: In the following questions, a statement of assertion is followed by a statement of reason. Mark the correct choice as:

(a) If both Assertion and Reason are true and Reason is the correct explanation of Assertion.

(b) If both Assertion and Reason are true but Reason is not the correct explanation of Assertion.

(c) If Assertion is true but Reason is false.

(d) If both Assertion and Reason are false.

1. **Assertion:** Chloroplasts mostly occur in mesophyll cells along their walls inside the leaves.
   Reason : The membrane system of chloroplast is responsible for trapping the light energy and also for the synthesis of ATP and NADPH.

2. **Assertion :** *Rhoeo* leaves contain anthocyanin pigments in epidermal cells.
   Reason : Anthocyanins are accessory photosynthetic pigments. **[AIIMS 2002]**

3. **Assertion:** Leaf colouration is due to the presence of four pigments - Chlorophyll a, chlorophyll b, xanthophylls and carotenoids.
   Reason : Chlorophyll b is the chief pigment associated with photosynthesis.

4. **Assertion:** Bacterial photosynthesis occurs by utilizing wavelength longer than 700 nm.
   Reason: Here reaction centre is B-890. **[AIIMS 2002]**

5. **Assertion :** There is a decrease in photosynthesis, if the photosynthetic cells are illuminated by light of P680 nm or more wavelength.
   Reason : In red drop phenomenon the rate of photosynthesis decreases.

6. **Assertion :** 6 molecules of CO_2 and 12 molecules of $NADPH^+ + H^+$ and 18 ATP are used to form one hexose molecule.
   Reason : Light reaction results in formation of ATP and $NADPH_2$.

7. **Assertion :** Cyclic pathway of photosynthesis first appeared in some eubacterial species.
   Reason : Oxygen started accumulating in the atmosphere after the non-cyclic pathway of photosynthesis evolved.

8. **Assertion :** Cyclic photophosphorylation synthesizes ATP.
   Reason : ATP synthesise in cyclic photophosphorylation is not associated with NADPH formation.

9. **Assertion :** Each molecule of ribulose-1, 5-bisphosphate fixes one molecule of CO_2.
   Reason : Three molecules of NADPH and two ATP are required for fixation of one molecule of CO_2.

10. **Assertion :**The stromal thylakoids are rich in both PS I and PS II.
    Reason : The granal membranes are rich in ATP synthetase.

11. **Assertion :**Cyclic photophosphorylation synthesizes ATP.
    Reason : ATP synthesise in cyclic hotophosphorylation is not associated with NADPH formation.

12. **Assertion :** Oxidative phosphorylation requires oxygen.
    Reason : Oxidative photophosphorylation occurs in mitochondria.

13. **Assertion :** Plants utilize 5-10 of the absorbed water in photosynthesis.
    Reason : Reduced leaf hydration decrease the photosynthesis.

14. **Assertion:** Six molecules of CO_2 are fixed to form a hexose.
    Reason: One molecule of CO_2 is fixed to produce 686 kcal in photosynthesis.

15. **Assertion:** 686,000 calories energy are produced in the formation of one molecule of glucose.
    Reason: The energy is provided by a total of 12 NADPH and 18 ATP.

16. **Assertion:** The stroma lamellae have both PS I and PS II.
Reason : The grana lamellae lack PS II as well as NADP reductase enzyme.

17. **Assertion:** The proton gradient is broken down due to the movement of protons across the membrane to stroma through the transmembrane channel of the F_0 of the ATP ase.
Reason: It is the breakdown of proton gradient that leads to release of energy.

18. **Assertion:** The splitting of water is associated with PS II.
Reason : Water is split into H^+, O_2 and electrons.

19. **Assertion :** Water splitting complex is associated with PS-II.
Reason : Water splitting complex and PS-II both are physically located on the outer side of the membrane of thylakoid.

20. **Assertion :** Cyclic pathway of photosynthesis first appeared in some eubacterial species.
Reason : Oxygen started accumulating in the atmosphere after the non-cyclic pathway of photosynthesis evolved.

21. **Assertion :** Rate of photosynthesis is dependent of duration of exposure of light.
Reason : At higher light intensities gradually rate of photosynthesis do not show further increase.

22. **Assertion:** C_3 plants respond to increased CO_2 concentration by increasing rate of photosynthesis.
Reason: The higher productivity of some greenhouse crops such as tomatoes and bell pepper is due to increased CO_2 concentration.

23. **Assertion:** The external factors that affect photosynthesis are number, size, age and orientation of leaves, mesophyll cells and chloroplasts and the amount of chlorophyll.
Reason: The internal factors that affect photosynthesis are availability of sunlight, temperature, CO_2 concentration and water.

24. **Assertion:** Sciophytes require lesser light intensity than heliophytes.
Reason: Sciophytes grow below the canopy of trees.

25. **Assertion :** The atmospheric concentration of CO_2 at which photosynthesis just compensates for respiration is referred to as CO_2 compensation point.
Reason : The CO_2 compensation point is reached when the amount of CO_2 uptake is less than that generated through respiration because the level of CO_2 in the atmosphere is more than that required for achieving CO_2 compensation point.
[AIIMS 2005]

26. **Assertion :** Under conditions of high light intensity and limited CO_2 supply, photorespiration has a useful role in protecting the plants from photo-oxidative damage.
Reason : If enough CO_2 is not available to utilize light energy for carboxylation to proceed, the excess energy may not cause damage to plants.
[AIIMS 2006]

27. **Assertion:** Tropical plants have a higher optimum temperature for photosynthesis than temperate plants.
Reason : The optimum temperature for photosynthesis of different plants depends on their habitat.

28. **Assertion :** Mitochondria helps in photosynthesis
Reason : Mitochondria have enzymes for dark reaction. **[AIIMS 1999]**

29. **Assertion :** Dark reaction is not entirely enzymatic reaction.
Reason : It occurs only in absence of light.
[AIIMS 2007]

30. **Assertion :** Dark reaction occurs only at night in the stroma of chloroplast.
Reason : CO_2 fixation occurs only during C_3 cycle.

31. **Assertion :** *Amaranthus* and sugarcane are called as Hatch & Slack plants.
Reason : One glucose is formed by fixation of 6 CO_2 in the plants.

32. **Assertion :** D.C.M.U. is a photosynthetic inhibitor.
Reason : D.C.M.U. inhibits photolysis of water.

33. **Assertion :** Photosynthetically C_4 plants are less efficient than C_3 plants.
Reason : The operation of C_4 pathway requires the involvement of only bundle-sheath cells.
[AIIMS 2006]

34. **Assertion :** C_4 Photosynthetic pathway is more efficient than the C_3 pathway.
Reason : Photorespiration is suppressed in C_4 plants.

35. **Assertion :** The movement of photosynthates is unidirectional.
Reason : Movement of photosynthates occurs with the water.

36. **Assertion :** C_4 pathway of CO_2 fixation is found in some tropical plants.
Reason : In this pathway, CO_2 is fixed by 3C compound.

37. **Assertion :** The concentration of O_2 in the atmosphere is inhibitory to photosynthesis.
Reason : Oxygen inhibitory effect is due to Warburg effect.

38. **Assertion :** CAM plants lack structural compartmentation of leaf, as found in C_4 plants.
Reason : Stomata of CAM plants are open during the day.

39. **Assertion :** Plants utilizing first RuBP in CO_2 fixation are called C_3 plants.
Reason : Plants utilizing first PEP in CO_2 fixations are called C_4 plants.

40. **Assertion :** CO_2 is transported from mesophyll cells to bundle sheath of chloroplasts in C_4 plants.
Reason : RuBP is called initial acceptor of CO_2 in C_2 plants.

41. **Assertion:** Dark reactions are called biosynthetic phase of photosynthesis.
Reason : Dark reactions do not directly depend on the presence of light but are dependent on the products of the light reaction i.e., ATP and NADPH.

42. **Assertion:** OAA is the first product of CO_2 fixation in C_3 pathway.
Reason : The first product of CO_2 fixation in C_4 pathway is PGA.

43. **Assertion:** The C_4 plants have a special type of leaf anatomy called Kranz anatomy.
Reason : Chloroplasts of bundle sheath cells have well developed grana and starch grains.

44. **Assertion:** The bundle sheath cells are rich in an enzyme phosphoenol pyruvate carboxylase (PEP case) in C_4 plants.
Reason : In C_4 plants, the mesophyll cells are rich in an enzyme Ribulose bisphosphate carboxylase-oxygenase (RuBisCO).

45. **Assertion:** Photorespiration does not occur in C_4 plants.
Reason : C_4 plants have a mechanism that increases the concentration of CO_2 at the enzyme site.

46. **Assertion:** The primary CO_2 acceptor in C_4 pathway is a 3-carbon molecule phosphoenol pyruvate (PEP).
Reason : The enzyme responsible for this fixation is PEP carboxylase or PEP case.

47. **Assertion:** Photorespiration is a wasteful process.
Reason : In photorespiratory pathway, there is no synthesis of sugars or ATP.

48. **Assertion :** C_3 pathway is more efficient than C_4 pathway.
Reason : Photorespiration does not occur in C_4 plant.

49. **Assertion :** Biosynthetic phase in photosynthesis is also called dark phase.
Reason : Biosynthetic phase in photosynthesis is also called Blackman's reaction.

50. **Assertion :** Photorespiration decreases the rate of photosynthesis.
Reason : Rate of respiration in C_3 and C_4 is same.

51. **Assertion :** In the photorespiration pathway, there is neither synthesis of sugar nor ATP formation takes place.
Reason : Release of CO_2 with ATP utilisation takes place in photorespiration.

52. **Assertion :** C_3-plants respond to lower CO_2 concentration by showing increased rate of photosynthesis.
Reason : C_4-plantd respond to higher CO_2 concentration by showing decreased rate of photosynthesis.

53. **Assertion :** Photorespiration decreases photosynthetic output.
Reason : In photorespiratory pathway, neither ATP nor NADPH is produced.

54. **Assertion :** Cyclic pathway of photosynthesis first appeared in some eubacterial species.
Reason : Oxygen started accumulating in the atmosphere after the non-cyclic pathway of photosynthesis evolved.

Solutions

1. **(b)** Chloroplasts function as the site of photosynthesis in eukaryotic photoautotrophs. Inside the leaves, the chloroplasts occur mostly in the mesophyll cells along their walls for easy diffusion of gases and receiving optimum quantity of incident light. Within the chloroplast there is the membranous system consisting of grana, the stroma lamellae, and the fluid stroma. The membrane system is responsible for trapping the light energy and also for the synthesis of ATP and NADPH.

2. **(c)** Anthocyanin pigments only give colouration since the epidermal cells mainly have potential colouring pigments. It is responsible for blue, red, pink and purple colours, observed in different parts of plants such as petals, stamens and fruits etc.

   Anthocyanins are also important for attracting insects for pollination and seed dispersal. Hence, anthocyanin pigments are not accessory photosynthetic pigments.

3. **(c)** Chlorophyll a is found in all photosynthetic plants except bacteria. Hence, it is called as universal photosynthetic pigment. It is also called primary photosynthetic pigment because it performs primary reaction of photosynthesis which involves conversion of light into chemical energy. Other photosynthetic pigments like chlorophyll b, carotenes and xanthophylls are called accessory pigments.

4. **(b)** In bacteria, photosynthesis utilizes light of wavelength more than 700 nm and their reaction centre is B-890.

5. **(b)** Although the efficiency of photosynthesis is uniform over most of the spectrum, it declines significantly in the red, *i.e.*, at wavelength of 680 nm and above. This phenomenon is called red drop. However, it was shown by Emerson that if light at 680 nm is supplemented with light of a shorter wavelength (< 600 nm), the quantum efficiency of photosynthesis in the red can be restored to normal.

6. **(b)** Six molecules of CO_2 enter Calvin cycle to produce one hexose molecule whereas 18 ATP, 12 $NADPH^+$ and H^+ molecules are used up. The light reaction of photosynthesis results in ATP and $NADPH_2$ formation.

7. **(b)** Cyclic pathway of photosynthesis appeared first in some eubacterial species. It is supposed to be the first evidence of production of ATP in the presence of light. During non-cyclic photophosphorylation photolysis of water takes place. Under the influence of light energy and the catalytic action of chlorophyll, water a substance of low energy value, is split up into oxygen and hydrogen. Oxygen is used in the chloroplast. Non-cyclic photophosphorylation is the only natural process which adds molecular oxygen to the atmosphere.

8. **(b)** In case of cyclic photophosphorylation, the electron, while passing between ferredoxin and plastoquinone and/or over the cytochrome complex the electron loses sufficient energy to form ATP from ADP and inorganic phosphate.

9. **(c)** Each molecule of ribulose-1, 5-biphosphate fixes one molecule of carbon dioxide with the addition of water, thereby resulting in the formation of two molecules of 3-phosphoglyceric acid (3-PGA). The fixation and reduction of one molecule of CO_2 requires three molecules of ATP and two of NADPH, coming from the photochemical reactions.

10. **(d)** The grana stacks of membranes are enriched in PS II and LHC (Light harvesting centre), while there is little ATP synthetase. On the other hand, a fraction of stroma thylakoids is rich in PS I and ATPase and poor in PS II and LHC.

11. **(b)** In case of cyclic photophosphorylation, the electron, while passing between ferredoxin and plastoquinone and/or over the cytochrome complex the electron loses sufficient energy to form ATP from ADP and inorganic phosphate.

12. (b) The synthesis of ATP *via* electron flow through the ETS, with oxygen as the terminal electron acceptor, is known as oxidative phosphorylation and takes place in mitochondria. In contrast to the oxidative phosphorylation of mitochondria, O_2 is not used in photophosphorylation of chloroplasts and $NADP^+$ is the last electron acceptor.

13. (d) Less than 1% of the total water absorbed is utilized in photosynthesis. The rest is lost in transpiration. Even a slight increase in transpiration reduces the leaf hydration that cuts down photosynthesis by causing stomatal closure and hence decreased CO_2 absorption, loss of leaf turgidity, reduced absorption of solar radiations and decrease in enzymatic activity.

14. (c) The overall equation of photosynthesis is
$CO_2 + 2H_2O + n(h\nu) \rightarrow (CH_2O)_6 + H_2O + O_2$
The standard free-energy change for the synthesis of hexose from CO_2 and H_2O is $\Delta G° = +686$ *kcal*. As six molecules of CO_2 are involved in forming one molecule of hexose, the energy input per CO_2 molecule will be 114 *kcal*.

15. (a) The energy balance of photosynthesis:
$$6CO_2 + 12H_2O \xrightarrow{light} C_6H_{12}O_6 + 6CO_2 + 6H_2O$$
represents a storage of 686,000 calories per mole. This amount of energy is provided by a total of 12 NADPH and 18 ATP molecules, which represent 750,000 calories. The efficiency reached by the PCR cycle is thus as high as 90% (686/750 × 100 = 90%).

16. (d) Thylakoid membranes possess photosynthetic pigments and coupling factors. Coupling factors are involved in ATP synthesis. Photosynthetic pigments include chlorophyll a, chlorophyll b, carotenes and xanthophylls. They occur in specific groups called photosystems (previously quantasomes). There are two photosystems. The grana lamellae have both PS I and PS II and the stroma lamellae lack PS II as well as NADP reductase enzyme.

17. (b) Electron transport in photosynthesis produces a proton gradient. The gradient develops inside the thylakoid lumen in chloroplasts. Proton pump is energised by electron flow. It creates a proton gradient or high concentration of H^+ in the lumen. The proton gradient is broken down due to movement of protons through transmembrane channels, CF_0 of ATPase. The breakdown of the gradient provides enough energy to cause a conformational change in the F_1 particle of the ATPase, which makes the enzyme synthesise several molecules of energy-packed ATP.

18. (b) The phenomenon of breaking up of water into hydrogen and oxygen in the illuminated chloroplast is called photolysis or photocatalytic splitting of water. Light energy, an oxygen evolving complex and an electron carrier are required. It is attached to the inner surface of the thylakoid membrane. The complex has four Mn ions. Light energised changes in Mn (Mn^{2+}, Mn^{3+}, Mn^{4+}) removes electrons from OH^- component of water forming oxygen.
The electrons released during photolysis of water are picked up by P_{680} photocentre of photosystem II.

19. (a) Water splitting complex is associated with PS-II, which itself is physically located on the inner side of the membrane of the thylakoid.

20. (b) Cyclic pathway of photosynthesis first appeared in some eubacterial species for ATP synthesis. Non-cyclic photophosphorylation is the only natural process, which adds oxygen to the atmosphere by photolysis of water. Non-cyclic photophosphorylation first appeared or originated in cyanobacteria.

21. (a) Rate of photosynthesis is dependent of duration of exposure of light. At higher light intensities, photosynthesis does not show further increase because at that level plant does not need sugar synthesis.

22. (b) Carbon dioxide is the major limiting factor for photosynthesis. The C_3 and C_4 plants respond differenly to CO_2 concentrations. At low light conditions neither group responds to high CO_2 conditions. At high light intensites, both C_3 and C_4 plants show increase in the rates of photosynthesis. The

fact that C_3 plants respond to higher CO_3 concentration by showing increased rates of photosynthesis leading to hihger productivity has been used for some greenhouse crops such as tomatoes and bell pepper. They are allowed to grow in carbon dioxide enriched atmosphere that leads to higher yields.

23. (d) Photosynthesis is under the influence of several factors, both interanl (plant) and external. The plant factors include the number, size, age and orientation of leaves, mesophyll cells and chloroplasts, internal CO_2 concentration and the amount of chlorophyll. The internal factors are dependent on the genetic composition and the growth of the plant. The external factors include the availability of sunlight, temperature, CO_3 concentration and water. As a plant photosynthesises, all these factors simultaneously affect its rate.

24. (a) Plants are categorised into two groups depending upon their inability or ability to tolerate high light intensity,shade plants (sciophytes) and sun plants (heliophytes). Sciophytes grow in poorly illuminated condition as below the canopy of tall plants in seek of shade. Heliophytes grow in the open.

25. (c) Compensation point is that value or point in the light intensity and atmospheric CO_2 concentration when the rate of photosynthesis is just equivalent to the rate of respiration in the photosynthetic organ. So that there is not net gaseous exchange.

26. (c) Photorespiration is the uptake of O_2 and release of CO_2 in light and results from the biosynthesis of glycolate in chloroplasts and subsequent metabolism of glycolate acid in the same leaf cell. During photorespiration loss of carbon takes place in the form of CO_2.

27. (a) The optimum temperature is 10°-25° C for C_3 plants and 30-45° C for C_4 plants. The temperature optimum for photosynthesis of different plants also depends on habitat that they are adapted to tropical plants have a higher temperature optimum than the plants adapted to temperate climates.

28. (d) Mitochondria helps in cellular respiration by transferring energy from organic compounds to ATP. Chloroplast helps in photosynthesis. Dark reaction takes part in the stroma of the chloroplast.

29. (a) During photosynthesis, assimilatory power ATP and $NADPH_2$ are produced which require light. This reaction is called light reactions or Hill's reaction. Assimilatory powers are required for the reduction of CO_2. This reaction is enzymatic and independent of light. It is called dark reaction which takes place in stroma of chloroplast. So, dark reaction is independent of presence or absence of light.

30. (d) Dark reaction is also known as light-independent phase. Unlike, light reaction, it does not require light as an essential factor. Thus, it can take place both in the presence or absence of light. The term dark reaction does not mean that it takes place only in dark period or at night. CO_2 fixation occurs in both C_3 and C_4 cycle. In C_3 cycle, CO_2 is added by the enzyme, RuBisco to a 5 carbon compound RuBP that is converted to 2 molecules of 3-carbon PGA. In C_4 cycle, the first product of CO_2 fixation (takes place in mesophyll) is a 4-carbon compound, oxaloacetic acid. It is seen in some tropical plants.

31. (b) *Amaranthus* sp and sugarcane are known as Hatch and Slack plants. In Hatch and Slack pathway, one glucose molecule is formed by fixation of $6CO_2$ in the plants.

32. (a) DCMU (Dichlorophenyl dimethyl urea) is a herbicide that can prevent non cyclic photophosphorylation and oxygen production. It inhibits photolysis of water.

33. (d) C_4 plants are more efficient in picking up CO_2 even when it is found in low concentration because of its high affinity for PEP. They show Kranz anatomy *i.e.* vascular bundle is surrounded by bundle sheath and mesopyll cells.

34. (a) C_4 photosynthetic pathway is more efficient than C_3 pathway as C_4 plants can pick up CO_2 even when it is found in low concentration. PEP enzymes show high affinity for CO_2. C_4 plants contain two types of chloroplast (Kranz anatomy) :

bundle sheath chloroplast and mesophyll chloroplast. Bundle sheath cells contain Calvin cycle enzymes. Due to high concentration of CO_2 in bundle sheath cells, RuBP carboxylase works only for Calvin cycle and not for photorespiration. Photorespiration is a wasteful process as it works to undo the act of photosynthesis in C_4 plants. No energy rich compound is produced in this process. When temperature increases, more and more photosynthetically fixed carbon is lost by photorespiration thus reducing the efficiency of C_3 plants.

35. **(a)** The movement of organic materials in the plant is bidirectional that is, substances are translocated in opposite directions in the stem simultaneously. The movement of photosynthates is independent of water translocation as it takes place through phloem whereas latter takes place through xylem.

36. **(b)** C_4 pathway found is in tropical angiosperms and is called as Hatch and Slack cycle. Here CO_2 is fixed by 3C compound (phosphoenol pyruvate, PEP).

37. **(a)** Small quantity of oxygen is essential for photosynthesis except in some anaerobic bacteria. The inhibition of photosynthesis at high O_2 levels may be due to

(i) Oxygen takes part in oxidation of photosynthetic pigments, intermediates and enzymes in the presence of strong light (photo-oxidation).

(ii) Oxygen is a strong quencher of excited state of chlorophyll.

(iii) It converts RuBP carboxylase to RuBP-oxygen. At a very high oxygen content the rate of photosynthesis begins to decline in all plants. The phenomenon is called Warburg effect (reduction due to photorespiration).

38. **(c)** CAM plants do not exhibit the structural compartmentation (C_3 and C_4 cycles taking place in different cells) of conventional C_4 plants. CAM plants fix CO_2 at night because their stomata are open at night and closed during the day.

39. **(b)** Plants that utilize primarily RuBP to fix CO_2, (which results in the formation of the three-carbon compound 3-PGA), are called C_3 plants. Hatch and Slack proposed a new pathway of CO_2 fixation *via* the carboxylation of PEP. Because the products are four-carbon compounds, plants exhibiting this pathway are referred to as C_4 plants.

40. **(c)** Malic acid or aspartic acid is translocated to bundle sheath cells through plasmodesmata. Inside the bundle sheath cells they are decarboxylated (and deaminated in case of aspartic acid) to form pyruvate and CO_2. CO_2 is again fixed inside the bundle sheath cells through Calvin cycle. RuBP of Calvin cycle is called secondary or final acceptor of CO_2 in C_4 plants.

41. **(b)** Photosythesis occurs in two phases: photochemical and biosynthetic. Photochemical phase is also called light or hill reaction. Biosynthetic phase is also called as dark or Blackmann's reaction. Dark reaction catalyses assimilation of CO_2 to carbohydrates. They occur in stroma or matrix of chloroplasts. These reactions do not require light directly but depend on assimilatory power (ATP and NADPH) produced during light reaction.

42. **(d)** CO_2 assimilation during photosynthesis is of two types, Calvin cycle or C_3 cycle and C_4 dicarboxylic acid cycle or C_4 cycle. The first product of CO_2 fixation in C_3 pathway is 3-phosphoglyceric acid (PGA) which is a 3-carbon compound and first product of CO_2 fixation in C_4 pathway is oxaloacetic acid (OAA) which is a 4-carbon compound.

43. **(c)** C_4 plants show 'kranz' type of anatomy. In 'kranz' anatomy, the mesophyll is undifferentiated and its cells occur in concentric layers around vascular bundles. The vascular bundles are surrounded by large sized bundle sheath cells which are arranged in wreath like manner in one to several layers. Chloroplasts of mesophyll cells are smaller, have well developed grana and they do not produce starch. Chloroplasts of bundle sheath cells are larger and agranal. Starch is often present.

44. **(d)** The primary CO_2 acceptor in C_4 cycle is a 3-carbon molecule phosphoenol pyruvate (PEP) present in the mesophyll cells. The enzyme responsible for this fixation is PEP carboxylase or PEP case. The mesophyll cells lack RuBisCO enzyme. The C_4 acid OAA is formed in the mesophyll cells. The CO_2 released in the bundle sheath cells enters the C_3 or the Calvin pathway, a pathway common to all plants. The bundle sheath cells are rich in an enzyme Ribulose bisphosphate carboxylase-oxygenase (RuBisCo), but lack PEPcase.

45. (a) In C_4 plants photorespiration does not occur beacuse they have a mechanism that increases the concentraion of CO_2 at the enzyme site. This takes place when the C_4 acid from the mesophyll is broken down in the bundle sheath cells to release CO_2. This results in increasing the intracellular concentration of CO_2. This ensures that the RuBisCO functions as a carboxylase minimising the oxygenase activity.

46. (b) Primary acceptor of CO_2 in C_4 plants is phosphoenol pyruvic acid (PEP). Carboxylation is catalysed by PEP carboxylase (PEP case). Carboxylation taking place with the help of PEP case is called beta carboxylation. First stable product in C_4 plant is OAA (oxaloacetic acid).

47. (a) Photorespiration is the light dependent process of oxygentation of ribulose biphosphate (RuBP) and release of carbon dioxide by the photosynthetic organs of a plant. In the photorespiratory pathway, there is neither synthesis of sugars, nor of ATP. Rather it results in the release of CO_2 with the utilisation of ATP. In the photorespiratory pathway there is no synthesis of ATP or NADPH. Therefore, photorespiration is a wasteful process.

48. (c) C_4 plants are more efficient than C_3 plants.

49. (b) The biosynthetic phase is also known as the dark phase or Blackman phase. Biosynthetic phase (Dark or Blackman's Reaction) C_3 (Calvin cycle) C_4 (dicarboxylic C_4 acid cycle) e.g., *Euphorbia corollata*, *Euphorbia maculata*. Grass *Alloteropsis semialata* has both C_3 and C_4 ecotypes (ecological variants).

50. (d) Photorespiration is a highly wasteful process because, it may drop down the photosynthesis up to 50%. Rate of respiration in C_3 and C_4 plants are not same as they have different types of leaf anatomy (arrangement of chloroplast).

51. (a) Photorespiration does not produce energy or reducing power. Rather, it consumes the energy further. It undoes the work of photosynthesis. It may reduce photosynthesis upto 50%. Therefore, photorespiration is a highly wasteful process. This happens only in C_3-plants.

52. (d) C_3-plants respond well to higher CO_2 concentration by showing increased rate of photosynthesis. C_4-plants respond to higher CO_2 concentration by showing increased rate of photosynthesis.

53. (a) In photorespiration, RuBisCo acts as an oxygenase enzyme instead of carboxylase enzyme. Active site of this enzyme is same for both of these activities. In C_3 plants, some O_2 always bind to RuBisCo.

$$\underset{(5C)}{\text{Ribulose}-1,5-\text{biphosphate}} + O_2 \xrightarrow[\text{Oxygenase}]{\text{RuBp}} \underset{(3C)}{\text{PGA}} + \underset{(2C)}{\text{Phosphoglycolate}}$$

Photorespiration does not produce energy or reducing power. Rather, it consumes energy. Further, it undoes the work of photosynthesis. There is 25% loss of fixed CO_2.

54. (b) Cyclic pathway of photosynthesis is appeared first in some eubacterial species. It is supposed to be the first evidence of production of ATP in the presence of light. During non-cyclic photophosphorylation photolysis of water takes place. Under the influence of light energy and the catalytic action of chlorophyll, water is split up into oxygen and hydrogen. Non-cyclic photophosphorylation is the only natural process which adds molecular oxygen to the atmosphere.

Chapter 14

Respiration in Plants

Directions: In the following questions, a statement of assertion is followed by a statement of reason. Mark the correct choice as:

(a) If both Assertion and Reason are true and Reason is the correct explanation of Assertion.

(b) If both Assertion and Reason are true but Reason is not the correct explanation of Assertion.

(c) If Assertion is true but Reason is false.

(d) If both Assertion and Reason are false.

1. **Assertion :** Stomata are absent in submerged hydrophytes.

   Reason : Respiration occurs by means of air chambers in submerged plants. **[AIIMS 1997]**

2. **Assertion :** Glycolysis is the first step of respiration in which glucose completely breaks into CO_2 and H_2O.

   Reason : In this process, there is net gain of twenty four molecules of ATP. **[AIIMS 2009]**

3. **Assertion :** Glycolysis occurs in cytoplasm.

   Reason : Enzymes for glycolysis are found in cytoplasm. It is common in aerobic/anaerobic respiration.

4. **Assertion :** Substrate level phosphorylation is present in glycolysis.

   Reason : Substrate level phosphorylation causes synthesis of ATP.

5. **Assertion:** Fructose-1, 6 diphosphate is converted into glyceraldehyde-3-phosphate and dihydroxy-acetone-3-phosphate.

   Reason: In the presence of enzyme aldolase, conversion of fructose-1,6 diphosphate into 3-phosphoglyceraldehyde and dihydroxyacetone-3-phosphate is facilitated.

6. **Assertion:** Plants do not have specialised respiratory organs.

   Reason: There is very little transport of gases from one plant part to another.

7. **Assertion:** The process of glycolysis is also known as EMP pathway.

   Reason: It is the only process of respiration in aerobic organisms.

8. **Assertion:** This conversion of 1,3-biphosphoglycerate (BPGA) to 3- phosphoglyceric acid (PGA) is an energy yielding step.

   Reason: By the formation of ATP, this energy is trapped.

9. **Assertion:** The incomplete oxidation of glucose into lactic acid or ethanol is fermentation.

   Reason: In only prokaryotes, it takes place under anaerobic condition.

10. **Assertion :** Banking industry makes use of yeasts such as *Saccharomyces cerevisiae.*

    Reason : Carbon dioxide produced during fermentation causes bread dough to rise by thermal expansion.

11. **Assertion:** During strenuous exercise, anaerobic respiration sometimes occurs in our skeletal muscles.

    Reason: Pyruvic acid is reduced to lactic acid in the presence of lactate dehydrogenase and in the absence of oxygen.

12. **Assertion :** In alcoholic fermentation, the hexose molecule is converted into glucose and fructose.

    Reason : Alcoholic fermentation is anaerobic respiration brought about by enzyme zymase.

13. **Assertion :** Under aerobic conditions, pyruvate gives rise to lactate.

    Reason : Under anaerobic condition, pyruvate gives rise to acetyl CoA.

14. **Assertion:** Both in aerobic and anaerobic conditions terminal oxidation occurs.

    Reason: Terminal oxidation stops at terminal step of respiration.

15. **Assertion:** The breaking of the C- C bonds of complex compound through oxidation within the cells and release of large amount of energy is respiration.
Reason: During respiration, the compounds that are oxidised are called respiratory substrates.

16. **Assertion:** In TCA cycle, the first step is the condensation of pyruvate with oxaloacetic acid and water.
Reason: This reaction is catalysed by enzyme pyruvate synthase.

17. **Assertion :** The product of the first reaction of the Kreb's cycle is citric acid, a six carbon compound.
Reason : The first reaction of the Kreb's cycle is the condensation of acetyl CoA with oxaloacetate.

18. **Assertion :** The inner membrane of mitochondria contains systems involving electron transport.
Reason : The mitochondrial matrix contains enzymes of Kreb's cycle.

19. **Assertion :** F_1 particles are present in the inner mitochondrial membrane.
Reason : An electron gradient formed on the inner mitochondrial membrane, forms ATP.

20. **Assertion :** In electron transport chain, there is a loss of energy at each step.
Reason : At each step of ETC, there are electron carriers.

21. **Assertion :** Both hexokinase and glucokinase require divalent cations Mg^{++} or Mn^{++}.
Reason : The divalent cations act as catalysts.

22. **Assertion :** Cytochromes are a group of copper containing electron transferring proteins.
Reason : The terminal cytochrome reacts with oxygen.

23. **Assertion:** The enzyme consists copper cytochrome oxidase.
Reason: Cyanide combine with copper of cytochrome oxidase, that prevents oxygen combining with it.

24. **Assertion:** The electron transport system (ETS) is the metabolic pathway through which the electron passes from one carrier to another.
Reason: ETS is present in the inner mitochondrial membrane.

25. **Assertion:** Complex II and complex III of ETS are NADH dehydrogenase complex respectively.
Reason: Cytochrome *c* acts as a mobile carrier for transfer of electrons between complex II and III.

26. **Assertion:** Pyruvic acid formed as a result of glycolysis, undergoes phosphorylation reaction to form acetyl CoA, during aerobic respiration.
Reason: During aerobic respiration of one molecule of glucose, there is net gain of 18 ATP molecules.

27. **Assertion:** In electron transport system the electrons are passed on to oxygen that results in the formation of H_2O.
Reason: Oxygen is the ultimate acceptor of electrons.

28. **Assertion:** Respiratory pathway is also an amphibolic pathway.
Reason: In respiration, there is breakdown of many substances (catabolism) and synthesis of many substances (anabolism) by respiratory intermediates.

29. **Assertion:** The energy currency of the cell is ATP.
Reason: ATP can be broken down to release energy wherever and whenever energy needs to be utilised.

30. **Assertion:** Oxidation of one molecule of NADH produces to 3 molecules of ATP, and that of one molecule of $FADH_2$ produces 2 molecules of ATP.
Reason: The number of ATP molecules synthesised depends on the nature of the electron donor.

31. **Assertion :** One way of indicating the ATP yield from oxidative phosphorylation is the P/O ratio.
Reason : The cell stores 40% of the chemical energy.

32. **Assertion :** During the hydrolysis of typical chemical bonds, about 3000 calories per mole are liberated.
Reason : ATP also yields about 3000 calories per mole after the release of any one of the two terminal phosphates.

33. **Assertion:** The RQ is equal to 1, when carbohydrates are used as substrate and are completely oxidised.
Reason: When proteins are used as substrate in respiration, the RQ is greater than 1.

Solutions

1. **(b)** Stomata are absent since gaseous exchange takes place through diffusion in submerged plants.
2. **(d)** Glycolysis is the process of breakdown of glucose or similar hexose sugar into two molecules of pyruvic acid through a series of enzyme mediated reactions, releasing energy (ATP) and reducing power ($NADH_2$). It is the first step of respiration, which occurs inside the cytoplasm and is independent of O_2. In glycolysis, two molecules of ATP are consumed during double phosphorylation of glucose to form fructose 1, 6 diphosphate. Four molecules of ATP are produced in the conversion of 1, 3-diphosphoglycerate to 3-phosphoglycerate and phosphenol pyruvate to pyruvate whereas, two molecules of $NADH_2$ are formed during oxidation of glyceraldehyde 3-phosphate to 1,3-diphosphoglycerate. Since, each NADH is equivalent to 3 ATP, so net gain in glycolysis is 8 ATP.
3. **(a)** Glycolyis occurs in cytoplasm as all necessary enzymes are found in it. This process is common in aerobic/anaerobic respiration. In this process, one glucose molecule is converted into 2 moles of pyruvic acid.
4. **(b)** One of the two phosphates of diphosphoglycerate is linked by high energy bond. It can synthesize ATP and form 3-phosphoglycerate. The enzyme is phosphoglycerate kinase. The direct synthesis of ATP from metabolites is called substrate level phosphorylation.

   During formation of phosphoenol pyruvate the phosphate radical pick up energy. It helps in the production of ATP by substrate level phosphorylation.
5. **(b)** In the presence of enzyme aldolase, fructose 1, 6-diphosphate is converted into a glyceraldehyde-3-phosphate and a dihydroxy acetone-3-phosphate molecules.

   $$\text{Fructose 1, 6-diphosphate} \xrightleftharpoons{\text{aldolase}} \text{3PGA} + \text{DiHAP}$$
6. **(a)** Unlike animals, plants have no specialised organs for gaseous exchange. Gaseous exchange in plants occurs by diffusion through stomata and lenticels. There are various reason for the absence of respiratory organs in plants. Each part of plant takes care of its own needs of gaseous exchange. There is little transport of gases from one part to another. Plants do not require much for gas exchange. All plant parts respire at rates far lower than animals. To take care of their own needs of gases during photosynthesis, leaves are well adapted. Moreover, leaves also utilise oxygen released during photosynthesis. In plants, cells are closely packed and located quite close to the surface of the plant.
7. **(c)** Glycolysis is also known as EMP pathway, as it was discovered by three German scientists-Gustav Embden, Otto Meyerhof and J. Parnas in 1930. In glycolysis, partial oxidation of glucose takes place that form two molecules of pyruvic acid. It occurs in the cytoplasm of the cell and is present in almost all living organisms. Aerobic respiration consists of diferent processes i.e., (i) glycolysis, (ii) oxidative decarboxylation of pyruvic acid, (iii) Krebs' cycle and (iv) terminal oxidation and oxidative phosphorylation.
8. **(b)** The conversion of 1, 3 -bisphosphoglycerate (BPGA) 3-phosphoglyceric acid (PGA) is an energy yielding step. One of the two phosphates of bisphosphoglycerate is linked by high energy bond. It can synthesise ATP and form 3-phosphoglycerate in the presence of enzyme phosphoglycerate kinase. The direct synthesis of ATP from metabolites is called substrate level phosphorylation.

   1, 3 bisphosphoglycerate + ADP

$\xrightarrow[+Mg^{2+}]{\text{Phosphoglycerate kinase}}$ 3-phosphoglycerate + ATP

9. (c) Fermentation is the incomplete oxidation of glucose under anaerobic conditions. In yeast the pyruvic acid is converted to CO_2 and ethanol. Other organisms like some bacteria produce lactic acid from pyruvic acid. In animal cells also, like muscles during exercise when oxygen is inadequate for cellular respiration, pyruvic acid is reduced to lactic acid in the presence of lactate dehydrogenase. Under anaerobic conditions fermentation takes place in many prokaryotes, unicellular eukaryotes and in germinating seeds.

10. (a) Baker's yeast (*Saccharomyces cerevisiae*) is added to flour during kneading. Yeast secretes enzymes like amylase (changes some starch to maltose), maltase (maltose to glucose) and zymase (glucose to ethyl alcohol and carbon dioxide). The dough swells up or leavens. Leavened dough is baked and both alcohol and carbon dioxide evaporate, the bread becomes soft and porous.

11. (a) In human body anaerobic respiration occurs in our skeletal muscles during strenous exercise. When oxygen is inadequate for cellular respiration pyruvic acid is reduced to lactic acid by lactate dehydrogenase. The reducing agent is NADH = H^+ which is reoxidised to NAD^+.

12. (a) Alcoholic fermentation is the respiration in absence of O_2. In this process, hexose molecule is changed to ethyl alcohol and CO_2. In presence of zymase enzyme. In this less amount of energy is released as compared to aerobic respiration.

13. (d) Under aerobic conditions, the products are pyruvate and coenzyme NADH. Pyruvate directly enters the mitochondrial matrix and is converted into acetyl-CoA. Under anaerobic conditions, pyruvate is used as a hydrogen acceptor and converted into lactate. In anaerobic conditions, pyruvate remains in the cytosol.

14. (d) Terminal oxidation is the name of oxidation found in aerobic respiration that occurs towards the end of catabolic process and involves the passage of both electrons and protons of reduced coenzymes to oxygen.

15. (b) Respiration is an energy releasing enzymatically controlled process that involves a step-wise oxidative breakdown of food substances inside living cells. Food reaches every cell of an organism for respiration to take place. During cellular respiration, the oxidation of food substances takes place. This process occurs in cytoplasm and mitochondria. During oxidation, chemical bonds (e.g., C - C bonds) are broken that releases energy and forms a number of biochemical intermediates. This energy is used in the synthesis of ATP. Those organic substances which are oxidised during respiration to liberate energy inside the living cells are respiratory substrate. The common respiratory substrates are carbohydrates, proteins, fats and organic acids. the most common respiratory substrate is glucose.

16. (d) The TCA cycle starts with the condensation of acetyl group with oxaloacetic acid (OAA) and water to yield citric acid. The reaction is catalysed by the enzyme citrate synthetase and a molecule of CoA is released.

$$\text{Acetyl CoA} + \text{OAA} + H_2O \xrightarrow[\text{Synthetase}]{\text{Citrate}} \text{Citrate} + \text{CoA}$$

17. (a) The first reaction of the Krebs cycle is the condensation of acetyl CoA (2 C compound) with oxaloacetate (4 C compound). Citric acid, a 6 carbon-compound is the first product of Krebs cycle.

18. (b) The inner membranes of mitochondria contain all systems involving electron transport. The mitochondrial matrix contains all the soluble enzymes of the citric acid or Kreb's cycle and those involved in the oxidation of fatty acids

19. (c) ATP synthase is located in F_1, or head piece of F_0- F_1 or elementary particles. The particles are present in the inner mitochondrial membrane. ATP synthase becomes active in ATP formation where there is a proton gradient having higher concentration of H^+ or protons on the F_0 side as compared to F_1 side.

20. (b) The passage of electrons from one enzyme or cytochrome to the next is a downhill journey with a loss of energy at each step. At each step the electron carriers include flavins, iron sulphur complexes, quinones and cytochromes.

21. (c) Both kinases require a divalent cation (Mg^{2+}or Mn^{2+}), which first combines with ATP to form the true substrate, $MgATP^{2-}$ or $MnATP^{2-}$.

22. (d) The cytochromes are a group of iron containing electron-transferring proteins of aerobic cells that act sequentially to transfer electrons from flavoprotein to molecular oxygen. The terminal cytochrome of the electron transport chain, which can react with oxygen, is called cytochrome oxidase.

23. (b) The final stage of respiratory chain involves cytochrome oxidase which consists copper. This stage can be specifically inhibited by cyanide or carbon monoxide. Cyanide combines with the copper, that prevents oxygen combining with it.

24. (c) Inner mitochondrical membrane contains groups of electron and proton transporting enzymes. In each group the enzymes are arranged in a specific series called electron transport chain (ETC) or mitochondrial respiratiory chain or electron transport system (ETS). An electron transport chain or system is a series of coenzymes and cytochromes that take part in the passage of electrons from one carrier to another. The passage of electrons from one enzyme or cytochrome to the next is a downhill journey with a loss of energy at each step.

25. (c) Complex II of ETS is succinate dehydroginase complex and complex III of ETS is cytochrome bc1 complex. Cytochrome c is a small protein which is attached to the outer surface of the inner mitochondrial membrane and acts as a mobile carrier for transfer of electrons between complex III and IV.

26. (d) During aerobic respiration, the final product of glycolysis is pyruvic acid which is transported from the cytoplasm into mitochondria and undergoes oxidative decarboxylation reaction to form acetyl CoA. Aerobic respiration is the complete oxidation of glucose into CO_2 and H_2O. In aerobic respiration of one molecule of glucose, its net gain is 36 ATP molecules.

27. (a) The last electron acceptor of respiratory chain is O_2. In electron transport system, electrons are passed on from one carrier to another and ultimately to oxygen and at the end of this chain, one molecule of water is produced as:

$$\frac{1}{2}O_2 + 2H^+ + 2e^- \rightarrow H_2O$$

28. (a) Amphibolic pathway is the pathway that functions for both catabolism and anabolism reactions. Respiratory pathway is mainly a catabolic process that serves to run the livng system by providing energy. The pathway produces a number of intermediates. Many of them are raw materials for building up both primary and secondary metabolites. Because the respiratory pathway is involved in both anabolism and catabolism, it would hence be better to consider the respiratory pathway as an amphibolic pathway rather than a catabolic one.

29. (a) The mechanism of breakdown of food materials within the cell to release energy, and the trapping of this energy for synthesis of ATP is cellular respiration. The energy released by oxidation in respiration is not used directly but is used to synthesise ATP, that is broken down whenever and wherever energy needs to be utilised. Hence, ATP acts as the energy currency of the cell. This trapped energy in ATP is utilised in various energy-requiring processes of the organisms.

30. (a) For the transfer of electrons from the substrates of Krebs' cycle, the ETS follows two routes.
Route 1 of ETS: The electrochemical gradient created as an electron pair passes from NADH to oxygen is sufficient to drive the synthesis of 3 ATP molecules.
Route 2 of ETS: The electron pair from $FADH_2$ passes over only a part of the electron transport chain. Therefore, fewer H^+ ions are added to the gradient. The smaller gradient generates only 2 ATP molecules for each pair of electrons.

31. (b) One way of indicating the ATP yield from oxidative phosphorylation is the P/O ratio, which is expressed as the moles of inorganic phosphate used per oxygen atom consumed. The cell stores 40% of the chemical energy liberated by the combustion of glucose in the form of ATP. The rest of the energy is dissipated as heat or used for other cell functions.

32. (c) During the hydrolysis of typical chemical bonds, about 3000 calories per mole are liberated. The release of any one of the two terminal phosphates of ATP yields about 7300 calories per mole, instead of the 3000 calories from common chemical bonds. The standard free energy of hydrolysis of ATP to ADP and phosphate is 7.30 K cal at pH 7.0 and temperature 37°C in the presence of excess Mg^{2+}.

33. (c) The respiratory quotient depends upon the type of respiratory substrate used during respiration. When carbohydrates are used as substrate and are completely oxidised, the RQ will be 1, because equal amounts of CO_2 and O_2 are evolved and consumed, respectively, as shown in the equation below:

$$C_6H_{12}O_6 + 6O_2 \rightarrow 6CO_2 + 6H_2O = \text{Energy}$$

$$RQ = \frac{6CO_2}{6O_2} = 1.0$$

Chapter 15

Plant Growth and Development

Directions: In the following questions, a statement of assertion is followed by a statement of reason. Mark the correct choice as:
(a) If both Assertion and Reason are true and Reason is the correct explanation of Assertion.
(b) If both Assertion and Reason are true but Reason is not the correct explanation of Assertion.
(c) If Assertion is true but Reason is false.
(d) If both Assertion and Reason are false.

1. **Assertion:** As a whole plant growth is indefinite.
Reason: Plants retain the capacity of continuous growth throughout their life.
2. **Assertion:** For the synthesis of protoplasm nutrients are required by plants which act as source of energy.
Reason: Water provides the medium for enzymatic activities needed for growth.
3. **Assertion:** Both at the root apex and the shoot apex, the constantly dividing cells show the meristematic phase of growth.
Reason: The cells of this region are rich in protoplasm and lacks nuclei.
4. **Assertion:** Primary growth of the plants leads to the elongation of the plants along their axis.
Reason: Root apical meristem and shoot apical meristem are responsible for primary growth of the plants.
5. **Assertion:** Sigmoid growth curve consists of four parts.
Reason: Lag phase is also known as grand phase of growth.
6. **Assertion:** Due to environment, the difference in shapes of leaves produced in air and those produced in water in buttercup represent the heterophyllous development.
Reason: The phenomenon of heterophylly is an example of plasticity.
7. **Assertion:** The sum of growth and differentiation is development.
Reason: Development in plants is under the control of extrinstic factors only.
8. **Assertion:** Secondary roots and shoots are plagiogeotropic.
Reason: Plagiogeotropic roots are those which develop at an angle of 45° from the vertical axis.
9. **Assertion :** Apical dominance is increased by removal of shoot tip.
Reason : Due to accumulation of auxin in lateral parts, growth is inhibited.
10. **Assertion:** F.W. Went isolated auxin from the timps of coleoptiles of wheat seedlings.
Reason: Ethylene delays the senescence.
11. **Assertion:** During Vietnam War, agent orange (a mixture of 2, 4-D and 2,4,5-T) was used .
Reason: 2,4-D and 2,4,5-T are used as herbicides.
12. **Assertion:** By suppressing the activity of lateral buds, auxins promote apical dominance.
Reason: In moriculture, periodic pruning of shoot tips is done to make mulberry plants bushy.
13. **Assertion** : Auxins help to prevent fruit and leaf drop at early stages.
Reason : Auxins promote the abscission of older mature leaves and fruits. **[AIIMS 2017]**
14. **Assertion :** The apical bud is the only source of auxins.
Reason : Removal of apical bud promotes lateral bud growth.
15. **Assertion :** Gibberellins induce flowering in long day plants.
Reason : Genetically tall plant become dwarf by application of Gibberellin.
16. **Assertion :** Stratification of seeds may promote their germination.
Reason : Stratification is promoted by gibberellin and cytokinins.

17. **Assertion:** Gibberellins are used in fruits like apple to elongate and improve its shape.
Reason: To speed up the malting process in brewing industry GA_3 is used.

18. **Assertion:** In plants, kinetin is found naturally.
Reason: Cytokinin breaks seed and bud dormancy.

19. **Assertion :** Cytokinis are anti-senescent.
Reason : Effects of cytokinins in antagonistic to ethylene.

20. **Assertion :** Ethylene causes climacteric ripening of fruits.
Reason : Climacteric fruits show a rise in respiration at the time of ripening.

21. **Assertion:** Abscisic acid (ABA) is also known as stress hormone.
Reason: ABA increases the tolerance of plants to various kinds of stresses.

22. **Assertion:** Flowering depends only on a combination of light and dark exposure in some plants.
Reason: The site of perception of light or dark duration are the shoot apices of plants.

23. **Assertion:** Photomodulation of flowering is regulated by phytochrome.
Reason: Active form of phytochrome (Pfr) directly induces floral induction in shoot buds.
[AIIMS 2015]

24. **Assertion:** "Touch" responses in *Mimosa* is an example of such movement
Reason: In the direction of stimulus, nastic movements occur.

25. **Assertion :** The pigment which causes photoperiodic stimulus is called phytochrome.
Statement 2 : Chemically phytochrome is a starch.

26. **Assertion :** Phototropism is a directional growth movement.
Statement 2 : Phototrophic movement occurs in the direction of light.

27. **Assertion :** Dark period plays more important part in flowering than light period.
Reason : Flowering occurs in short-day plant if the dark period is interrupted by light break.

28. **Assertion :** Phytochrome exists in two forms P_r and P_{fr}.
Reason : P_r form stimulates and P_{fr} form inhibit flowering.

29. **Assertion :** Floral initiation is done by florigen.
Reason : Floring is translocated from flowers to leaves.

30. **Assertion :** Vernalization is a treatment to plant given artifically.
Reason : Vernalization is perceived by whole plant.

31. **Assertion :** Vernalization is acceleration of subsequent flowering by low temperature treatment.
Reason : Site of vernalization is apical meristem.
[AIIMS 2015]

32. **Assertion:** The promotion of flowering by a period of low temperature is vernalisation.
Reason: It prevents precocious reproductive development late in the growing season.

Solutions

1. (a) The shoot tip tissues in plants are meristematic.
2. (b) Nutrients are raw materials required for synthesis of protoplasm as well as source of energy. It should be rich in nitrogenous components to increase the synthesis of protoplasm and carbohydrates for energy and cell wall synthesis. All types of micronutrients and macronutrients should be available for proper growth. Water is required for cell elongation, maintenance of turgidity of growing cells and for providing medium for enzyme action. Even slight deficiency of water reduces growth. It may, however, promote differentiation. Water stress completely stops growth.
3. (c) The root apex, shoot apex and many other regions consists meristematic tissue. By mitotic divisions of the meristematic cells new cells are produced. These cells have cellulosic cells walls, contains large nucleus and rich in protoplasm. It is called the phase of cell formation or cell division.
4. (a) Growth is unique in plants because plants retain the capacity for unlimited growth throughout their life. These ability of the plants is due to the presence of meristems at certain locations in their body. The cells of such meristems have the ability to divide and self-perpetuate. The root apical meristem and shoot apical meristem are indeterminate meristems, because these meristems continue thier activity throughout life of the plant. Root apical meristem and shoot apical meristem cause primary growth of plants and also causes the elongation of the plants along their axis.
5. (c) An S-shaped or sigmoid curve is obtained, if total growth is plotted against time. It consists of four parts-lag phase, log phase, phase of diminishing growth and stationary phase. Growth is slow in the lag phase, rapid during log or exponential phase, slow again during the phase of diminishing growth. During the stationary phase growth stops completely. Log phase is also called as grand phase of growth due to fast growth in this phase.
6. (b) During different phases of growth as well as in response to environment different structures are developed. To cope up with the changes in environment. The plant organs also change their structures, which is called plasticity. Heterophylly is the occurrence of different types of leaves on the same plant in different growth phases or under different environmental conditions. In case of environmental plasticity shown by aquatic butter cup *Ranunculus flabellaris*, the submerged leaves are highly dissected while the emerged leaves are broad and lobed.
7. (c) In the life of a plant, growth, differentiation and development are closely related events. Development is sum of growth and differentiation. Development in plants is under control of both intrinsic and extrinsic factors. Intrinsic factors include intracellular genetic factors and intercellular factors growth regulators. Extrinsic factors are light, temperature, water, oxygen and nutrition, etc.
8. (a) Secondary roots and shoots are plagiogeotropic i.e., they grow to a position at an oblique angle (45°) to the gravitational force. Root and stem branches lie at an angle other than 90° to the direction of gravity.
9. (d) Removal of shoot tip increases the lateral dominance not apical dominance. Accumulation of auxin in the lateral part elongates the cells and increases growth.
10. (d) F.W. Went isolated auxin from tips of coleoptiles of oat seedlings. Ethylene promotes senescence and abscission of plant organs especially of leaves and flowers.
11. (b) The first selective herbicides to be discovered and used widely were 2,4-D and its derivatives and are very potent auxins. 2,4-D and 2,4,5-T destroy dicot weeds. They block their sieve elements and disturb mitosis. The plant is ultimately destroyed. Agent orange, which was used in the war in Vietnam as a defoliant is an effective mixture of free 2,4-D and the N-butyl ester of 2,4,5-T.

12. (a) Auxin is produced by shoot tip that acts as a growth promoter for apical bud and inhibit the growth of lateral buds. When a terminal bud is removed, the nearest axillary buds begin to grow and the plant branches rapidly. In case of mulberry plants, pruning is done to remove apical dominance and causes more branching of the main body of the plant.

13. (b) Auxin delays abscission of young leaves and fruits. Its effect is through non-formation of abscission zone below a leaf or fruit. Abscission zone cuts off nutrients and water supply. However, auxin promotes the abscission of mature or older leaves and fruits.

14. (d) The apical bud is not the only source of auxins. Young developing leaves also produce auxins and it has been shown that auxins from this source may inhibit lateral bud growth. When the apical bud is removed, the lateral buds sprout. However, if a paste of auxin is painted on the cut end of the decapitated shoot, the lateral buds remain inhibited, as if the apical bud is present.

15. (c) Application of GA can induce flowering in long day plants. It has no favourbale effect on size of flower and fruit in certain plants. The genetically dwarf plants can be made tall by application of GA.

16. (b) Stratification of seeds may affect the disappearance of inhibitors and the buildup of germination promoters such as the gibberellins and cytokinins. Natural stratification occurs when seeds shed in the fall are covered with cold soil, debris and snow. In artificial stratification, layers of seeds are alternated with layers of moistened *Sphagnum* sand or some other appropriate material and stored at low temperatures.

17. (b) Gibberellins are applied to increase the number and size of several fruits e.g., grape, tomato. Size and shape of apple frutis is enhanced by application of GA_4 and GA_7 mixture. Gibberellins (e.g., GA_3) increase the yield of malt from barley grains i.e., malting.

18. (d) The first cytokinin was discovered from degraded autoclaved Herring sperm DNA. It is called kinetin (6-furfuryl amino-purine). Kinetin does not occur naturally and is a synthetic hormone. Cytokinins help to overcome the apical dominance. It is the ethylene that breaks seed and bud dormancy.

19. (b) When cytokinins are added directly to the abscission layer, senescence of the zone is retarded. They delayed the degradation of protein and chlorophyll of the plant parts and hence delay senescence. As they act as anti senescent, they act as antagonistic to ethylene which accelerate senescence.

20. (b) In most fruits, the rate of respiration will undergo a sharp rise and then fall near the end of ripening. Kidd and West termed this phenomenon "climacteric rise". The climacteric acts as a trigger that sets in progress those changes that rapidly transform the fruit from an unripe to a ripe condition. Finally, application of ethylene to unripe fruit will bring on a premature climacteric and accelerate ripening.

21. (a) Abscisic acid increases resistance of plants to cold and other types of stresses like drought and water logging etc. It is therefore also known as stress hormone.

22. (d) To induce flowering, some plants require a periodic exposure to light. It is now also known that not only the duration of light period but the duration of dark period is also of equal importance. Hence, it shows that flowering in certain plants depends not only on a combination of light and dark exposures but also their relative durations. These response of plants to periods of day/night is termed photoperiodism. The shoot apices modify themselves into flowering apices prior to flowering, shoot apices cannot percieve photoperiods by themselves. The leaves are the site of perception of light/dark duration.

23. (a) Phytochrome is a receptor pigment that is present in leaves. They are responsible for flowering in plants. These are two types P_r (Red light) and P_{fr}(far-red light) P_{fr} are responsible for flowering in LDP.

24. (c) Nastic movements are non-directional movements in which the response is determined by the structure of the responsive organ and not the direction of the stimulus. "Touch" responses in

Mimosa are an example of movements that do not necessarily occur towards or away from the stimulus. The movement occurs due to turgor changes in the cells of pulvinus or swollen area lying at the base of the petiole, pinnae and pinnules.

25. (c) Phytochrome is a pigment involved in the perception of photoperiodic stimuli controlling flowering, seed germination and other morphogenetic phenomena. It is a protein with a chromophore (pigment-coloured portion) prosthetic group (*e.g.*, Chromoprotein).

26. (a) Phototropism is a paratonic directional growth movement of curvature which is induced and determined by the direction of light stimulus. Shoots grow towards the source of light hence called positively phototrophic while roots grow away from the source of light hence called negatively phototrophic.

27. (c) It has been demonstrated that flowering in plant is more of a response to the dark period than to the light period. In short day plants, plants can flower in complete darkness if supplied with exogenous nutrients. Flowering is prevented in them if dark period below the critical level is interrupted by a flash of light. Interruption of light by dark inhibits flowering under normal photoperiods.

28. (c) Light energy becomes effective when it is absorbed by a pigment. These pigments are called phytochromes. It occurs in two forms namely P_r and P_{fr}. The two forms are interconvertible. The P_r form absorbs red light of 660 nm and changed to P_{fr}. The P_{fr} form absorbs far red light of 730 nm and changed to P_r. The P_r form stimulates whereas P_{fr} form inhibit flowering. The P_r form stimulates whereas P_{fr} form inhibit flowering. P_{fr} form of phytochrome is the active form. The P_r form is not considered to be active.

29. (c) Cajlakhjan, working on floral initiation, coined the term florigen for the flowering hormone thought to be present in photoinduced leaves and plants. It is supposed that leaves prepare a special compound A in receiving CO_2. A in turn produces B in dark and is followed by formation of C (florigen). The florigen translocates from vegetative meristems to floral initiation.

30. (b) Many plants do not come to flower before they experience a low temperature. These plants remain vegetative during the warm season, receive low temprature during winter, grow further and then bear flowers and fruits. Vernalization is, therefore, a process of shortening of the juvenile or vegetative phase and hastening flowering by a previous cold treatment. The stimulus of vernalization is perceived only by the meristematic cells, *e.g.*, shoot tip, embryo tips, root apex, developing leaves etc.

31. (b) The physiological mechanism of flowering in plants is controlled by two factors— light period and low temperature. The cold treatment of plants to induce flowering is called vernalization. Term vernalization was first given by T.D.Lysenko(1928). As a result of vernalization a flowering hormone called vernaline is formed. Site of vernalization is apical meristem.

32. (b) There are plants for which flowering is either quantitatively or qualitatively dependent on exposure to low temperature. This is termed as vernalisation. Late in the growing season, it prevents precocious reproductive development and enables the plant to have sufficient time to reach maturity. Vernalisation refers specially to the promotion of flowering by a period of low temperature. Some important food plants, wheat, barley, rye have two kinds of varieties: winter and spring varieties. The spring varieties are planted in spring. They come to flower and bear fruits prior to end of growing season. If the winter varieties are sown similarly, they fail to flower and produce fruits before the end of growing season. They are planted in autumn, that form seedlings in which form they cover winter. The seedlings resume growth in spring, and bear flowers and fruits in summer.

Chapter

16

Digestion and Absorption

Directions: In the following questions, a statement of assertion is followed by a statement of reason. Mark the correct choice as:

(a) If both Assertion and Reason are true and Reason is the correct explanation of Assertion.

(b) If both Assertion and Reason are true but Reason is not the correct explanation of Assertion.

(c) If Assertion is true but Reason is false.

(d) If both Assertion and Reason are false.

1. **Assertion:** Thick layers of muscles are present in the wall of alimentary canal.
Reason: These muscles help in the mixing of food materials with the enzymes coming from different glands in the alimentary canal.

2. **Assertion:** Human beings have two sets of teeth during their life.
Reason: Human beings have thecodont dentition.

3. **Assertion:** Oesophagus pierces the diaphragm and enters the abdominal cavity.
Reason: Peristaltic movement starts from oesophagus.

4. **Assertion :** Chewing is one of the important process of digestion in animals.
Reason : It helps in enzyme action.

5. **Assertion :** Presence of HCl in stomach is necessary for the process of digestion.
Reason : HCl kills and inhibits the growth of bacteria in the stomach.

6. **Assertion:** Absorption of digested food mainly occurs in the stomach.
Reason: Stomach produces the hormone secretin and the intrinsic factor and it liquifies ingested food.

7. **Assertion:** The sight, smell and presence of food in the oral cavity can stimulate secretion of saliva.
Reason: The activities of gastro-intestinal tract are only under neural control for proper coordination of different parts.

8. **Assertion:** Gastrectomy can lead to iron-deficiency or anaemia.
Reason: HCl of gastric juice converts Fe^{3+} into Fe^{2+} which makes iron absorbable.

9. **Assertion :** HCl in the gastric juices maintain strong pH (1.5-2.5) in the stomach but does not digest the walls of stomach and duodenum.
Reason : Protection to intestinal wall and stomach from the enzymatic actions is provided by the mucous secreted by goblet cells, bicarbonates from pancreas, mucous and bicarbonates from Brunner's gland.

10. **Assertion :** The main part of carbohydrate digestion takes place in small intestine.
Reason : Herc, pancreatic amylase converts carbohydrates into lactose.

11. **Assertion :** Pancreatic amylase digest starch to maltose.
Reason : Pancreatic amylase breaks the peptide bond of protein.

12. **Assertion :** Trypsin helps in digestion of blood of predator animals.
Reason : Trypsin hydrolyses fibrinogen.

13. **Assertion :** Lipases of bile help in the emulsification of fats.
Reason : Lipases can break large fat droplets into smaller ones. **[AIIMS 2011]**

14. **Assertion :** Starch is hydrolysed by ptyalin to maltose.
Reason : Sucrase hydrolyses sucrose to lactose. **[AIIMS 2016]**

15. **Assertion:** Blood sugar level falls rapidly after hepatectomy.
Reason: The glycogen of the liver is the principal source of blood sugar.

16. **Assertion:** Arachidonic acid is an unsaturated fatty acid.
Reason: There are present one or more double bonds between carbon atoms in unsaturated fatty acids.

17. **Assertion:** Rumen of alimentary canal of ruminant animals harbour numerous bacteria and protozoa.
Reason: Bacteria and protozoa help in the secretion of gastric juice in the rumen.

18. **Assertion:** Wall of small intestine consists of many tube like glands.
Reason: These glands secrete enzymes DNAse and RNAse into the intestinal juice.

19. **Assertion:** In alcoholic fermentation, the hexose molecule is converted into glucose and fructose.
Reason: Alcoholic fermentation is anaerobic respiration that is brought about by the activity of enzyme catalase.

20. **Assertion:** Insulin is secreted by α-cells of islets of langerhans of pancreas.
Reason: Insulin promotes conversion of sucrose to glycogen.

21. **Assertion:** Carbohydrates are more suitable for the production of energy in the body than proteins and fats.
Reason: Carbohydrates can be stored in the tissues as glycogen for use in the production of energy, whenever necessary.

22. **Assertion:** The amino acid glycine comes under the category of non-essential amino acids.
Reason: This is due to the fact that it can not be synthesised in the body.

23. **Assertion:** In alcoholic drink, alcohol is converted into glucose in the liver.
Reason: Liver cells are able to produce glucose from alcohol by fermentation.

24. **Assertion:** Adult human being is not perfect in digestion of milk.
Reason: With age, man produces little or no lactase in the intestinal juice.

25. **Assertion:** Volume and fluidity of intestinal contents have increased in a person.
Reason: The person drank sea water.

26. **Assertion:** Pancreas is a heterocrine gland.
Reason: Endocrine part secretes insulin and glucagon and exocrine part secretes an acidic pancreatic juice containing enzymes.

27. **Assertion:** Trypsinogen is activated by enterokinase into active trypsin which in turn activates other enzymes in the pancreatic juice.
Reason: The pancreatic juice contains inactive enzymes which are activated by intestinal juice.

28. **Assertion:** Starch in the chyme are hydrolyzed by pancreatic amylase into glucose molecules.
Reason: About 70 per cent of the starch is hydrolyzed in oral cavity by salivary amylase.

29. **Assertion:** Mucosal epithelium of gut has goblet cells which secrete mucus.
Reason: Mucus in the gastric and pancreatic juice protects the mucosa layer from excoriation by acidic secretion.

30. **Assertion:** Bile helps in emulsification of fat.
Reason: Bile salts help in incorporating fatty acids and glycerol into water soluble droplets called chylomicrons.

31. **Assertion:** Bile is not a true digestive juice.
Reason: Bile lacks digestive enzymes.

32. **Assertion:** Fat is restricted in the diet of a person who has undergone an operation to remove gall bladder.
Reason: Gall bladder stores lipases which are released in small intestine for digestion.

33. **Assertion** : Liver and pancreas are the largest digestive glands of our body. Pancreas is the second largest gland after liver.
Reason : Pancreas is considered a mixed gland as it functions both as exocrine and endocrine.

34. **Assertion** : In human gut, small intestine is the longest part of digestive system.
Reason : Different type of food like proteins, fats and carbohydrates are digested completely in this longest part of human alimentary canal.

35. **Assertion** : Absorption of water from the small intestine helps in maintaining the osmotic balance with the blood.
Reason : More than 90% of the water is absorbed from the small intestine by osmosis and the process associated with absorption of electrolytes or salts like Na^+ and K^+ and digested food to balance the osmotic concentration with blood.

36. **Assertion** : In the condition of obstructive jaundice, large amounts of unabsorbed fats are eliminated out of the body.
Reason : Entry of bile into the small intestine is prevented during obstructive jaundice.
[AIIMS 2009]

37. **Assertion** : Water and electrolytes are almost fully absorbed in the large intestine.
Reason : In large intestine, haustral contractions (slow segmenting movements) roll the forming faeces over and over, causing absorption of water and electrolytes. **[AIIMS 2017]**

38. **Assertion:** Caecum is a small blind sac which hosts some symbiotic micro-organisms.
Reason: *Escherichia coli* in return produces vitamin B_{12}, vitamin K, thiamine and riboflavin.

39. **Assertion:** Products of digestion are absorbed in the large intestine.
Reason: The mucosal lining of large intestine forms finger-like foldings called villi which aid in absorption.

40. **Assertion :** Diarrhoea is the abnormal frequent movement of bowel and increased liquidity of faeces that may be caused by microorganisms, stress and milk sugar intolerance.
Reason : Mild diarrhoea is caused by taking active trophozoites deposited on the food items by files. Causal parasite is *Trichomonas hominis* of large intestine. Chyme passes rapidly through the small intestine and faeces in the large intestine. So, there is not enough time for the absorption of water and electrolytes by colon.

41. **Assertion :** Scurvy is caused by deficiency of vitamin C.
Reason : Deficiency of ascorbic acid causes scurvy. **[AIIMS 2001]**

42. **Assertion:** Minerals are not biologically active substances.
Reason: Some individuals suffer from anaemia due to deficiency of copper.

43. **Assertion:** Sea-faring fishermen sometimes eat raw fish.
Reason: They can be deficient of Vitamin B_1.

Solutions

1. (d) Thick layers of muscles are present in the alimentary canal. These muscles facilitate the movement of food particles through alimentary canal. Large food particles are broken down into small, semi liquid particles by the action of these muscles. Later, these help in the forward flow of food materials and mixing of enzymes coming from different glands related to alimentary canal.
2. (b) Majority of mammals including human beings possess two sets of teeth during their life, a set of permanent or adult teeth. This type of dentition is called diphyodont. Human beings also have thecodont dentition, i.e., teeth are embedded in the sockets of the jaw bones.
3. (b) Oesophagus is a long and thin tube that pierces the diaphragm and enters the abdominal cavity. In oesophagus, voluntary muscle fibres are present in the anterior 1/3 and involuntary muscle fibres are present in posterior 2/3. Peristaltic movement of contraction and relaxation of muscles starts from oesophagus.
4. (a) Chewing food helps in ptyalin action (ptyalin or salivary amylase is a starch hydrolysing enzyme present in the saliva of human), because it mixes the food with saliva. It also breaks food particles into smaller particles with greater surface area exposed to enzyme action. It also starts starch digestion in mouth.
5. (b) Presence of hydrochloric acid in stomach is necessary for digestion because acidic medium activates the action of gastric juice. HCl maintains a strong acidic pH of about 1-2 in the stomach. At this acidic pH, inactive pepsinogen is spontaneously hydrolysed to active pepsin and inactive pro-rennin is converted to active rennin. Pepsin and rennin digest proteins to peptones and proteoses. In addition, HCl helps to kill and inhibit the growth of bacteria and other harmful organisms that may enter in the stomach along with the food.
6. (d) Absorption takes place in small intestine as it offers large surface area for absorption. Stomach produces the hormone gastrin and intrinsic factor.
7. (c) The activities of the gastro-intestinal tract are under neural and hormonal control for proper coordination of different parts. The sight, smell and /or the presence of food in the oral cavity can stimulate secretion of saliva. Gastric and intestinal secretions are also similarly stimulated by neural signal. The muscular activities of different parts of the alimentary canal can also be moderated by neural mechanisms, both local and through CNS. Hormonal control of the secretion of digestive juices is carried out by local hormones produced by gastric and intestinal mucosa.
8. (a) HCl of gastric juice converts Fe^{3+} into Fe^{2+} which makes the absorption of iron possible. Non-secretion of HCl (achlorhydria) because of gastrectomy (partial or full surgical removal of stomach) can lead to iron-deficiency or anaemia.
9. (a) HCI present in the gastric juices maintains a strong pH in stomach. But the wall of stomach is not digested with its action because goblet cells secretes mucous which lubricates the innermost layer continuously in the stomach and intestine. The wall is also protected by the bicarbonates of pancreatic juices and Brunner's gland.
10. (c) In small intestine, pancreatic amylase converts starch and dextrins into maltoses and small intestine is main site for digestion of carbohydrates.
11. (c) Pancreatic amylase is a starch splitting enzyme similar to ptyalin by hydrolysing starch and glycogen to maltose, isomaltose and limit dextrins.

12. (a) Trypsin is protein digesting enzyme present in the intestine of animals. Though it cannot digest casein (a milk protein), in predator animals drinking the blood of their prey, trypsin hydrolyses fibriongen of blood into fibrin, leading to blood coagulation thus, help in blood digestion. It also activates other pancreatic proteases.

13. (d) It is not lipases but the bile salts which are responsible for the emulsification of fats. Bile salts are steroids secreted by the liver in the bile. In the intestinal lumen, they reduce the surface tension of fat dropletes, causing their breakdown into many smaller ones. A stable fine emulsion of fat is thereby formed. On the other hand, lipases are the enzymes which hydrolyse fats and oils. Lipases can digest fat in significant amounts only when large fat droplets are broken into tiny droplets to form a fine emulsion. Emulsificaion of fats by bile salts thus, increases the lipase action on fats.

14. (c) Sucrase hydrolyses sucrose to glucose and fructose.

15. (a) In liver, glycogen a reserve food material is changed into glucose (glycogenolysis) and released into blood. Under abnormal conditions, liver can convert proteins and fats into glucose by complex chemical reactions i.e. called gluconeogenesis. Thus, due to hepatectomy, blood sugar level falls rapidly.

16. (a) Fatty acids which lack any double or triple bond in their hydrocarbon chain are known as saturated fatty acids. Example, lauric acid, myristic acid, palmitic acid, stearic acid etc. In contrast to saturated fatty acids, unsaturated fatty acids have one or more double bonds between carbon atoms at fixed place along with the hydrocarbon chain. Example, palmitoleic acid, oleic acid, linoleic acid, linolenic acid, arachidonic acid etc.

17. (c) Ruminant animals such as cattle, buffalo, sheep, goat and camel have a compound stomach, which consists of four chamber, *viz*, rumen, reticulum, omasum and abomasum. Rumen is the first and the largest of the four chambers. Rumen and reticulum harbour numerous bacteria and protozoa, which carry out extensive fermentation of cellulose. So, these two chambers function as sites for cellulose digestion in ruminants. The gastric juice containing enzymes and HCl is secreted only by the fourth chamber i.e., Abomasum.

18. (c) Numerous tube like glands are present in the wall of small intestine which secrete intestinal juice into the intestinal lumen. This juice contains a number of enzymes like enterokinase, aminopeptidases, dipeptidases, maltase, lactase, lipase etc. for digesting various types of food. On the other hand, the enzymes RNAse and DNAse are present in the pancreatic juice. These enzymes are secreted by the pancreas and are drained into the small intestine via hepato pancreatic duct.

19. (b) Alcoholic fermentation is anaerobic respiration in the absence of O_2. In this process, hexose molecule is changed to ethyl alcohol and CO_2 in the presence of zymase enzyme. In this, less amount of energy is released as compared to aerobic respiration.

20. (d) Insulin is secreted by β-cells of islets of langerhans. It helps in conversion of glucose into glycogen decreasing blood sugar level. This is called glycogenesis.

21. (b) Carbohydrates are more suitable for the production of energy in the body than proteins and fats, because carbohydrate molecules contain relatively more oxygen than the others, and consequently, require less molecules of oxygen for their oxidation. In other words, for each litre of oxygen consumed, carbohydrates yield far more energy than proteins or fats. Carbohydrates are also stored in the tissue as glycogen for use in the production of energy, when necessary. Glycogen is the stored fuel particularly in such tissues as skeletal muscles which then have to work with a supply of oxygen far lower than their immediate need.

22. (c) Non essential amino acids are those amino acids which need not be supplied in the diet because they can be synthesised by

the body, particularly from carbohydrate metabolites. Glycine is one such non essential amino acid. On the contrary, essential amino acids are those amino acids which can not be synthesised in the animal body and must be supplied with food in adequate amounts. Out of twenty amino acids, eight are considered essential in human diet.

23. **(d)** In liver, alcohol is oxidised into acetaldehyde which is further oxidised into acetate. The latter is converted to acetyl coenzyme A which is used in Krebs' cycle. Ethyl alcohol → Acetaldehyde → Acetate → Acetyl Co A → $CO_2 + H_2O$

24. **(a)** The human being is the only mammal who ingests significant amount of lactose in milk. Curiously, many human adults can not digest milk, because with age they produce little or no lactose in the intestinal juice. In such persons, the lactose of milk remains undigested and is fermented in the intestine producing gases and acids. This results in flatulence, intestinal cramps and diarrhoea.

Adult human
↓
Less or no lactase
↓
Lactose remains undigested
↓
Undigested substances fermented
↓
Produce gas, acids, intestinal cramps, diarrhoea

25. **(a)** If sea water is drunk, its Mg^{2+} ions increase the solute concentration in the intestinal lumen because Mg^{2+} is absorbed very slowly. On the contrary, Mg^{2+} draws water from the blood to the intestinal lumen by osmosis. So, water is not gained, but is lost from the blood on drinking sea water. Thus, there occurs increase in the fluidity and volume of intestinal contents. In the same way, this consequently stimulates intestinal peristalsis and evacuation of fluid faeces.

26. **(c)** The pancreas is compound (both exocrine and endocrine) elongated organ situated between the limbs of the 'U' shaped duodenum. The exocrine portion secretes an alkaline pancreatic juice containing enzymes and the endocrine portion secretes hormones, insulin and glucagon.

27. **(a)** Pancreatic juice consists of various types of inactive protein digestive enzymes such as trypsinogen, chymotrypsinogen, procarboxypeptidase and proelastase. Out of these, trypsinogen is activated into trypsin due to the activity of enzyme enterokinase. Trypsin further results in the activation of other inactive enzymes.

28. **(d)** About 30 per cent of starch is hydrolyzed in the oral cavity by salivary amylase into a disaccharide-maltose. The pancreatic juice contains starch digesting-enzyme, called pancreatic α-amylase which converts starch into maltose, isomaltose and α-dextrins. Intestinal juice or succus entericus contains maltase, isomaltase, sucrase (invertase), lactase and α-dextrinase which act on disaccharides produced by the action of amylases to form the simple absorbable form glucose.

29. **(b)** Mucosal epithelium has goblet cells which secrete mucus that helps in lubrication. The mucus in gastric and pancreatic secretion plays an important role in lubrication and protection of mucosa epithelium from excoriation by highly acidic HCl.

30. **(c)** Bile is a watery fluid mixture containing bile pigments, bile salts, cholesterol, phospholipids, etc. Bile salts break the large fats into smaller ones forming small, spherical, water soluble molecules called micelles.

31. **(a)** Bile contains bile pigments (billirubin and biliverdin), bile salts, cholesterol and phospholipids but no enzymes. Hence, it is not regarded as true digestive juice.

32. **(c)** The gall bladder stores bile which is released for the emulsification of fats thus, helping in fat digestion.

33. **(b)** Pancreas is a mixed (compound) gland. It is present inferior to the stomach in the bend of proximal part of the small intestine (duodenum). It is both exocrine and endocrine gland. Digestive secretion is secreted by the exocrine part, which is

poured into the small intestine. Liver is the largest gland in human body.

34. **(a)** Small intestine of the human gut is a narrow long tube. Because of its small diameter, it is called small intestine. Its length is according to the height of individual. It is the major site of digestion and absorption of different type of food. Digestion and absorption of various food is carried out in a particular part of small intestine, like absorption of iron takes place in proximal part of duodenum. Food digestion starts from oral cavity in humans, which continues in stomach and is digested completely in small intestine. Undigested and unabsorbed food (faeces) is transferred to long intestine where the water and some vitamins are absorbed.

35. **(a)** Absorption of water takes place by osmosis from the lumen of the small intestine through its epithelial cells and into blood stream through villi. This absorption of water is concerned with the salt absorption and digested food, which in turn, maintains an osmotic balance with blood running in the whole body.

36. **(a)** In the condition of obstructive jaundice, the entry of bile into the small intestine is prevented due to an obstruction in the bile duct. As we know that bile salts helps in the digestion of fats by emulsification and also in their absorption by the formation of water soluble droplets called micelles from where fatty acids, glycerides, sterols and fat soluble vitamins are absorbed into the intestinal cells. Therefore, in the absence of bile, the fats remain unabsorbed and consequently are eliminated out of the body in the faeces.

37. **(a)** Water and electrolytes are completely absorbed in the large intertine due to the haustral contractions

38. **(a)** Caecum forms the niche of a complex community of micro-organisms. These are found to live in a mutualistic relationship with humans within their gut by synthesizing various important components like vitamin B_{12}, vitamin K, thiamine, riboflavin as well as metabolizing sterols, bile acids and xenobiotics.

39. **(d)** The innermost layer lining the lumen of the alimentary canal is the mucosa. This layer forms small finger-like foldings called villi in the small intestine. Villi help in increasing absorptive surface of the small-intestine. They are supplied with a network of capillaries and a large lymph vessel called the lacteal. Because of these modifications, about 90% of absorption of all nutrients occurs in the small intestine.

40. **(a)** Diarrhoea is an abnormal frequent movement of bowl. Excessive liquidity and frequency of faeces discharge is caused by active trophozoites present on uncovered food (contaminated by flies). Its causal organism is *Trichomonas hominis*. However, it is also caused by intolerance with some eatables like milk. In this disorder, food is not stored for required time in the parts of the alimentary canal for digestion and absorption.

41. **(a)** Deficiency of ascorbic acid/vitamin C causes scurvy.

42. **(d)** Minerals take part in biological reactions and are thus biologically active. Anaemia is caused by deficiency of iron.

43. **(a)** Sea faring fisherman suffer from paralysis because raw fish muscles contain an enzyme which destroys Vitamin B_1.

Chapter 17 Breathing and Exchange of Gases

Directions: In the following questions, a statement of assertion is followed by a statement of reason. Mark the correct choice as:

(a) If both Assertion and Reason are true and Reason is the correct explanation of Assertion.
(b) If both Assertion and Reason are true but Reason is not the correct explanation of Assertion.
(c) If Assertion is true but Reason is false.
(d) If both Assertion and Reason are false.

1. **Assertion :** Most fish when out of water, die of suffocation.
   Reason : Atmospheric air contains far less oxygen content than the dissolved oxygen in water.
2. **Assertion :** Gill-lamellae in aquatic animals help in exchange of gases.
   Reason : Each gill lamella carries many blood capillaries.
3. **Assertion :** In mammals, complex respiratory system has developed.
   Reason : Mammalian skin is impermeable to gases.
4. **Assertion :** Insects develop a complex system of air tubes called trachea for respiratory purpose.
   Reason : Exchange through body surface is not possible in insects.
5. **Assertion :** Coughing and sneezing are necessary.
   Reason : Coughing and sneezing are reflex actions
6. **Assertion :** Aerobic animals are not truely aerobic.
   Reason : They produce lactic acid anaerobically.
7. **Assertion :** If there is no air in trachea, it will not collapse.
   Reason : Trachea is having the cartilagenous ring.
8. **Assertion :** Inspiration occurs due to muscular relaxation.
   Reason : During inspiration, the diaphragm and external intercostal muscle contract simultaneously.
9. **Assertion :** Aerobic respiration involves the exchange of respiratory gases twice.
   Reason : Exchange occurs from lung to heart and then heart to lung.
10. **Assertion:** Alveoli are the primary sites for exchange of gases.
    Reason: All factors in our body are favourable for diffusion of O_2 from alveoli to tissues and that of CO_2 from tissues to alveoli.
11. **Assertion:** Tracheae, primary, secondary and tertiary bronchi are supported by incomplete cartilaginous rings.
    Reason: These rings of cartilage make the wall non-collapsible.
12. **Assertion:** Respiratory rhythm centre is moderated by pneumotaxic centre, located in the medulla region of the brain.
    Reason: Pneumotaxic centre controls the switch 'ON' point of inspiration.
13. **Assertion:** Excessive inflation of the lungs is prevented by Hering-Breuer reflex.
    Reason: On overstretching of the lungs, the stretch receptors send impulses along the vagus nerve to stimulate the expiratory centre.
14. **Assertion:** The lungs are situated in thoracic chamber which is anatomically an air-tight chamber.
    Reason: Such an arrangement is essential to avoid any change in pulmonary volume.
15. **Assertion:** Vocal cords consist of three pairs of mucous membrane that extend into the lumen of the larynx.
    Reason: Only two pairs of cords are responsible for production of sound.
16. **Assertion :** During inspiration, pressure of air falls in the thorax.
    Reason : There is a rise in volume of thorax during inspiration.

17. **Assertion :** Vital capacity is higher in athletes than non-athletes.
Reason : Vital capacity is about 3.5-4.5 litres in a normal adult person.

18. **Assertion :** Forceful expiration occurs through expiratory muscles.
Reason : Expiratory muscles expire quickly.

19. **Assertion :** Histamine is involved in allergic and inflammatory reactions.
Reason : Histamine is a vasodilator.

20. **Assertion :** Blood of insects is colourless.
Reason : The blood of insect does not play any role in transport of oxygen.

21. **Assertion :** Oxyhaemoglobin dissociates near the organ tissue due to Bohr effect and oxygen is released.
Reason : Increased CO_2 concentration reduces the affinity of haemoglobin for oxygen.
[AIIMS 2010]

22. **Assertion:** Inspiration occurs when there is a negative pressure in the lungs with respect to the atmospheric pressure.
Reason: During inspiration, a decrease in pulmonary volume increases the intra-pulmonary pressure than atmospheric pressure which forces the air from outside to move into the lungs.

23. **Assertion:** The role of oxygen in the regulation of respiratory rhythm is quite insignificant.
Reason: Increased pCO_2 and H^+ concentration inputs from chemoreceptors can activate respiratory rhythm centre to make necessary adjustments.

24. **Assertion:** 70 percent of CO_2 formed from catabolism is trapped as bicarbonate in the RBCs at the tissue level.
Reason: At tissue level, carbonic anhydrase in RBCs facilitates the formation of CO_2 and H_2O from bicarbonate.

25. **Assertion:** Chloride shift is exchange of Cl^- of plasma and HCO_3^- of RBCs.
Reason: Chloride shift mainatins an acid base balance between the RBCs and plasma.

26. **Assertion:** Carbonic anhydrase is present in the erythrocytes.
Reason: In erythrocytes carbon dioxide combines with water and is transported.

27. **Assertion :** Symptoms of emphysema develops when a person living on plains ascends and stays on a mountain.
Reason : Air pressure and partial pressure of oxygen falls with the rise in altitude.

28. **Assertion :** Severve Acute Respiratory Syndrome (SARS) originated in China.
Reason : China is the most populated country of the world. **[AIIMS 2003]**

29. **Assertion :** Many visitors to the hills suffer from skin and respiratory allergy problems.
Reason : Conifer trees produce a large quantity of wind-borne pollen grains. **[AIIMS 2003]**

Solutions

1. **(c)** Although atmospheric air contains far more oxygen content than the water (air contains 21% oxygen and water contains 0.5-0.9% oxygen by volume depending on the temperature), still most fish when out of water die of suffocation due to lack of oxygen. When fish is taken out of water the gills stick together thereby reducing the surface area. Reduced surface area lowers gas exchange and so death occurs.
2. **(a)** Gills are the main respiratory organs of aquatic animals. Each gill bears rows of comb-like, soft, thin gill-filament, each gill-filament bears many flat, parallel membrane-like gill-lamellae. Each gill lamella carries many blood capillaries. Water taken through the mouth, is made to flow from the pharynx in a single direction between the gill lamella. This greatly helps in the gaseous exchange across the lamellar membrane between the capillary blood and the flowing water.
3. **(b)** Mammalian skin is impermeable so that water loss through it, is minimised. But mammals need far more oxygen to maintain their high metabolic rates than lower animals; so they need a more extensive respiratory surface. Thus a complex respiratory system has evolved in mammals to meet this need. The mammalian respiratory system consists of the nasal cavity, nasopharynx, larynx, trachea, bronchi, bronchiole and lungs.
4. **(a)** As the integument of insect is thick and impermeable to minimise lose of body water, they can not carry out gas exchange through their body surface. To overcome this difficulty they have developed a complex system of air tubes called trachea to reach the air directly near the tissue cells. Each trachea communicates with the exterior through openings in the body wall.
5. **(b)** Coughing and sneezing should to take place because these reactions serve to keep the air passages free from foreign matter. Coughing is a reflex action under nervous control. The minute receptors found in the wall of trachea, bronchi, bronchioles and alveoli are highly sensitive to foreign matter (smoke, dust etc.) Like coughing, sneezing is also a reflex action triggered because of irritation to nasal passages. In this, sensory impulses travel from nasal passages to the medulla through trigeminal nerves. The reaction involves the same series of events as in cough reflex, but the air explodes out both through nose and mouth, expelling the foreign matter from nasal passages.
6. **(a)** In most animals, tissue oxidation are carried out by aerobic respiration. But sometimes in aerobically respiring animals, anaerobic metabolism take place in certain tissues like skeletal muscles which do not immediately get as much oxygen as in necessary for metabolize glucose during vigorous movements.
7. **(a)** There is no air in trachea, it does not collapse due to the presence of C-shaped narrow cartilagenous ring or discs.
8. **(a)** Inspiration is the result of muscular contraction. The diaphragm and external intercoastal muscle contracts simultaneously. The lateral thoracic wall moves outward and upward.
9. **(c)** Aerobic respiration involves the exchange of respiratory gases at two places in muticellular animals-one between the body surface and surrounding medium, the other between the individual cells and the extracellular fluid. Lungs are involved in the first step of exchange, but not the heart.
10. **(b)** The solubility of the gases as well as the thickness of the membranes involved in diffusion are important factors that affect the rate of diffusion. A gradient of partial pressure is present for oxygen from alveoli to blood and blood to tissue. Similarly, a gradient of CO_2 is present in the opposite direction i.e., from tissues to blood and blood to alveoli. The pO_2 in alveoli is higher (104 mm Hg) than that in deoxygenated blood in the capillaries arising from pulmonary arteries (95 mm Hg), therefore, oxygen diffuses from the alveoli to the blood. Similarly, the partial pressure of carbon dioxide (pCO_2) is higher in deoxygenated blood (45 mm Hg) than that in alveoli (40 mm Hg), therefore carbon dioxide passes from the blood to the alveoli. It is further dependent on the solubility of the diffusing

gases. As the solubility of CO_2 is 20-25 times higher than that of O_2, the amount of CO_2 that can diffuse through the diffusion membrane per unit difference in partial pressure is much higher compared to that of O_2. Therefore, all the factors in our body are favourable for diffusion of O_2 from alveoli to tissues and that of CO_2 from tissues to alveoli.

Alveolus is the primary site of exchange as it has an extensive network of blood capillaries and consists of squamous epithelium. Due to very intimate conact of blood capillaries with the alveoli, the exchange of gases takes place easily.

11. **(a)** The cartilage rings are present in the trachea to prevent it from collapsing. This enables the lumen of trachea to stay open during breathing.
12. **(d)** Pneumotaxic centre in the pons region of the brain can moderate functions of the respiratory rhythm centre. Neural signals from this centre can reduce the duration of inspiration and thereby alter the respiratory rate. A chemosensitive area is situated adjacent to the rhythm centre to make necessary adjustments in the respiratory process. Receptors associated with aortic arch and carotid artery also can recognize changes in CO_2 and H^+ concentration and send necessary signals to the rhythm centre for remedial actions. The role of oxygen in the regulation of respiratory rhythm is quite insignificant.
13. **(c)** In the walls of bronchi and bronchioles stretch receptors are located and are stimulated by overstretching of the lungs. Nerve impulses are sent along the vagus nerve to inhibit the inspiratory area. The result is that expiration begins. Therefore, it is mainly a protective mechanism for preventing excessive inflation of the lungs.
14. **(c)** The lungs are situated in the thoracic chamber which is anatomically an air-tight chamber. The thoracic chamber is formed dorsally by the vertebral column, ventrally by the sternum, laterally by the ribs and on the lower side by the dome-shaped diaphragm. The anatomical setup of lungs in thorax is such that any change in the volume of the thoracic cavity will be reflected in the lung (pulmonary) cavity. Such an arrangement is essential for breathing, as we cannot directly alter the pulmonary volume.
15. **(d)** Inside the larynx are present two pairs of vocal cords. One pair is of false vocal cords which has little to do with sound production and the second inner pair is true vocal cords. When air is forced through the larynx, it causes vibration of the true vocal cords and sound is produced. The pitch of sound is determined by the tension on the vocal cords-the greater the tension, the higher the pitch.
16. **(a)** During inspiration (breathing in) the pressure of air falls in the thorax because of increase in its volume which is brought about by the contraction of diaphragm and inspiratory muscles. Since lungs are situated in the thorax, therefore a fall of pressure in thorax also lowers the pressure inside lungs, due to which air from outside rushes into the lungs through nostrils, trachea and bronchi.
17. **(b)** If a person first inspires with his maximum effort and then expires also with maximum effort the volume of air breathed out is called the vital capacity. An athlete requires more oxygen during exercise on a regular basis. This gradual effort of an athlete to meet his oxygen demand ultimately increases the vital capacity.
18. **(c)** In forceful expiration requiring effort, a different group of intercostal and some abdominal muscles contract to reduce the volume of thorax more than that in ordinary respiration. So, a larger volume of air is breathed out, such muscles are called expiratory muscles.
19. **(a)** Histamine is a derivative of the amino acid histidine produced by damaged cells of vertebrates. When released, it has the effect of dilating capillaries and lowering blood pressure. Histamine is involved in allergic and inflammatory reactions.
20. **(b)** Blood is colourless in insects. Insects have tracheal respiration. It is carried on by an extensive system of inter-communicating tubes called tratrachea.
21. **(a)** Bohr's effect is the effect of CO_2 on oxyhaemoglobin. Body tissues obtain oxygen from oxyhaemoglobin because of its dissociation caused by low O_2 and high CO_2 concentration. The increased CO_2 concentration reduces the affinity of haemoglobin for oxygen.

22. (c) The movement of air into and out of the lungs is carried out by creating a pressure gradient between the lungs and the atmosphere. Inspiration occurs when the pressure within the lungs (intra-pulmonary pressure) is less than the atmospheric pressure, i.e., there is a negative pressure in the lungs with respect to atmospheric pressure. Inspiration is initiated by the contraction of diaphragm which increases the volume of thoracic chamber in the antero-posterior axis. The contraction of external intercostal muscles lifts up the ribs and the sternum causing an increase in the volume of the thoracic chamber in the dorso-ventral axis. The overall increase in the thoracic volume causes a similar increase in pulmonary volume. This increase in pulmonary volume decreases the intra-pulmonary pressure, which becomes less than the atmospheric pressure forcing the air from outside to move into the lungs.

23. (a) Pneumotaxic centre in the pons region of the brain can moderate functions of the respiratory rhythm centre. Neural signals from this centre can reduce the duration of inspiration and therby alter the respiratory rate. A chemosensitive area is situated adjacent to the rhythm centre to make necessary adjustments in the respiratory process. Receptors associated with aortic arch and carotid artery also can recognize changes in CO_2 and H^+ concentration and send necessary signals to the rhythm centre for remedial actions. The role of oxygen in the regulation of respiratory rhythm is quite insignificant.

24. (c) RBCs contain a very high concentration of carbonic anhydrase enzyme which facilitates the following reaction in both directions.

$$CO_2 + H_2O \underset{}{\overset{\text{Carbonic anhydrase}}{\rightleftharpoons}} H_2CO_3 \underset{}{\overset{\text{Carbonic anhydrase}}{\rightleftharpoons}} HCO^-_3 + H^+$$

At the tissue site where partial pressure of CO_2 is high due to catabolism, CO_2 diffuses into blood (RBCs and plasma) and forms HCO_3^- and H^+. At the alveolar site where pCO_2 is low, the reaction proceeds in the opposite direction leading to the formation of CO_2 and H_2O.

25. (b) Chloride shift is the movement of chloride ions (Cl^-) into red blood cells. Carbon dioxide reacts with water to form carbonic acid in the red blood cells. The carbonic acid then dissociates into hydrogen carbonate ions (HCO_3^-) and hydrogen ions (H^+). The plasma membrane is relatively permeable to negative ions. Therefore, the hydrogen carbonate ions diffuse out of the cell into the plasma, leaving the hydrogen ions, which create a net positive charge; this is neutralized by the diffusion of chloride ions from the plasma into the cell.

26. (a) Carbonic anhydrase enzyme found in R.B.Cs catalyzes the interconversion of CO_2 and H_2CO_3. It plays an important role in respiration by influencing CO_2 transport in the blood.

27. (a) When a person living on plains ascend and stays on a mountain above 8000 feet from the sea level, he develops symptoms of mountain sickness which includes breathlessness, headache, dizziness, irritability, nausea, vomiting, mental fatigue and a bluish ting on the skin, nails and lips. The rise in altitude, consequently lowers the partial pressure of oxygen. This lowers the alveolar partial pressure of oxygen causes reduction in the diffusion of oxygen from the alveolar air to the blood. so oxygenation of blood is decreased progressively, which produces the symptoms of mountain sickness, Emphysema.

28. (b) The world health organization (WHO) reported China as the origin place of SARS. Several other countries have reported SARS cases after travel to China and its nearby areas/countries in Asia or close contact with a person affected with SARS. Microbiologists of Hongkong Central University initially detected a virus corona virus as causative agent of SARS. It is very known fact that the China is the most populated country. This fact cannot be correlated with SARS

29. (b) The skin problem could be due to pollen allergy and respiratory problem could be due to the decrease in oxygen content, since the atmosphere becomes thin as one goes up the hill.

Chapter

18

Body Fluids and Circulation

Directions: In the following questions, a statement of assertion is followed by a statement of reason. Mark the correct choice as:

(a) If both Assertion and Reason are true and Reason is the correct explanation of Assertion.

(b) If both Assertion and Reason are true but Reason is not the correct explanation of Assertion.

(c) If Assertion is true but Reason is false.

(d) If both Assertion and Reason are false.

1. **Assertion :** WBCs accumulate at the site of wounds by diapedesis.
Reason : It is the sqeezing of leucocytes from the endothelium. **[AIIMS 2002]**

2. **Assertion:** In most of the mammal RBCs are devoid of nucleus.
Reason: Red colour is filled in the entire cytoplasm of RBCs, iron containing complex protein called haemoglobin.

3. **Assertion:** In lymphatic system, lymph is known as tissue fluid.
Reason: It comprises of plasma proteins, RBCs and WBCs.

4. **Assertion:** Type 'O' blood group individuals are called 'universal donors'.
Reason: RBCs of 'O' blood group consists both 'A' and 'B' surface antigens.

5. **Assertion (A)** : Blood coagulates in uninjured blood vessels.
Reason (R) : Uninjured blood vessels release an anticoagulant heparin. **[AIIMS 2007]**

6. **Assertion:** Fibrins are produced by the conversion of inactive fibrinogens in the plasma, in the presence of enzyme thrombin.
Reason: Plasma without fibrinogen and blood corpuscles is called serum.

7. **Assertion:** The clotting process can occur in the absence of all cellular elements except platelets.
Reason: Activated platelets release vitamin K.

8. **Assertion :** Prothrombinase enzyme act as antiheparin.
Reason : Heparin prevent coagulation of blood in blood vessels. **[AIIMS 2010]**

9. **Assertion :** Blood is coloured in the insects.
Reason : Insect blood has no role in O_2 transport. **[AIIMS 2012, 2013]**

10. **Assertion :** When there is a fall in the blood pressure due to loss of blood volume, this is compensated by vasoconstriction of veins.
Reason : Veins hold the extra amount of blood which can be shifted to the arteries as required. **[AIIMS 2010, 2015]**

11. **Assertion:** Sympathetic nerves can increase the strength of ventricular contraction neural signals.
Reason: To increase the cardiac output parasympathetic neural signals synergistically act with sympathetic neural signal.

12. **Assertion:** Open circulatory system is more efficient than closed circulatory system.
Reason: In closed circulatory system rather than in open circulatory system, the blood flow is slow.

13. **Assertion:** In amphibians and reptiles, double circulation is incomplete.
Reason: Unlike in birds and mammals, in amphibian and reptiles, the left atrium receives oxygenated blood and right atrium receives deoxygenated blood.

14. **Assertion:** Left atrium possesses the thickest muscles.
Reason: Left atrium receives blood from the lungs.

15. **Assertion:** In the human heart, there is no mixing of oxygenated and deoxygenated blood.
Reason: Presence of valves in the heart allows the movement of blood in one direction only.

16. Assertion: Atria act as primer pumps that increase the ventricular pumping.
Reason: Through the atria about 80 percent of the blood flows directly into ventricles.

17. Assertion : Heart of fish contains only deoxygenated blood.
Reason : Oxygenated blood does not return back to the heart in fishes.

18. Assertion : Closed circulatory system is more effective than open type.
Reason : The closed circulatory system considerably enhances the speed, precision and efficiency of circulation.

19. Assertion : Heart valves resemble swing doors in action.
Reason : Valves are present in the heart chamber, at the opening of the heart into large arteries and veins.

20. Assertion : Blood pressure is arterial blood pressure.
Reason : It is measured by sphygmomanometer. **[AIIMS 2010]**

21. Assertion : The muscle fibres of SA node possess the muscle fibres.
Reason : Due to this fact, it can initiate excitory waves at the highest rate

22. Assertion : Blood pressure is arterial blood pressure.
Reason : Blood pressure is measured by sphygmomanometer. **[AIIMS 2000]**

23. Assertion : Smaller the organism higher is the rate of metabolism per gram weight.
Reason : The heart rate of a six month old baby is much higher than that of an old person. **[AIIMS 2007]**

24. Assertion: Sino-atrial node (SAN) is also known as the pacemaker.
Reason: The maximum number of action potentials is generated by SAN and is responsible to initiate and maintain the rhythmic contractions of the heart.

25. Assertion: The cardiac output of an athlete man and of an ordinary is the same.
Reason: It is impossible to alter the stroke volume as well as heart rate.

26. Assertion: When a person is performing normal work. On an average, his heart beat is 72-75 heart beats per minute.
Reason: One heart beat is completed in 0.8 second.

27. Assertion: At a very slow velocity, blood flows in the lacunae and sinuses of prawn.
Resaon: This occurs because of the absence of heart in the prawn.

28. Assertion: The enlarged Q and R waves indicate myocardial infarction.
Reason: In the normal recording of ECG, any deviation indicates possible abnormality or disease.

29. Assertion : Lub is a heart sound which is produced during each cardiac cycle.
Reason : It is associated with the closure of the tricuspid and bicuspid valves. **[AIIMS 2016]**

30. Assertion : Electrocardiogram is record or electrical activity of the heart which shows certain waves called P, Q, R, S and T waves.
Reason : It gives important information concerning the spread of excitation to the different parts of heart and it is of value in the diagnosis of cases of abnormal cardiac rhythm and myocardial damage.

31. Assertion : EEG is of immense diagnostic value in the cardiac diseases.
Reason : Defects in cardiac functions can be reflected in changes in the pattern of electrical potentials recorded in the EEG.

32. Assertion : Persons suffering from haemophilia fail to produce blood clotting factor VIII.
Reason : Prothrombin producing platelets in such persons are found in very low concentration.

33. Assertion : The increased permeability of the lymph capillaries is easily altered.
Reason : The increased permeability of the capillary walls leads to oedema or swelling.

34. Assertion : An artificial pacemaker can replace the sinoatrial node of heart.
Reason : This is because, an artificial pacemaker is capable of stimulating the heart electrically to maintain its beats.

35. Assertion : Atherosclerosis is a disease charaterized by the thickening of arterial walls.
Reason : Deposition of cholesterol and triglycerides in the arterial walls causes atherosclerosis.

36. Assertion : Saline water is not given to patients of hypertension.
Reason : Saline water can cause vomiting and may drop blood pressure suddenly causing cardiac arrest.

Solutions

1. **(b)** During wound, germs are removed by the process of phagocytosis by WBC. WBCs accumulate at the site of wound by diapedesis. It is the squeezing of leucocytes out from the endothelium of capillaries to fight against foreign agent.

2. **(b)** Matured mammalian RBCs lacks cell organelles including nucleus, mitochondria, ribosomes, centrioles and endoplasmic reticulum. It increases the surface area of RBCs and enables them to contain more haemoglobin. Thus, almost entire cytoplasm is filled with haemoglobin.

3. **(c)** Lymphatic system comprises of lymph, lymphatic capillaries, lymphatic vessels, lymphatic nodes and lymphatic ducts. Lymph is a transparent fluid derived from blood and other tissues, that accumulates in the interstitial spaces as the interstitial fluid. It also contains leucocytes, mainly the lymphocytes. This fluid has a composition similar to that of plasma, except that it is low in proteins.

4. **(c)** If a blood transfusion is made between an incompatible donor and recipient, reaction of antigens on the cells and antibodies in the plasma will produce clots that will clog the capillaries. Type O blood group individuals are without A and B antigens on their RBCs, but consists antibodies for both these antigens in their plasma. Hence, these persons can donate blood to anyone. O blood group is the most important blood group for transfusion.

5. **(d)** When an injury is caused to a blood vessel, bleeding starts which is stopped by blood clotting. At the site of injury blood platelets release platelet factor - 3 and injured tissues release thromboplastin. The two combine to form prothrombinase enzyme which converts prothrombin to thrombin. The latter stimulates formation of fibrin thread or clot. Blood contains an anticoagutant heparin which prevents blood clotting in uninjured vessels.

6. **(c)** A coagulam is mainly formed of a network of threads called fibrins in which dead and damaged formed elements of blood are trapped. Fibrins are produced by the conversion of inactive fibrinogens in the plasma by the enzyme thrombin. Thrombins, in turn are formed from another inactive substance present in the plasma called prothrombin. An enzyme complex, prothrombinase, is required for the above reaction.

   The clot seals the wound and stops bleeding. After its formation, clot starts contracting and a pale yellow fluid, the serum, oozes out. This serum is blood plasma minus fibrinogen and blood corpuscles.

7. **(c)** Activated platelets are essential for blood clotting because several of the cascade reactions occurs on the surface of platelets. When an injury is caused, the blood platelets release certain chemicals that are called platelet factors (e.g., thromboplastin). These factors combine in presence of calcium ions (Ca^{2+}) and form prothrombinase which in turn catalyze the formation of thrombin from prothrombin. Thrombin acts as an enzyme, which helps in the formation of fibrin molecules. Fibrin is an essential component of blood clotting. Vitamin K is essential for production of prothrombin. Prothrombin and many plasma clotting factors are produced in the liver. The liver requires vitamin K to produce prothrombin and several other clotting factors.

8. **(b)** Prothrombinase enzyme is necessary for blood clotting. It acts as antiheparin. Coagulation of blood in vessels is prevented by heparin, a quick acting anticoagulant. It inhibits conversion of prothrombin to thrombin and is used in open-heart surgery.

9. **(b)** Insect blood is colourless and does not play any role in transport of oxygen. Insects have tracheal respiration.

10. (a) When the blood pressure of an individual decreases due to loss of blood volume, then vasoconstriction of veins occurs. This shifts the little amount of blood from veins to arteries.

11. (c) Through the sympathetic nerves (part of ANS) neural signals can increase the rate of heart beat, the strength of ventricular contraction and thereby the cardiac output. On the other hand, parasympathetic neural signals (another component of ANS) decrease the rate of heart beat, speed of conduction of action potential and thereby the cardiac output.

12. (d) The closed circulatory system is more efficient than the open circulatory system because in open circulatory system, open spaces and channels the blood flows through whereas in closed circulatory system, the blood flows through proper blood vessels. Also, in closed circulatory system arterial musculature and precapillary sphincters regulate the flow of blood, due to the volume of blood flowing through a tissue or an organ may be regulated according to needs. Moreover in closed circulatory system, the blood flows far more rapidly in closed blood vesssels than in wide open channels and body cavities. Thus, blood takes much shorter time to circulate through the closed system than in open circulatory system.

13. (c) Amphibians and the reptiles (except crocodiles) consists a 3-chambered heart with two atria and a single ventricle, whereas crocodiles, birds and mammals possess a 4-chambered heart with two atria and two ventricles. In amphibians and reptiles, the left atrium receives oxygenated blood from the gills/lungs/skin and the right atrium gets the deoxygenated blood from other body parts. However, they get mixed up in the single ventricle that pumps out mixed blood (incomplete double circulation). In birds and mammals, oxygenated and deoxygenated blood received by the left and right atria respectively passes on the ventricles of the same sides. The ventricles pump it out without any mixing up, i.e., two separate circulatory pathways are present in these organisms, hence, these animals have double circulation.

14. (d) Left ventricle has thickest muscles because it pumps the blood to the whole body.

15. (b) In the human heart, there is no mixing of deoxygenated and oxygenated blood due to the presence of inter - atrial and inter - ventricular septum. These septa completely divide the atria and ventricles into right and left and thus avoid mixing of blood. The presence of valves that prevents the backflow of the blood. The two atria are separated from the ventricles by membranous valves. The valve separating the right atrium from the right ventricle is known as the right atrioventricular valve or tricuspid valve (as it is made of three flaps or cusps). The valve separating the left atria and the left ventricle is called left atrioventricular valve or the bicuspid valve or the mitral valve (since it is made of two flaps). They allow the flow of blood from atria to ventricles and not in the backward direction. At the base of the aorta are present three membranous, pocket-shaped semilunar valves. These valves check the return of the blood to the ventricle.

16. (a) From the great veins into the atria; blood normally flows continuously about 80 per cent of the blood flows directly through the atria into the ventricles, even before the atria contract. Then, atrial contraction usually leads to an additional 20 per cent filling of the ventricles. Therefore, the atria simply functions as primer pumps that increase the ventricular pumping effectiveness as much as 20 per cent.

17. (a) The heart is a pumping organ for blood circulation which consists of chambers communicating with each other. In fishes the heart is two-chambered, consisting of an auricle and a ventricle. An accessory chamber called sinus venosus is also present which serves as a reservoir and opens anteriorly into auricle through the sino - atrial aperture. Fish heart contains and pumps only deoxygenated blood

because after getting oxygenated from gills, the blood doesn't return back to the heart. Instead, it is supplied directly to the various parts of the body.

18. (a) There are some reasons behind the effectiveness of closed circulatory system over the open type. These are -

(i) The blood flows more rapidly in closed blood cavities

(ii) It takes much shorter time to circulate through the closed system and return to the heart.

(iii) This quickens the supply and removal of materials to and from the tissues by the blood.

(iv) In the closed system, the arteriolar diameter can be regulated to alter the blood flow, so the volume of blood flowing through a tissue or organ may be regulated according to its needs. No such regulation is possible in open type.

19. (b) The valve present in heart when pushed by blood in the right direction causes the flaps of the valve to swing apart and allow the blood to flow through, but when pushed in the opposite direction, the flaps close sharply to block the passage through the valve. Thus these valves resemble swing doors in action. Hence, the valves of the heart maintain unidirectional flow of blood and prevent it's regurgitation in the opposite direction.

20. (b) Blood pressure is the arterial blood pressure taken in left brachial artery and the instrument used to measure blood pressure is sphygmomanometer.

21. (d) SA node and AV node are the contraction node. SA node possess the highest rhythmicity among all cardiac muscle fibres and can initiate excitory wave at highest rate.

22. (b) Blood pressure is the arterial pressure of blood exerted on the wall of arteries with each heart beat. It is measured from the brachial artery in the elbow pit. It is expressed as

$$= \frac{\text{systolic pressure (mm/Hg)}}{\text{diastolic pressure (mm/Hg)}}$$

Arterial (superficial; arteries) blood pressure is measured by sphygmomanometer.

23. (b) The basal metabol rate is defined as the energy requirement of human body at rest. BMR of smallest animals are generally higher then larger animals. Peoples with higher metabolism means that they have higher heart rate. Heart rate of baby is 70-190 times/minute, whereas adults (including serious) is 60-100 times/ minute.

24. (a) In the myogenic heart, contraction is initiated by specialized muscles. The SAN can generate the maximum number of action potentials, i.e., 70-75 min^{-1}, and is responsible for initiating and maintaining the rhythmic contractile activity of the heart. Therefore, it is called the pacemaker. The SAN controls the heart beat because its rate of rhythmical discharge is faster than that of any other part of the heart. Therefore, the SAN is virtually always the pacemaker of the normal heart.

25. (d) The stroke volume multiplied by the heart rate (no. of beats per min.) gives the cardiac output. Therefore, the volume of blood pumeped out by each ventricle per minte and averages 5000 mL or 5 litres in a healthy individual is called cardiac output. The body has the ability to alter the stroke volume as well as the heart rate and thereby the cardiac output. For example, the cardiac output of an athlete will be much higher than that of an ordinary man.

26. (a) One heart beat completes in 0.8 – 0.83 second. therefore, there are 60/0.8 or 60/ 0.83, i.e., 72 – 75 heart beats per minute on an average when a person is performing normal work.

27. (c) Lacunae and sinuses are the open spaces and channels that are present in the tissues of prawn. Prawn possesses a heart which pumps the oxygenated blood into some arteries, which directly open into the lacunae and sinuses. The tissues are thus in direct contact with blood. A sufficiently high blood pressure, however, cannot be maintained in the open lacunae and sinuses inspite of the pumping action of the heart. So, blood flows at a very slow velocity in the lacunae and sinuses.

28. (a) A normal electrocardiogram (ECG) is consists of P wave, a QRS wave (complex) and a T wave. The ECGs obtained from different individuals have roughly the same shape and any deviation from this shape shows a possible abnormality or disease. For example, the enlarged Q and R waves indicate a myocardial infarction, enlargement of the P wave shows enlargement of the atria. T wave is flat when the heart muscles receive insufficient oxygen as in atherosclerotic heart disease.

29. (b) Lub and dub are two heart sounds, which occur due to the closure of cuspid valves and semilunar valves respectively. Lub is the first heart sound which is formed due to closure of atrioventricular valves at the beginning of ventricular systole. It is low pitched of long duration (0.15 sec).

30. (a) ECG consists of P-wave, QRS wave and T-wave. ECG gives important information concerning the spread of excitation to the different parts of heart and in the diagnosis of abnormal cardiac rhythm and myocardial damage.

31. (d) EEG is an index of the brain functions. EEG or electroencephalogram represents the spontaneous electrical activity of the brain as recorded from the electrodes placed on the scalp. EEG wave pattern obtained shows certain characterstic feature of the brain like the frequency amplitude of the signals of brain. Thus, any deviation from the normal caused either due to brain disease or change in the physiological state of the brain can be easily detected by EEG.

32. (a) Haemophilia is caused by lack of activity of blood clotting factor VIII or IX and they show platelet function disorder.

33. (b) The permeability of the lymph capillaries is easily altered. It may be explained by giving examples. For instance, in an infected wound, bacteria release chemicals which increase the permeability of the capillaries in the region, resulting in a local swelling. A swelling appears even in an uninfected injury because an injured tissue can somehow affect capillary permeability. The high permeability makes the lymph capillaries most likely route for the spread of microorganisms and cancer cells in the body.

34. (a) An artificial pacemaker is a therapeutic instrument which is implanted in the heart of patients to generate the heart beat. A pacemaker is used when the normal heart rate of 72-80 drops down to abnormally low levels like 30-40 due to diseases or operations and threatens the life of the patient. Sometime, the SA node may become damaged or defective. It then fails to generate cardiac impulses at the normal rate. The heart beats become abnormally slow and irregular, and ventricles fail to pump the required amount of blood. This is remedied by the surgical grafting of artificial pacemaker instrument in the chest of the patient. The artificial pacemaker stimulates the heart electrically at regular intervals to maintain its beats. Thus it replaces the SA node as the originator of the cardiac impulse.

35. (a) Atherosclerosis refers to the deposition of fatty substances specially cholesterol and triglycerides in the tunica of internal and smooth muscles of medium sized and large arteries. Such a deposition is called atherosclerotic or atheromatous plaque. Gradually these plaques grow. As a result, the lumen of the artery decreases and the flow of the blood is reduced.

36. (c) Saline water is not given to a patient of hypertension because it may cause rise in the blood pressure which may be fatal to patient.

Chapter 19

Excretory Products and their Elimination

Directions: In the following questions, a statement of assertion is followed by a statement of reason. Mark the correct choice as:
(a) If both Assertion and Reason are true and Reason is the correct explanation of Assertion.
(b) If both Assertion and Reason are true but Reason is not the correct explanation of Assertion.
(c) If Assertion is true but Reason is false.
(d) If both Assertion and Reason are false.

1. **Assertion :** Aquatic mammals like whales and seals are said to be ureotelic animals.
Reason : It is because of the fact that their main nitrogenous waste product is urea.
2. **Assertion:** Sharks are said to be ammonotelic animals.
Reason: Sharks have a ability to retain considerable amounts of ammonia in vertebrates.
3. **Assertion:** Ammonia should be removed from the body as rapidly as it is formed.
Reason: In water, ammonia is insoluble.
4. **Assertion:** Both ammonia and urea are excreted by earthworms.
Reason: Excretion in earthworm depends on the environment.
5. **Assertion:** In birds and reptiles, main excretory product is the combined form of urine and faeces.
Reason: Birds and reptiles consists no separate chamber for excretion of urine and faeces.
6. **Assertion:** Comparative to uric acid, urea is a more toxic excretory substance.
Reason: Birds and insects are uricotelic animals.
7. **Assertion:** The primary excretory organ in vertebrates is referred to as liver.
Reason: Liver helps kidneys urine secretion.
8. **Assertion :** Urinary bladder and ureters are lined by transitional epithelium.
Reason : Ureters carry the urine to urinary bladder where it is stored temporarily.
9. **Assertion :** In vertebrates, the liver is also referred as an accessory excretory organ.
Reason : Liver helps kidneys in the secretion of urine.
10. **Assertion :** If human urine is allowed to stand for some time, it smells strongly of ammonia.
Reason : Main constituent of human urine is ammonia. **[AIIMS 2013]**
11. **Assertion :** Kidneys maintain the osmotic concentration of the blood.
Reason : Kidneys eliminate either hypotonic or hypertonic urine according to the need of the body.
12. **Assertion :** During physiology of excretion, deamination does not take place in liver.
Reason : Deamination is a process to make use of excess of amino acids which cannot be incorporated into protoplasm. **[AIIMS 2001]**
13. **Assertion:** According to their relative position in the cortex, nephrons are of two types cortical and juxtamedullary.
Reason: Juxtamedullary nephrons have short loop of Henle whereas cortical nephrons have long loop of Henle.
14. **Assertion:** In cortical nephrons, vasa recta is absent or highly reduced.
Reason: Cortical nephrons are mainly concerned with concentration of urine.
15. **Assertion:** Homeostasis is a process of maintaining a constant internal environment.
Reason: Kidneys are excretory and homeostatic organs.
16. **Assertion:** Nephron is the functional unit of excretory organs of lobsters.
Reason: The filtration of blood takes place in the malpighian body (the glomerulus and Bowman's capsule).
17. **Assertion :** Renal threshold of glucose is said to be 180 mg per 100 ml.
Reason : Glucose starts appearing in the urine when its blood level exceed 180 mg per 100 ml of blood.
18. **Assertion :** Kidneys maintain the osmotic concentration of the blood.
Reason : Kidneys eliminate either hypotonic or hypertonic urine according to the need of the body.

19. **Assertion :** In the descending limb of loop of Henle, the urine is hypertonic, while in ascending limb of loop of Henle, the urine is hypotonic.
Reason : Descending limb is impermeable to Na^+, while ascending limb is impermeable to H_2O.
20. **Assertion :** The glomerular filtrate resembles the protein free plasma in composition and osmotic pressure.
Reason : The glomerular capillary wall and inner membrane of Bowman's capsule are impermeable to large molecules.
21. **Assertion :** Secreting hypotonic urine is effective in reducing urinary loss of water.
Reason : Hypotonic urine is more concentrated and higher in osmotic pressure than the blood.
22. **Assertion :** Ultrafiltration takes place in presence of effective filtration pressure.
Reason : In ultrafiltration process, blood is filtered in Bowman's capsule, filtered fluid contain protein & blood corpuscles also. **[AIIMS 2010]**
23. **Assertion:** Tubular secretion takes part in the removal of foreign bodies, ions and molecules from the body.
Reason: As much as 99 percent of the material in the filtrate is reabsorbed from the body due to tubular secretion.
24. **Assertion:** In producing a concentrated urine the Henle's loop and vasa recta play a significant role.
Reason: Henle's loop and vasa recta helps in the counter current arrangement.
25. **Assertion:** Glomerular filtration needs expenditure of energy by kidney.
Reason: Glomerular filtration takes place because pressure in the Bowman's capsule is higher than the pressure in glomerular capillaries.
26. **Assertion:** The pH and ionic balance of blood is maintained by DCT and collecting duct.
Reason: DCTs of many nephrons open into a collecting duct.
27. **Assertion:** For the regulation of glomerular filtration rate (GFR), the kidneys have built in mechanisms.
Reason: ANF mechanism is one such efficient mechanism.
28. **Assertion:** Deamination take place in liver cells, during the physiology of excretion.
Reason: Deamination is a process to make use of excess of amino acids that cannot be incorporated into the protoplasm.
29. **Assertion:** For long periods, camel can go without water.
Reason: Camels stores water in the pouches of their rumen and fat in their hump.
30. **Assertion:** Mammals, living in deserts contain more concentrated urine.
Reason: They consists very long loop of Henle in their nephrones.
31. **Assertion (A) :** When the urine moves through the descending limb, it become hypertonic and as it passes through the ascending limb of Henle's loop it becomes hypotonic.
Reason (R) : The descending limb is permeable to sodium ions, while the ascending limb is impermeable to sodium ions.
32. **Assertion :** Hemodialysis can save and prolong the life of uremic patients.
Reason : Waste products like urea can be removed from the blood by the process of hemodialysis.
33. **Assertion :** Aldosterone is a steroid hormone and is important in the control of sodium and potassium ion concentration in mammals.
Reason : It upgrades sodium ion concentration in the ECF by promoting reabsorption of sodium ions from renal tubules and excretion of potassium ions in urine. **[AIIMS 2007]**
34. **Assertion:** Renin secretion stimulation will increase the volume of the extracellular fluid (ECF).
Reason: The increase in ECF occurs due to decreased active reabsorption of Na^+.
35. **Assertion:** The amount of water in the urine is controlled by antidiuretic hormone (ADH).
Reason: ADH determines the permeability of the collecting duct to water.
36. **Assertion:** Angiotensin II increases the glomerular blood pressure thereby GFR.
Reason: To release renin, angiotensin II activates the JG cells.
37. **Assertion :** During micturition, urine is prevented from flowing back into the ureters.
Reason : Urethral sphincters relax during micturition.
38. **Assertion:** Diabetes insipidus is featured by excessive urination and too much thirst of water.
Reason: The posterior lobe of pituitary gland secretes anti-diuretic hormone (ADH).
39. **Assertion:** Phenylketonuria is a recessive hereditary disease which is caused by the body's failure to oxidize an amino acid phenylalanine to tyrosine, due to defective enzyme.
Reason: It results in the presence of phenylalanine acid in the urine.
40. **Assertion:** Vasopressin increases the water permeability of distal convoluted tubule.
Reason: In absence of ADH, water re-absorption is considerably reduced.

Solutions

1. (a) Ureotelism is defined as the urinary elimination of nitrogen mainly as urea. Aquatic mammals like whales and seals are said to be ureotelic animals because their major nitrogenous waste product is urea. As a matter of fact, ammonia is the basic nitrogenous catabolite of protein but since ammonia is highly toxic to the animals, therefore, its concentration must be kept very low in the blood.

2. (d) Sharks are ureotelic, they are not ammonotelic animals. Ureotelic animals excrete urea instead of ammonia as the major nitrogenous waste product. These include man and all other mammals, terrestrial and semi-aquatic amphibians such as toads and frogs, cartilaginous fishes (elasmobranchs) such as sharks and sting rays. Sharks need to avoid water loss from body, thus they cannot excrete ammonia, as it requires enough water to be eliminated. In order to retain so much urea in their blood, their blood osmotic pressure approaches that of sea water. This minimises water loss from their body to adjust to the concentrated saline water of the sea.

3. (c) Ammonia is a type of the basic nitrogenous catabolite of proteins, that is highly soluble in water and highly toxic to the animal. Therefore, its concentration must be kept very low in the blood. Due to this ammonia should be removed as rapidly from the body as it is formed. A large volume of water is required by the animals to dissolve ammonia and remove it from the body. So, its elimination in urine involves considerable loss of water from the body.

4. (a) When sufficient water is available, earthworms excrete ammonia. Because a large volume of water is needed by the animal to dissolve ammonia and eliminate it from, the body. Whereas in drier environment the animal removes urea as it needs only considerable amount of water for the excretion of urea because urea is very soluble in water.

5. (a) In birds and reptiles, ureters and the rectum open into a common sac is known as the cloaca (as there is no chamber for urine and faces) for these two that stores both, and reabsorbs water from them and ultimately excretes these white and brownish black material along with aqueous fluid.

6. (b) Urea is more toxic than uric acid and less toxic to ammonia.
Ammonia > Urea > Uric acid
Urea formation takes place in kidneys.

7. (d) In vertebrates, accessory excretory organs are the lungs, liver and skin are referred as because besides the urinary system, these organs also participate in the removal of waste products from the body. The liver helps in the excretion of cholesterol, bile pigments (bilirubin and biliverdin), inactivated products of steroid hormones, some vitamins and many drugs. These are carried by the bile to the intestine and are eliminated with the faeces. It has no role in urine secretion.

8. (b) Urinary bladder and ureters of excretory system are lined by transitional epithelium because it is a stretchable epithelium, hence the urinary bladder and ureters may be considerably stretched without getting torn when they are filled with urine. Ureters are thin muscular tubes which emerge from the hilum of each kidney. Urine enters the ureters from the renal pelvis and is conducted along the ureters by peristaltic waves on their walls. Ureters from both the kidneys finally open into urinary bladder which is a hollow muscular sac. In this way urine from both the kidneys is drained into the urinary bladder which stores it temporarily.

9. (c) In vertebrates, the lungs, liver & skin are referred as accessory excretory organs because besides the urinary system these

organs also participate in the removal of waste products from the body. The liver is the principal organ for the excretion of cholesterol, bile pigments (bilirubin and biliverdin) and inactivated products of steroid hormones, some vitamins and many drugs. It secretes these substances in the bile and indirectly helps by formation of urea through amino acids in ornithine cycle. They are carried by the bile to the intestine and are ultimately eliminated with the faeces. It has no role in secretion of urine.

10. (c) Urea is the chief nitrogenous constituent of human urine, though it possesses small amount of ammonia. But when the urine is allowed to stand for sometime, bacterial degradation occurs and it leads to the production of ammonia from urine, and thus smells strongly.

11. (a) Kidneys play an essential role in maintaining the concentration and osmotic pressure of blood. When water intake of an aminal is very high, the urine excreted has to be hypotonic i.e., dilute and lower in osmotic pressure than their blood in order to remove the excess of water contrary to this, when there is a threat of excessive water loss from the body; the urine needs to be hypertonic more concentrated and higher in osmotic pressure than their blood, to reduce the loss of water with urine. In this way, the osmotic concentration of the blood is maintained.

12. (d) Deamination is the process of converting amino acid to keto acid with the release of NH_3. It occurs in the liver.

13. (c) The nephrons are of two types on the basis of location. In majority of nephrons, the loop of Henle is too short, that extends only little into the medulla. These nephrons are called cortical nephrons and form 85% of the total nephrons. In some of the nephrons, the loop of Henle is very long and runs deep into the medulla. these nephrons are called juxtamedullary nephrons ehich form 15% of the total nephrons.

14. (c) Cortical nephrons are situated in the renal cortex and consists of short loop of Henle and no vasa recta. Hence, they are not involved in concentration of urine. They control plasma volume when water supply is normal.

15. (b) The term homeostasis (homeios same; stasis = standing) was introduced by Walter Cannon in 1932. It maintains the stability of the cell environment and this way provides the organism with a degree of independence of the environment; in order to achieve stability, mammals have two kidneys that perform excretory fuction and maintain urea level in blood.

16. (d) Nephron is the principal functional unit of the kidney of vertebrates. Its number reaches to one million in each kidney. Filtration of blood takes place in the Malpighian body, later is composed of a tuft of capillaries called the glomerulus, and is together with the cupped end of the renal tubules, is called Bowman's capsule.

17. (a) Renal thereshold of a substance is at its highest concentration in the blood, up to which it is totally reabsorbed from the glomerular filtrate. Renal threshold of glucose is about 180 mg per 100 ml. It is totally reabsored and does not appear in the urine so long as its blood level does not exceed 180 mg. But when its blood level exceeds 180 mg, some of the filtered glucose is left unabsorbed in the tubules and consequently appears in the urine. Some substances which are either totally reabsorbed actively or most of their amounts are reabsorbed actively are called high threshold substances. High threshold substances are excreted in the urine only when their blood concentration is considerably high, for example glucose and amino acids.

18. (a) Kidneys play an essential role in maintaining the concentration and osmotic pressure (osmoconcentration) of blood. When water intake of an animal is very high, the urine excreted has to be hypotonic i.e., dilute and lower in osmotic pressure than their blood in order to remove the excess of water. Contary to this, when there is a threat of excessive water loss from the body; the urine needs to be hypertonic more concentrated and higher in osmotic pressure than their blood, to reduce the loss of water with urine. In this way, the osmotic concentration of the blood is maintained.

19. (a) Descending limb is permeable to water but not to Na^+. Consequently water moves out into interstitium and concentration of Na^+ in tubular filtrate rises making the filtrate hypertonic. Ascending loop is impermeable to water but permeable to Na^+ and makes the filtrate hypotonic.

20. (a) Glomerular filtrate is the protein free fluid which is filtered from the blood of glomerular capilaries to the lumen of the Bowman's capsule. This process is called glomerular filtration. About one-fifth of the total volumne of plasma flowing through the kidneys is filtered out as the glomerular filtrate. The filtration occurs across the membrane made to the glomerular capillary wall and the inner memrane of the Bowman's capsule. The pores of this following membrane are impermeable to large molecules or particles. Large particles like blood cells and protein macromolecules do not normally enter into the glomerular filtrate. But smaller molecules like glucose, urea, creatinine, amino acids and mineral salts are filtered into the Bowman's capsule in concentrations more or less similar to their respective concentrations in the plasma. The filtrate therefore almost resembles the protein free plasma in composition and osmotic pressure.

21. (d) When there is a threat of excessive water loss from the body of the animal, then the urine excreted needs to be hypertonic and not hypotonic. Mammals and birds can excrete hypertonic urine which is more concentrated than their blood. Isotonic glomerular filtrate is first filtered into the Bowman's capsules of nephrons in kidney. The tublues of nephrons then reabsorb a large volume of water from the glomerular filtrate not accompained by the reabsorption of proportionate amounts of solutes. This leaves the urine more concentrated than the blood which in very effective in reducing the urinary loss of water.

22. (c) Ultrafiltration takes place in renal corpuscle of uriniferous tubule. It takes place in presence of effective filtration pressure. During the process, blood is filtered and contains only blood plasma – proteins. The filtered blood entering into Bowman's capsule is called glomerular filtrate.
Glomerular filtrate = Blood – (Blood corpuscles + plasma proteins)

23. (c) Such chemicals in the blood that are not removed by filtration from the glomerular capillaries are removed by a the process of urine formation called tubular secretion. These chemicals are removed from the blood by both passive and active transports in the peritubular capillaries to the nephron tubule.
The chemicals removed by tubular secretion include foreign bodies and ions and ions and molecules that are toxic at elevated levels.

24. (a) Mammals are able to produce concentrated urine. the Henle's loop and vasa recta play a significant role in this. In opposite directions filtrate flows in the two limbs of Henle's loop and thus forms a counter current. The flow of blood through the two limbs of vasa recta is also in a counter current pattern. The proximity between the Henle's loop and vasa recta, as well as the counter current in them helps in maintaining an increasing osmolarity towards the inner medullary interstitum, interstitial gradient present helps in an easy passage of water from the collecting tubule thereby concentrating the filtrate (urine). Human kidneys can produce urine nearly four times concentrated than the initial filtrate formed.

25. (d) Glomerular filtration occurs due to the pressure of the blood flowing in the glomerular capillaries is higher than the pressure of the filtrate in Bowman's capsule, In other words, blood pressure drives glomerular filtration, and because the process takes advantage of a pressure

gradient, glomerular filtration does not need the expenditure of energy by kidney cells.

26. **(b)** DCT has ability of reabsorption of HCO_3^- and selective secretion of hydrogen and potassium ions and NH_3 in order to maintain the pH and sodium-potassium balance in blood. Collecting ducts thus play an important role in the maintenance of pH and ionic balance of blood. DCTs of many nephrons open into a straight tube called collecting duct, many of which converge and open into renal pelvis through medullary pyramids in the calyces.

27. **(c)** For the regulation of glomerular filtration rate, the kidneys have built-in mechanisms. One such efficient mechanism is known as renin-angiotensin mechanism and is carried out by juxtaglomerular apparatus (JGA). JGA is a special sensitive region formed by cellular modifications in the distal convoluted tubule and the afferent arteriole at the location of their contact. A fall in GFR can stimulate the JG cells to release renin which can stimulate the glomerular blood flow and thereby the GFR back to normal. An increase in blood flow to the atria of the heart can cause the release of Atril Natriuretc Factor (ANF). This causes vasodilation (dilation of blood vessels) and thereby decrease the blood pressure. ANF mechanism, therefore, acts as a check on the renin-angiotensin mechanism.

28. **(b)** Deamination is a process to make use of excess of amino acid that cannot be incorporated into the protoplasm by elimination or protein or aminoacids or amino group from carboxyl group with the formation of ammonia and keto acid.

29. **(c)** For long periods, camels have the ability to withstand water deprivation. But they do not store any water in the pouches of their rumen. The fat of hump is not particularly useful as a source of water because respiration must be enhanced to oxidise fat to produce water and this enhances respiratory loss of moisture. They reduce urinary loss of water by secreting small volume of the urine much more hypertonic than the human urine. They lose far less water in the sweat, because they sweat only when their body temperature rises by as much as 60 °C. Moreover, compared to all other mammals. These factors are mainly responsible for the camel's ability to go without water for long periods.

30. **(a)** The functional unit of kidney is called as nephron. Latter contains a tubular region is present between proximal and distal convoluted tubule, the loop of Henle. The length of loop of Henle is proportional to the concentration of urine. The mammals (chordates) living in desert consists longer loop of Henle in their nephrons. So, these animals contain more concentrated urine.

31. **(a)** The descending limb of loop of Henle is permeable of water but almost impermeable to electrolytes. This concentrates the filtrate as it moves down. The ascending limb is impermeable to water but allows transport of electrolytes actively or passively. Therefore, as the concentrated filtrate passes upward, it gets diluted due to the passage of electrolytes to the medullary fluid.

32. **(a)** The blood urea level rises abnormally (uremia) in patients suffering from renal failures. In uremia patients, an artificial kidney is used for removing accumulated waste products like urea from the blood by a process called hemodialysis. In this way, hemodialysis saves and prolongs the life of many uremic patients.

33. **(a)** Aldosterone is one of the important mineralocorticoids in humans secreted by adrenal cortex. Its main function is to regulate sodium content of the body . It increases sodium ion concentration in the blood by absorbing sodium ions from renal tubules. Excessive production of aldosterone causes a disease aldosteronism. Its symptoms include high blood pressure, high blood volume.

34. **(c)** Renin is a type of proteolytic enzyme, that is secreted into the blood by juxtaglomerular cells of the kidney under the control of the sympathetic nervous system. The only known physiological effect of renin is to stimulate formation of angiotensin I from its plasma substrate, angiotensinogen. In turn, angiotensin I, appears to serve only a specific substrate for angiotensin converting enzyme (ACE), a peptidase that converts angiotensin I to angiotensin II. Angiotensin II, stimulates the secretion of aldosterone from the zona glomerulosa of the adrenal cortex. Aldosterone promotes reabsorption of Na^+ ions by epithelial cells of the collecting duct. Retaining Na^+ raises the osmotic pressure of blood and reduces water loss from the body. Hence, causing an increase in extracellular fluid (ECF) volume.

35. (a) Osmoreceptors in the body are activated by changes in blood volume, body fluid volume and ionic concentration. An excessive loss of fluid from the body can activate these receptors that stimulate the hypothalamus to release antidiuretic hormone (ADH) or vasopressin from the neurohypophysis. It facilitates water reabsorption from latter parts of the tubule, thereby preventing diuresis. An increase in body fluid volume can switch off the osmoreceptors and suppress the ADH release to complete the feedback.

36. (c) Angiotensin II acts as a powerful vasoconstricort, increases the glomerular blood pressure and thereby GFR. Angiotensin II also activates the adrenal cortex to release aldosterone. Aldosterone leads to reabsorption of Na^+ and water from the distal parts of the tubule. This also leads to an increase in blood pressure and GFR.

37. (b) The act of releasing the urine is called micturition. Besides functioning as a temporary reservoir of urine, the urinary bladder also evacuates the urine by the process of micturition at suitable intervals. When enough urine has accumulated in the bladder to distend the bladder and raise its pressure sufficiently, a spontaneous nervous activity (reflex) is initiated; this causes the smooth muscles on the bladder wall to contract and the urethral sphincters, which guard the urethra, to relax. Urine consequently flows from the bladder through the urethra to the exterior. But it is prevented from flowing back into the ureters, because the terminal part of each ureter passes obliquely through the bladder wall and is consequently closed due to compression by the contracting bladder muscles.

38. (b) Antidiuretic hormone (ADH) or vasopressin is secreted from posterior pituitary gland. It is stimulated in response to a fall in the water content of blood plasma, that leads to an increase in the permeability to water of the distal and collecting tubules of the nephron. Deficiency or hyposecretion of ADH results in diabetes insipidus. Diabetes insipidus is characterised by micturating dilute urine several times a day that results in excessive thirst (polydipsia) and dehydration.

39. (a) Phenylketonuria results when there is a deficiency of liver enzyme phenyl alanine hydroxylase that converts phenyl alanine into tyrosine. It results with a high level of phenyl alaine in blood, tissue fluids and urine.

40. (b) ADH is secreted by pituitary gland. It increases the water permeability of distal convoluted tubules and collecting tubules, hence, plays a significant role in water re-absorption. Its absence will reduce water reabsorption which may lead to water diuresis or diabetes insipidus.

Chapter 20

Locomotion and Movement

Directions: In the following questions, a statement of assertion is followed by a statement of reason. Mark the correct choice as:

(a) If both Assertion and Reason are true and Reason is the correct explanation of Assertion.

(b) If both Assertion and Reason are true but Reason is not the correct explanation of Assertion.

(c) If Assertion is true but Reason is false.

(d) If both Assertion and Reason are false.

1. **Assertion :** There are similarities between the locomotion of unicellular organisms and multicellular animals.

   Reason : Ciliary, flagellar and amoeboid movements occur in unicellular organisms.

2. **Assertion:** Muscle fibre is a syncitium.

   Reason: Muscle fibre has a large number of parallelly arranged myofilaments in the sarcoplasm.

3. **Assertion:** Visceral muscles are smooth in appearance.

   Reason: Many muscle cells assemble in a branching pattern to form a visceral muscle.

4. **Assertion:** Locomotion in *Hydra* is carried out by two types of contractile cells.

   Reason: Muscle fibres are lacking in *Hydra*.

5. **Assertion:** The portion of the myofibril between two successive 'Z' lines is considered as the functional unit of contraction called sarcomere.

   Reason: During contraction, 'I' bands get reduced whereas 'A' bands retain the length, thereby causing shortening of the sarcomere.

6. **Assertion :** Extra oxygen consumption in human body is known as oxygen debt.

   Reason : The extra oxygen is required by the body to oxidise the accumulated lactic acid produced during strenous exercise.

7. **Assertion :** Biceps and triceps are called antagonistic muscles.

   Reason : This is due to the fact that they contract and relax together.

8. **Assertion :** Muscle contraction force increases with rise in strength of stimulus.

   Reason : This is due to increased contraction of individual muscle fibres with increase in stimulus strength.

9. **Assertion:** Fatigue is inability of muscle to relax.

   Reason: It is due to lactic acid accumulation by repeated contractions. **[AIIMS 1998]**

10. **Assertion :** The phase of muscle contraction occurs when myosin binds and releases actin.

    Reason : Muscle contraction is initiated by a signal sent by the peripheral nervous system via motor neuron. **[AIIMS 2016]**

11. **Assertion:** Mechanism of muscle contraction is explained by sliding-filament theory.

    Reason: Contraction of muscle fibre takes place by the sliding of thick filaments over the thin filaments.

12. **Assertion:** On stimulation, a muscle cell releases calcium ions (Ca^{2+}) from sarcoplasmic reticulum.

    Reason: By reacting with a protein complex, Ca^{2+} uncover active sites on the actin filaments.

13. **Assertion:** A person becomes fatigue very soon during exercise.

    Reason: Muscle fibres undergo oxygen debt during exercise.

14. **Assertion:** Red muscles depend on anaerobic process for energy.

    Reason: Red muscles have few number of mitochondria in them.

15. **Assertion:** Rapid spasm in muscle is termed as tetany.

    Reason: Tetany is usually caused by an increase in the blood calcium level.

16. **Assertion:** Human has dicondylic skull.
Reason: Skull articulates with superior region of the vertebral column with the help of two occipital condyles.
17. **Assertion:** Radius is shorter than ulna.
Reason: It has large olecranon process.
18. **Assertion:** Bone has very hard matrix whereas cartilage has pliable matrix.
Reason: Bone has calcium salts in its matrix whereas cartilage has chondroitin salts in its matrix.
19. **Assertion:** First seven pairs of ribs are called true ribs.
Reason: These ribs are not connected ventrally to the sternum.
20. **Assertion :** Ball and socket joints are the most mobile joints.
Reason : Synovial fluid is present here.
21. **Assertion :** Triceps is said to be an extensor muscle for elbow joint.
Reason : Triceps relaxes during extension of forearm at the elbow joint.
22. **Assertion:** The joint between atlas and axis is an example of gliding joint.
Reason: Gliding joint allows movement primarily in one plane.
23. **Assertion:** Fibrous joints play a significant role in locomotion.
Reason: Fibrous joints have fluid-filled cavity between the articulating surfaces of the two bones.
24. **Assertion :** Arthritis or inflammation of a joint makes the joint painful.
Reason : Some toxic substances are deposited at the joint.
25. **Assertion :** Inflammation of a skeletal joint may immobilize the movements of the joint.
Reason : Uric acid crystals in the joint cavity and ossification of articular cartilage leads to this. **[AIIMS 2006]**

Solutions

1. **(b)** Main movement found in unicellular organisms are ciliary, flagellar and amoeboid movements. In multicellular animals also, phagocytes migrate through tissues by amoeboid movements. Ciliary movement of cells lining the upper respiratory tract, fallopian tubes and vasa efferentia of testes transport, respectively dust particles, ova and sperms in specific direction in those organs. Mammalian sperms move into the female reproductive tract by flagellar movements.
2. **(b)** Muscle fibre is a syncitium as the sarcoplasm contains many nuclei.
   A characteristic feature of the muscle fibre is the presence of a large number of parallelly arranged filaments in the sarcoplasm called myofilaments or myofibrils. Each myofibril has alternate dark and light bands on it.
3. **(c)** Visceral muscles are located in the inner walls of hollow visceral organs of the body like the alimentary canal, reproductive tract, etc. They do not exhibit any striation and are smooth in appearance. Hence, they are called smooth muscles (nonstriated muscle). Many cardiac muscle cells assemble in a branching pattern to form a cardiac muscle.
4. **(a)** As muscle fibres are lacking in *Hydra*, the animal uses two types of contractile cells for this purpose. Processes of these cells run in the body wall both along the long axis of the body and arround the central body cavity. Contraction and relaxation of these cells respectively, shorten and elongate these processes. They consequently cause all types of movement of *Hydra* including shortening, elongation and also bending of body and tentacular movement. Locomotion is carried out by somersaults looping.
5. **(b)** Each myofibril contains actin and myosin filaments which give it striated appearance due to dark and light bands. The light bands are made of actin and are called I-bands or isotropic band, whereas the dark bands are called 'A' or anisotropic bands and contain myosin. Both the proteins are arranged as rod-like structres, parallel to each other and also to the longitudinal axis of the myofibrils. In the centre of each 'I' band is an elastic fibre called 'Z' line which bisects it. The portion of the myofibril between two successive 'Z' lines is considered as the functional unit of contraction and is called a sarcomere. During contraction, the 'Z' lines attached to the actins are pulled inwards thereby causing a shortening of the sarcomere, i.e., contraction. Hence, during shortening of the muscle, i.e., contraction, the 'I' bands get reduced, whereas the 'A' bands retain the length.
6. **(b)** During strenous exercise, the muscle does not get sufficient oxygen to meet its energy needs immediately. So, it contracts anaerobically and accumulates lactic acid. During recovery, the oxygen consumption of the muscle by far exceeds than in the resting state. The extra oxygen consumed during recovery is called oxygen debt of the muscle.
7. **(c)** Antagonistic muscles are those muscles which contract to produce opposite movements at the same joint. When a muscle contracts to produce a movement, its antagonist must relax to allow that movement to take place. Biceps and triceps are called antagonistic muscles. Because during flexion at the elbow, biceps contracts and triceps relaxes; during extension at the same joint, triceps contract and biceps relax.
8. **(c)** The muscle fibre always contracts with the maximum force and this force doesn't rise on increasing the strength of the stimulus. If the stimulus is of strength below the threshold, then the muscle fibre doesn't

contract at all. This is known as all or none law. But the entire muscle doesn't obey this law, it means that force of contraction of muscle increase with rise in strength of the stimulus. This is due to the fact that the strength of the threshold stimulus varies from muscle fibre to muscle fibre in a muscle.

9. **(a)** Due to the accumulation of lactic acid, muscles do not respond to a stimuli after a prolonged previous activity.

10. **(c)** The phase of muscle contraction occurs when myosin binds and releases actin. Muscle contraction is initiated by a signal sent by the central nervous system via a motor neuron. A motor neuron along with the muscle fibres connected to it constitutes a motor unit.

11. **(c)** Mechanism of muscle contraction is best explained by the sliding filament theory which states that contraction of a muscle fibre takes place by the sliding of the actin filaments over the thick myosin filaments.

12. **(b)** A neural signal on reaching the neuromuscular junction releases a neurotransmitter (acetylcholine) which generates an action potential in the sarcolemma. This spreads through the muscle fibre and causes the release of calcium ions from sarcoplasmic reticulum into the sarcoplasm. Increase in Ca^{2+} level leads to the binding of calcium with a subunit of troponin on actin filaments and thereby, removing the mask of active sites for myosin.

13. **(b)** During strenuous exercise, the muscle does not get sufficient oxygen to meet its energy requirement immediately. So, muscle contracts in the absence of oxygen. But it gets fatigued sooner in the absence of oxygen as the metabolic products of cellular respiration mainly lactic acid accumulates. This accumulation of lactic acid leads to muscle fatigue.
After strenuous exercise, the oxygen consumption of muscle exceeeds. The extra oxygen consumed during recovery is called oxygen debt of the muscle. It is used in oxidizing the accumulated lactic acid aerobically and in restoring the depleted creatine phosphate and ATP in the muscle fibre. A small part of oxygen debt also goes to myoglobin which binds and stores oxygen for future use.

14. **(d)** Muscle contains a red coloured oxygen storing pigment called myoglobin. Myoglobin content is high in some of the muscles which gives a reddish appearance to them. Such muscles are called the red fibres. These muscles also contain plenty of mitochondria which can utilise the large amount of oxygen stored in them for ATP production. These muscles, therefore, can also be called aerobic muscles.

15. **(c)** Tetany is a spasm and twitching of the muscles, particularly of face, hands and feet. Rapid spasms (wild contractions) in muscle is due to low Ca^{2+} in body fluid which may be due to underactive parathyroid gland.

16. **(a)** Skull has two occipital condyles, with the help of these two condyles, skull is connected by first vertebra of vertebral column, i.e., Atlas, this type of skull is called dicondylic skull which is present in humans.

17. **(b)** Ulna is longer than radius. Its upper end has a larger olecranon process that forms the eminence of our elbow. The head of the radius articulates with the humerus.

18. **(a)** Bone is hard as its matrix has an inflexible material, the ossein. Matrix and of the bone also contains calcium and magnesium salts which also adds in building rigidity of the tissue. Cartilage is soft and pliable as its matrix has a flexible material, the chondrin. Matrix of the cartilage chiefly consists of chondroitin sulphate, that is capable of withstanding considerable pressure.

19. **(c)** First seven pairs of ribs are called true ribs. Dorsally, they are attached to the thoracic vertebrae and ventrally connected to the sternum with the help of hyaline cartilage.

20. **(b)** Synovial fluid is a thick sticky fluid of egg white consistency, secreted by synovial membranes into the synovial cavity. Though the presence of synovial fluid is one of the reasons behind the mobility of the joints, but the most accurate reason is

the arrangement of the bones at the joint, the spheroidal ball-like end of one bone articulates here with the cup-shaped depression in another. This allows the bone with the ball head to move freely in many planes. Shoulder joints and hip joints are the ball-and-socket joints.

21. **(c)** Movements are produced at joints by contraction of skeletal muscles inserted into articulating bones. The contraction of an extensor muscle extends a joint, hence causing extension of the limb. Contraction of triceps brings about the extension of forearm at the elbow joint hence, it is said to be the extensor muscle for elbow joint.

22. **(d)** A gliding joint permits back -and -forth and side-to-side movements. No rotation or twisting is possible because the bones are packed closely together or held in place by ligaments. Gliding joints are found between the carpal bones and between the tarsal bones. A pivot joints allows movement primarily in one plane. In a pivot joint, rounded or pointed bone fits into a shallow depression in another bone. The joint between the atlas and axis is an example of pivot joint.

23. **(d)** Fibrous joints do not allow any movement. This type of joint is found in flat skull bones which fuse end-to end with the help of dense fibrous connective tissues in the form of sutures to form the cranium.

24. **(c)** Arthritis or inflammation of a joint makes the joint painful and may even immobilise the movements at the joint. This may result from a lack of the synovial fluid at the joint. The ossification of the articular cartilage, deposition of uric acid crystals in the joint cavity or other changes occur at the joint.

25. **(a)** Painful inflammation of the synovial membrane of the joints results in stiffening of joints and painful movement. Uric acid accumulation in the joints can lead to painful movement of joint.

Chapter

21

Neural Control and Coordination

Directions: In the following questions, a statement of assertion is followed by a statement of reason. Mark the correct choice as:

(a) If both Assertion and Reason are true and Reason is the correct explanation of Assertion.

(b) If both Assertion and Reason are true but Reason is not the correct explanation of Assertion.

(c) If Assertion is true but Reason is false.

(d) If both Assertion and Reason are false.

1. **Assertion :** Nerve conduction is the one way conduction.
   Reason : Nerve impulse is transmitted from dendrite terminals to axon terminals.
2. **Assertion :** The chemical stored in the synaptic vesicles are termed as neurotransmitters.
   Reason : Synaptic vesicles release these chemicals in the synaptic cleft.
3. **Assertion :** The imbalance in concentration of Na^+, K^+ and proteins generates resting potential.
   Reason : To maintain the unequal distribution of Na^+ & K^+, the neurons use electrical energy.
4. **Assertion :** Transmission of nerve impulse across a synapse is accomplished by neurotransmitters.
   Reason : Transmission across a synapse usually requires neurotransmitters because there is a small space, *i.e.*, synaptic cleft, that separates one neuron from another. **[AIIMS 1999]**
5. **Assertion :** The axonal membrane of the neuron is more permeable to sodium ion (Na^+) and nearly impermeable to potassium (K^+).
   Reason : In a resting state, neuron conducts impulses. **[AIIMS 2016]**
6. **Assertion:** Electrical synapses are rare in our system.
   Reason: Impulse transmission across an electrical synapse is slower than that across a chemical synapse.
7. **Assertion:** Multipolar neurons have two or more axons and one dendrite.
   Reason: Multipolar neurons are found usually in the embryonic stage.
8. **Assertion:** Myelinated nerve fibres are present in spinal and cranial nerves.
   Reason: Myelinated nerves conduct impulses more rapidly than unmyelinated nerves.
9. **Assertion:** The resting membrane of the neuron exhibit polarity of charges.
   Reason: The outer surface of the axonal membrane possesses a negative charge while its inner surface becomes positively charged.
10. **Assertion:** Nerve fibre can become excited through touch, smell, pressure and chemical changes and there is a change in polarity.
    Reason: It is called action potential.
11. **Assertion :** The membrane of a neuron is polarised.
    Reason : Ion channels on the neural membrane are selectively permeable to different ions.
12. **Assertion :** The presynaptic neuron transmits an impulse (action potential) across the synaptic cleft to the postsynaptic neuron.
    Reason : For the transmission of impulses at synapse, chemicals called neurotransmitters are responsible.
13. **Assertion :** Neurons are excitable cells.
    Reason : The membrane of neurons in a depolarised state is responsible for excitability.
14. **Assertion :** Neurons regulates the endocrine activity but not vice-versa.
    Reason : Endocrine gland regulates neural activity and neural activity regulates endocrine gland.
15. **Assertion :** During physical exercise, the demand of oxygen is increased, which compels the lungs and heart to increase the rate of respiration and to increase the blood flow for proper supply of oxygen respectively.
    Reason : Coordination is the process through which two or more organs interact and complement the functions of each other.

16. **Assertion :** Cerebrospinal fluid is present throughout the central nervous system.
Reason : CSF has no such function.
17. **Assertion :** The brain stem contains centres for controlling activities.
Reason : Brain stem is very sensitive.
18. **Assertion :** Medulla oblongata causes reflex actions like vomiting, coughing and sneezing.
Reason : It has many nerve cells which control autonomic reflexes.
19. **Assertion :** A cerebellum is related with skillful voluntary movement and involuntary activity like body balance, equilibrium, *etc.*
Reason : It is a part of hind brain and is situated behind the pons. **[AIIMS 2010]**
20. **Assertion:** The PNS comprises of all the nerves of the body associated with CNS.
Reason: PNS is the site of information processing and control.
21. **Assertion:** Medulla contains centres which control respiration, cardiovascular reflexes and gastric secretions.
Reason: Medulla contains several neurosecretory cells which secrete hormones.
22. **Assertion:** Anterior lobe of pituitary is attached to hypothalamus by a vein.
Reason: This attachment is done through a portal vein.
23. **Assertion:** All motor neurons are efferent neurons.
Reason: Motor neurons conduct nerve impulses from the spinal cord to the brain.
24. **Assertion:** Some areas of the brain and spinal cord look white.
Reason: This is because cell bodies of neurons are situated in those areas.
25. **Assertion:** The peripheral nervous system includes nerves coursing between the central nervous system and different parts of the body.
Reason: In man, only peripheral nervous system is present.
26. **Assertion:** Spinal cord has a column of both grey and white matter.
Reason: Grey matter forms the central spinal canal.
27. **Assertion :** Neuroglial cells are known as the packing cells of brain.
Reason : A type of neuroglial cells forms the myelin sheath around axon.
28. **Assertion :** Cerebral cortex appears white.
Reason : It is because of the myelin sheath covering of the tracts.
29. **Assertion:** Association areas are neither clearly sensory nor motor in function.
Reason: Association areas are responsible for complex functions like intersensory associations, memory and communication.
30. **Assertion:** Reflex arc comprises of at least one afferent neuron, one efferent neuron and a part of PNS.
Reason: The efferent neuron receives signal from a sensory organ and transmits the impulse via a ventral nerve root into the PNS.
31. **Assertion:** Rabies is an acute infectious disease of warm blooded mammals characterized by involvement of central nervous system resulting in paralysis and finally death.
Reason: This is caused due to neurotropic filterable bacteria in saliva of rabid animals.
32. **Assertion :** Humans can sense changes in the environment.
Reason : Sensory organs detect all types of changes in environment.
33. **Assertion :** Tongue is a gustatoreceptor.
Reason : Receptors for gustatory sensations are located in the taste bud.
34. **Assertion :** Vitamin A deficiency produces night blindness.
Reason : Photosensitive pigment rhodopsin is synthesised from vitamin A.
35. **Assertion :** Circular smooth muscles of iris contract when bright light falls on the eye.
Reason : Pupil gets constricted by the contraction of circular smooth muscles of iris.
36. **Assertion:** Visual acuity is the greatest at fovea.
Reason: The fovea is a thick area of the retina where both rods and cones are present.
37. **Assertion :** Astigmatism is due to uneven curvature of lens.
Reason : It is treated with cylindrical lenses. **[AIIMS 2007]**
38. **Assertion:** Choroid layer is thick over the posterior two-third of the eye ball but it becomes thin in the anterior part.
Reason: Choroid layer lacks blood vessels. It forms ciliary body in the anterior part of the eye ball.

39. **Assertion:** When all the three types of cones are stimulated equally, a mosaic of red, green and blue lights is produced.
Reason: Twilight or scotopic vision is produced by cones.

41. **Assertion:** Sparrows possess poor night vision.
Reason: Sparrows eyes are made up of ommatidia.

42. **Assertion:** The eye is said to have power of accomodation.
Reason: Ciliary muscles alters the shape of the lens for near or far vision during accomodation.

43. **Assertion :** Cerebral cortex has high concentration of neuron cell bodies in it.
Reason : The cerebral cortex is referred to as the white matter of the brain.

44. **Assertion :** Iris muscles show both dilation as well as constriction of pupil.
Reason : It is sympathetic and parasympathetic nervous system which have antagonistic functions.

45. **Assertion:** The inner ear contains three ossicles (malleus, incus and stapes) which are attached to one another in a chain-like fashion.
Reason: The stapes is attached to the tympanic membrane and the malleus is attached to the oval window of the cochlea.

46. **Assertion :** The auditory ossicles help in hearing.
Reason : Auditory ossicles maintain the balance of air pressure between two sides of the eardrum.

47. **Assertion:** Vestibular apparatus helps us in maintaining balance of body and posture.
Reason: Due to the arrangement of semicircular canals of vestibular apparatus, movement of head in any direction will stimulate sensory cells to maintain dynamic equilibrium.

40. **Assertion:** The space between the cornea and the lens is called the vitreous chamber.
Reason: The space between the lens and reatina is called the aqueous chamber.

48. **Assertion:** The Eustachian tube helps in equalising the pressures on either sides of the ear drum.
Reason: The Eustachian tube connects the middle ear cavity with the pharynx.

49. **Assertion:** After hearing a sound, nerve impulse passes from neurons to the brain.
Reason: The neurons which pass nerve impulses from the body organ to the brain is called afferent neuron.

50. **Assertion :** Organ of Jacobson is well developed in snakes.
Reason : It is responsible for smell.

Solutions

1. (c) Nerve impulses are always transmitted across a synapse from the axon terminals of one neuron to the dendrite/cell body of the next neuron but never in the reverse direction. Since the neurotransmitter is present only in the axon terminals and not in the dendrite or cell body, it cannot be released from the dendrite or cell body even if the impulse reaches there.
2. (b) The axon terminal of the neuron contains many membrane bound vesicles called synaptic vesicle, in its cytoplasm. Within these vesicles , chemical substances such as adrenaline and acetylcholine remain stored. These chemicals are called neurotransmitters because they help to transmit nerve impulses across the synapses. When a nerve impulse passes the axon terminal, its synaptic vesicles release their stored chemicals to the synaptic cleft. These diffuse through the cleft to reach the membrane of the next neuron, stimulating the latter. This causes the nerve impulse to be transmitted along the next neuron.
3. (c) To maintain the unequal distribution of Na^+ and K^+ ion, the neurons use chemical energy in the form of ATP to actively transport Na^+ ion out of cell and more K^+ inside the cell.
4. (a) Transmission of nerve impulse across synapses is accomplishe by neurotransmitter because synapses comprises of a synaptic cleft between the end of one nerve fibres and the beginning of the next.
5. (d) The axonal membrane of neuron is more permeable to potassium ions (K^+) and nearly impermeable to sodium ions (Na^+). In a resting state, neuron does not conduct any impulse as the fluids outside the cell membrane carry a relatively high positive charge while the fluids inside the cell membrane carry a less positive, or relatively negative charge.
6. (c) There are two types of synapses, namely, electrical synapses and chemical synapses. At electrical synapses, the membranes of pre- and post-synaptic neurons are in very close proximity. Electrical current can flow directly from one neuron into the other across these synapses. At a chemical synapse, the membranes of the pre- and post-synaptic neurons are separated by a fluid-filled space called synaptic cleft. Chemicals called neurotransmitters are involved in the transmission of impulses at these synapses. Impulse transmission across and electrical synapse is always faster than that across a chemical synapse. Electrical synapses are rare in our system.
7. (d) Based on the number of axons and dendrites, the neurons are divided into three types, i.e, multipolar (with one axon and two or more dendrites; found in the cerebral cortex), bipolar (with one axon and one dendrite, found in the retina of eye) and unipolar (cell body with one axon only; found usually in the embryonic stage).
8. (b) Myelinated nerve fibres are present in spinal and cranial nerves. Unmyelinated nerve fibre is enclosed by a Schwann cell that does not form a myelin sheath around the axon, and is commonly found in autonomous and the somatic neural systems. The conduction of impulses is faster in myelinated nerve fibre (or medullated nerve fibre) because when an impulse travels along a medullated nerve fibre, it does not proceed uniformly along the length of the axis cylinder, but jumps from one node of Ranvier to the next. This is called the saltatory conduction of impulses.
9. (c) When a neuron is not conducting any impulse, i.e., resting, the axonal membrane is comparatively more permeable to potassium ions (K^+) and nearly impermeable to sodium ions (Na^+). Similarly, the membrane is impermeable to negatively charged proteins present in the axoplasm. Consequently, the axoplasm inside the axon contains high concentration of K^+ and negatively charged proteins and low concentration of Na^+. These ionic

gradients across the resting membrane are maintained by the active transport of ions by the sodium-potassium pump which transports 3 Na^+ outwards for 2 K^+ into the cell. As a result, the outer surface of the axonal membrane possesses a positive charge while its inner surface becomes negatively charged and therefore, is polarised.

10. **(b)** Action potential occurs in response to stimulation of nerve fibre as a result of various stimuli like touch, smell, pressure and chemical changes.

11. **(a)** The plasma membrane of the neuron is polarised due to the high out flow of Na^+ ions to outside and low intake of K^+ ion. Na^+ ions outflow by the ion channel of plasma membrane and K^+ ions inflow by it. This creates a difference in the positive potential across the plasma membrane. The membrane is less positive inside which is normally termed as negative inside w.r.t. outside.

12. **(b)** Signals from the axon terminal of presynaptic neuron are transmitted to the dendrites of the postsynaptic neuron with the help of chemicals known as neurotransmitters.

13. **(a)** Neurons are excitable cells. Excitability is the ability of nerve cells to generate an electrical impulse in response to stimulus. When a nerve fibre receives stimulus, the potential across the membrane is reversed at the point of excitation. It means, the inner side of plasma membrane of the cell becomes more positively charged with respect to the outer side of plasma membrane. This change in polarity is called action potential. This condition of reverse polarity is said to be depolarised.

14. **(c)** The autonomous nervous system regulates the secretion of glands, whereas the glands do not regulate the nervous system.

15. **(a)** Coordination between organs/organ system, is the key for better functioning of our body. In case of physical exercise, the increased demand of oxygen initiates a cascade, which coordinates lungs, heart and blood vessels of the body to fulfil the demand.

16. **(c)** An extracellular fluid called cerebrospinal fluid is present throughout the central nervous system. It affords some protection to central nervous system from injury and shock.

17. **(b)** The brain stem consists of pons varoli, medulla oblongata, mid brain and diencephalon. It is the connection between brain and spinal cord. It contains centres for controlling many vital activities, *e.g.* respiratory centres, vasomotor centres, salivary centres etc. It also carries nerve tracts between the spinal cord and the higher brain structure.

18. **(a)** Medulla oblongata consists of accumulation of nerve cells act as vital centres of many autonomic reflexes like vomiting, coughing and sneezing.

19. **(b)** Hind brain consists of cerebellum located dorsally to medulla oblongat and pons varoli. It contains centres for maintenance of posture and equilibrium of the body and for the muscle tone. All activities of the cerebellum are involuntary but may involve learning in their early stages.

20. **(c)** The CNS includes the brain and the spinal cord and is the site of information processing and control. The PNS comprises of all the nerves of the body associated with the CNS.

21. **(c)** The medulla contains centres which control respiration, cardiovascular reflexes and gastric secretions. The hypothalamus is the basal part of diencephalon (forebrain) which contains several groups of neurosecretory cells called nuclei that produce hormones. These hormones regulate the synthesis and secretion of pituitary hormones.

22. **(b)** Anterior lobe of pituitary is called pars distalis. It is attached to hypothalamus by hypophyseal portal vein. This portal vein is called hypothalamo – hypophyseal portal vein.

23. **(c)** The neurons and nerve fibres which conduct nerve impulse from the Central Nervous System (CNS) to the peripheral organs and tissues are called efferent neurons and efferent nerve fibres respectively. Some of the neurons and nerve fibres conduct nerve impulses to the

muscles and gland to stimulate or inhibit their activities. Many of these nerve fibres cause movements of muscles. So, such neurons and nerve fibres are known as motor neurons and motor nerve fibres, respectively. The motor nerve fibres are the axons of motor neurons. All motor neurons are efferent neurons, because they conduct impulses from the CNS system to the peripheral tissues *viz*, muscles and gland.

24. (c) The brain and the spinal cord constitute the central nervous system. The areas of the CNS where the cell bodies of the neurons are situated, look grey and constitute the grey matter. Other areas look white and constitute the white matter of the CNS. The white matter contains only nerve fibres cruising from or to the nerve cells in the grey matter. It looks white due to the presence of myelin around the myelinated fibres. In most parts of the brain, the grey matter containing the nerve cells is situated on the surface while the white matter made of fibres is located deep inside the brain; but in the spinal cord, the grey matter is internal and white matter occurs outside.

25. (c) The nervous system of human comprises of Central Nervous System – brain and spinal cord.
Peripheral Nervous System – consists of nerves present between brain and body parts.

26. (b) The spinal cord extends downwards from the brain stem. The grey matter from a column running along the central part of the spinal canal (= neurocoel, lined with ciliated ependymal epithelium), containing the cerebrospinal fluid, running along the central part of the grey matter. Grey matter is composed of nerve cells, bodies, dendrites and synapses. The white matter forms an outer column surrounding the grey matter at its centre.

27. (a) Neuroglial cells are the packing and supporting cells found in brain and spinal cord. They are of three types, astrocytes, oligodendrocytes and microglia. Astrocytes are responsible for separation of two neurons by insulation. Oligodendrocytes are a category of glial cells that form myelin sheath around the axon. Microglia are phagocytic as well as scavengers. They engulf microbes and cellular debris. Nearly 50% of all brain cells are neuroglia. Schwann cells are the neuroglial cell, which are present in PNS.

28. (d) The layer of cells which covers the cerebral hemisphere is called cerebral cortex and is thrown into prominent folds. The cerebral cortex is referred to as the grey matter due to its greyish appearance. The neuron cell bodies are concentrated here giving the colour.

29. (a) The cerebral cortex contains motor areas, sensory areas and large regions that are neither clearly sensory nor motor in function. These regions are called as the association areas which are responsible for complex functions like intersensory associations, memory and communication. Association area is concerned with the reception of sensory impulses and start of motor impulses.

30. (d) The reflex pathway comprises at least one afferent neuron (receptor) and one efferent (effector or excitor) neuron appropriately arranged in a series. The afferent neuron receives signal from a sensory organ and transmits the impulse via a dorsal nerve root into the CNS (at the level of spinal cord). The efferent neuron then carries signals from CNS to the effector. The stimulus and response thus, forms a reflex arc.

31. (c) Rabies is an overwhelming encephalomyelitis and includes severe headache and high fever with excitement and depression. This disease occurs by a virus called rhabdovirus.

32. (a) The sensory organs detect all types of changes in the environment and send appropriate signals to the CNS, where all the inputs are processed and analysed. Signals are then sent to different parts of the brain. This is how we can sense changes in the environment.

33. (a) Tongue is also called as gustatoreceptor, i.e., it is a receptor for taste. The receptor for gustatory sensation are located in taste buds on tongue.

34. (a) The light sensitive inner layer of eyeball

called retina contain photoreceptors *viz.* rod and cone cells which convert the energy of specific wavelengths of light into action potentials of nerve fibres. Rods are sensitive even to dim light and consequently enable to see in dim light and at night. They contain a purple coloured photosensitive pigment, called rhodopsin. Rhodopsin consists of the protein scotopsin and retinene, a derivative of vitamin A which is required for proper vision and is required for the regeneration of rhodopsin after it has been exposed to light.

35. (b) It is a pigmented, muscular, opaque diaphragm which extends from the ciliary body in front of a biconvex transparent lens. Iris has a small central aperture called pupil. Light passing through cornea enters through the pupil to fall on the lens behind it. The iris has two sets of smooth muscles arranged circularly and radially around the pupil. The pupil gets constricted by the contraction of circular muscles to reduce the amount of light falling on the lens. On the contrary, the pupil gets dilated by the contraction of radial muscles to increase the amount of light falling on the lens.

36. (c) The fovea is a thinned-out portion of the retina where only the cones are densely packed. It is the point where the visual acuity (resolution) is the greatest.

37. (b) Astigmatism is a kind in defect of vision in which the image of an object is distorted. It is because all the light rays do not come to focus on retina due to abnormal curvature of the lens . It can be corrected by wearing cylindrical lenses.

38. (d) The middle layer, choroid, contains many blood vessels and looks bluish in colour. the choroid layer is thin over the posterior two-third of the eye ball, but it becomes thick in the anterior part to form the ciliary body.

39. (d) In the human eye, there are three types of cones which possess their own characteristic photopigments that respond to red, green and blue lights. The sensations of different colours are produced by various combinations of these cones and their photopigments. When these cones are stimulated equally, a sensation of white light is produced. The daylight (photopic) vision and colour vision are functions of cones and the twilight (scotopic) vision is the function of the rods.

40. (d) The space between the cornea and the lens is called the aqueous chamber and contains a thin watery fluid called aqueous humor. The space between the lens and the retina is called the vitreous chamber and is filled with a transparent gel called vitreous humor.

41. (c) Animals, like sparrows, which are active only in day time, have mostly cone cells in their retina and therefore, they possess poor night vision.

Ommatidia are the elongated tube like units of a compound eye present in higher invertebrates like prawns, crabs and insects.

42. (b) The lens in resting eye focusses parallel rays from distant objects (more than 6 m away) on the retina. But to increase the power of the lens for focussing divergent rays from near object on the retina, a reflex called accomodation is needed. The eye has got the property to form images of both near and far objects on the retina by changing the convexity of the lens. This is known as the power of accomodation.

43. (c) The layer of cell which covers the cerebral hemispheres is called cerebral cortex and is thrown into prominent folds. It is referred to as the grey matter. It is called grey matter due to its greyish appearance. Neuron cell bodies are concentrated here to give it the greyish appearance.

44. (a) Autonomic nervous system includes sympathetic nervous system and parasympathetic nervous system which have anutagonistic functions. Iris muscles, under sympathetic nervous syetem dilates pupil, while under parasympathetic nervous system constricts pupil.

45. (d) The middle ear contains three ossicles called malleus, incus and stapes which are attached to one another in a chain-like fashion. The malleus is attached to the tympanic membrane and the stapes is attached to the oval window of the cochlea. The ear ossicles increase the efficiency of transmission of sound waves to the inner ear.

46. (c) Auditory ossicles are the three small bones present in the cavity of the middle ear. These are hammer like malleus, anvil-like incus and stirrup-like stapes. Sound waves reach the ear drum through the external auditory canal and vibrates the ear drum. The vibrations of the latter are transmitted by the auditory ossicles to the fluid endolymph which fills the internal ear. The auditory ossicles also increase the force of vibrations by approximately ten times.

47. (a) The inner ear contains a complex system called vestibular apparatus, located above the cochlea. The vestibular apparatus is composed of three semi-circular canals and the otolith organ consisting of the saccule and utricle. Each semi-circular canal lies in a different plane at right angles to each other. The membranous canals are suspended in the perilymph of the bony canals. The base of canals is swollen and is called ampulla, which contains a projecting ridge called crista ampullaris which has hair cells. The saccule and utricle contain a projecting ridge called macula. The crista and macula are the specific receptors of the vestibular apparatus responsible for maintenance of balance of the body and posture. Cristae detect turning or rotational movements of the head (angular acceleration).Maculae detects changes in the head (or body) with respect to gravity (static equilibrium) and movement in one direction (linear acceleration). Since the three semicircular ducts are arranged in three different planes, movement of the head in any direction will stimulate the sensory cells of atleast one crista.

48. (a) The eustachian tube connects the middle ear cavity with the nasopharynx. It aerates the middle ear system and clears mucus from the middle ear into the nasopharynx. Opening and closing functions of the eustachian tube are physiologically and pathologically important. Normal opening of the eustachian tube equalizes atmospheric pressure in the middle ear; closing of the eustachian tube protects the middle ear from unwanted pressure fluctuations and loud sounds.

49. (b) Activity of sense organs is related with two types of neurons (afferent and efferent). The neurons which pass nerve impulses from the body organ to the brain is called afferent neuron. The neurons which pass nerve impulses from the brain to the body organs are called efferent neurons.

50. (a) Jacobson's organ is an auxiliary olfactory sense organ that is found in many animals. It is well developed in snakes and lizards but less developed in human beings.

Chapter 22 Chemical Co-ordination and Integration

Directions: In the following questions, a statement of assertion is followed by a statement of reason. Mark the correct choice as:

(a) If both Assertion and Reason are true and Reason is the correct explanation of Assertion.
(b) If both Assertion and Reason are true but Reason is not the correct explanation of Assertion.
(c) If Assertion is true but Reason is false.
(d) If both Assertion and Reason are false.

1. **Assertion :** Failure of secretion of somatotropin from an early age causes dwarfism in the patient.
   Reason : Somatotropin hormone stimulates the body growth and elongation of long bones.
2. **Assertion:** Neurohypophysis is under the direct regulation of the hypothalamus.
   Reason: Neurohypophysis stores and releases two hormones called oxytocin and vasopressin which are actually synthesized by the hypothalamus.
3. **Assertion:** Failure of secretion of hormone vasopressin causes diabetes mellitus in the patient.
   Reason: Vasopressin increases the volume of urine by increasing the reabsorption of water from the urine.
4. **Assertion :** The person with diabetes insipidus feels thirsty.
   Reason : A person with diabetes insipidus suffers from excess secretion of vasopressin. **[AIIMS 2010]**
5. **Assertion :** Diabetes insipidus is marked by excessive urination and too much thirst of water.
   Reason : Anti-diuretic hormone (ADH) is secreted by the posterior lobe of pituitary gland.
6. **Assertion:** Oxytocin is also known as Anti Diuretic hormone (ADH).
   Reason: It can cause an increase in the renal reabsorption of water. **[AIIMS 2004]**
7. **Assertion:** Melatonin influences the menstrual cycle, pigmentation and defense capability.
   Reason: It plays an important role in the regulation of diurnal rhythm of our body.
8. **Assertion :** The tadpoles become giant tadpoles when fed on thiourea.
   Reason : Thiourea is an antithyroid substance.
9. **Assertion:** Thyroid hormones promote physical growth and development of mental faculties.
   Reason: Hypothyroidism in adults causes retarded sexual development.
10. **Assertion :** Hormone calcitonin has antagonistic effect to that of parathormone.
    Reason : Calcitonin decreases blood calcium level while parathormone increases blood calcium level. **[AIIMS 2009]**
11. **Assertion:** PTH is a hypercalcemic hormone.
    Reason: It stimulates the process of bone resorption.
12. **Assertion:** Immune response of old persons become weak.
    Reason: Thymus degenerates in old individuals.
13. **Assertion:** Adrenal medulla is called the gland for 'fight, fright and flight'.
    Reason: The hormones adrenaline and noradrenaline help the body to combat against stress and emergency conditions.
14. **Assertion:** Adrenal medullary hormones help in combating stress.
    Reason: Both adrenaline and noradrenaline act on same organs and produce similar effects.
15. **Assertion:** Adrenal cortex is not vital for survival and may be removed without subsequently leading to death.
    Reason: It secretes a number of steroid hormones which have only cummulative effects on the hormones of other glands.
16. **Assertion:** Cortisol produces anti-inflammatory reactions and suppresses the immune response.
    Reason: It stimulates gluconeognesis, lipogenesis, and proteogenesis.

17. **Assertion:** Androgens stimulate muscular growth.
Reason: These produce anabolic effects on protein and carbohydrate metabolism.

18. **Assertion :** Aldosterone increases the volume of blood and other extracellular fluids.
Reason : The secretion of aldosterone is stimulated by a fall in the circulating volume of blood.

19. **Assertion :** Our body secretes adrenaline in intense cold.
Reason : Adrenaline raises metabolic rate.
[AIIMS 2006]

20. **Assertion:** A tumor of adrenal cortex may cause Addison's disease.
Reason: This happens due to over secretion of cortisol by the tumor.

21. **Assertion:** Insulin forms a hormone receptor complex which regulates gene expression.
Reason: It is a peptide hormone which can easily pass cell membrane to interact with hormone-receptor complex.

22. **Assertion:** Insulin is an anabolic hormone.
Reason: A fall in blood amino-acids also increases insulin secretion.

23. **Assertion:** Insulin stimulates glycogenolysis and gluconeogenesis resulting in hyperglycemia.
Reason: Prolonged hyperglycemia leads to complex disorder called diabetes insipidus.

24. **Assertion :** Females have less stature than males after puberty.
Reason : This happens because of the presence of hCG in the blood of females.

25. **Assertion :** Mammary glands are apocrine glands.
Reason : The distal part containing secretory granules break down and leaves as a secretion.
[AIIMS 2009]

26. **Assertion:** Oxytocin is called as 'milk-ejection hormone'.
Reason: Oxytocin acts on the smooth muscles of our body and stimulates their contraction.

27. **Assertion:** FSH is also known as interstitial cell stimulating hormone.
Reason: It is because of the fact that FSH stimulates the interstitial cells of testis.

28. **Assertion:** The estrogen level falls after menopause.
Reason: Estrogen is synthesized and secreted mainly by uterine lining.

29. **Assertion:** Prolactin is also called the 'milk ejection hormone'.
Reason: It stimulates the smooth muscle contractions of the mammary glands.

30. **Assertion:** Renal cells are involved in stimulating the formation of RBCs.
Reason: The juxtaglomerular cells of kidney produce erythropoietin.

Solutions

1. (a) The somatotropin (STH), also called growth hormone (GH) is secreted by the anterior lobe of pituitary gland. Somatotropin stimulates body growth by stimulating retention of proteins and calcium in the body, synthesis and deposition of proteins in tissues, growth and elongation of long bones, and proportionate growth of muscles and visceral organs. The failure of secretion of growth hormone from an early age stops the growth of long bones and of the body prematurely; this makes the patient dwarf and the condition is called dwarfism.

2. (c) Neurohypophysis also known as posterior pituitary stores and releases two hormones called oxytocin and vasopressin which are actually synthesized by the hypothalamus and are transported axonally to neurohypophysis. Therefore, the posterior pituitary is under the direct neural regulation of the hypothalamus.

3. (d) Vasopressin or anti-diuretic hormone (ADH) reduces the volume of urine by increasing the reabsorption of water from the urine in the distal convoluted tubules, collecting tubules and collecting ducts in the kidney. It does so by rendering the walls of these tubules leads to diabetes insipidus (increased urination). Although the volume of urine is increased. No glucose appears in the urine of such patients.

   Diabetes mellitus is a disease which is caused due to the failure of insulin hormone secretion by the pancreatic islets. The osmotic effect of glucose in the urine considerably increases the volume of urine, due to which thirst is also enhanced. In extreme cases, the patient suffers from coma and may die.

4. (c) Vasopressin or antidiuretic hormone is secreted by posterior pituitary gland. The deficiency of vaopressin results in a disorder known as diabetes insipidus. The main symptoms of diabetes insipidus are increase in thirst and increase in urination.

5. (b) Diabetes insipidus (DI) occurs when the kidneys are unable to conserve water as they perform their function of filtering blood. The amount of water conserved is controlled by antidiuretic hormone (ADH) also called vasopressin which is secreted by posterior lobe of pituitary gland. Diabetes inspidus is characterised by excessive urination and thirst. This problem appears due to the increase in permeability of collecting tubules.

6. (d) The hormone vasopressin (also known as antidiuretic hormone, ADH) reduces the volume of urine by increasing the reabsorption of water from the urine in the distal convoluted tubules, collecting tubules and collecting ducts in the kidney. It does so by rendering the walls of those tubules permeable to water. Failure of secretion of vasopressin leads to a reduced renal reabsorption of water and a consequent elimination of a large volume of very dilute (hypotonic) urine. Oxytocin is another hormone released by the posterior lobe of the pituitary gland. Oxytocin contracts the mammary glands, smooth muscles of uterus. Uterine contractions, stimulated by oxytocin at the end of pregnancy, help in the child-birth or parturition, hence also called birth hormone.

7. (b) Melatonin concentration in the blood follows a diurnal (day-night) cycle as it rises in the evening and through the night and drops to a low around noon. Because of this light mediated response, the pineal gland may act as a kind of 'biological clock' which may produce circadian rhythms (variations following a 24 hour cycle). In addition, melatonin also influences metabolism, pigmentation, the menstrual cycle as well as our defence capability.

8. (a) The thyroid gland secretes thyroxine and triiodothyronine hormone. One of their functions is stimulation of tissue differentiation. Because of this action, they promote metamorphosis of tadpoles into adult frogs. Feeding of anti-thyroid substances like thiourea to tadpoles, delays

their metamorphosis. As they continue to grow without metamorphosis, they become giant tadpoles.

9. (b) Thyroid hormones stimulate protein synthesis and, therefore, promote growth of the body tissues (physical development). They also regulate the development of mental faculties. Hyperthyroidism in adults causes myxoedema. This disease is characterized by puffy appearance due to accumulation of fat in the subcutaneous tissue because of low metabolic rate. The patient lacks alertness, intelligence and initiative. He also suffers from slow heart beat, low body temperature and retarded sexual development.

10. (a) Calcitonin or thyrocalcitonin is secreted by parafollicular cells of thyroid stroma. It retards bone dissolution and stimulates excretion of calcium in urine. Thus, it lowers calcium level in extra cellular fluid (ECF). Parathormone is secreted by chief cells of parathyroid gland and is also known as Collip's hormone. It maintains blood calcium level by increasing its absorption from food in intestine and its reabsorption from nephrons in the kidney. Maintenance of proper calcium level is in fact, a combined function of parathormone and calcitonin. When calcium level falls below normal parathormone maintains it by promoting its absorption, reabsorption and also by demineralisation of bones. When blood calcium level exceeds above normal then calcitonin hormone increases excretion of calcium in urine.

11. (a) Parathyroid hormone (PTH) increases the Ca^{2+} levels in the blood. PTH acts on bones and stimulates the process of bone resorption (dissolution/demineralisation). PTH also stimulates reabsorption of Ca^{2+} by the renal tubules and increases Ca^{2+} absorption from the digested food. It is, thus, clear that PTH is a hypercalcemic hormone, i.e., it increases the blood Ca^{2+} levels. Along with calcitonin, it plays a significant role in calcium balance in the body.

12. (a) Thymus plays a major role in the development of the immune system. This gland secretes the peptide hormones called thymosins. Thymosins play a major role in the differentiation of T-lymphocytes, which provide cell-mediated immunity. In addition, thymosins also promote production of antibodies to provide humoral immunity. Thymus is degenerated in old individuals resulting in a decreased production of thymosins. As a result, the immune responses of old persons become weak.

13. (a) Adrenaline or epinephrine dilates (widens) arterioles in the skeletal muscles and constricts (narrows) those in the skin and abdominal viscera. It increases the rate and force of heart beats and arterial blood pressure by enhancing the cardiac output. Adrenaline relaxes the smooth muscles of gastro-intestinal tract, and urinary bladder and bronchioles and contracts the sphincters of gastrointestinal tract and bladder. It increases blood sugar and blood lactic acid levels and also increases heat production, metabolic rate and body temperature. Noradrenaline or norepinephrine constricts arterioles in general or increases the total peripheral resistance against the flow of blood. The coordinated actions of both adrenaline and noradrenaline, thus help the body to react under stress conditions.

14. (b) The adrenal medulla secretes two hormones called adrenaline or epinephrine and noradrenaline or norepinephrine. Adrenaline and noradrenaline are rapidly secreted in response to stress of any kind and during emergency situations and are called emergency hormones or hormones of fight. These hormones increase alertness, pupillary dilation, piloerection, sweating, etc. Both the hormones increase the heart beat, the strength of heart contraction and the rate of respiration. They also stimulate the breakdown of glycogen resulting in an increased concentration of glucose in blood. In addition, they also stimulate the breakdown of lipids and proteins. Both the hormones act on the same organs and produce similar effects on them e.g., accelerate heart beat, raise blood pressure, slow peristalsis, etc.

15. (d) The outer part of adrenal gland is called adrenal cortex. This part of adrenal is vitally important for life and its destruction or

removal kills the animal. It secretes a number of steroid hormones which are broadly classified into three groups, viz. glucocorticoids, mineralocorticoids and sex corticoids. Glucocorticoids regulate the metabolisms of carbohydrate, fats and proteins. Mineralocorticoids regulate the balance of water and electroytes in our body. Sex corticoids stimulate the development of external sex characters.

16. (c) The adrenal cortex produces glucocorticoids which stimulates gluconeogenesis, lipolysis and proteolysis, and inhibit cellular uptakes and utilization of amino acids. In our body, cortisol is the main glucocorticoid; cortisol produces anti-inflammatory reactions and suppresses the immune response.

17. (a) Androgens produce anabolic (synthetic) effects on protein and carbohydrate metabolism. This anabolic effect causes greatly increased deposition of protein everywhere in the body, but especially in the muscles. Androgens, therefore, stimulate muscular growth.

18. (b) Aldosterone is a mineralocorticoid secreted from the outermost cellular layer (called zona glomerulosa) of the adrenal cortex. The mineralocorticoids regulate the metabolism of sodium and potassium. Their secretion is stimulated by a fall in plasma Na^+ concentration, or a rise in plasma K^+ concentration, or a fall in circulating volume of blood. Aldosterone reduces the elmination of Na^+ in the urine, sweat, saliva and bile by enhancing the active reabsorption of this ion from those fluids. It also increases the elimination of K^+ in those fluids in exchange of the reabsorbed Na^+. By retaining more Na^+ in the blood, it increases the reabsorption of water from the urine by the osmotic effect of Na^+. Due to the same reason, it increases the volume of blood and other extracellular fluids.

19. (a) Adrenaline is an emergency hormone whose concentration increases under stress conditions. Adrenaline is secreted from adrenal medulla. It initiates many bodily responses, including the stimulation of heart action and an increase in blood pressure, metabolic rate, and blood glucose concentration.

20. (d) A destruction of adrenal cortex by diseases like tuberculosis produces Addison's disease, due to the deficiency of glucocorticoids and mineralocorticoids which are secreted by the adrenal cortex regions zona fasciculata and zona glomerulosa respectively. Symptoms of Addison's disease include a bronze-like pigmentation of skin, low blood sugar, low plasma Na^+, high plasma K^+, increased urinary Na^+, nausea, vomiting and diarrhoea.

Cortisol is a glucocorticoid which regulates the metabolisms of carbohydrates, fats and proteins. A tumor of the adrenal cortex may secrete too much cortisol to produce Cushing's syndrome. High blood sugar, appearance of sugar in the urine, obesity, wasting of limb muscles, rise in plasma Na^+, fall in plasma K^+, rise in blood volume and high blood pressure are observed in the patient suffering from Cushing's syndrome.

21. (c) Insulin is a peptide hormone which is water soluble. Water soluble hormones require extracellular receptors that generate second messengers for carrying out their activity. Insulin binds to its specific receptor molecule located on the plasma membrane to form the hormone receptor complex, (HRC) which in turn generates second messengers that regulate cellular mechanism. Water soluble hormones (e.g., amino acid derivatives, peptides and protein hormones) do not enter the target cell.

22. (c) Insulin is an anabolic hormone. It increases the synthesis of fat in the adipose tissue from fatty acids as well as glucose. It promotes protein synthesis in tissues from amino acids. It reduces catabolism of proteins, breakdown and oxidation of fats by decreasing the enzmes which induce gluconeogenesis. Insulin increases the utilization of glucose in tissues and facilitates the storage of glucose as glycogen. A rise in blood glucose level and blood amino acids stimulates both synthesis and the secretion of insulin.

23. (d) Insulin plays a major role in the regulation of glucose homeostasis. Insulin mainly acts on hepatocytes and adipocytes (cells of

adipose tissue), and enhances cellular glucose uptake and utilisation. As a result, there is a rapid movement of glucose from blood to hepatocytes and adipocytes resulting in decreased blood glucose level (hypoglycemia). Insulin stimulates conversion of glucose to glycogen (glycogenesis) in the target cells. Glucagon is a hyperglycemic hormone. Glucagon acts mainly on the liver cells (hepatocytes) and stimulates glycogenolysis which also contributes to a complex disorder called diabetes mellitus.

24. **(c)** Males have more stature than females because of the action of male sex hormone-testosterone which is secreted by testis in males. Body starts secreting testosterone from the age of puberty. Its secretion is under the influence of Luteinizing Hormone (LH) of the anterior lobe of pituitary gland. Testosterone controls the development of secondary sexual characters in males like hoarseness of voice, development of facial hairs, bone growth, calcium retention, closing of epiphysial cartilage. The total quantity of bone matrix increases. The pelvic outlet is narrowed and lengthened. The strength of the pelvic bones increases to carry more loads. That is why males have more stature than females after puberty when this hormone is present in the blood. hCG (Human Chorionic Gonadotropin) is the hormone secreted by human placenta during pregnancy. hCG enlarges the corpus luteum in the mother's ovary and stimulates it to secrete progesterone.

25. **(a)** Based on the mode of secretion, the glands are of three types : mesocrine, apocrine and holocrine. Mammary glands that are present in mammals to feed the young ones with milk are the example of apocrine glands. In apocrine glands, the secretion accumulates as secretory granules in the distal part of the cell. This part later breaks down and leaves as a secretion.

26. **(b)** Oxytocin acts on the smooth muscles of our body and stimulates their contraction. In females, it stimulates a vigorous contraction of uterus at the time of child birth, and milk ejection from the mammary gland during suckling.

27. **(d)** LH (luteinizing hormone) is also known as Interstitial Cell Stimulating Hormone (ICSH). It stimulates the interstitial cells of leydig (testis) to secrete the male sex hormone testosterone and other androgen to regulate the secondary sexual characteristics.

The follicle stimulating hormone (FSH) is secreted by anterior pituitary. It stimulates the testes in the males to produce sperms and the ovaries in the female to produce ova. It also stimulates ovaries to secrete female sex hormones called estrogens.

28. **(c)** Estrogen is synthesized and secreted mainly by the growing ovarian follicles. Menopause is the time in a woman's life when the ovaries cease to produce an egg every month. Therefore, menstruation ceases gradually. During this condition ovaries fail to respond or may be resistant to FSH. In this case, FSH levels are very high and the estrogen level very low. This may happen because both the ovaries by menopause have run out of ovarian follicles. So, menopause may begin when no follicles, there is a reduced supply of estrogen and progesterone.

29. **(d)** Oxytocin hormone is also known as 'milk ejection hormone' because oxytocin induces contractions of the mammary gland muscles and helps in the flow of stored milk from the mammary glands to the mouth of the suckling infant. Oxytocin contracts the smooth muscles of uterus and mammary glands. Uterine contractions, stimulated by oxytocin at the end of pregnancy, help in child-birth. That is why, it is also called 'birth hormone'.

Prolactin or lactogenic hormone or luteotrophic hormone (LTH) is secreted by the anterior pituitary which helps in the growth of mammary glands during pregnancy and initiates the secretion of milk after child-birth.

30. **(a)** The Juxtaglomerular cells of kidney produce erythropoietin which is responsible for stimulating the formation of RBCs.

Chapter 23

Reproduction in Organisms

Directions: In the following questions, a statement of assertion is followed by a statement of reason. Mark the correct choice as:

(a) If both Assertion and Reason are true and Reason is the correct explanation of Assertion.
(b) If both Assertion and Reason are true but Reason is not the correct explanation of Assertion.
(c) If Assertion is true but Reason is false.
(d) If both Assertion and Reason are false.

1. **Assertion:** Asexual reproduction is also known as blastogenesis.
Reason: There is no formation and fusion of gametes in asexual reproduction.
2. **Assertion:** Asexual reproduction involves formation of clones of an organism.
Reason: Clones are morphologically and genetically similar individuals.
3. **Assertion:** Algae and fungi switch to asexual method of reproduction before the onset of adverse conditions.
Reason: Asexual reproduction may introduce variations and leads to the formation of many clones.
4. **Assertion:** The life span of plants is greater than animals.
Reason: Plants continue their growth at their tips.
5. **Assertion:** Organisms that reproduce by binary fission are immortal.
Reason: Such organisms have special kind of rejuvenation capability.
6. **Assertion:** Several seed bearing plants propagate vegetatively.
Reason: Sweet potatoes undergo vegetative propagation by means of root tubers.
7. **Assertion:** Specialised plant structures such as rhizomes, tubers, corms, bulbs, etc., are excellent methods of a sexual reproduction.
Reason: They are common means of propagation in most of monocot families.
8. **Assertion:** The main function of stem is reproduction.
Reason: Stem does not bear leaves to manufacture food for plants.
9. **Assertion:** Rhizomes, tubers and corms are excellent methods of sexual reproduction.
Reason: Autogamy is transfer of pollen from anther of one flower to stigma of another.
10. **Assertion:** A plant can be retained and multiplied indefinitely without any change or variation through asexual reproduction.
Reason: Asexual reproduction does not involve meiosis and syngamy.
11. **Assertion :** Runners are grown above the ground horizontally or prostrate develop at the base of erect shoots.
Reason : Runners bear nodes and internodes.
12. **Assertion :** Sponges are less specialized ones.
Reason : Sponges show a high power of regeneration.
13. **Assertion :** Angiospermic flowers perform the function of sexual reproduction.
Reason : The male and female reproductive structures are found in the flowers.
14. **Assertion :** Many plants are propagated vegetatively even though they bear seeds.
Reason : Potatoes multiply by tubers, apple by cutting.
15. **Assertion :** Leaves of *Bryophyllum, Begonia* help in vegetative multiplication.
Reason : Leaves of these plants possess adventitious buds. **[AIIMS 2014]**
16. **Assertion:** Grafting is cannot be usually performed in monocots.
Reason: Successful grafting requires that cambia of both stock and scion fuse and form new vascular tissues.
17. **Assertion:** Offsprings formed by asexual reproduction are called clones.
Reason: Clones are morphologically similar.
18. **Assertion:** Vegetative reproduction is a kind of asexual reproduction in plants.
Reason: The vegetative propagules give rise to offspring.

19. **Assertion:** Isogametes are formed in majority of sexually reproducing organisms.
Reason: Morphologically distinct type of gametes are called isogametes.
20. **Assertion:** Algae and fish produce a large number of gametes.
Reason: They show internal fertilization.
21. **Assertion:** Chances of survival of young ones is greater in viviparous organisms.
Reason: All mammals are viviparous.
22. **Assertion:** The development of embryo from the zygote is called embryogenesis.
Reason: Cell divisions increase the number of cells in the developing embryo.
23. **Assertion:** Parthenogenesis does not play any role in organic evolution.
Reason: In parthenogenesis females develop new organisms without fertilization.
24. **Assertion:** Reproduction by zoospores occur in some higher fungi.
Reason: Zoospores are non-motile and non-flagellated spores.
25. **Assertion:** Asparagus can be vegetatively propagated with the stem.
Reason: It has unbranched swollen, underground stems with circular nodes that have buds for growth of daughter plants.
26. **Assertion:** The zygote developed from sexual reproduction is diploid.
Reason: In sexual reproduction, haploid gametes fuse and form zygote.
27. **Assertion:** Unisexual flowers should either be staminate or pistillate.
Reason: They are found in monoecious and dioecious plants as well.
28. **Assertion:** Red flowers are more frequently pollinated by honey bees.
Reason: Honey bees mainly visit flower for pollen grains.
29. **Assertion:** Viviparous animals provide better protection to the young ones.
Reason: The young ones, in viviparous animals are delivered after a certain stage of growth by the females.
30. **Assertion:** All organisms that reproduce sexually exhibit processes that are fundamentally similar.
Reason: In sexual reproduction, the sequence of events is pre-fertilisation, fertilisation and post -fertilisation.
31. **Assertion:** A large number of gametes are produced by organisms that exhibit external fertilization.
Reason: It helps to increase the chances of syngamy and produce a large number of offsprings ensure survival.
32. **Assertion:** Zygote is the link between two generations.
Reason: Zygote is the product of two gametes and producer of next generation.
33. **Assertion:** Zygote is formed inside the ovule in flowering plants.
Reason: The ovule develops into seed after fertilisation.
34. **Assertion:** Reproduction enables the continuity of the species for generations.
Reason: Reproduction is a biological process in which an organism gives rise to young ones similar to itself.
35. **Assertion:** It is difficult to define vegetative, reproductive and sensecent phases in perennial plant species.
Reason: Perennial plants have very short life span.
36. **Assertion:** Some female animals permit copulation only during oestrous cycle.
Reason: Oestrous cycle is observed in non-primate mammals.
37. **Assertion:** *Cucurbita* is a monoecious plant.
Reason: Both male and female flowers are present on the same plant.
38. **Assertion:** Endosperm in gymnosperms is haploid as it is formed before fertilization.
Reason: Endosperms is formed post-fertilization in angiosperms and is diploid.
39. **Assertion:** Gametes formed by sexual reproduction are haploid in nature.
Reason: Dioecious plants are those that have their reproductive structures on different plants.
40. **Assertion:** Papaya is a dioecious plant.
Reason: Dioecious plants are those that have their reproductive structures on different plants.
41. **Assertion:** In external fertilisation, syngamy occurs inside the female.
Reason: The offsprings produced are vulnerable to predators.
42. **Assertion:** Plants of new genetic sequence are not produced in apomixis.
Reason: Two individual of same genetic sequence meet.
43. **Assertion:** Water hyacinth is an invasive aquatic plant which spreads all over the water in a short period of time.
Reason: Water hyacinth can reproduce vegetatively.

Solutions

1. **(b)** Blastogenesis development of an organism from non-sexual reproductive units like buds fragments etc. In asexual reproduction there is no formation and fusion of gametes.

2. **(b)** The reproduction is known as asexual reproduction, when an offspring is produced by a single parent without the involvement of gamete formation. As a result, the offspring that are produced are not only similar to one another but are also exact copies of their parent. Such a group of morphologically and genetically similar individuals are called clones.

3. **(d)** Algae and fungi multiply asexually during favourable conditions but gametes are formed during unfavourable conditions. The gametes fuse to form zygotes which often develop a thick wall to become zygospores. The later are dispersed. Under favourable conditions zygospore germinates to form new organism. Sexual reproduction induces variations which may help in survival of organism.

4. **(a)** The plant at their tips possess meristematic tissues which help them to grow throughout their lives even though the rest of their bodies is mainly made up of sclerenchyma, xylem and cork.

5. **(b)** In binary fission, the reproductive unit is comprised of the parent body as a whole, which gives rise to two daugther cells upon completion of the process. There are, however, no remnants and thus, the parent body cannot be said to be dead. The parent continues its life in the form of two daughter cells and hence, organisms undergoing binary fission are regarded immortal.

6. **(b)** Formation of new plants by means of vegetative units as tubers, buds, rhizomes is called vegetative propagation. It is useful for producing large number of offsprings within a short time and for preserving qualities such as disease resistance. In sweet potato, root tubers take part in vegetative propagation.

7. **(a)** Asexual reproduction produces individuals that are genetically identical to the parent plant. Roots such as corms, stem tubers, rhizomes, and stolon undergo vegetative reproduction. They are usually found in monocotyledonous families.

8. **(d)** Stems have four main functions which are: Support for the elevation of leaves, flowers and fruits. The stems keep the leaves in the light and provide a place for the plant to keep its flowers and fruits. Transport of fluids between the roots and the shoots in the xylem and phloem.

9. **(d)** Asexual reproduction produces individuals that are genetically identical to the parent plant. Roots such as corms, stem tubers, rhizomes, and stolon undergo vegetative reproduction. Self-pollination occurs when pollen from one flower pollinates the same flower or other flowers of the same individual.

10. **(a)** In asexual mode of reproduction, the genetic constituent remains the same. So the offspring and parents are morphologically and genetically same.

11. **(b)** Runners are special, narrow, green, above ground horizontal or prostrate branches which develop at the bases of erect shoots.

12. **(b)** Sponges are non-motile animals attached to some solid support. The body design involves very minimal differentiation and division into tissues.

13. **(a)** Angiospermic flowers possess male and female sex organs and perform the sexual reproduction.

14. **(a)** Vegetative reproduction is asexual type of reproduction potato, sugarcane, apple, etc., are multiplied by asexual means.

15. **(a)** Vegetative propagation through leaves takes place in *Bryophyllum* and *Begonia*. The leaf in the plant is broad and has notches at its margins. Buds arise from notches and these buds are called epiphyllous buds.

16. **(a)** Grafting only works with dicots and gymnosperms, and not with monocots.

Monocots do not have a vascular cambium, which is needed for the process to work.

17. (b) Clones are genetically and morphologically similar to parent. Off spring are formed by a sexual reproduction.

18. (b) Vegetative reproduction is a kind of asexual reproduction in plants where offsprings are formed by vegetative propagules like tuber, sucker, runner, etc.

19. (d) In certain algae, the two gametes are so similar in appearance that they are called homogametes or isogametes. Therefore, it is not possible to differentiate them into male and female gametes. However, in most of the sexually reproducing organisms the gametes are of two morphologically dissimilar type, hence they are known as heterogametes or anisogametes.

20. (c) In most aquatic organisms, such as a majority of algae and fishes as well as amphibians, syngamy occurs in the external medium (water) i.e, outside the body of the organism. This type of gametic fusion is called external fertilisation. Organisms exhibiting external fertilisation show great synchrony between the sexes and release a large number of gametes into the surrounding medium (water) in order to enhance the chances of syngamy. A major disadvantage is that the offspring are extremely vulnerable to predators threatening their survival upto adulthood.

21. (c) The zygote develops into a young one inside the body of the female organism in viviparous animals. After attaining a certain stage of growth, the young ones are delivered out of the body of the female organism. The chances of survival of young ones is greater in viviparous organisms because of proper embryonic care and protection. All mammals are not viviparous; some are egg-laying, i.e., oviparous e.g., duck -billed *platypus*.

22. (b) Embryogenesis refers to the process of development of embryo from the zygote. During embryogenesis, zygote undergoes cell divison (mitosis) and cell differentiation. While cell divisions increase the number of cells in the developing embryo; cell differentiation helps groups of cells to undergo certain modifications to form specialised tissues and organs to form an organism.

23. (a) Parthenogenesis is the development of an egg (ovum) into a complete individual without fertilization. Parthenogenesis occurs in its natural course in many invertebrates like insects, arachnids, some vertebrates and some birds (e.g., turkeys). Parthenogenesis eliminates variations in a population so it does not play any role in organic evolution.

24. (d) The zoospores are special kind of motile and flagellated spores produced inside the zoosporangia. They are generally naked (witout cell wall). The flagella helps to swim in aquatic habitats for proper dispersal. The reproduction by zoospores occurs in some lower fungi phycomycetes *e.g., Albugo, Phytophthora, etc. and some algae (e.g., Chlamydomonas Ulothrix).*

25. (d) Asparagus has fleshy roots which develop adventitious buds. These take part in vegetative propagation and develop into new plants under suitable conditions.

26. (a) Gametes are haploid irrespective of whether the structures or cells producing them are haploid or diploid. It is due to meiosis which occurs in the life of all sexually reproducing organisms. The strucutre formed by the fusion of gametes is always diploid.

27. (b) In angiosperms, the unisexual male flower bears stamens (staminate) and the unisexual female flower bears pistil (pistillate). Monoecious refers to a condition in flowering plants where both male and female flowers are present in the same plant, while dioecious refers to them being present in separate individuals.

28. (d) Bees utilize ultraviolet radiations for the purpose of observation. They are primarily attracted to yellow, blue and purple flowers. Red flowers are seldom visited by honey bees as red appears black in ultraviolet radiation. Honey bees visit flowers for both nectar and pollen grains.

29. (a) The zygote develops inside the body of the female in viviparous animals which is delivered only after it has undergone certain amount of growth. The offsprings

have a better chance of surival in viviparous animals.

30. (b) These events may be grouped into three stages: The pre-fertilization, fertilization and the post-fertilization events. In the first stage of sexual reproduction, "meiosis", the number of chromosomes is reduced from a diploid number (2n) to a haploid number (n). During "fertilization", haploid gametes come together to form a diploid zygote and the original number of chromosomes is restored.

31. (a) Organisms that undergo external fertilisation are often vulnerable to predators and productions of a large number of offsprings helps the species to continue even after predation.

32. (a) Zygote is the product of two gametes and if it survives it will then produce the gamete (male or female gamete) for next generation.

33. (a) In flowering plants the zygote is formed inside the ovule and the zygote then develops into embryo and the ovule into seed.

34. (a) Reproduction is a biological process in which an organism produces young ones like itself. It is one of the most important characteristics of the living organisms. Reproduction mainatins the continuity of species by producing the same form over generations.

35. (c) Perennial plants live for many years i.e., they have a very long life span. Hence, it becomes very difficult to define and study their vegetative, reproductive and sensecent phases.

36. (b) In non-primate mammals like cows, sheep, rats, deer, dogs, tiger, etc., cyclical changes during reproduction and are called oestrous cycle. It consists of a short period of oestros or heat (e.g., 12–24 hours in cow) followed by an oestrous or passive period. Sex urge is increased and the female permits copulation only during oestrous period.

37. (a) In higher organisms, sex organs develop, which differentiate male and female organisms. When both male and female flowers are present on the same plant, it is called monoecious plant. e.g., Maize, coconut and cucurbits.

38. (c) The endosperm in angiosperms is of a special type formed post-fertilization as a product of fusion of a male gamete with the diploid secondary nucleus present in the central cell, and is thus triploid in nature.

39. (a) Meiocytes (gamete mother cell) are specialised cells in diploid organisms that undergo meiosis to form haploid gametes. Gametes have only one set of chromosomes.

40. (a) Dioecious is the term used to describe unisexual condition, e.g. papaya and *Marchantia*.

41. (d) External fertilisation is the type of fertilisation that occurs outside female body. The offsprings develop outside and are thus exposed to environmental pressures and predators, e.g., bony fish and frog.

42. (b) Apomixis is an asexual reproduction that occurs without fertilization and not involving meiosis. One example of apomixis is the apomictic parthenogenesis. It its one in which the egg cell is produced through mitosis. It then develops directly into an embryo without the prior fertilization. The offspring from apomictic parthenogenesis would therefore be full clones of the maternal parent. The apomictic parthenogenesis is in contrast to another form of parthenogenesis, which is automictic parthenogenesis. The latter involves meiotic division and therefore produces haploid gametes. The resulting offspring would therefore be half clones of the mother in contrast to the offspring of apomictic parthenogenesis that are full clones of the mother. Apomixis is more common in plants.

43. (a) The aquatic plant 'water hyacinth' is one of the most invasive weeds found growing wherever there is standing water. It drains oxygen from the water, which leads to death of other aquatic forms of life. It can propagate vegetavtively at a phenomenal rate and spread all over the water body in a short period of time, hence it is very difficult to get rid off.

Chapter 24 Sexual Reproduction in Flowering Plants

Directions: In the following questions, a statement of assertion is followed by a statement of reason. Mark the correct choice as:
(a) If both Assertion and Reason are true and Reason is the correct explanation of Assertion.
(b) If both Assertion and Reason are true but Reason is not the correct explanation of Assertion.
(c) If Assertion is true but Reason is false.
(d) If both Assertion and Reason are false.

1. **Assertion :** Autogamy is a transfer of pollen grains from an anther to the stigma of the same flower on the same plant.
Reason : Xenogamy is pollination between two flowers on different plants.
2. **Assertion :** Insects visit flower to gather honey.
Reason : Attraction of flowers prevents the insects from damaging other parts of the plant. **[AIIMS 2004]**
3. **Assertion :** Pollen mother cells (PMCs) are the first male gametophytic cells.
Reason : Each PMC gives rise to two pollens. **[AIIMS 2009]**
4. **Assertion :** Chasmogamous flowers require pollinating agents.
Reason : Cleistogamous flowers do not expose their sex organs. **[AIIMS 2012]**
5. **Assertion:** Gynoecium consists of pistil.
Reason: It represents the male reproductive part in flowering plants.
6. **Assertion:** Flowers are the structures related to sexual reproduction in flowering plants.
Reason: Various embryological processes of plants occur in a flower.
7. **Assertion:** Geitonogamy is genetically similar to autogamy.
Reason: The pollen grains come from same plant.
8. **Assertion:** Cleistogamous flowers produce assured seed set in the absence of pollinators.
Reason: These flowers do not open at all.
9. **Assertion:** A typical microsporangium of angiosperms is generally surrounded by four wall layers.
Reason: The outer three wall layers perform the function of protection and help in dehiscence of anther to release the pollen.
10. **Assertion:** Exine of a pollen grain is made up of sporopollenins which are resistant to high temperatures, strong acids or alkali as well as enzymatic degradation.
Reason: Sporopollenins are absent in the region of germ pores.
11. **Assertion:** An angiospermous flower represents the modified condensed shoot which performs the function of sexual reproduction.
Reason: The fertile leaves of the shoot become modified into microsporophylls and magasporophylls which bear ovules and anthers respectively.
12. **Assertion:** Although geitonogamy is functionally cross-pollination involving a pollinating agent, genetically it is similar to autogamy since the pollen grains come from the same parent.
Reason: In getionogamy, pollen grains from the anthers of one flower are transferred to the stigma of another flower borne on the same plant.
13. **Assertion:** The pre-pollination growth of male gametophyte occurs inside the microsporangium whereas the rest of the growth occurs over the female reproductive organs.
Reason: Growth of the entire female gametophyte occurs inside the megaspora-ngium.
14. **Assertion:** Hydrophily is a major mode of pollination in most of the aquatic plants in angiosperms.
Reason: Almost all the aquatic dicot and monocot plants require water for the transport of male gametes and for fertilisation.

15. **Assertion:** Pollen grains from male parent are mostly transferred to the stigma in the female parent by some external agency.
Reason: This is because the male flowers or male organs have no internal device to reach the female organs in another flower.

16. **Assertion:** In angiosperms, the male gametophyte is the pollen grain.
Reason: Pollen grain contains stigma, style and ovary.

17. **Assertion:** Xenogamy is pollination between two flowers on different plants.
Reason: Pollination between two flowers on the same plant is autogamy.

18. **Assertion:** Anemophilous plants have to produce enormous quantities of pollen.
Reason: Because during the transit of pollen through a wind, a considerable amount of pollen is lost.

19. **Assertion:** Tapetum helps in the dehiscence of microspores from tetrad.
Reason: It shows callose activity.

20. **Assertion:** Megaspore mother cell undergoes meiosis to produce four haploid gametes.
Reason: Megaspore mother cell is $2n$, meiosis gives haploid structure.

21. **Assertion:** Megaspore mother cell undergoes meiosis to produce four megaspores.
Reason: Megaspore mother cell and megaspore both are haploid.

22. **Assertion:** Meiosis is the cell division which occurs in sexually reproducing organisms.
Reason: Meiotic cell division results into two cells having exactly same genetic make up.

23. **Assertion :** If pollen mother cells has 42 chromosomes, the pollen has only 21 chromosomes.
Reason : Pollens are formed after meiosis in pollen mother cell. **[AIIMS 1997]**

24. **Assertion:** In a microsporangium, the tapetal cells possesss little cytoplasm and generally have a single prominent nucleus.
Reason: During microsporogenesis, the microspore mother cells (MMCs) undergo mitotic divisions to produce haploid microspore tetrads.

25. **Assertion:** In most angiosperms, microspores of a tetrad grow and separate from one another shortly after meiosis.
Reason: In the members of familes Orchidaceae and Asclepiadaceae, all the pollen grains of a sporangium remain united to form a compact structure called pollinium.

26. **Assertion :** Double fertilization is characteristic feature of angiospersms.
Reason : Double fertilization involves two fusions. **[AIIMS 2016]**

27. **Assertion :** The ovary forms fruit after fertilization.
Reason : The ovary forms parthenocarpic fruits without fertilization.

28. **Assertion :** The two cotyledons in seed are embryonic leaves.
Reason : The embryo contains radicle and plumule.

29. **Assertion :** The largest cell of the embryo sac is central cell.
Reason : It consists of a fused nuclei.

30. **Assertion :** Endosperm is a nutritive tissue and it is triploid.
Reason : Endosperm is formed by fusion of secondary nucleus to second male gamete. It is used by developing embryo.

31. **Assertion :** The megaspore mother cell divides meiotically to produce four spores.
Reason : Megaspore mother cells are haploid and megaspore is diploid.

32. **Assertion :** Nuclear endosperm is formed by subsequent nuclear division without wall formation.
Reason : Coconut is an example of such endosperm, where the endosperm remains nuclear throughout the development of the fruit.

33. **Assertion:** The method of development of embryo sac from a single functional megaspore is termed as monosporic development.
Reason: In monosporic type of embryo sac development, usually the megaspore which is situated towards micropylar end remains functional.

34. **Assertion:** The suspensor serves as the main nutritive tissues for the embryo during embryo development in dicots.
Reason: The last cell of the suspensor at the end adjacent to the embryo is known as haustorium.

35. **Assertion:** The embryo capable of germination should have well-developed radicle plumule and one or two cotyledons.
Reason: In Orobanchaceae and Orchidaceae the embryo never differentiates a true radicle, plumule and cotyledons, but can germinate.

36. **Assertion:** Proembryo is restricted to 2-celled stage.
Reason: It has one basal and one apical cell.
37. **Assertion:** Anatropous type of ovule is most common.
Reason: Anatropous ovule resembles a horse-shoe.
38. **Assertion:** Megaspore mother cell undergoes meiotic division.
Reason: All four megaspores form female gametophyte.
39. **Assertion:** The chalazal cells of the embryo sac are called central cell.
Reason: They play nutritive role for embryo sac.
40. **Assertion:** The largest cell of the embryo sac is central cell.
Reason: It consists of a fused nuclei.
41. **Assertion:** Synergids play an important role in directing pollen tube growth.
Reason: Because synergids secrete some chemotropically active substance.
42. **Assertion:** The two sperms in a pollen tube often change their shape.
Reason: The sperms are released in the synergid as intact cells but only their nuclei migrate.
43. **Assertion:** In apomixis, plants of new genetic variations are not produced.
Reason: In apomixis, reductional division takes place.
44. **Assertion:** Apomixis is a form of asexual reproduction that mimics sexual reproduction in plants.
Reason: Apomixis involves the production of seeds without the fusion of gametes.
45. **Assertion:** The pollen sterility has been attributed to the malfunctioning of tapetum.
Reason: Premature degeneration of the tapetum deprives the developing spores of its nutrition.
46. **Assertion:** Self-incompatibility is a genetic mechanism which prevents pollen from the same flower or other flowers of the same plant from fertilizing the ovules by inhibiting pollen germination or pollen tube growth in the pistil.
Reason: In gametophytic self-incompatibility, the incompatibility reaction is determined by the genotype of the sporophytic tissue of the plant frome which the pollen is derived.
47. **Assertion:** Endosperm development precedes embryo development in angiosperms.
Reason: Double fertilization ensures that the nutritive tissue is formed only when the formation of embryo has taken place so that the energy spent on the formation of endosperm does not get wasted.
48. **Assertion:** Coconut water represents the cellular endosperm and the surrounding white kernel represents the free-nuclear endosperm in Cocos nucifera.
Reason: PEN undergoes a number of free nuclear divisions all of which are subsequently followed by wall formation.
49. **Assertion:** Ex-albuminous seeds do not possess any residual endosperm, as it is compeltely consumed during embryo development.
Reason: Wheat, castor, pea and groundnut are all the examples of ex-albuminous seeds.
50. **Assertion:** Formation of nucellar endosperm occurs by subsequent nuclear division without wall formation.
Reason: Coconut is an example of such endosperm, where the endosperm remains nuclear throughout the development of the fruit.
51. **Assertion:** Cellular endosperm is formed by both nuclear division and wall formation.
Reason: It lacks haustoria.
52. **Assertion:** Non-albuminous seeds have no residual endosperm.
Reason: The endosperm is completely consumed during embryo development.
53. **Assertion:** Mango is a true fruit.
Reason: The thalamus also contributes to formation of fruit in false fruits.
54. **Assertion:** Some fruits are seedless or contain non-viable seeds.
Reason: They are produced without fertilisation.
55. **Assertion:** The first step in artificial hybridisation is removal of anthers.
Reason: It prevents contamination of anthers.
56. **Assertion:** Endosperm development proceeds embryo development.
Reason: It assures nutrition to developing embryo.

Solutions

1. (c) Based on the destination of pollen grains, two types of pollination are recognised. When pollen grains are transferred from an anther to the stigma of the same flower the process is called self-pollination or autogamy. Cross-pollination is further classified depending on whether the pollination has occurred between two flowers on the same plant (geitonogamy) or between two flowers on different plants (xenogamy).
2. (d) Honey bee visit flowers to gather nectar and turn it into honey. Visiting of insects for nectar helps in pollination.
3. (d) Primary sporogenous cell gives rise to microspore mother cells or pollen mother cells (PMCs). They are sporophytic in nature *i.e.*, diploid. These cells undergo meiosis (reduction division) which gives rise to 4 microspores or pollens and this formation of microspores or pollens is called microsporogenesis. Microspores represent the beginning of the gametophytic phase and they are haploid in nature.
4. (b) The majority of angiosperms bear chasmogamous flowers, which means the flowers expose their mature anthers and stigma to the pollinating agents. There is another group of plants which set seeds without exposing their sex organs. Such flowers are called cleistogamous and the phenomenon is cleistogamy.
5. (c) The gynoecium represents the female reproductive part of the flower consisting of pistil.
6. (a) Embryological processes occur in ovary, which is a part of flower.
7. (a) Geitonogamy is functionally cross-pollination involving pollinating agent, genetically it is similar to autogamy since the pollen grains come from the same plant.
8. (a) Cleistogamous flowers do not open at all thus ensuring fertilisation and hence produce assured seed-set even in the absence of pollinators.
9. (b) A typical microsporangium consists of two parts, outer wall and central homogeneous sporogenous tissue. Microsporangial wall has four types of layers– epidermis, endothecium, 1–3 middle layers and tapetum. The outer three wall layers perform the function of protection in the young anther and mechanism of dehiscence in the ripe anther.
10. (b) Wall of a pollen grain consists of two layers– outer exine and inner intine. Exine is the hard outer layer which is made up of sporopollenin. Sporopollenin is one of the most resistant organic material known. It can withstand high temperature, strong acids or alkali and is not degraded by enzymes. Because of the presence of sporopollenin, pollen grains are well preserved as fossils. At certain places, the exine is thin or absent, these areas may have thickened intine or deposition of callose. They are called germ pores (if rounded) or germinal furrows (if elongated). Sporopollenin is absent in the region of germ pores or germinal furrows.
11. (c) A flower is a modified condensed shoot specialised to carry out the function of sexual reproduction in angiosperms. Like a branch, it arises in the axil of a small leaf like structure called bract. The receptalce (thalamus or torus) of a flower supports all the floral appendages (i.e., sepals, petals, stamens and carpels). The receptalce consists of several crowded nodes which are separated by condensed internodes. The fertile leaves of the shoot become microsporophylls (stamens) and megasporo phylls (carpels) which bear anthers and ovules respectively. The anthers produce pollen grains and the ovules possess eggs.
12. (a) Geitonogamy is a type of pollination in which pollen grains of one flower are transferred to the stigma of another flower belonging to either the same plant or genetically similar plant. It usually occurs

in plants which show monoecious condition (unisexual male and female flowers borne on the same plant. Thus, geitonogamy is functionally cross pollination as it involves pollinating agent to carry out pollination, but genetically it is similar to autogamy (self-pollination) since the pollen grains come from the genetically same plant.

13. (b) Pollen grain or microspore is the first cell of male gametophyte generation and represents immature male gametophyte generation and represents immature male gametophyte. Development of male gametophyte is precocious, that is, it begins inside the microsporangium or pollen sac. The pollen grain is shed at 2 or 3 celled stage. The liberated pollen grains are transferred to the receptive surface of the carpel (i.e., stigma) through pollination. Growth of the pollen grain further occurs over the female reproductive organs. Female gametophyte or embryo sac is an oval multicellular haploid structure which is embedded in the nucellus towards micropylar end of the ovule (or integumented megasporangium). Whole of the development of female gametophyte occurs inside the megasporangium.

14. (d) Hydrophily is the mode of pollination which is accomplished through the agency of water. Pollination by water is quite rare in flowering plants and is limited to only about 30 genera, mostly monocotyledons e.g., *Vallisneria, Zostera, Ceratophyllum,* etc. In many aquatic plants with emergent flowers, pollination occurs by wind or insects, e.g., Lotus, Water Lily, Water Hyacinth, etc.

15. (a) Internal copulatory organs are absent in plants and thus the aid of an external agency is required for the transfer of pollen grains from the anther to the stigma.

16. (c) Pollen grain does not contain the stigma, style and ovary. It is female gametophyte (gynoecium) which contains stigma, style and ovary.

17. (c) Two types of pollination are recognised based on the destination of pollen grains. When pollen grains are transferred from an anther to the stigma of the same flower, the process is called self pollination or autogamy. Cross-pollination is further classified depending on whether the pollination has occurred between two flowers on the same plant (geitonogamy) or between two flowers on different plants (xenogamy).

18. (a) Wind pollinated or anemophilous plants produce a large amount of pollen to compensate for the loss of pollen grains during transfer.

19. (a) In *Tradescantia bracteata,* it has been shown that the plasmodial cytoplasm derived from the tapetum has callose activity. Shortly before callose degradation starts the cytoplasm of tapetal cells show certain vesicles which are probably associated with callose activity. This suggests that sporophytic tissue, presumably tapetum, is involved in the synthesis of callose enzyme for the release of microspores in a tetrad by degrading the callose wall.

20. (a) Megaspore mother cell is diploid and after meiosis four haploid megaspores are formed.

21. (c) Megaspore mother cell is diploid and megaspore is haploid.

22. (c) In meiotic cell division the resultant cell does not have the exact genetic make up due to the process of crossing over. Crossing over takes place in the meiotic cell division only.

23. (a) Pollen mother cells undergo meiosis and produce pollen grains. The pollen grains have haploid number of chromosomes.

24. (d) Tapetum is the innermost wall layer of a microsporangium. It nourishes the developing pollen grains. The tapetal cells enlarge radially and become filled with dense protoplasmic contents as well as nutrients. Tapetal cells are generally multinucleate or their nucleus becomes polyploid due to endoploidy. Microsporogenesis refers to the process of formation of haploid microspores (or pollen grains) from a microspore mother cell (MMC) or pollen mother cell (PMC_ through meiosis (and not mitosis).

25. (b) In most angiosperms, microspores (pollen grains) of a tetrad grow and separate from one another shortly after meiosis. However, in some plants the spores tend to remain together in tetrads for longer periods and develop into pollen grains (*e.g., Drimys, Drosera*). In many members of families Orchidaceae and Asclepiadaceae, all the microspores in a sporangium remain united to form a pollinium.

26. (b) Double fertilization is a characteristic feature of angiosperms. It involves two fusions in which one female gametes fuse with egg cell to form zygote and other male gamete fuses with the diploid secondary nucleus to produce triploid primary endosperm nucleus.

27. (b) After fertilization the ovary begins to grow and gradually matures into the fruit. In some cultivated varieties of oranges, banana, grapes, apples, pineapples and some other fruits the ovary may grow into the fruit without fertilization. Such a fruit is seedless or with immature seeds and is known as the parthenocarpic fruits.

28. (b) In angiosperms, cotyledons are embryonic leaves. Embryo also has radicle and plumule which gives rise to root and shoot respectively.

29. (b) The central cell is the largest cell of the embryo sac. It has a highly vacuolate cytoplasm which is rich in reserve food and golgi bodies. In the middle the cell contains two polar nuclei which have large nucleoli. The polar nuclei fuse to form a single diploid secondary or fusion nucleus.

30. (a) In angiosperm, triploid endosperm is formed by fusion of secondary nucleus and second male gamete. This tissue is used by developing embryo.

31. (c) The megaspore mother cell is diploid. This divides by meiotic division and produce four haploid megaspores.

32. (c) In nuclear type of endosperm the division of the primary endosperm nucleus and a few subsequent nuclear division are not accompanied by wall formation. So numerous nuclei are freely suspended in its sap. In coconut, the primary endosperm nucleus undergoes a number of free nuclear divisions. When the fruit is about 50 mm long before the embryo sac gets filled with a clear fluid in which float numerous nuclei of various sizes. At a later stage (about 100 mm long fruit) the suspension shows in addition to free nuclei, several cells each enclosing variable number of nuclei. Gradually these cells and free nuclei start setting at the periphery of the cavity and layers of cellular endosperm start appearing. In mature coconuts the liquid endosperm becomes milky and it does not contain free nuclei or cell.

33. (c) In monosporic (*Polygonum*) type of development of embryo sac, only one megaspore situated towards chalazal end remains functional. The remaining three megaspores gradually degenerate and finally disappear. The functional haploid megaspore enlarges in size and, by means of three successive mitotic divisions, gives rise to an eight-nucleate embryo sac. This type of embryo sac development occurs in a majority of flowering plants and the common example is *Polygonum*.

34. (d) During embryo development in dicots, the suspensor cell divides transversely a few times to produce a filamentous suspensor of 6-10 cells. The first cell of suspenor towards the micropylar end becomes swollen and functions as haustorium whereas the last cell of suspensor at the end adjacent to the embryo is known as hypophysis. The function of the suspensor is to anchor the embryo to the embryo sac and push it deep into the endoperm so that the embyo lies in a nutritionally favourable environment.

35. (b) Embryo generally possesses an embryonic root (radicle) a embryonic shoot (plumule) and one or two cotyledons irrespective of its mode of development a nature. Some groups of plants however, are characterised by the presence of reduced embryos, lacking the differentiation of these organs, for example, the plants of Balanophoraceae, Orchidaceae, Orobanchceae.

36. (a) From the 2-celled stage until the initiation of organs the embryo is commonly called proembryo. In the majority of angiosperms the zygote divides transversely, resulting in small apical cell towards the interior of the embryo sac and a large basal cell.

37. (c) The ovules where the micropyle comes to lie close to the funiculus due to unilateral growth of the ovule are called anatropous. This is the most common type of ovule in angiosperms. The curvature of the ovule also affects the nucellus in a way that the later becomes horse shoe-shaped the ovule is called amphitropous.

38. (c) One hypodermal nucellar cell of the micropylar region differentiates the sporogenous cell. It forms a diploid megaspore mother cell or megasporocyte. The megaspore mother cells undergo meiosis and forms a row of four haploid megaspores. Only the chalazal megaspore remains functional Megaspore enlarges and gives rise to female gametophyte, also called embryo sac.

39. (b) The three chalazal cells of the embryo sac are called antipodal cells. They are the vegetative cells of the embryo sac which may degenerate soon or take part in absorbing nourishment from the surrounding nucellar cells. Internally they are connected with the central cell by means of plasmodesmata.

40. (b) The central cell is the largest cell of the embryo sac. It consists of a highly vacuolate cytoplasm which is rich in reserve food and Golgi bodies. In the middle the cell contains two polar nuclei which have large nucleoli. The polar nuclei fuse to form a single diploid secondary or fusion nucleus.

41. (a) Synergids are special type of cells found in the embryo sac which direct the growth of the pollen tube towards the egg cell for fertilization by the sperm cell.

42. (b) Each pollen grain contains a vegetative cell, and a generative cell that divides to form two sperm cells. The vegetative cell then produces the pollen tube, a tubular protrusion from the pollen grain, which carries the sperm cells within its cytoplasm. The sperm cells are the male gametes that will join with the egg cell and the central cell in double fertilization. The two sperms in a pollen tube often change their shape.

43. (c) Apomixis is the type of asexual reproduction in which development of reproductive propagules takes place without meiosis and syngamy. There are two kinds of apomixis (asexual reproduction) in flowering plants: Agamospermy and vegetative propagation. Agamospermy is further divided into three types:

(i) Adventive Embryony: Formation of embryo directly from the diploid sporophytic cells (nucellus integument) of ovule (other than zygote) is called adventives embryony, e.g., Citrus.

(ii) Parthenogenesis: Formation of embryo from unfertilized egg.

(iii) Apospory and apogamy: Formation of embryo from any other cell of embryo sac (other than egg) without fertilization.

During embryogenesis, an embryo develops from zygote inside the embryo sac and the embryo sac becomes an endosperm. Apomictic embryo, if develops, increases the number of embryos inside the seed. Occurrence of more than one embryo in a seed is called polyembryony.

44. (a) Apomixis is a mode of reproduction in some plants which results in the formation of seeds without gametic fusion. It is a form of asexual reproduction. In plants, apomixis commonly mimics sexual reproduction but produces seeds without fertilization, e.g., some species of Asteraceae and grasses. There are several methods of apomictic development in seeds.

45. (a) Tapetum acts as a nourishing tissue for the developing microspores. If degeneration of tapetum occurs earlier than usually the spores are deprived of nutrition and as a result the pollen grains released are sterile.

46. (c) Self-incompatibility is the inability of pollen from a flower to germinate on the stigma of the same flower (or other flower of same plant). Two categories of self-incompatibility have been recognized depending on the origin of factors determining the mating types :

(i) Gametophytic self-incompatibility (GSI). The incompatibility process is determined by the genotype of male gametophyte (pollen) itself, e.g., Liliaceae, Poaceae, Solanaceae.

(ii) Sporophytic self-incompatibility (SSI). The incompatibility process is controlled by the genotype of the sporophytic tissue of the plant from which the pollen is derived, e.g., Asteraceae, Brassicaceae.

47. **(a)** During double fertilization occurs in angiosperms, one male gamete fuses with the egg to form the diploid zygote (syngamy or generative fertilization). the diploid zygote finally develops into embryo. The other male gamete fuses with the two polar nuclei (or secondary nucleus) to form the triploid primary endosperm nucleus, PEN (triple fusion or vegetative fertilization). Double fertilization ensures that the nutritive tissue is formed only when the formation of embryo has taken place by fertilization of the oosphere or egg so that the energy spent on the formation of endosperm does not go waste in case the fertilization fail.

48. **(d)** In *Cocos nucifera* (coconut), the coconut water is free-nuclear endosperm and the surrounding kernel represents the cellular endosperm. The primary endosperm nucleus (PEN) first undergoes a number of free nuclear divisions without wall formation to form a large number of free nuclei (free nuclear endosperm).

49. **(c)** In some seeds, the endosperm persists in the seed as food storage tissue. Such seeds are called endospermic or albuminous, e.g., Castor, Maize, Wheat, Barley, rubber, coconut. In others, the endosperm is completely eaten up by the growing embryo. The food for later development of embryo is then stored in cotyledons which become massive. Such seeds are non-endospermic or ex-albuminous, e.g., Pea, Gram, Bean, Groundnut.

50. **(c)** The division of the primary endosperm nucleus and a few subsequent nuclear division are not accompanied by wall formation in nucellar type of endosperm. So numerous nuclei freely suspended in its sap. In coconut, the primary endosperm nucleus undergoes a number of free nuclear divisions. When the fruit is about 50 *mm* long before the embryo sac gets filled with a clear fluid in which float numerous nuclei of various sizes. At a later stage the suspension shows in addition to free nuclei, several cells each enclosing variable number of nuclei.

51. **(c)** Cellular endosperm is characterized by the absence of free nuclear stage. The division of the primary endosperm nucleus and a few subsequent nuclear division are regularly followed by wall formation. The occurrence of haustoria is a common feature of this type of endosperm. The haustoria may be micropylar or chalazal. Occasionally, both types of haustoria are present in the same plant.

52. **(a)** In non-albuminous seeds the endosperm is fully consumed by the developing embryo and thus no residue is left.

53. **(b)** In false fruits the thalamus also contributes to fruit formation, e.g. apple, cashew nut, etc.

54. **(a)** parthenocarpic fruits are seedless because there is no fertilisation.

55. **(c)** Emasculation is done in hybridisation and female flower is bagged to prevent contamination.

56. **(a)** Endosperm is source of nutrition for the developing embryo, thus the nature ensures that endosperm is formed before starting the process of embryogenesis.

Chapter 25

Human Reproduction

Directions: In the following questions, a statement of assertion is followed by a statement of reason. Mark the correct choice as:

(a) If both Assertion and Reason are true and Reason is the correct explanation of Assertion.
(b) If both Assertion and Reason are true but Reason is not the correct explanation of Assertion.
(c) If Assertion is true but Reason is false.
(d) If both Assertion and Reason are false.

1. **Assertion :** In human male, testes are extra-abdominal and lie in scrotal sacs.
Reason : Scrotum acts as thermoregulator and keeps testicular temperature lower by 2°C for normal spermatogenesis.
2. **Assertion :** Testicular lobules are the compartments present in testes.
Reason : These lobules are involved in the process of fertilization. **[AIIMS 2016]**
3. **Assertion :** Interstitial cell is present in the region outside the seminiferous tubule called interstitial spaces.
Reason : Interstitial cells provide nutrition to the sertoli cells. **[AIIMS 2016, 2017]**
4. **Assertion:** The testes are situated outside the abdominal cavity within the scrotum.
Reason: Muscles in scrotum helps to maintain low temperature of testes, necessary for spermatogenesis.
5. **Assertion:** The bulbourethral gland is a male accessory gland.
Reason: Its secretion helps in the lubrication of the penis, thereby facilitating reproduction.
6. **Assertion:** Each seminiferous tubule is lined on its inside by three type of cells.
Reason: These cells are male germ cells, Sertoli cells and Leydig cells.
7. **Assertion:** In human male, there are perianal glands near the anus.
Reason: Perianal glands secretes sex-attractant pheromone which initiates sexual desire in human.
8. **Assertion:** Testes are located in the scrotum, outside the coelom.
Reason: A vaginal coelom partly surrounds the testes in the scrotum.
9. **Assertion:** Fimbriae are finger-like projections of the infundibulum part of oviduct which is closest to ovary.
Reason: They are important for collection of ovum after ovulation from ovary.
10. **Assertion:** Finger-like projections appear on the trophoblast called chorionic villi after implantation.
Reason: Chorionic villi are surrounded by the uterine tissue and maternal blood.
11. **Assertion:** Infundibulum is a funnel shaped part closer to ovary.
Reason: The edges of infundibulum helps in collection of the ovum after ovulation.
12. **Assertion:** The female external genitalia includes mons pubis, labia majora and labia minora.
Reason: The glandular tissue of each breast is divided into 5-10 mammary lobes.
13. **Assertion:** Vagina acts as copulation canal and fertilization canal.
Reason: Both insemination and fusion of gametes occur in the vagina of female.
14. **Assertion:** In the testis, spermatogenesis occurs in the seminiferous tubules and testosterone secretion takes place from the sertoli cells.
Reason: Testosterone brings growth and maturation of primany sex organs and also development of accessory sex characters.
15. **Assertion:** Spermatogenesis starts at the age of puberty.
Reason: There is a siginificant increase in level of gonadotropin releasing hormone at puberty.
16. **Assertion:** Human male ejaculates about 200 to 300 million sperms during coitus.
Reason: Only few reach the isthmus ampullary junction for process of fertilisation.
17. **Assertion:** The sperm head contains a cap-like structure called acrosome.
Reason: Acrosome is filled with enzymes that help in fertilisation of the ovum.

18. **Assertion:** A drop in temperature does not affect spermatogenesis.
Reason: During temperature drop, the smooth muscles contract and bring the testes closer to the pelvic cavity.
19. **Assertion:** The human male ejaculates about 50-100 million sperms during a coitus.
Reason: For normal shape and size.
20. **Assertion:** The type B spermatogonia undergo mitosis to form primary spermatocyte.
Reason: Primary spermatocyte completes the first meiotic division leading to secondary spermatocytes.
21. **Assertion:** The middle piece is called as power house of the sperm.
Reason: The numerous mitochondria coiling around axial filament produce energy for the movement of the tail.
22. **Assertion:** The regions outside the seminiferous tubules are called interstitial spaces, which contain Leydig cell.
Reason: Leydig cells synthesise and secrete testicular hormones called androgens.
23. **Assertion:** Primary spermatocytes of testes are haploid.
Reason: These are formed by meiosis-I in the spermatogonia.
24. **Assertion:** Stem cells possess the property of totipotency.
Reason: These cells can give rise to any type of cells.
25. **Assertion :** At puberty, human male develops secondary sexual characters.
Reason : At puberty, there is decreased secretion of testosterone in male.
26. **Assertion :** Head of sperm consists of acrosome and mitochondria.
Reason : Acrosome contains spiral row of mitochondria. **[AIIMS 2014]**
27. **Assertion:** In a Graafian follicle, the primary oocyte and the follicular cells may be regarded as sibling cells.
Reason: Both arise from the same parent cell the oogonium by mitotic division.
28. **Assertion:** The shape of the uterus is like an inverted pear.
Reason: The inner glandular layer that lines the uterine cavity is called as myometrium.
29. **Assertion:** Fallopian funnel of oviduct has finger-like fimbriae.
Reason: Graafian follicle of ovary is with secondary oocyte hanging in cavity called antrum.
30. **Assertion:** Production of FSH increases, while that of LH decreases in the ovulation phase.
Reason: Due to decrease in the level of LH, ovulation (releasing of ova) takes place.
31. **Assertion:** Graafian follicle ruptures at the mid of menstrual cycle releasing the ovum.
Reason: Both LH and FSH attain a peak level at the middle of cycle.
32. **Assertion:** Progesterone is required for maintenance of the endometrium.
Reason: Endometrium is essential for implanation of embryo.
33. **Assertion:** The endometrium undergoes cyclical changes during menstrual cycle.
Reason: The myometrium exhibits strong contractions during delivery of the baby.
34. **Assertion:** Menstrual phase is also called shedding tears of lost ovum.
Reason: In the menstrual phase, cast of endometrial lining along with ovum takes place due to reduced titre of oestrogen and progesterone.
35. **Assertion :** Penetration of sperm into ovum is a chemical process.
Reason : Acrosome of sperm secretes a lytic enzyme hyaluronidase which dissolves vitelline membrane of ovum.
36. **Assertion :** Size of breasts increases at puberty in human female.
Reason : Prolactin secretion starts at puberty.
37. **Assertion :** During fertilization only head of spermatozoa enters egg.
Reason : If several spermatozoa hit the egg at same time, all can enter the egg.
38. **Assertion :** Corpus luteum degenerates in the absence of fertilization.
Reason : Progesterone level decreases.
[AIIMS 2009]
39. **Assertion :** Mammalian ova produces hyaluronidase.
Reason : The eggs of mammal are microlecithal and telolecithal. **[AIIMS 2009]**
40. **Assertion:** Ovum retains most of the contents of the primary oocyte and is much lartger than a spermatozoa.
Reason: Ovum requires energy to go about in search of a spermatozoa for fertilisation.

41. **Assertion:** Not all copulation leads to pregnancy.
Reason: Fertilisation can only occur if the ovum and sperms are transported simultaneously to the ampullary isthmic junction.
42. **Assertion :** Implantation is the process of attachment of blastocyst on uterine endometrium.
Reason : Implantation is controlled by trophoblast and occurs by decidual cell reaction.
43. **Assertion:** Placenta is an endocrine gland.
Reason: It secretes many hormones essential for pregnancy.
44. **Assertion:** A woman passes out hCG in the urine during pregnancy.
Reason: The presence of hCG in urine is the basis for pregnancy test.
45. **Assertion:** Breast feeding during initial period of infant growth is recommended.
Reason: Colostrum contains several antibodies, essential to render immunity in newborns.
46. **Assertion:** During pregnancy, the levels of hormones like estrogens and progesterone are increased.
Reason: The increased production of these hormones is essential for foetal growth.
47. **Assertion:** Vigrous contraction of the uterus at the end of pregnancy causes expulsion.
Reason: The stimulatory reflex between the uterine contraction and oxytocin results in weakening contractions.
48. **Assertion:** There is generally monospermy in most of animals.
Reason: Vitelline membrane of ovum checks polyspermy.
49. **Assertion:** All Metatherian are placental mammals.
Reason: All placental mammals have menstrual cycle.
50. **Assertion:** Placenta in addition to connection with mother and foetus, is a ductless gland.
Reason: It releases human gonadotropins.
51. **Assertion :** Embryonic development proves inter-relationship and common ancestory of metazoans.
Reason : It involves similar sequence of five dynamic processes during development.
52. **Assertion :** In morula stage, cells divide without increase in size.
Reason : Zona pellucida remains undivided till cleavage is complete. **[AIIMS 1997]**
53. **Assertion:** The embryo with 8 to 16 blastomeres is called a morula.
Reason: The morula continues to divide and transforms into trophoblast.
54. **Assertion:** Cleavage is also called fractionating process.
Reason: In cleavage, number of blastomere increases but size of blastomere decreases.
55. **Assertion:** Gastrular movements are morphogenetic.
Reason: During gastrulation, cells move in masses and towards definite direction.
56. **Assertion:** Cleavage in human zygote is holoblastic.
Reason: Human egg contains abundant yolk in ooplasm.
57. **Assertion:** Holoblastic cleavage with almost equal sized blastomeres is a characteristic of placental animals.
Reason: Eggs of most mammals, including human, are of centrolecithal type.
58. **Assertion:** Parturition is induced by neural signal in maternal pituitary.
Reason: At the end of gestation period, the maternal pituitary releases prolactin which causes uterine contractions.
59. **Assertion:** Twins may arise from a single egg or from two eggs.
Reason: One egg gives rise to identical twins by separation of blastomeres and two eggs produce non-identical twins.
60. **Assertion :** Death is one of the important regulatory process on earth.
Reason : It avoids over-crowding caused by continuous reproduction. **[AIIMS 2002]**
61. **Assertion :** Old age is not an illness. It is a continuation of life with decreasing capacity for adaptation.
Reason : Cessation of mitosis is a normal genetically programmed event. **[AIIMS 2006]**
62. **Assertion :** Senescence is the time when age associated defects are manifested.
Reason : Certain genes may be undergoing sequential switching on and off during one's life. **[AIIMS 2005]**
63. **Assertion:** In humans, the gamete contributed by the male determines whether the child produced will be male or female.
Reason: Sex in humans is a polygenic trait. Depending upon a cumulative effect of some genes on X-chromosome.

Solutions

1. (a) In human male, one pair testes are present in thin walled skin pouches called scrotal sac (so are extra abdominal) hanging from lower abdominal wall between the legs. Scrotal sac act as thermoregulators and keeps the testicular temperature 2°C lower than body temperature for normal spermatogenesis, as high abdominal temperature kills the spermatogenic tissue.

2. (d) Testicular lobules are the compartments present in the testes that are not involved in the process of fertilization as whole. Fusion of male and female gametes is called fertilization.

3. (c) Leydig cells, also known as interstitial cells, are found adjacent to the seminiferous tubules in the testicle. They produce testosterone in the presence of luteinizing hormone (LH).

4. (a) The testes are situated outside the abdominal cavity within a pouch called scrotum. The scrotum helps in maintaining low temperature of the testes (2-2.5 °C) lower than the normal internal body temperature which is necessary for spermatogenesis.

5. (a) Bulbourethral gland, also called Cowper's Gland, either of two pea-shaped glands in the male are located beneath the prostate gland at the beginning of the internal portion of the penis. These are responsible for adding fluids to semen during the process of ejaculation, thereby facilitating the process of reproduction.

6. (d) Each seminiferous tubule is lined on its inside by two types of cells called male germ cells (spermatogonia) and sertoli cells. The male germ cells undergo meiotic divisions finally leading to sperm formation, while sertoli cells provide nutrition to the germ cells. The regions outside the seminiferous tubules called interstitial spaces, contain small blood vessels and interstitial cells or Leydig cells. Leydig cells synthesise and secrete testicular hormones called androgens.

7. (d) Perianal gland are found in rabbit not in human beings. These are a pair of dark elongated scent glands lying behind the cowper's glands. These are sex attractant secreting glands, its smell serves as sex attractant for the female.

8. (c) Vaginal coelom partly surrounds the testes in scrotum in a wrong statement because vagina is the part of external genitalia (vulva) in the female reproductive system and scrotum is a sac like structure in which testes are suspended.

9. (b) The ends of the fallopian tubes close to the ovaries are covered with finger like projections called fimbriae. Each of these fimbriae are covered with tiny hair like projections called cilia. When an egg cell is released from the ovary, it is swept into the fallopian tube by the cilia of the fimbriae.

10. (b) After implantation, finger-like projections appear on the trophoblast called chorionic villi which are surrounded by the uterine tissue and maternal blood. The chorionic villi and uterine tissue become interdigitated with each other and jointly form a structural and functional unit between developing embryo (foetus) and maternal body called placenta.

11. (b) In human females, each fallopian tube extends from the periphery of each ovary to the uterus, the part closer to the ovary is the funnel shaped infundibulum. The edges of the infundibulum possess finger-like projections called fimbriae which help in collection of the ovum after ovulation.

12. (c) The female external genitalia include mons pubis, labia majora, labia minora, hymen and clitoris. Mons pubis is a cushion of fatty tissue covered by skin and pubic hair. The labia majora are fleshy patches of tissue, which extend down the mons pubis and surrounds the vaginal opening. The labia minora are paired folds of tissue under the

labia majora. A functional mammary gland is characteristic of all female mammals. The mammary glands are paired structures (breasts) that contain glandular tissue and variable amount of fat. The glandular tissue of each breast is divided into 15-20 mammary lobes containing clusters of cells called alveoli.

13. **(d)** Vagina is the tubular female copulatory organ. Passageway for menstrual flow as well as birth canal. Vagina receives semen from male during mating but fertilization (fusion of gametes) occurs in fallopian tube.

14. **(d)** In the testis, spermatogenesis occurs in the seminiferous tubules and testosterone secretion takes place in the interstitial cells. Testosterone brings growth and maturation of secondary sex organs. It also brings about development of secondary sex characters.

15. **(a)** Spermatogenesis starts at the age of puberty due to significant increase in the Gonadotropin Releasing Hormone (GnRH).

16. **(a)** The male releases large number of sperms inside female reproductive tract to increase chances of fertilisation.

17. **(b)** Acrosome contains enzymes that help the sperm penetrate the ova during the fertilisation process.

18. **(a)** The normal temperature of the testes in the scrotum is about 2-2.5 °C lower than the internal body temperature. When the body is chilled, the smooth muscle contracts and brings the testes closer to the pelvic cavity. This movement towards the pelvic cavity allows the testes to absorb heat from the rest of the body so that the sperrm cells do not become chilled and get optimum temperature for spermatogenesis.

19. **(d)** The human male ejaculates about 200 to 300 million sperms during a coitus out of which, at least 60 percent sperms must have normal shape and size and atleast 40 percent of them must show vigorous motility for normal fertility.

20. **(b)** Type B spermatogonia undergo mitosis to produce diploid intermediate cells called primary spermatocytes. These cells further undergo first meiotic or reductional division to give rise to haploid secondary spermatocytes.

21. **(a)** The middle piece of human contains mitochondria coiled round the axial filament called mitochondrial spiral. They provide energy for the movement of the sperm. So it is called as the 'power house of the sperm'.

22. **(b)** Each testicular lobule contains one to three highly coiled seminiferous tubules in which sperms are produced. Each seminiferous tubule is lined on its inside by two types of cells called male germ cells (spermatogonia) and sertoli cells. The male germ cells undergo meiotic divisions finally leading to sperm formation, while sertoli cells provide nutrition to hte germ cells. The regions outside the seminiferous tubules called interstitial spaces, contain small blood vessels and interstitial cells or Leydig cells. These cells synthesise and secrete testicular hormones called androgens.

23. **(d)** Primary spermatocytes of testes are diploid and formed by mitotic division in the spermatogonium.

24. **(a)** Stem cells have the property to give rise to any type of cell/tissue.

25. **(c)** Puberty in human male is controlled by male sex hormone testosterone which is secreted by interstitial or leydig cells of testes. So, secondary sexual characters develop and at puberty, secretion of testosterone is increased.

26. **(c)** Head of a sperm has acrosome but the spiral row of mitochondria are present in the mid (connecting) piece of the sperm.

27. **(a)** Primary oocyte and follicle cells both arise from the Graafian follicle by mitosis cell division. Hence, these are regarded as the sibling cells.

28. **(c)** The uterus is single and it is also called womb. The shape of the uterus is like an inverted pear. The wall of the uterus has three layers, external thin membranous perimetrium, middle thick layer of smooth myometrium and inner glandular layer of endometrium.

29. **(b)** Infundibulum is funnel shaped end of fallopian or oviduct. The funnel is called oviducal funnel or fallopian funnel. Its free

end bears a number of finger like processes called fimbriae, but graafian follicle of ovary is with secondary oocyte hanging in cavity, called antrum.

30. (c) In fertility phase/ovulation, production of FSH decrease, while that of LH increases. It causes ovulation. The ovum is drawn into fallopian tube. It is viable for two days when fertilisation can occur. Ovulation takes place between 10th-14th day.
Two characteristics of the fertility phase that help in fertilisation are :
(i) Uterine movement help in the spread of sperms in female reproductive tract.
(ii) Ciliary movements in the epithelium of fallopian tubes for bringing in the ovum.

31. (a) Graafian follicle is formed due to increase in FSH and ruptures due to rise in level of LH during middle of menstrual cycle.

32. (b) Progesterone prepares the uterus for pregnancy. After ovulation occurs, the ovaries start to produce progesterone needed by the uterus. Progesterone causes the uterine lining or endometrium to thicken. This helps to prepare a supportive environment in the uterus for a fertilized egg.

33. (b) The wall of the uterus has three layers of tissue. The external thin membranous perimetrium, middle thick layer of smooth muscle, myometrium and inner glandular layer called endometrium that lines the uterine cavity. The endometrium undergoes cyclical changes during menstrual cycle while the myometrium exhibits strong contraction during the delivery of the baby.

34. (a) Menstrual phase is the phase of menstrual flow which continues for 3-5 days and involves discharge of blood along with casting off endometrial lining due to reduced titre of both estrogen and progesterone. Menstrual phase is also called funeral of unfertilized egg or shedding tears of lost ovum. First day of menstrual phase is also considered to be first day of menstrual cycle.

35. (a) Penetration of sperm is a chemical mechanism. In this, acrosome of sperm undergoes acrosomal reaction and releases certain sperm lysins, which dissolve the egg locally and make the path for the penetration of sperm lysins which are acidic proteins. These sperms lysins contain a lysing enzyme hyaluronidase which dissolves the hyaluronic acid polymers in the intercellular spaces which holds the granulosa cells of corona radiata together; corona penetrating enzyme and acrosin. Then it dissolves the zona pellucida. Only sperm nucleus and middle piece enters the ovum.

36. (b) In female, breasts size increases after puberty under the stimulation of estrogen. Size of breasts is further increased during pregnancy and after childbirth under the stimulation of prolactin hormone.

37. (c) During fertilization, only one sperm head enters into ovum and remaining parts of body degenerates. If several spermatozoa hit the egg at same time, even then only one can get entry into egg because after entry of one sperm, the egg becomes impervious to other sperms.

38. (b) In female, graafian follicle forms corpus luteum after ovulation. The cells of corpus luteum are called luteal cells. The cytoplasm of luteal cells have yellow granules called lutein which secrete the hormone progesterone to maintain pregnancy if fertilization takes place. In the absence of fertilization, corpus luteum degenerates and forms corpus albicans and there is decrease in progesterone level as well.

39. (d) Hyaluronidase, a hydrolytic enzyme is an acrosomal content in mammalian sperm. It helps at the time of fertilization during the penetration of the sperm into the ovum. Based on the amount of yolk, mammalian eggs are alecithal means egg without yolk. Microlecithal eggs contain very little yolk *e.g.*, sea urchin, starfish. On the basis of distribution of yolk telolecithal eggs are those eggs in which the yolk, is concentrated towards the vegetal pole and cytoplasm and nucleus lie near the animal pole, *e.g.*, birds and reptiles.

40. (c) Sperm needs energy to move about in female tract, so that fertilisation of ova takes place.

41. (a) All copulation do not lead to fertilisation as the synchronisation of sperm and ova reaching the fallopian tube is important.

42. (b) The process of attachment of the blastocyst (mammalian blastula) on the endometrium of uterus is called implantation.

43. (b) Placenta is an endocrine gland that is present only during pregnancy. It is responsible for production of various hormones like human Chorionic Gonadotropin (hCG), estrogen, progesterone, human placental lactogen (hPL).

44. (b) The chorionic cells secrete a hormone called human Chorionic Gonadotropin (hCG), which resembles and takes over the job of pituitary LH during pregnancy. hCG maintains the corpus luteum and stimulates it to secrete progesterone.

45. (a) Colostrum is rich in antibodies, which is essential for new born babies.

46. (b) During pregnancy, the levels of hormones like estrogen, progestrogens, cortisol, prolactin, thyroxine, etc., are increased several folds in the maternal blood. Increased production of these hormones is essential for supporting the foetal growth, metabolic changes in the mother and maintenance of pregnancy.

47. (c) Vigorous contraction of the uterus at the end of pregnancy causes parturition. Parturition is induced by a complex neuroendocrine mechanism. The signals for parturition originate from the fully developed foetus and the placenta which induce mild uterine contractions called foetal ejection reflex.

48. (b) Entrance of a single sperm into an oocyte is called monospermy generally found in most of animals. Cortical granules are extruded in the perivitelline space by exocytosis and some of these are attached along inner surface of vitelline membrane which now thickens and becomes impervious to any other sperm entry. It is now called fertilization membrane. It prevents polyspermy.

49. (b) Metatherians are pouched mammals or marsupials, whereas eutherians are placental mammals with well developed placenta

50. (a) Placenta is a ductless endocrine gland which produces various hormones like human Chorionic Gonadotropin (hCG), estrogen, progesterone, human placental lactogen (hPL).

51. (a) Embryonic development includes a definite series of phases which are fundamentally similar in all sexually reproducing organisms, and transform a one-celled zygote to a multicellular and fully formed developmental stage till hatching or birth. Such a remarkable similarity of embryonic development proves that all metazoans are interrelated and have common ancestory. Embryonic development involves five dynamic changes and identifiable processes which are - gametogenesis, fertilization, cleavage, gastrulation and organogenesis.

52. (a) Morula involves cleavage of cells till 32 cell stage is formed. It is still surrounded by zona pellucida.

53. (c) Cleavage starts as the zygote moves through the isthmus of the oviduct towards the uterus and forms 2, 4, 8, 16 daughter cells called blastomeres. The embryo with 8 to 16 blastomeres is called a morula. The morula continues to divide and transforms into blastocyst as it moves furither into the uterus.

54. (a) During cleavage, there is no growth during interphase so the size of blastomeres becomes gradually smaller. Cleavage is thus called fractionating process. In morula stage, the cells divide without any increase in size because in cleavage there is increase in number of blastomeres but decrease in size of blastomeres.

55. (a) Gastrulation is a process by which blastocyst is changed into a gastrula larva with three primary germ layers. In this, cells of the blastodermic vesicle visibly move in small masses to their final and predetermined positions. These movements are interdependent and are called morphogenetic movements.

56. **(c)** Human egg contains very less ooplasm, hence, called alecithal egg.

57. **(c)** Holoblastic cleavage is found in the eggs, which are microlecithal (little yolk). In them, the cleavage is complete and thus, is called holoblastic cleavage. Human eggs are microlecithal not centrolecithal.

58. **(d)** The process of delivery of foetus (childbirth) is called parturition. Parturition is induced by a complex neuroendocrine mechanism. The signals for parturition originate from the fully developed foetus and the placenta which induces mild uterine contractions called foetal ejection reflex. This triggers release of oxytocin from the maternal pituitary. Oxytocin acts on the uterine muscles and causes stronger uterine contractions which in turn stimulate further secretion of oxytocin. The stimulatory reflex between the uterine contractions and oxytocin secretion continues resulting in stronger and stronger contractions. This leads to expulsion of the baby out of the uterus through the birth canal.

59. **(a)** Twins are of two types:

(i) Identical Twins (maternal twins): One egg gives rise to identical twins by complete separation of blastomere.

(ii) Non-identical Twins (Fraternal Twins): Two eggs fertilized by two sperms give rise to non-identical twins.

60. **(a)** Death is the ultimate goal of every organism. This is caused by the wear and tear of organs which constitute the body of a living being.

61. **(c)** Old age is the progressive deterioration in the structure and functioning of cells, tissues and organs and cessation of immune system.

62. **(a)** According to programmed senescence theory of ageing, ageing is a result of switching on and off of certain genes. B and T- lymphocytes undergo programmed cell death called apoptosis.

63. **(c)** In human, the gamete contributed by male- determines the sex of a child. Sex in human is a polygenic trait depending upon a cumulative effect of some genes present on Y-chromosome and not on X-chromosome.

Chapter 26

Reproductive Health

Directions: In the following questions, a statement of assertion is followed by a statement of reason. Mark the correct choice as:

(a) If both Assertion and Reason are true and Reason is the correct explanation of Assertion.

(b) If both Assertion and Reason are true but Reason is not the correct explanation of Assertion.

(c) If Assertion is true but Reason is false.

(d) If both Assertion and Reason are false.

1. **Assertion:** A person should be considered reproductively healthy if they have healthy reproductive organs but are emotionally imbalanced.
   Reason: This statement about reproductive health was given by WHO.
2. **Assertion:** Family planning is an action plan to attain reproductive health among people.
   Reason: Improved programmes covering reproduction related areas were propagated by RCH to create awareness among people.
3. **Assertion:** Reproductive and Child Healthcare Programmes is for reproduction related areas.
   Reason: It deals with creating awareness among various reproduction related aspects.
4. **Assertion:** A wide range of contraceptive methods are available for family planning.
   Reason: Natural method includes condoms, diaphragms, etc., while barrier methods use of included method like periodic abstinence, lactational amenorrhea, etc.
5. **Assertion:** Introduction of sex education in schools should be encouraged.
   Reason: This will encourage children to believe in myths about sex related aspects.
6. **Assertion:** Amniocentesis is often missemployed.
   Reason: Amniocentesis is meant for determining the genetic disorders in the foetus, but it is being used to determine the sex of the foetus, leading to death of the normal female foetus.
7. **Assertion:** Natality increases both population density and population size.
   Reason: Natality increases the number of individuals in an area by births.
8. **Assertion:** Saheli, the new oral contraceptive for the females, contains a steroidal preparation.
   Reason: It is "once in a day" pill with very few side effects.
9. **Assertion:** Rapid decline in death rate, MMR and IMR have lead to a staggering rise in population.
   Reason: Such an alarming growth rate has lead to an absolute scarcity of even the most basic requirements, i.e. food and shelter.
10. **Assertion:** Zero population growth should be achieved as early as possible to control human population.
    Reason: This as requires not two children per couple but a lilttle more.
11. **Assertion:** Periodic abstinence is a method in which couples avoid from coitus from day 17 to 27 of menstrual cycle.
    Reason: It is a very effective method and 100% sure of birth control.
12. **Assertion:** There is chance of fertilisation during 10 -17 days menstrual cycle.
    Reason: Ovulation occurs during these days.
13. **Assertion:** Contraceptives are methods to prevent unwanted pergnancies.
    Reason: Unwanted pregnancies can only be prevent by using oral contraceptives.
14. **Asertion:** Barrier methods prevent physical meeting of sperms and ova.
    Reason: This prevents conception.
15. **Assertion:** Reusable contraceptives are not full proof method of contraceptions.
    Reason: Diaphragms, cervical caps and vaults are barrier methods which prevent conceptions by blocking entry of sperms through cervix. They are reusable.

16. **Assertion:** Diaphragms, cervical caps and vaults are barriers made of rubber.
Reason: They are inserted into the male reproductive tract during coitus.

17. **Assertion :** Copper-T is an effective contraceptive device in human females.
Reason : Copper-T prevents passage of sperms from vagina upwards into fallopian tubes. **[AIIMS 2011, 2014]**

18. **Assertion :** Cu-T and Cu-7 do not suppresses sperm-motility.
Reason : Hormones released by them do not affect sperm motility. **[AIIMS 2009]**

19. **Assertion:** Pills are very effective contraceptive methods with lesser side effects.
Reason: Pills inhibit ovulation and implantation as well as retard entry of sperms.

20. **Assertion:** Use of condom is a protection against AIDS and sexual diseases besides checking pregnancy.
Reason: Certain contraceptives are planted under the skin of the upper arm to prevent pregnancy.

21. **Assertion:** In barrier methods, ovum and sperms are prevented from physical meetings.
Reason: Barriers, methods are used during coitus, to prevent the entry of ejaculated semen into the female reproductive tract.

22. **Assertion:** Sterilization is a terminal method used only for males.
Reason: These techniques are highly effective and their reversibility is very good.

23. **Asertion:** A surgical method of contraception is sterilisation.
Reason: It blocks gamete transport and thereby prevents conception.

24. **Assertion:** Chances of conception are almost nil as long as the mother breast-feeds the child fully.
Reason: This method is based on the fact that ovulation do not occur during the period of intense lactation.

25. **Assertion:** A small part of the vas deferens is removed or tied up in vasectomy.
Reason: In tubectomy, a small part of the fallopian tube is removed or tied up.

26. **Assertion:** Second trimester abortions are much more complicated.
Reason: The foetus becomes intimately associated with the maternal tissues after 12 weeks.

27. **Assertion:** Syphilies, gonorrhoea and AIDS are STDs.
Reason: These diseases are transmitted through sexual intercourse.

28. **Assertion :** HIV infection can be avoided by use of condoms.
Reason : Condoms secrete anti-viral interferons. **[AIIMS 2014]**

29. **Assertion:** STDs are transmitted through sexual intercourse.
Reason: STDs can be prevented by using barrier contraceptives like condoms.

30. **Assertion:** Infertility is the inability to produce children inspite of unprotected sex.
Reason: Infertile couples could have children using assisted reproductive technologies (ART).

31. **Assertion:** Intra cytoplasmic sperm injection (ICSI) is a procedure to form an embryo in vitro.
Reason: Sperm is directly injected into the ovum.

32. **Assertion:** IVF in fertilization is carried out outside the body of woman.
Reason: The zygote upto 8 blastomeres could be transferred into the fallopian tube.

33. **Assertion:** Both male and female can be infertile.
Reason: Infertility can result due to any fertility related disorder.

34. **Assertion:** In zygote intra fallopian transfer the zygote is transferred to the fallopian tubes of the female.
Reason: ZIFT is a in vivo fertilisation method.

35. **Assertion:** Artificial insemination is method of introduction of semen inside the female.
Reason: This technique is used in those cases where males have low sperm count.

36. **Assertion:** IUT is the transfer of embryo with more than 8 blastomeres into the fallopian tubes.
Reason: This is a very popular method of forming embryos in-vivo.

37. **Assertion :** Test-tube baby has raised several legal problems.
Reason : It involves in vitro fertilization followed by embryo transfer.

38. **Assertion:** Biologically, woman is superior to man.
Reason: A woman provides nutrition to developing foetus during gestation and also nourishes the baby on her milk after birth.

Solutions

1. **(d)** A person is reproductively healthy if he/she is capable of producing offsprings.
2. **(b)** Family planning helps in maintaining reproductive health.
3. **(a)** The Reproductive and Child Health (RCH) Programme was launched in October 1997. The main aim of the programme is to reduce infant, child and maternal mortality rates.
4. **(c)** Natural methods work on the principle of avoiding chances of meeting of ovum and sperm, e.g. periodic abstinence, lactiational amenorrhea. In barrier methods, ovum and sperm are prevented from physically meeting with help of a barrier, e.g. condoms, cervical caps, etc.
5. **(c)** Introduction of sex education in schools should be encouraged to provide right information to the young children and to discourage them from believing in myths and having misconceptions about sex-related aspects. Proper information about reproductive organs, adolescence and related changes, safe and hygienic sexual practices, sexually transmitted diseases (STDs), AIDS, etc., would help people, especially those in the adolescent age group to lead a reproductively healthy life.
6. **(a)** Amniocentesis (amniotic fluid test or AFT) is a medical procedure used in prenatal diagnosis of chromosomal abnormalities and fetal infections, and also for sex determination, in which a small amount of amniotic fluid, which contains foetal tissues, is sampled from the amniotic sac surrounding a developing foetus, and then the foetal DNA is examined for genetic abnormalities.
7. **(a)** Natality is generally expressd as number of birth per 1,000 individuals of a population per year. It increase the population size and population density.
8. **(d)** Saheli - the new oral contraceptive for the females contains a non-steroidal preparation. It is a 'once a week' pill with very few side effects and high contraceptive value.
9. **(b)** There is rapid decline in Infant Mortality Rate (IMR) and Maternal Mortality Rate (MMR) The recent World Bank data puts the MMR for India reported in 2015 at 174 per 100, 000 live births, which is a significant decline from the 215 figure that was reported in 2010.
10. **(a)** Two children per couple holds good for zero population growth. But in large democratic countries like India, it will take little more.
11. **(d)** Periodic abstinence is a natural method in which the couples avoid or abstain from coitus from day 10 to 17 of the menstrual cycle when ovulation could be expected. The effectiveness of this method is limited because only a few women have reuglar menstrual cycles and the actual time of ovulation can be produced as the ovulation in humans occurs about 14 days before the onset of the next menstruation.
12. **(a)** Ovulation is likely to occur between 10-17 days of menstrual cycle.
13. **(c)** Contraceptives can be broadly grouped into natural, barrier, IUDs, oral contraceptives, injectables, implants and surgical methods.
14. **(a)** Barrier methods include the diaphragm, cervical cap, male condom, and female condom and spermicidal foam, sponges, and film. Unlike other methods of birth control, barrier methods these are used only during sexual intercourse.
15. **(b)** Reusable contraceptives do not guarantee prevention from accidental pregnancy.
16. **(c)** Diaphragms, cervical caps and vaults are barriers made of rubber that are inserted into the female reproductive tract to cover the cervix during coitus. They prevent conception by blocking the entry of sperms throug the cervix. They are reusable.

17. (c) Intrauterine device (IUD) Copper-T is plastic or metal object placed in the uterus by a doctor. Copper-T prevent the fertilization of the egg or implantation of the embryo.

18. (d) Cu-7 and Cu-T are intrauterine contraceptive devices for females. They suppress the sperm motility. Their mode of action is different. Cu-T and Cu-7 discharge 50-75 micrograms of ionic copper into the uterus daily. These copper ions interfere with life-sustaining functions that regulate implantation in the uterus. No any hormone is released by them.

19. (b) Oral administration of small doses of either progestogens or progestogen-estrogen combinations is a contraceptive method used by the females called as pills. They inhibit ovulation and implantation as well as alter the quality of cervical mucus to prevent/retard entry of sperms. Pills are very effective with lesser side effects and are well acccepted by the females.

20. (b) It is a simple but effective method and has no side effect. It checks pregnancy by preventing deposition of semen in the vagina. Condom should be used regularly and put on before starting coital activity, otherwise sperm containing lubricating fluid may be left in the vagina. Condom is also a safeguard against infection of AIDS and sexual diseases (STDs).

Certain contraceptives, such as progestin, minipil or progestogen in combination with estrogen are also used by the females as injection or implants under the skin of the upper arm.

21. (a) In barrier methods, ovum and sperms are prevented from physically meeting with the help of barriers, such methods are available for both males and females. Condoms are barriers made of thin rubber/latex sheath that are used to cover the penis in the male or vagina and cervix in the female, just before coitus so that the ejaculated semen would not enter into the female reproductive tract. This can prevent conception.

22. (d) Sterilization, is generally advised for the male/female partner as a terminal method to prevent further pregnancies. Sterilization procedure in the male is called 'vasectomy' and that in the female, 'tubectomy'. In vasectomy, a small part of the vas deferens is removed or tied up through a small incision. In tubectomy, a small part of the fallopian tube is inserted through vagina. These techniques are highly effective but their reversibility is very poor.

23. (a) The permanent birth control method for women that most people are familiar with is tubal ligation (tubectomy). And for men, it's vasectomy. Both are surgical methods that permanently prevent pregnancy.

24. (a) Lactational amenorrhea (absence of menstruation) method is based on the fact that ovulation and therefore the cycle do not occur during the period of intense lactation following parturition. Therefore, as long as the mother breast-feeds the child fully, chances of conception are almost nil.

25. (b) Surgical intervention blocks gamete transport and thereby prevents conception. Sterilization procedure in the male is called 'vasectomy' and in the female, it is 'tubectomy'. In vasectomy, a small part of the vas deferens is removed or tied up through a small incision on the scrotum whereas in tubectomy, a small part of the fallopian tube is removed or tied up through a small incision in the abdomen or through vagina.

26. (a) MTP is comparatively safe upto 12 weeks (the first trimester) of pregnancy. It becomes more risky after the first trimester period of pregnancy as the foetus becomes intimately associated with the maternal tissues.

27. (a) Diseases or infections which are transmitted through sexual intercourse are collectively called sexually transmitted disease (STD). Gonorrhoea, syphilis, genital herpes, chlamydiasis, genital warts, trichomoniasis, hepatitis-B and HIV leading to AIDS are some of the common STDs.

28. (c) The use of condoms has been shown to decrease the transmission of AIDS because condoms is contraceptic.

29. (a) Sexually transmitted diseases (STDs) are infections that are commonly spread by sex, especially vaginal intercourse, anal sex or oral sex. The causes of STDs are bacteria, parasites, yeast, and viruses.

30. (b) Infertility is a failure to conceive within one or more years of regular unprotected sex. The couples can be assisted to have children through certain special techniques called the assisted reproductive technologies (ART). The applications of reproductive technology are (i) Test tube baby, (ii) Artificial insemination technique (AIT), (iii) Gamete intra Fallopian transfer (GIFT), (iV) Intracytoplasmic sperm injection (ICSI).

31. (b) Intra cytoplasmic sperm injection (ICSI) is a specialised procedure to form an embryo in the laboratory in which a sperm is directly injected into the ovum.

32. (b) In IVF, the fusion of ovum and sperm is done outside the body of woman, to form a zygote which is allowed to divide to form embryo. This embryo is implanted in the uterus where it develops into a foetus which in turn develops into a child. This is called as a test tube baby. In this method, ova from the wife/donor female and sperms from the husbands/donor male are induced to form zygote in the laboratory. The zygote is allowed to divide forming 8 blastomeres. The zygote or early embryo is transferred into the fallopian tube (ZIFT– zygote Intra Fallopian Transfer).

33. (b) Infertility can also refer to the biological inability of an individual to contribute to conception, or to a female who cannot carry a pregnancy to full term.

34. (c) ZIFT is a in vitro fertilisation method, in which zygote is transferred in the fallopian tube of the female.

35. (a) Artificial insemination (AI) or intrauterine insemination (IUI) is way of treating infertility. It involves direct insertion of semen into a woman's womb. The sperm used in artificial insemination may be provided by either the woman's husband or partner (partner sperm) or by a known or anonymous sperm donor.

36. (d) In IVF method, popularly known as test tube baby programme, ova from the wife/ donor (female) and sperms from the husband/donor (male) are collected and introduced to form zygote under simulated conditions in the laboratory. The zygote or early embryos (with upto 8 blastomeres) could be transferred into the fallopian tube (ZIFT) and embryos with more than 8 blastomeres into the uterus (IUT). This is in vitro fertilization (IVF-fertilization outside the body in almost similar conditions as that in the body) followed by embryo transfer (ET).

37. (b) In very rare cases, a surrogate mother may have to be used to bring up in vitro fertilized ovum to maturity. Though biological realization of a test tube baby is a remarkable achievement, it has raised several ethical and legal problems like the right over the child.
The technique of in-vitro fertilization followed by the embryo-transfer in the uterus of the normal female to start the development and finally leading to normal birth, is called test tube baby.

38. (a) Woman plays an important role in the continuity of the family and human race. She provide nutrition to the foetus in her womb about nine months through placenta. Even after birth, she nourishes the infant on her milk. Hence, biologically woman is superior to man.

Chapter 27 Principles of Inheritance and Variation

Directions: In the following questions, a statement of assertion is followed by a statement of reason. Mark the correct choice as:

(a) If both Assertion and Reason are true and Reason is the correct explanation of Assertion.
(b) If both Assertion and Reason are true but Reason is not the correct explanation of Assertion.
(c) If Assertion is true but Reason is false.
(d) If both Assertion and Reason are false.

1. **Assertion :** Mendel was successful in his hybridization.
   Reason : Garden pea proved ideal experimental material.
2. **Assertion:** Mendel used true-breeding pea lines for artificial pollination experiments for his genetic studies.
   Reason: For several generations, a true-breeding line shows the stable trait inheritance and expression.
3. **Assertion:** On true breeding lines, Mendel conducted cross pollination experiments.
   Reason: For several generations, true breed line have stable trait inheritance.
4. **Assertion :** Cross of F_1 individual with recessive homozygous parent is test cross.
   Reason : No recessive individual are obtained in the monohybrid test cross progeny.
5. **Assertion:** The progeny produced have both the characters of parents.
   Reason: The process by which characters pass from parent to progeny is known as inheritance.
6. **Assertion:** The progeny in F_2-generation traits were identical to their parental type.
   Reason: The progeny show no blending of traits.
7. **Assertion:** Genes pass from one generation to another.
   Reason: The unit of inheritance are genes.
8. **Assertion :** In a monohybrid cross, F_1 generation indicate dominant characters.
   Reason : Dominance occurs only in heterozygous state.
9. **Assertion:** In monohybrid cross, at F_2 stage, both parental traits are expressed in 3 : 1 proportion.
   Reason: At F_2 stage, the contrasting parental traits show blending.
10. **Assertion:** The cross between the F_1 progeny and either of the parent types is a test cross.
    Reason: The cross between F_1 progeny and the double recessive genotype is back cross.
11. **Assertion :** A pair of contrasting characters is termed as allele.
    Reason : Only one gene of an allele is expressed in an individual.
12. **Assertion :** In *Mirabilis*, selfing of F_1 pink flower plants produces same phenotypic & genotypic ratio.
    Reason : Flower colour gene shows incomplete dominance.
13. **Assertion:** Gametes receives only one allele of a gene.
    Reason: During gamete formation, mitosis takes place leads to formation of haploid cells.
14. **Assertion:** In F_2 generation of plant Mirabilis jalapa, the pink coloured flowers appear.
    Reason: This is observed due epistatic suppression of white colour alleles in one of parental flowers by red colour alleles.
15. **Assertion:** A good example of multiple alleles is ABO blood group sytem.
    Reason: When I^A and I^B alleles are present together in ABO blood group sytem, they both express their own types.
16. **Assertion:** By means of dihybrid cross, the law of independent assortment can be studied.
    Reason: The law of independent assortment is applicable only to linked genes.

17. **Assertion:** In *Cucurbita pepo,* variety of fruit is result of recessive epistasis.
Reason: In recessive epistatsis, a recessive gene at one locus enhances the expression of another gene, at a different locus.

18. **Assertion:** The F_1-generation resembles both the parents in codominance.
Reason: An example is different type of red blood cells that determine ABO blood grouping in humans.

19. **Assertion** : A women can go to the court if a man refuses to own his child. He has blood group B and women has A while child has O.
Reason : Genetically she is right he can be father of the child.

20. **Assertion:** Behaviour of chromosome is parallel to gene.
Reason: Genes are located on the chromosome.

21. **Assertion:** Some genes together passes from one generation to another.
Reason: The genes are located closely on a chromosome.

22. **Assertion:** Pairing and separation of pair of chromosomes results in the segregation of a pair of factors they carried.
Reason: On non-homologous chromosomes, two alleles of a gene pair are located on similar sites.

23. **Assertion:** On the position of centromere the shape of chromosomes is based.
Reason: The chromosome bends in the region of centromere during anaphase.

24. **Assertion:** Heterochromatin is genetically inactive.
Reason: Heterochromatin lacks genes.

25. **Assertion:** Kinetochore takes part in the movement of chromosomes.
Reason: It consists points for attachment of microtubules.

26. **Assertion:** Short palindromic sequence is recognized by restriction endonuclease which cuts at specific sites.
Reason: When a restriction endonuclease acts on Palindrome, it cleaves both the strands of DNA molecules.

27. **Assertion:** The lampbrush chromosomes are known as diplotene chromosomes bivalents.
Reason: During diplotene, the number of loops is maximum.

28. **Assertion:** Through banding technique human chromosomes have been studied.
Reason: Though banding technique banding technique is useful.

29. **Assertion** : The genetic complement of an organism is called genotype.
Reason : Genotype is the type of hereditary properties of an organism. **[AIIMS 1999]**

30. **Assertion** : In case of incomplete linkage, linked gene show new combination along with parental combination.
Reason : In case of incomplete linkage, linked genes are separated by crossing over.
[AIIMS 2000]

31. **Assertion:** In plants, somaclonal variations may be present that is produced from callus.
Reason: Due to recombination during meiosis somaclonal variations are caused.

32. **Assertion:** Generally, hybrids are back crossed.
Reason: To increase the traits of the parent back cross is done.

33. **Assertion:** A gene may consists several allelomorphs.
Reason: In more than one ways, wild form can mutate.

34. **Assertion** : In birds, the chromosome composition of the egg determines the sex.
Reason : Female birds are heterogametic.

35. **Assertion** : Most of experiments regarding sex determination were done on *Drosophila*.
Reason : It is fruit fly.

36. **Assertion** : In humans, most sex-linked genes are present on the X-chromosome.
Reason : X-chromosome contains a large number of genes with major effects on phenotype.

37. **Assertion** : In humans, the gamete contributed by the male determines whether the child produced will be male or female.
Reason : Sex in humans is a polygenic trait depending upon a cumulative effect of some genes on X-chromosome and some on Y-chromosome. **[AIIMS 2005]**

38. **Assertion:** Insects have female homogametic.
Reason: In insects males shows XX sex chromosome and females shows XY sex chromosome.

39. **Assertion:** When white eyed, yellow bodied drosophila females were hybridized with red eyed, brown-bodied males; and F_1 progeny was intercrossed, F_2 ratio deviated from 9 : 3 : 3 : 1.
Reason: When two genes in a dihybrid are on the same chromosome, the proportion of parental gene combinations are much higher than the non-parental type.

40. **Assertion:** In pigeons, males are homogametic and females are heterogametic.
Reason: In pigeons, males have ZZ sex chromosomes and females have ZW sex chromosomes.

41. **Assertion:** The maximum frequency of recombination, that can result from crossing over between linked genes, is 50 percent.
Reason: Higher frequency of crossing over is shown in linked genes if distance between them is longer.

42. **Assertion** : The linked genes tend to get inherited together.
Reason : The link between them fails to break.

43. **Assertion:** Mustard gas acts as a mutagen.
Reason: It transfers alkyl groups to the bases in DNA.

44. **Assertion:** To study mutation, haploids are used.
Reason: Most of the mutations are recessive.

45. **Assertion** : The banding pattern of the chromosome can be studied by dyes as quinacrine, mustard dye of Giemsa.
Reason : These patterns are used for finger printing to study even genetic defects.

46. **Assertion** : The percentage frequency with which a gene successfully manifests its phenotypic effect is called expressivity.
Reason : The extent or intensity of phenotypic expressions of certain genes may vary in different individuals due to environmental influences.

47. **Assertion** : In a diploid organism only dominant mutations will show their effect immediately, recessive mutations do not influence the traits immediately.
Reason : The recessive mutants accumulate in gene pool and once the recessive mutations has established homozygous state it is exposed to natural selection.

48. **Assertion** : Muton gene has fewer nucleotides than a cistron.
Reason : Benzer coined the term muton to the smallest unit of genetic material capable of mutational change.

49. **Assertion** : The phenomenon of a single gene influencing more than one character is pleiotropism.
Reason : The gene responsible for phenylketonuria affects a number of abnormal phenotypic traits.

50. **Assertion** : There are cows of two colour coats.
Reason : It is a case of mutation.

51. **Assertion** : Translocation heterozygotes are generally semisterile.
Reason : During meiosis in a translocation heterozygote 50% of gametes carry deficiencies and duplications.

52. **Assertion** : Polyploidy is multiplication of chromosome number.
Reason : Polyploidy increase the tolerance of plants towards climatic extremes.

53. **Assertion:** Aneuploidy may be of hypoploidy or hyperploidy type.
Reason: Monosomy lacks one pair of chromosomes. **[AIIMS 2011]**

54. **Assertion** : Haemophilia never occurs in women.
Reason : Gene for haemophilia is located on X chromosome.

55. **Assertion** : Haemophilia is a recessive sex linked disease.
Reason : Haemophilia occurs due to mutation of a structural gene on chromosome 15. **[AIIMS 2007]**

56. **Assertion** : Persons suffering from haemophilia fail to produce blood clotting factor VIII.
Reason : Prothrombin producing platelets in such persons are found in very low concentration. **[AIIMS 2008]**

57. **Assertion** : Haemophilia is a sex-linked disorder.
Reason : It never occurs in females as this disorder is associated with genes of 'Y' chromosome.

58. **Assertion** : Haemophilia is a genetic disorder generally found in males.
Reason : Haemophilia is a sex-linked trait and the gene for haemophilia is located on the Y-chromosome.

59. **Assertion** : Sickle-cell anaemia is a genetically determined disorder affecting many new born babies.

Reason : It is caused by heterozygosity for allele Hb^S producing a single amino acid substitution in the α-chain of the normal haemoglobin molecule determined by allele Hb^A.

60. **Assertion:** Females, homozygous for genes present on the X chromosomes do not express a trait more markedly than do hemizygous males.

Reason: The mechanism of dosage compensation accounts for effective dosage genes in males and females.

61. **Assertion:** Sickle-cell anaemia is an autosome-linked recessive disorder which can be transmitted if for the gene both parents are heterozygous.

Reason: In sickle-cell anaemia, haemoglobin molecule undergoes polymerisation under low oxygen tension which causes the change in shape of RBC.

62. **Assertion:** Sickle-cell anaemia is an autosome linked recessive trait.

Reason: A single allele of a gene controlls this disorder.

63. **Assertion:** For every cell, tissue and organ of a person, the DNA fingerprint is the same.

Reason: For treatment of inherited disorders like Huntigton's disease, Alzheimer's and Sickle cell anaemia DNA fingerprint is used.

64. **Assertion** : Phenylketonuria is an inborn error of metabolism.

Reason : Phenylalanine is not converted into alanine in individuals suffering from this disease.

65. **Assertion:** In case of phenylketonuria, phenylpyruvic acid is excreted through urine.

Reason: Enzyme phenylalanine hydroxylase is absent in the affected individual.

66. **Assertion** : Phenylketonuria is a recessive hereditary disease caused by body's failure to oxidize an amino acid phenylalanine to tyrosine, because of a defective enzyme.

Reason : It results in the presence of phenylalanine acid in urine. **[AIIMS 2000]**

67. **Assertion:** An additional copy of chromosome number 21 causes down syndrome.

Reason: Aneuploidy occurs from an extra copy of chromosome.

68. **Assertion:** Due to absence of any one of the X and Y sex chromosome Turner's syndrome is caused.

Reason: Such individuals show masculine as well as feminine development.

Solutions

1. **(b)** Mendel chose garden pea as plant material for his experiments, since it had the following advantages:
   (i) Well defined characters.
   (ii) Bisexual flowers.
   (iii) Predominantly self-fertilization.
   (iv) Easy hybridization.
   Besides these features, garden pea, being self-fertilized, had pure lines due to natural self-fertilization for a number of years. Therefore, any variety used was pure for the characters it carried. Mendel's success was mainly based on the fact that he considered a single character at one time.
2. **(a)** On garden pea for many years mendel carried out hybridization experiments. He performed various types of cross breeding and then allowed the offspring for self breeding. He selected varieties and used pure lines of ture breeding lines, i.e., they produce offspring resembling the parents. these lines show the stable trait inheritance and expression for several generations making them suitable for genetic studies.
3. **(a)** True breeding lines have inheritance of pure characters for several generations.
4. **(c)** In the monohybrid test cross progeny both heterozygous and recessive individuals are obtained in 1 : 1 ratio.
5. **(b)** According to Mendelian inheritance, genes come in different varieties called alleles. Somatic cells contain 2 alleles with one allele provided by each parent of an organism.
6. **(a)** Both the characters appear during the formation of F_2-generation, so no blending occurs.
7. **(b)** Chromosomes carry gene that passes on the traits of parents to the offsprings during genetic recombination.
8. **(c)** Monohybrid cross is a cross between two organisms of a species which is made to study the inheritance of a single pair of alleles or factors of a character. Dominant character is one of a pair of alleles which can express itself whether present in homozygous or heterozygous state. In F_1, generation, the generation of hybrids produced from a cross between the genetically different homozygous individuals called parents the progenies are heterozygous dominant.
9. **(c)** Both the parental traits of a character in F_2 generation are expressed in the ratio of three dominant to one recessive. Whereas, in F_1 generation only one of the parental traits is expressed and the other lies hidden or unexpressed. However, in the hybrid there is no mixing of two characters. At the time formation of gamete, two factors separate or segregate and passes into different gametes, that hence have one factor of a pair. During fertilization, gametes fuse randomly so that factors come together in new generation and freely express themselves.
10. **(d)** Back cross is a cross of F_1 hybrid with either of the two parents. When F_1 offsprings are crossed with the dominant parents, all the F_2 generation offsprings develop dominant character. On the other hand, when F_1 hybrids are crossed with recessive parent, individuals with both the phenotypes appear in equal proportions.
    Crossing of F_1 individual with dominant phenotype with its homozygous recessive parent is called test cross. It is used to determine whether the individuals exhibiting dominant characters are homozygous or heterozygous.
11. **(c)** An allele is an alternative form of a gene one member of a pair that is located at a specific position on a specific chromosome. Diploid organisms, for example, humans, have paired homologous chromosomes in their somatic cells, and these contain two copies of each gene.
12. **(a)** F_2 phenotypic and genotypic ratio in monohybrid cross involving incomplete dominance is

1 :	2 :	1
RR	Rr	rr
(red)	(pink)	(white)

13. **(c)** Meiosis is the process by which gametes are formed and during this process only one variant of gene pass to the gamete.
14. **(c)** In *Mirabilis jalapa* (four o'clock) have two types, of flower colour in pure state: red

and white. When the two types of plants are crossed, the hybrid or plants of F_1 generation produce pink flowers. If the latter are selfed, the plants of F_2 generation are of three types-red, pink and white flowered in the ratio of 1 : 2 : 1. Due to incomplete dominance of red (dominant) over white (recessive), the pink colour apparently appears. Thus, pink is differentiated from red and white.

15. (b) In the ABO system, consists four blood groups A, B, AB and O. ABO blood groups are controlled by gene I. The gene has three alleles I^A, I^B and i. This phenomenon is known as multiple allelism. I^A and I^B are completely dominant over i. When I^A and I^B are present together, they both express themselves and produce AB blood group. This phenomenon is known as codominance.

16. (c) The law of independent assortment states that two factors of each character separate or assort independent of the factors of other characters at the time of gamete formation and get randomly rearranged in the offspring producing both parental and traits of new combinations. The principle of law of independent assortment is applicable to only those factors or genes that are either located distantly on the same chromosome or occur on different chromosomes. Actually, a chromosome bears hundred of genes. All the genes of factors present on a chromosome are inherited together except when crossing over takes place.

17. (d) Fruit colour of summer squash *(Cucurbita pepo)* is governed by a gene that produces yellow colour in dominant state (Y) and green colour in recessive state (YY). There is a non-pigment forming epistatic gene that in dominant state (W-_ produces white colour (W-Y-, W- yy) while in recessive state it allows the yellow (wwY-_ and green (wwyy) expression. This shows dominant epistasis where a dominant epistatic allele suppresses the expression of a non allellic gene whether the latter is dominant or recessive.

18. (b) When two alleles for trait are equally expressed with neither being recessive or dominant, is known as codominance. As for example– A person with type AB blood, that means both A and B alleles are equally expressed.

19. (a) In ABO blood group system, the classification of human blood is based on the inherited properties of red blood cells (erythrocytes) as determined by the presence or absence of the antigens A and B, which are carried on the surface of the red cells. One parent with A and another with B can produce a child with A, B, AB or O blood types.

20. (d) Frequent separation does not occur in linked gene. They remain together because linked gene live very closely to each other.

21. (a) A chromosome consists of a single, very long DNA helix on which thousands of genes are encoded. The region of the chromosome at which a particular gene is located is called its locus. Gene is basic unit of hereditary.

22. (c) According to the chromosomal theory of inheritance, the chromosomes possess Mendalian factors or genes. The chromosomes segregate and during meiosis assort independently and recombine in zygote during fertilization. Chromosomes, like genes occur in pairs. The two alleles of a gene pair lies on homologous sites on homologous chromosomes.

23. (a) For a chromosome, the position of centromere is fixed. It may be located at the centre (metacentric chromosome), near the centre (submetacentric) subterminal (acrocentric chromosome) or terminal (telocentric chromosome) position. During anaphase the chromosome bends in the region of centromere. On the basis of the position of centromere, an anaphasic chromosome can have V-shape, L-shape, J-shape or I-shape.

24. (c) Genetic analyses shows that heterochromatin is genetically inactive. Most of the genes of eukaryotes that have been extensively characterized lies in euchromatic regions of the chromosomes. The earlier belief that their is lack of genes in heterochromatic regions is not correct, because genes could be located in heterochromatic regions in several cases like *Drosophila* and tomato. In heterochromatic region the genes perhaps become active for a short period.

25. (a) The surface of centromere consists a special trilaminar plate called kinetochore. It has points for attachment of microtubules. Microtubules produce chromosome fibres or tactile fibrils that is required for the movement of chromosomes during anaphase.

26. (b) All restriction enzymes do not cut at palindromic sequences. A lot of them do though, simply because it is more effective. Recognising a palindromic sequence enables them to cut both strands of DNA at the "same" site, because the strand will have the same sequence only in different directions at that site.

27. (b) The lampbrush chromosomes are highly elongated special kind of synapsed mid-prophase or diplotene chromosome bivalents which have already undergone crossing over. It takes place in diplotene stage of most animal oocystes, spermatocytes of many and even giant nucleus of unicellular alga *Acetabularia*. In meiosis, the number of pairs of loops gradually increase till it reaches maximum is diplotene.

28. (a) Chromosomes are stained with special fluoroscent dyes that have differential affinity for different parts of the chromosomes. It brings about specific banding pattern in which bands are segments of stained chromosomes that appear lighter, darker or stained in comparison to adjacent parts. This technique of staining chromosome is highly useful in knowing various types of chromosomal aberrations or abnormalities like additions, deletions and inversions.

29. (a) Genotype is the hereditary properties of an organism and genetic complement of organism is called genotype.

30. (a) In case of incomplete linkage, the linked gene shows new combination along with parental combination due to crossing over between chromatids.

31. (a) The cells of the plants regenerated from callus that show heritable variation for both qualitative and quantitative traits, such a variation is called somaclonal variation. these variations occurs as a result of chromosome structural changes, gene mutations, plasmagene mutations, gene amplification, altered expression of multigene families, transposable elements or mitotic crossing over.

32. (a) Back cross is a cross that is performed between hybrid and one of its parents. In plant breeding, to increase the traits of that parent back cross is performed after few times in order.

In order to obtain its disease resistance. For example, a crop plant is crossed with a wild variety. In the process most good traits or the crop plant get diluted. In order to transfer the good traits back into it. The hybrid is, therefore, repeatedly crossed with parent crop plant.

33. (a) According to Mendel's inheritance concept, each gene had two alternative forms or allelomorphs, one being dominant and the other recessive. Practically, the wild form can mutate in several ways. The mutant produce can also mutate is several ways. It can also mutate once again to give rise to another mutant form. Therefore, a gene can have more than two allelomorphs. These allelomorphs make multiple alleles series.

34. (a) In most birds, the females are heterogametic (designated as Z W) and males are homogametic (designated as Z Z). The females produce two types of eggs (A + Z) and (A + W). The male gametes or sperms are of one type (A + Z), 1 : 1 sex ratio is produced in the offspring.

35. (b) Fruit fly, *Drosophila* is a tiny fly about 2 mm size which is often found hovering over ripe fruits like mango and banana. *Drosophila* is suitable as experimental material because :-

(i) It is easy to grow in laboratory on a culture medium supported with yeast.
(ii) The fly has a short life span.
(iii) Numerous generations can be obtained in a year.
(iv) Females are easily distinguishable from the males.
(v) Presence of polytene chromosomes can indicate different types of chromosome aberrations.

36. (a) Most sex - linked genes in male heterogametic animals are present on the X- chromosome. Some animals however, may carry a few genes on the Y chromosome that produce visible effects on the phenotype of the organism. Y linkage is very rare in higher animal, particularly mammals. X linkage, on the other hand, is very common in all mammals that have been studied, the mammalian X chromosome contains a larger number of genes with major effects on phenotype.

37. **(c)** In humans, sex of a child depends upon the gametes produced by the male (X, Y).

38. **(c)** In insects, males only have one X chromosomes while females have two (XX) chromosomes i.e. homogametic.

39. **(a)** In Drosophila, on X chromosome the genes for body and eye colour are located. When two genes in a dihybrid cross are situated on the same chromosome, the proportion of parental gene combination are higher than non-parental type. This takes place due to physical association or linkage of the two genes while non-parental gene combinations due to recombination between two genes. Thus, linkage and recombination deviates the ratio from Mendalian ratio of a dihybrid cross, (9 : 3 : 3: 1).

40. **(a)** In pigeons, ZW-ZZ type of sex determination mechanism is found. In this type, the male has two homomorphic sex chromosomes (ZZ) and is homogametic, and the female has two heteromorphic sex chromosomes (ZW) and is heterogametic. Thus, there are two types of eggs with Z and with W and only one type of sperms, i.e., each with Z.

41. **(b)** During sexual reproduction, genetic markers located on the same chromosome tend to remain together, a phenomenon is called linkage. If two genes are linked completely, all gametes would carry the parental combinations and no recombinants would be produced. This in sharp contrast to the 50% recombinant gametes a characteristic of independent assortment. Hence, frequency that can result from crossing over between linked genes is between 0–50%. Strength of the linkage between two genes is inversely proportional to the distance between the two, i.e., two linked genes that show higher frequency of crossing over, if the distance between them is higher and lower frequency if the distance is small.

42. **(a)** When two genes are located on the same chromosome they are called linked genes because they tend to be inherited together. They are an exception to Mendel's law of Segregation because these genes are not inherited independently.

43. **(a)** Mustard gas was the first chemical mutagen discovered. During World war II, C. Auerbach and her associates first discovered the mutagenic effects of mustard gas and related compounds. These compounds are examples of a large class of chemical mutagens that transfer alkyl (CH_3^-, $CH_3CH_2^-$ etc.) groups to the bases in DNA, thus are known as alkylating agents.

44. **(a)** Mutations may be either recessive or dominant. In haploid organisms, like viruses and bacteria, both recessive and dominant mutations can be seen by their effects on the phenotype of the organisms in which they originated. Therefore, in several crops desirable mutants have been isolated among haploids derived in culture.

45. **(a)** Cytogenetic analyses are almost always based on examination of chromosomes fixed during mitotic metaphase. Chromosome banding has since become a standard and indispensible tool for cytogenetic analysis and several banding techniques have been developed : **Q banding** : chromosomes are stained with a fluorescent dye such as quinacrine. **G banding** : produced by staining with Geimsa after digesting the chromosomes with trypsin. **C banding** : chromosomes are treated with acid and base, an then stained with Giesma stain.

46. **(b)** Expressivity describes the phenomenon of differing clinical features or phenotype among individuals carrying the same gene allele or genotype. Variable expression of a phenotype may be influenced by other genetic variations, epigenetic factors, or environment.

47. **(a)** For a recessive allele to produce a recessive phenotype, the individual must have two copies, one from each parent. An individual with one dominant and one recessive allele for a gene will have the dominant phenotype. For a recessive mutation to give rise to a mutant phenotype in a diploid organism, both alleles must carry the mutation. However, one copy of a dominant mutant allele leads to a mutant phenotype. Recessive mutations inactivate the affected gene and lead to a loss of function.

48. **(b)** Muton are elements within a gene that can undergo a mutation and lead to the production of mutant phenotype. The term "muton" is a unit of mutation. It is the largest element in a gene which encodes a polypeptide during protein synthesis. The term "cistron" is a unit of function. Benzer coined the terms cistron (unit of function), recon (unit of recombination) and muton (unit of mutation).

49. **(a)** In pleiotropism, a single gene affects a number of phenotypic traits in the same organism. Phenylketonuria is one of the most widely cited examples in pleiotropy in humans. Phenylketonuria is a genetic disorder inherited from a person's parents. It is due to mutations in the PAH gene which results in low levels of the enzyme phenylalanine hydroxylase.

50. **(c)** Codominance is observed when two different alleles of a specific single-gene trait are both expressed simultaneously. It follows non-mendelian inheritance patterns. Codominance is generally observed in case of coat color of organisms. One such example is the coat color observed in cow.

51. **(a)** When two non-homologous chromosomes mutate by exchanging parts, the resulting chromosomal rearrangements are translocations. Translocations are diagnosed genetically by semi-sterility and by the apparent linkage of genes known to be on separate chromosomes. A heterozygous translocation shows 50 percent sterility and linkage of genes on the chromosome involved in the translocation.

52. **(b)** Polyploidy is the heritable condition of possessing more than two complete sets of chromosomes. Polyploidization with environmental change or stress, and that has led to an increased recognition of its short-term adaptive potential.

53. **(c)** Aneuploidy can be either due to loss of one or more chromosomes (hypoploidy) or due to addition of one or more chromosomes to complete chromosome complement (hyperploidy). Hypopliody is mainly due to loss of a single chromosomes, monosomes $(2n-1)$ or due to loss of one pair of chromosomes, nullisomes $(2n-2)$.

54. **(c)** Haemophilia never occurs in women because it is a recessive gene disease if both the sex chromosome X^hX^h, it will be lethal i.e. such female die before birth. Its gene is never found on chromosome Y.

55. **(c)** Haemophilia also known as bleeder disease is an example of recessive sex linked inheritance in human beings. It is masked in heterozygous condition. The person suffering from this disease lack factors VIII and IX responsible for blood clotting. A small cut may lead to bleeding till death. Men are affected by this disease while women are the carriers.

Mutation of a structural gene on chromosome number 15 causes Marfan syndrome. This disease results in formation of abnormal form of connective tissues and characteristic extreme loosseness of joints.

56. **(c)** Haemophilia bleeding disorder is a group of hereditary genetic disorders that impair the body's ability to control blood clotting or coagulation. In its most common form, Hemophilia A, clotting factor VIII is absent. In Haemophilia B, factor IX is deficient. Factor VIII participates in blood coagulation; it is a cofactor for factor IXa which, in the presence of Ca^{+2} and phospholipids forms a complex that converts factor X to the activated form Xa. Defects in this gene results in hemophilia A, a common recessive X-linked coagulation disorder. Prothrombin producing platelets in such persons are not found in very low concentration.

57. **(c)** Haemophilia is an inherited bleeding disorder where the blood doesn't clot properly. They are typically inherited from one's parents through an X chromosome. Males can have a disease like hemophilia if they inherit an affected X chromosome that has a mutation in either the factor VIII or factor IX gene. Females can also have hemophilia, but this is much rarer.

58. **(c)** Haemophilia is a sex linked disease in which the patient continues to bleed even from a minor cut since he or she does not possess the natural phenomenon of blood clotting. Haemophilia is genetically due to the presence of a recessive gene h, carried by X-chromosome.

59. (c) Sickle cell anemia is a disease in which your body produces abnormally shaped red blood cells. The cells are shaped like a crescent or sickle. The gene defect is a known mutation of a single nucleotide (A to T) of the β-globin gene, which results in glutamic acid (Glu) being substituted by valine (Val) at position 6.

60. (a) Males have only one X chromosome and females have two X chromosomes. Thus, a dosage compensation mechanism must be present through which the effective dosage of genes of the two sexes is made equal. This is achieved by inactivation of one X chromosome in females which gets condensed and become heteropyknotic. Since only one X chromosome is needed for normal metabolism in cells of females, in some cells, the other X chromosome has the ability of being heterochromatic and euchromatic in others. Therefore, dosage compensation regulates the level of enzyme in males and females.

61. (b) An autosome linked recessive trait, sickle cell anaemia that can be transfered from parents to the offspring, if both the partners are carrier for the gene (or heterozygous). The defect is caused by the substitution of Glutamic acid (Glu) by Valine (Val) at the sixth position of the beta globin chain of the haemoglobin molecule. Results due to the single base substituiton at the sixth codon of the beta globin gene from GAG to GuG, the substitution of amino acid in the globin protein occurs. The mutant molecule of haemoglobin under low oxygen tension undergoes polymerisation causing the change in the shape of the RBC from biconcave disc to elongated sickle likes structure.

62. (c) Sickle-cell anaemia is inherited from parents of an individual in an autosomal recessive trait mutation is present in both alleles father and mother.

63. (c) DNA fingerprinting is a method used to identify an individual from a sample of DNA by looking at unique patterns in their DNA. The test is used to determine whether a family relationship exists between two people, to identify organisms causing a disease, and to solve crimes. Only a small sample of cells is needed for DNA fingerprinting. A drop of blood or the root of a hair contains enough DNA for testing.

64. (c) Phenylketonuria is an inborn, autosomal, recessive metabolic disorder in which the homozygous recessive individual lacks the enzyme phenylalanine hydroxylase needed to change phenylalanine (amino acid) to tyrosine (amino acid) in liver. It results in hyperphenylalaninemia which is characterised by accumulation and excretion of phenylalanine, phenylpyruvic acid and related compounds.

65. (a) Phenylketonuria is an inherited error of metabolism caused by a deficiency of enzyme phenylalanine hydroxylase. It is an autosomal recessive trait. It is a hereditary human condition that results from the inability to convert phenylalanine into tyrosine. This leads to over production of phenylalanine and its conversion to phenylpyruvic acid and other derivatives. Due to poor absorption by kidneys, these are then excreted in urine.

66. (b) Phenylketonuria is an recessive autosomal gene disorder. It occurs due to the absence of enzyme phenylalanine hydroxylase which changes phenylalanine to tyrosine.

67. (a) Aneuploidy is the presence of an abnormal number of chromosomes in a cell, for example a human cell having 45 or 47 chromosomes instead of the usual 46. Aneuploidy is an error in cell division that results in the "daughter" cells having the wrong number of chromosomes. Chromosomes in Down syndrome is the most common human condition due to aneuploidy. Down syndrome also known as trisomy 21, is a genetic disorder caused by the presence of all or part of a third copy of chromosome 21.

68. (d) Due absence of X chromosome Turner's syndrome occurs. Individuals having a single X chromosome 2A + XO (45) have female sexual differentiation but ovaries are rudimentary. Other associated phenotypes of this condition are short stature, webbed-neck, broad chest, lack of secondary sexual characteristics and sterility. Thus, any change in the copies of the sex chromosomes may disrupt the genetic information which is necessary for normal sexual development.

Chapter

28

Molecular Basis of Inheritance

Directions: In the following questions, a statement of assertion is followed by a statement of reason. Mark the correct choice as:

(a) If both Assertion and Reason are true and Reason is the correct explanation of Assertion.
(b) If both Assertion and Reason are true but Reason is not the correct explanation of Assertion.
(c) If Assertion is true but Reason is false.
(d) If both Assertion and Reason are false.

1. **Assertion :** In a DNA molecule, A–T rich parts melt before G–C rich parts.
   Reason : In between A and T there are three H–bond, whereas in between G and C there are two H-bonds. **[AIIMS 2010, 2015]**
2. **Assertion:** The two chains of DNA have anti-polarity.
   Reason: In one chain of DNA, ribose sugar at 5' end consists of a free phosphate moiety while at the other end the ribose has a free 3' OH group.
3. **Assertion:** Adenine cannot pair with cytosine.
   Reason: Adenine and cytosine do not have a perfect match between hydrogen donor and hydrogen acceptor sites. Hence, they cannot pair.
4. **Assertion:** The sugar phosphate backbone of two chains in DNA double helix show anti-parallel polarity.
   Reason: The phosphodiester bonds in one strand go from a 3' carbon of one nucleotide to a 5' carbon of adjacent nucleotide, whereas those in complementary strand go vice versa.
5. **Assertion:** DNA is considered to be better genetic material than RNA for most organisms.
   Reason: 2'-OH group present in DNA makes it labile and less reactive.
6. **Assertion :** Histones are basic proteins of major importance in packaging of eukaryotic DNA. DNA and histones comprise chromatin forming the bulk of eukaryotic chromosome.
   Reason : Histones are of five major types $H_1, H_2A\ H_2B, H_3$ and H_4. **[AIIMS 2000]**
7. **Assertion :** DNA is associated with proteins.
   Reason : DNA binds around histone proteins that form a pool and the entire structure is called a nucleosome. **[AIIMS 2013]**
8. **Assertion:** Histones are basic in nature.
   Reason: Histones are rich in the amino acids lysine and arginine.
9. **Assertion:** DNA acts as a genetic material in all organisms.
   Reason: It is a single-stranded biomolecule.
10. **Assertion:** In Griffith's experiment, a mixture of heat-killed virulent bacteria R and live non-virulent bacteria S, lead to the death of mice.
    Reason: 'Transforming principle' got transferred from heat killed R strain to S strain and made it virulent.
11. **Assertion:** Template or antisense strand, having $3' \rightarrow 5'$ polarity takes part in transcription.
    Reason: Non-template or sense strand, having $5' \rightarrow 3'$ polarity, does not take part in transcription.
12. **Assertion:** The uptake of DNA during transformation is an active, energy requiring process.
    Reason: Transformation occurs only in those bacteria, which possess the enzymatic machinery involved in the active uptake and recombination.
13. **Assertion:** Killer strain of *Paramecium aurelia* can kill sensitive strain.
    Reason: If sensitive strain is provided kappa particle, it becomes killer.
14. **Assertion:** Scaffold proteins are nonhistone chromosomal proteins.
    Reason: They are rich in lysine and arginine.
15. **Assertion:** Viruses having RNA genome have shorter life span and mutate faster.
    Reason: RNA is unstable and thus mutates faster.

16. **Assertion:** Replication on one strand of DNA is continuous and on another is discontinuous.
Reason: The DNA polymerase works in 3' → 5' direction.

17. **Assertion:** The mechanism of DNA replication is semiconservative in nature.
Reason: Each of the complementary strands of the parental double helix is conserved during the process.

18. **Assertion:** Synthesis of daughter or new strand occurs continuously along the parent 3' → 5' strand.
Reason: DNA polymerase can polymerise nucleotides in 3' → 5' direction on 5' → 3' strand.

19. **Assertion:** One of the two strands of DNA is called sense strand and other is called antisense strand.
Reason: Sense strand of DNA forms complementary RNA.

20. **Assertion:** The nitrogen bases of the two chains of DNA are held together by hydrogen bonds.
Reason: Both chains of DNA are antiparallel.

21. **Assertion** : Replication and transcription occurs in cytoplasm.
Reason : mRNA is transferred from the nucleus into the cytoplasm where ribosomes and amino acids are available for protein synthesis.

22. **Assertion** : Central dogma is the flow of information from DNA to mRNA and then decoding the information present in mRNA in the form of protein.
Reason : In retroviruses, reverse of central dogma occurs.

23. **Assertion** : One gene is required for one enzyme.
Reason : Genes express themselves through synthesis of enzymes.

24. **Assertion** : An mRNA has both initiation codon and termination codon.
Reason : It specifies only a single polypeptide or number of them.

25. **Assertion** : UAA, UAG and UGA terminate protein synthesis.
Reason : They are not recognised by tRNA.

26. **Assertion** : The tRNA molecules possess anticodons.
Reason : It needs the message in form of codon.

27. **Assertion:** mRNA attaches to ribosome through its 3' end.
Reason: The mRNA has F-capsular nucleotide and bases of lagging sequence. **[AIIMS 2002]**

28. **Assertion:** A single mRNA strand is capable of forming a number of different polypeptide chains.
Reason: The mRNA strand has terminator codons.

29. **Assertion:** mRNA has some untranslated regions that are not translated.
Reason: UTRs are required for efficient translation.

30. **Assertion:** Eukaryotic mRNA requires post-transcription processing for formation of functional mRNA.
Reason: Eukaryotic transcripts possess extra non-functional segments called introns.

31. **Assertion:** A change in nitrogen base at the third position of a codon causes change in the expression of the codon.
Reason: A codon is mostly read by all the three nitrogen bases.

32. **Assertion:** Untranslated regions are sequences of RNA before initiation codon and after termination codon.
Reason: Untranslated regions provide stability to mRNA and also increase translational efficiency.

33. **Assertion:** The predominant site for control of gene expression in prokaryotes is transcription initiation.
Reason: The activity of RNA polymerase is regulated by accessory proteins, which affect recognition of start sites.

34. **Assertion:** Initiation step of protein synthesis in prokaryotes and eukaryotes has several differences.
Reason: They both form *m*RNA-*t*RNA complex with smaller subunit of ribosome.

35. **Assertion:** Polycistronic mRNA, found in prokaryotes, specify a number of polypeptides.
Reason: Monocistronic mRNA, found in eukaryotes, specify only a single polypeptide.

36. **Assertion:** tRNA recognises its corresponding codon in mRNA.
Reason: For each codon, there is an individual tRNA.

37. **Assertion:** A monocistronic *m*RNA can produce several types of polypeptide chains.
Reason: The terminator codon is present on the *r*RNA.

38. **Assertion:** Regulator and operator genes are not associated with constitutive genes.
Reason: Constitutive genes need not be repressed.

39. **Assertion:** In transcription, the strand with 3'→5' polarity acts as the template strand.
Reason: The RNA polymerase catalyses the polymerisation in only one direction that is 5'→3'.

40. **Assertion :** Genetic code is universal.
Reason : Genetic code is same for all organisms.

41. **Assertion :** The genetic codes are commaless.
Reason : Genetic codes are overlapping.

42. **Assertion:** When the DNA sequences of two people are cut using the same restriction enzyme, the length and number of fragments obtained are different for both.
Reason: DNA sequence is arranged tandemly in many copy numbers which varies from chromosome to chromosome in an individual, showing high degree of polymorphism.

43. **Assertion:** Repetitive sequences make up very large portion of human genome.
Reason: Repetitive sequences do not have direct coding functions in the genome.

44. **Assertion:** DNA polymerase-I acts as proofreader.
Reason: DNA polymerase-I removes mismatched nucleotides.

45. **Assertion:** *r*RNA is the most abundant RNA.
Reason: *r*RNA is a constituent of ribosomes.

46. **Assertion:** Ribosomes protect *m*RNA from ribonuclease.
Reason: *m*RNA is located in the gap between the two ribosomal subunits.

47. **Assertion:** In prokaryotes, there are three initiation factors used for protein synthesis.
Reason: All the initiation factors have their own functions.

48. **Assertion :** Comparative biochemistry provides a strong evidence in favour of a common ancestry of living beings.
Reason : Genetic code is universal.

49. **Assertion:** RNA produced during transcription in eukaryotic cells cannot be straight away used in photosynthesis.
Reason: RNA splicing phenomena helps in the removal of exons.

50. **Assertion :** A gene is a section of DNA that codes for a defined biochemical function.
Reason : The nature of the protein, therefore, depends upon genetic makeup.

51. **Assertion :** The genetic code is degenerate.
Reason : Most amino acids are coded by more than one codon.

52. **Assertion :** A number of different polypeptide chains can be formed from a single mRNA strand.
Reason : The mRNA strand has terminator codons.

53. **Assertion:** An organism with lethal mutation may not even develop beyond the zygote.
Reason: All types of gene mutations are lethal. **[AIIMS 2006]**

54. **Assertion:** Polytene chromosomes have a high amount of DNA.
Reason: Polytene chromosomes are formed by repeated replication. **[AIIMS 2006]**

55. **Assertion:** Lac operon is a repressible operon.
Reason: The product of gene activity stops the activity of the lac operon.

56. **Assertion:** hnRNA is larger than mRNA.
Reason: hnRNA has non-translating introns which are not required for translation.

57. **Assertion:** The bacteria and other prokaryotes show high adaptability to the changing environment.
Reason: Member of kingdom Monera are efficient in regulating gene expression.

58. **Assertion:** DNA is found in mitochondria and chloroplast are called prochromosome.
Reason: They are similar to prokaryotic chromosome.

59. **Assertion :** Prokaryotic DNA is similar to mitochondrial DNA.
Reason : Mitochondrial are proved to have evolved from the prokaryotes.

60. **Assertion:** Heterochromatin is transcripationally inactive.
Reason: Heterochromatin is densely packed.

61. **Assertion :** Crick suggested for the first time requirement of 'adaptor' molecule for translation with polynucleotide chain having 75-85 bases.
Reason : It will synthesize inducible enzymes.

62. Assertion : The expression of cellular genetic information in unidirectional.

Reason : Cancer virus goes topsy-turvy, therefore, reverse transcription allows a sequence of RNA to be retrieved and used as genetic information.

63. Assertion: *Agrobacterium tumefaciens* is popular in genetic engineering because this bacterium is associated with the roots of all cereal and pulse crops.

Reason: A gene incorporated in the bacterial chromosomal genome gets automatically transferred to the crop with which the bacterium is associated.

64. Assertion : DNA fingerprinting is applied in paternity testing in case of disputes.

Reason : It employs the principle of polymorphism in DNA sequences as the polymorphisms are inheritable from parent to children.

65. Assertion: Gel electrophoresis and elution are two important processes.

Reason: After staining with ethidium bromide it has to be exposed to U.V. light.

Solutions

1. (c) In a DNA molecule, A-T rich parts melt before G-C rich parts because there are two H-bond between A and T whereas in between G and C, there are three H-bond.
2. (a) The two chains of DNA have anti-parallel polarity this is because one chain has free phosphate moiety at 5'-end of the sugar and another chain has free phosphate moiety at 3'-end.
3. (a) In DNA, the code letters are A, T, G, and C, which stand for the chemicals adenine, thymine, guanine, and cytosine, respectively. In base pairing, adenine always pairs with thymine, and guanine always pairs with cytosine.
4. (a) The backbone of a DNA chain or strand is built up of alternate deoxyribose sugar and phosphoric acid groups. The phosphate group is connected to carbon 5' of the sugar residue of its own nucleotide and carbon 3' of the sugar residue of the next nucleotide by (3' $\rightarrow$ 5') phosphodiester bonds. The two DNA chains are antiparallel, that is, they run parallel but in opposite directions. In one chain the direction is 5' $\rightarrow$ 3' while in the opposite one, it is 3' $\rightarrow$ 5'.
5. (c) The genetic material should be stable enough not to change with different stages of life cycle, age or with change in physiology of the organism. The DNA strands being complementary, if separated by heating come together only when appropriate conditions are provided. Further, 2'-OH group present at every nucleotide in RNA is a reactive group and makes RNA labile and easily degradable. RNA is also now known to be catalytic, hence reactive. Therefore, DNA chemically is less reactive and structurally more stable when compared to RNA. Therefore, among the two nucleic acids, DNA is a better genetic material.
6. (a) Histones are basic proteins found in the eukaryotic chromosomes. These are rich in the amino acids lysine and arginine. Histonie proteins are basic proteins consisting of 5 types – H_1, H_2A, H_2B, H_3, H_4. DNA is coiled around it. It exists as octamers linked with H_1.
7. (a) A chain of DNA has 140 base pairs, make $1\frac{3}{4}$ turns and twist around a histone octamer forming nucleosome. The core of nucleosome consists of 4 histones H_2A, H_2B, H_3 and H_4.
8. (a) Histones contain a large proportion of the positively charged (basic) amino acids, lysine and arginine in their structure. DNA is negatively charged due to the phosphate groups on its backbone.
9. (d) DNA is the hereditary material found in the nucleus of eukaryotic cells and the cytoplasm of prokaryotic cells that determines the composition of the organism. There is another type of genetic material found in cells and viruses known as ribonucleic acid (RNA). DNA is double stranded as well as single stranded biomolecule.
10. (d) When bacteria *Streptococcus pneumoniae* are grown on a culture plate, some produce smooth shiny colonies (S) while others produce rough colonies (R). This is because the S strain bacteria have a mucous (polysaccharide) coat, while R strain does not. Mice infected with the S strain (virulent) die from pneumonia infection but mice infected with the R strain do not develop pneumonia. In Griffith's experiment, some 'transforming principle', transferred from the heat-killed S strain, had enabled the R strain to synthesize a smooth polysaccharide coat and become virulent which must be due to the transfer of the genetic material. This is known as transformation.
11. (b) Strand of DNA which has 3' $\rightarrow$ 5' polarity is called template strand or master strand or antisense, or (-) strand. The other strand which has a polarity of 5' $\rightarrow$ 3' is displaced during transcription. This non-template strand which does not take part in transcription is also called sense or coding strand or plus (+) strand because genetic code present in this strand is similar to genetic code (based on mRNA) except that uracil is replaced by thymine.

12. (a) Transformation does not involve passive entry of DNA molecules through permeable cell walls and membranes. It does not occur 'naturally' in all species of bacteria, only in those species possessing the enzymatic machinery involved in the active uptake and recombination processes. Even in these species, all cells in a given population are not capable of active uptake of DNA. Only competent cells, which possess a so – called competence factor are capable of serving as recipients in transformation.
13. (b) *Paramecium aurelia* has two strains : killer and sensitive. The killer strain is able to kill the sensitive strain protist by means of chemical paramecin, secreted by minute cytoplasmic particles called kappa particle. The sensitive strain protists do not have kappa particles. The sensitive strain can also become killer if it receives sufficient kappa particles.
14. (c) Structural nonhistone chromosomal proteins are called scaffold proteins as they constitute the core axis of the chromosome. They contain very little lysine and arginine but instead possess abundant tyrosine and tryptophan types of amino acids.
15. (a) Unlike DNA, RNA is usually single-stranded. Additionally, RNA contains ribose sugars rather than deoxyribose sugars, which makes RNA more unstable and more prone to degradation. RNA is synthesized from DNA by an enzyme known as RNA polymerase during a process called transcription. Viruses having RNA have shorter life span and mutate at faster rate.
16. (a) The DNA polymerase works in the 3' $\rightarrow$ 5' direction thus continuously synthesising the strand having polarity 5' $\rightarrow$ 3'.
17. (a) DNA replication is semiconservative, a type of replication in which one strand of the daughter duplex is derived from the parent while the other strand is formed new. This is carried out by the separation of two strands. The separated strands function as templates. The new strands built up over the templates of old strands will have complementray base pairs (A opposite T and G opposite C). The two daughter DNA molecules thus, formed will be carbon copies of the parent molecule but shall have one new strand and one old strand.
18. (c) DNA-polymerase can polymerise nucleotides only in 5' $\rightarrow$ 3' direction on 3' $\rightarrow$ 5' strand because it adds them at the 3' direction on 3' $\rightarrow$ 5' strand because it adds them at the 3' end. Replication over the two templates proceeds in opposite directions. One strand with polarity 3' $\rightarrow$ 5' forms its complementary strand continuously because 3' end of latter is always open for elongation. It is called leading strand. Replication is discontinuous on the other template with polarity 5' $\rightarrow$ 3' because only a short segment of DNA strand can be built in 5' $\rightarrow$ 3' direction due to exposure of a small stretch of template at one time. Short segments of replicated DNA are called Okazaki fragments. DNA strand built up of Okazaki fragments is called lagging strand. As one strand grows continuously while the other strand is formed discontinuously, DNA replication is semidiscontinuous.
19. (b) Only one of the two strands of DNA possesses correct hereditary information. It is known as sense strand. Its complementary strand is called antisense strand. Antisense RNA that is made from the DNA strand that is complementary to the sense strand of the DNA.
20. (b) The nitrogen bases of DNA are of two types namely (i) pyrimidines and (ii) purines. The nitrogen bases of the two chains formed complementary pairs with purine of one and pyrimidine of the other held together by hydrogen bonds. The two chains are antiparallel with 5' $\rightarrow$ 3' orientation of one and 3' $\rightarrow$ 5' orientation of the other.
21. (d) Replication and transcription occur in the nucleus whereas translation occurs in cytoplasm. mRNA is transferred from the nucleus as it is needed in the formation of proteins (amino acid), rRNA, tRNA and mRNA.
22. (b) Biosynthesis of protein is under direct control of DNA in most cases or else under the control of genetic RNA where DNA is absent. Sequences of bases in a particular segment of a polynucleotide chain will determine the sequence of amino acids in a particular polypeptide. The relationship is popularly known as central dogma. Flow of information is one way, *i.e.*, from DNA, information is transferred to RNA (mRNA)

and from RNA to protein. Temin (1970) reported that retroviruses operate a central dogma reverse or teminism inside host cells. Genomic RNA of these viruses first synthesizes DNA through reverse transcription. DNA then transfers information to messenger RNA which takes part in translation of the coded information to form polypeptide.

$$DNA \xrightarrow{\text{transcription}} RNA \xrightarrow{\text{translation}} proteins$$

(i) One way flow of information (central dogma)

$$DNA \underset{\longleftarrow}{\xrightarrow{\text{transcription}}} RNA \xrightarrow{\text{translation}} proteins$$

(i) Reverse flow of transcription information

23. (a) Genes control various traits in an organism through a controlled exercise on the developmental processes. Such a control is due to synthesis of proteins, which is under direct control of genes. Some of these proteins synthesized by genes are enzymes and control biosynthetic pathways. Based on their work, Beadle and Tatum proposed a concept called one gene-one enzyme hypothesis. Such a hypothesis means that if in a biosynthetic pathway several steps are involved, each step is controlled by a specific enzyme, which is synthesized under the control of a specific gene.

24. (b) mRNA is a long RNA. It gets attached to ribosome. mRNA has methylated region at the 5' terminus. It functions as a cap for attachment with ribosome. Cap is followed by an initiation codon (AUG) either immediately or after a small non coding region. Then there is coding region followed by termination codon (UAA, UAG or UGA). There is then a small non coding region and poly A area at the 3' terminus. An mRNA may specify only a single polypeptide or a number of them. The former is called monocistronic while the latter is known as polycistronic.

25. (a) Synthesis of polypeptide terminates when a nonsense codon of mRNA reaches the A - site. There are three nonsense codons - UAA, UAG and UGA. These codons are not recognised by any of the tRNAs. Therefore, no more aminoacyl tRNA reaches the A- site. The P-site tRNA is hydrolysed and the completed polypeptide is released in the presence of release factor. Thus termination occurs.

26. (b) tRNA has anticodons which read the message expressed in the form of codons in mRNA and occupy a specific place on mRNA. tRNA also recognises the amino acids.

27. (d) mRNA is attached to the ribosome by means of protein ribophorin I & II. The sequence of nucleotides on mRNA is called codon.

28. (b) A single mRNA strand is capable of forming different polypeptide chains because it has different reading frame (the way through which reading of mRNA by tRNA occurs).

29. (b) In molecular genetics, the 5' untranslated region (5' UTR) (leader sequence or leader RNA) is the region of an mRNA that is directly upstream from the initiation codon. This region is important for the regulation of translation of a transcript by differing mechanisms in viruses, prokaryotes and eukaryotes. The three prime untranslated regions (3'-UTR) is the section of messenger RNA (mRNA) that immediately follows the translation termination codon. An mRNA molecule is transcribed from the DNA sequence and is later translated into protein.

30. (a) In eukaryotes, the monocistronic structural genes have interrupted coding sequences i.e., the genes in eukaryotes are split. The Coding sequences or expressed sequences are defined as exons. They are said to be those sequence that appear in mature or processed RNA. The exons are interrupted by introns or intervening sequences which do not appear in nature or processed RNA. The exons are interrupted by introns or intervening sequences which do not appear in mature or processed RNA. Thus, post-transcription processing, which involves splicing of introns and fusion of exons, is required to form functional mRNA.

31. (d) According to Wobble hypothesis, only the first two position of triplet codon on mRNA have a precise pairing with the bases of the tRNA anticodon. The pairing of the third position bases of the codon may be ambiguous, and varies according to the

nucleotide present in this position. Thus, a single tRNA type is able to recognize two or more codons differing only in the third base. The same is called wobble position.

32. (b) A translational unit in mRNA is the sequence of RNA that is flanked by the start codon (AUG) and the stop codon and codes for a polypeptide. An mRNA has some additional sequences that are not translated and are referred as untranslated regions (UTR). The UTRs are present at both 5'-end (before start codon) and 3'-end (after stop codon). They are required for efficient translation process.

33. (a) In prokaryotes, control of the rate of transcriptional initiation is the predominant site for control of gene expression. In a transcription unit, the activity of RNA polymerase at a given promoter is in turn regulated by interaction with accessory proteins, which affect its ability to recognize start sites. These regulatory proteins can act both positively (activators) and negatively (repressors).

34. (b) The differences between initiation step of protein synthesis in eukaryotes and prokaryotes are :

(i) In prokaryotes initiation factors are three – IF_1, IF_2 and IF_3. Eukaryotes have at least ten initiation factors – eIF_1, eIF_2, eIF_3, eIF_4A, eIF_4B, eIF_4C, eIF_4D, eIF_4F, eIF_5 and eIF_6.

(ii) In eukaryotes, formylation of methionine does not take place. In prokaryotes, *t*RNA is charged with formylated methionine.

(iii) The larger subunit of ribosome combines with 40S – *m*RNA – $tRNA^{Met}$ (in case of prokaryotes, 30S) complex to form intact ribosome. It requires initiation factor IF1 in prokaryotes and factors eIF1, eIF4 (A, B, C) in eukaryotes.

35. (b) When a paritcular gene codes for a mRNA strand it is said to be monocistronic or monogenic. When several genes (cistrons) are transcribed into a single mRNA molecule, it is described as polycistronic or polygenic. Monoistronic mRNA codes for one complete protein molecule while polycistronic mRNA codes for a number of protein molecules. Prokaryotic mRNA are polycistronic. Eukaryotic mRNA are monocistronic.

36. (c) tRNA has an anticodon loop which has 7 bases, out of which three bases form anticodon for recognising and attaching to the codon of mRNA. Since there are 61 codons specifying amino acids, the cell should contain 61 different tRNA molecules, each with a different anticodon. Actually, however, the number of tRNA molecule types discovered is much less than 61. This implies that the anticodons of some tRNAs read more than one codon on mRNA.

37. (d) Eukaryotic *m*RNA is called monocistronic i.e., formed from one gene. These have been described to contain only 1 initiation site, who gave one *m*RNA-one polypeptide chain hypothesis.

The terminator codon is present on *m*RNA molecule, which stops the formation of a polypeptide chain at that point, the three termination codons are UGA, UAA and UAG

38. (a) Regulator gene controls the operator gene in cooperation with a chemical compound called inducer present in the cytoplasm. The regulatior gene codes for and produce a protein substance called repressor. The repressor substance combines with the operator gene to repress its function. Therefore, it is called regulator gene.

The constitutive genes keep on functioning all the time. They need not be repressed. Therefore, the regulator and operator genes are not associated with them.

39. (a) During transcription, only one of the two DNA strands is copied. This is called the template strand because it acts as a template for the mRNA that is being assembled by the ribosome. The template strand has 3'-5' polarity. The non-template strand is known as the coding strand. Because the coding strand and the mRNA formed from the template strand are both complementary to the template strand, they will have the same sequence. RNA polymerase also known as DNA-dependent RNA polymerase, is an enzyme that produces primary transcript RNA.

40. (a) The genetic code is applicable universally, *i.e.*, a codon specifies the same amino acid from a virus to a tree or human being. The major exception to the universality of the code occurs in mitochondria of humans, yeast and several other species, where UGA is a tryptophan codon.

41. (c) A commaless genetic code means that no punctuations are needed between any two words. The genetic code is non-overlapping. In actual practice six bases code for not more than two amino acids.

42. (a) In satellite DNA, repetition of bases is in tandem. Depending upon length, base composition and numbers of tandemly repetitive units, satellite DNAs have subcategories like microsatellites and minisatellites. Satellite DNAs show polymorphism. The mutations in the noncoding sequences have piled up with time and form the basis of DNA polymorphism (variation at genetic level arises due to mutations). DNA polymorphism is the basis of genetic mapping of human genome as well as DNA fingerprinting. DNA of each organism has specific sequences that can be cleaved by restriction enzymes to produce fragments of different lengths. These fragments are called restriction fragments. Occurrence of different length of DNA sequence cleaved at restriction sites is referred to as restriction fragment length polymorphism (RFLP).

43. (b) Repeated or repetitive sequences make up a large portion of human genome. These sequences are nucleotide sequences that are repeated many times, sometimes hundred to thousand times. They have no direct coding function but provide informations as to chromosome structure, dynamics and evolution.

44. (a) DNA polymerase I can also remove thymine dimers produced due to UV irradiation and fill the gap due to excision. The newly formed segment is sealed by DNA ligase.

45. (b) The amount of *r*RNA is 70-80% of total RNA. It is a constituent of ribosomes. RNAs of eukaryotes are of four types –28 S, 18 S, 5.8 S and 5 S. Prokaryotic ribosomes have three types of RNAs –23 S, 16 S amd 5 S.

46. (a) The *m*RNA is located in the gap between the two ribosomal subunits, as a result of which the ribosome protects a stretch of 25 nucleotides of the *m*RNA from degradation by ribonuclease.

47. (a) In prokaryotes, three initiation factors are present – IF_1, IF_2, IF_3. All three factors are essential for initiation when natural *m*RNA are used as templates. IF_3 binds to the 30 S ribosomal subunit and is required for its binding to the *m*RNA starting site. IF_3 also functions as a ribosome dissociation factors. IF_2 binds the initiator *f*Met- *t*RNA and carries it to the ribosome (together with GTP) in response to the first AUG codon. IF_1 participates in the interaction between IF_2 and the initiator *t*RNA.

48. (a) The genetic code, the three-letter codons direct the assembly of exactly the same amino acids in nearly every organism on earth. Bacteria, plants and you all use exactly the same genetic code. That's why it is said that the genetic code is universal. The biochemistry of all living things on earth is incredibly similar, showing that all of earth's organisms share a common ancestry.

49. (c) Splicing is the editing of the nascent precursor messenger RNA (pre-mRNA) transcript into a mature messenger RNA (mRNA). After splicing, introns are removed and exons are joined together (ligated).

50. (a) A section of DNA that codes for one particular protein is called a gene. Each chromosome contains thousands of different genes.

51. (a) Phenomenon in which more than one codon encodes a single amino acid is called degeneracy of genetic code.

52. (b) A single mRNA strand is capable of forming different polypeptide chains because it has different reading frame (the way through which reading of mRNA by tRNA).

53. (c) Organisms with lethal mutation bear lethal genes that result in the death of the individual which carries them. The completely lethal genes usually cause death of the zygote. Mutation is a sudden heritable change in the sequence of gene occuring on the chromosomes. Mutation may be beneficial, normal, sublethal or lethal.

54. (a) Polytene chromosomes show endomitosis and they have high DNA content.

55. (d) An operon is a part of genetic material (or DNA)which acts as a single regulated unit having one or more structural genes, an

operator gene, a promoter gene, a regulator gene, a repressor inducer or corepressor (from outside). Lac operon is an inducible operon. An inducible operon system is a regulated unit of genetic material which is switched on in response to the presence of a chemical.

56. **(a)** hnRNA contains some introns. Introns are the intervening sequences, which do not code for proteins. Before translation, they have to be removed. That's why, hnRNA is larger than mRNA.

57. **(a)** To a considerable degree, the adaptability of bacteria and other prokaryotes depends on their ability to "turn on" and "turn off" the expression of specific sets of genes in response to environmental changes. Regulatory mechanisms of this type are very important in microorganisms because of the frequent exposure of these organisms to sudden changes in environment. They provide microorganisms with a great deal of "plasticity", an ability to rapidly adjust their metabolic processes in order to achieve maximum growth and reproduction under highly variable environmental conditions.

58. **(a)** Prokaryotic chromosome (prochromosome) consists of a naked double strand of DNA, that is DNA is not associated with histone proteins. DNA is not linear but is circular with no free ends. DNAs of mitochondria and chloroplast resembles prokaryotic chromosome and are, therefore, called organelle prochromo-some.

59. **(b)** The endosymbiotic theory postulates that the several key organelles of eukaryotes had originated as symbiosis between separate single-called organisms. According to this theory, mitochondria, plastids (e.g., chloroplasts), and possibly other organelles represent formerly free-living bacteria that were taken inside the other cells as an endosymbiont. Molecular and biochemical evidence suggested that the mitochondrion is developed form proteobacteria (in particular, rickettsiales, close relatives) and the chloroplast from cyanobacteria.

60. **(a)** Euchromatin is prevalent in cells that are active in the transcription of many of their genes while heterochromatin is most abundant in cells that are less active or not active. Heterochromatin is a tightly packed form of DNA, which comes in multiple varieties.

61. **(c)** Crick, in his adaptor hypothesis, proposed that small RNA molecules would be the adaptors that could be charged with amino acids by specific enzymes and that could identify the codons (triplets of nucleotides) of the mRNA by base-pairing. These adaptors could thus participate in incorporating the amino acids into a growing polypeptide. Subsequently these adaptors were identified and are now known as the tRNA molecules. A transfer RNA is an adaptor molecule composed of RNA, typically 76 to 90 nucleotides in length.

62. **(a)** Genetic information flows unidirectional, from DNA to protein and with messenger RNA (mRNA) as intermediate. Cancer virus goes topsy-turvy, sequence of RNA to be retrieved and used as genetic information.

63. **(d)** *Agrobacterium tumefacines* is a rod shaped free living bacteria it cause infection only in broad leave dicot plant through the wound site and transfer the tumor inducing gene to host plant and cause tumor. This spontaneous transfer of gene occurs only by the *Agrobacterium.*

64. **(a)** DNA fingerprinting is a test to identify and evaluate the genetic information, called DNA (deoxyribonucleic acid), of a person's cells. The first methods for finding out genetics used for DNA profiling involved RFLP(Restriction fragment length polymorphism) analysis. DNA is collected from cells, such as a blood sample, and cut into small pieces using a restriction enzyme (restriction digest). This generates thousands of DNA fragments of differing sizes as a consequence of variations between DNA sequences of different individuals. The fragments are then separated on the basis of size using gel electrophoresis.

65. **(b)** Gel extraction or gel isolation is a technique used to isolate a desired fragment of intact DNA from an agarose gel through agarose gel electrophoresis. The basic principle behind DNA recovery from agarose gel involves a sequence of bind, wash, and elute steps.

Chapter 29

Evolution

Directions: In the following questions, a statement of assertion is followed by a statement of reason. Mark the correct choice as:

(a) If both Assertion and Reason are true and Reason is the correct explanation of Assertion.
(b) If both Assertion and Reason are true but Reason is not the correct explanation of Assertion.
(c) If Assertion is true but Reason is false.
(d) If both Assertion and Reason are false.

1. **Assertion :** According to big-bang hypothesis about 20 billion years ago universe was a big ball of only neutrons.
Reason : Movement of these particles is known to generate tremendous heat which caused explosion due to temperature and pressure changes.

2. **Assertion :** Big-bang theory is based on studies of Sir James Jeans.
Reason : He gave the theory of steady state.

3. **Assertion :** Milky way is the galaxy in the universe.
Reason : Our Earth is part of milky way.

4. **Assertion :** The primitive atmosphere was reducing once *i.e.*, without oxygen.
Reason : In the primitive atmosphere, oxygen was involved in forming ozone. **[AIIMS 2009]**

5. **Assertion :** Organic compounds first evolved in earth required for origin of life were protein and nucleic acid.
Reason : All life forms were in water environment only. **[AIIMS 2016]**

6. **Assertion:** Theory of chemical evolution proposed that life comes from pre-existing non-living organic molecules.
Reason: The primitive earth conditions led to production of organic molecules.

7. **Assertion:** Louis Pasteur showed that in flask open to air, new living organisms appeared in the heat killed yeast culture.
Reason: Life arises from pre-existing life.

8. **Assertion:** Primitive atmosphere was of reducing type.
Reason: First hydrogen atoms combined with all oxygen.

9. **Assertion :** Stanley Miller could work on experimental evidence of origin of life because of Harold Urey.
Reason : H. Urey was geochemist, cosmochemist and teacher of S. miller.

10. **Assertion :** Darwin's finches show a variety of beaks suited for eating large seeds, flying insects and cactus seeds.
Reason : Ancestral seed-eating stock of Darwin's finches radiated out from South America main land to different geographical areas of the Galapagos Islands, where they found competitor-free new habitats.

11. **Assertion :** Coacervates are believed to be the precursors of life.
Reason : Coacervates were self-duplicating aggregates of proteins surrounded by lipid molecules. **[AIIMS 2004]**

12. **Assertion:** The first cells used RNA as their hereditary molecule.
Reason: DNA evolved from RNA.

13. **Assertion :** The first molecules formed for replicating cells were most probably RNA.
Reason : This was proved by origin of ribozyme T. Cech in *Tetrahymena.*

14. **Assertion:** We have lost all the direct evidence of origin of life.
Reason: The persons responsible for protecting evidences were not skilled. **[AIIMS 1998]**

15. **Assertion :** The earliest organisms that appeared on the earth were non-green and presumably anaerobes.
Reason : The first autotrophic organisms were the chemoautotrophs that never released oxygen. **[AIIMS 2006]**

16. **Assertion:** Earth is billions of years old.
Reason: This inference has been established by radioisotope dating methods.

17. **Assertion:** Analogous structures are different in appearance with same function.
Reason: Divergent evolution leads to analogy.
18. **Assertion:** Thorns and tendrils of *Bougainvillea* and cucurbita represent homology.
Reason: Homologous organs have similar functions but are different in their structural details and origin.
19. **Assertion:** Moths living in the industrial areas became dark to match body color to the tree trunks.
Reason: Smoke from industries covers the moths, making them appear dark.
20. **Assertion:** The embryos of fish, salamander, tortoise, chick and a man, of same age resemble one another closely.
Reason: Ontogeny recapitulates phylogeny.
21. **Assertion:** Cell like aggregates of complex organic compounds are called coacervates.
Reason: Coacervates have power to grow and divide.
22. **Assertion :** From evolutionary point of view, human gestation period is believed to be shortening.
Reason : One major evolutionary trend in humans has been the larger head undergoing relatively faster growth rate in the foetal stage.
[AIIMS 2004]
23. **Assertion :** Natural selection is the outcome of difference in survival and reproduction among individuals that show variation in one or more traits.
Reason : Adaptive forms of a given trait tend to become more common; less adaptive ones become less common or disappear.
[AIIMS 2004, 2012]
24. **Assertion:** Lichens act as pollution indicators.
Reason: Lichens will not grow in areas that are polluted.
25. **Assertion:** Adaptive ability is inherited from generation to generation.
Reason: Some organisms are better adapted to survive in a hostile environment.
26. **Assertion:** Darwin's finches of Galapagos Islands have different types of modified beaks according to their food habits.
Reason: Adaptive radiation leads to development of different functional structure from a common ancestral form.
27. **Assertion:** Disruptive radiation leads to development of different functional structure from a common ancestral form.
Reason: This type of selection favours average sized individuals.
28. **Assertion:** Homologous organs have common ancestry and similar function.
Reason: Analogous organs have unlike origin and dissimilar function.
29. **Assertion :** *Ginkgo biloba* is a living fossil.
Reason : Organism which have persisted and remain unchanged for the past several million years while their relatives disappeared.
[AIIMS 2000]
30. **Assertion:** Animals adopt different strategies to survive in hostile environment.
Reason: Praying mantis is green in colour, which allows it to merge with plant foliage.
31. **Assertion:** Whales and mammals share similarites in the pattern of bones of forelimbes.
Reason: These organisms developed along different directions due to adaptions to different needs.
32. **Assertion:** Hugo de Vries said mutations cause speciation.
Reason: Mutations are slow changes.
33. **Assertion:** Microspheres are believed to be the precursors of life.
Reason: Microspheres are self-duplicating aggregates of proteins surrounded by lipid bilayer.
34. **Assertion:** Genetic drift refers to changes in the allele frequency occurring by chances.
Reason: Sampling errors often lead to the elimination of certain alleles and fixation of others, reducing genetic variability.
35. **Assertion:** Evolutionary trend is continuous change of character in a lineage.
Reason: Lineage is an evolutionary sequence arranged in linear order.
36. **Assertion:** The theory of survival of the fittest is widely misunderstood.
Reason: Evolution does not always increase the chances of a species survival and species do not survive when such chances happen rapidly.
37. **Assertion:** Mutations cause evolution.
Reason: Ancon sheep and hornless cattle are developed by inducing mutation.

38. **Assertion :** Oxidizing atmosphere came about 3.6 billion years ago.
Reason : Fossils, stromatolites suggest the dominance of oxygenic cyanobacteria from that age.

39. **Assertion :** Mutations are important for the survival of a species.
Reason : A living species that would suppress mutation process might gain a temporary advantage in an unchanged environment.

40. **Assertion :** The process of speciation occurs only in allopatric populations.
Reason : The sympatric species can arise either to changes in the chromosome number or due to introgressive hybridization and polyploidy.

41. **Assertion :** The establishment of reproductive isolation is an event of biological significance.
Reason : In the absence of reproductive isolation species can merge back into single population.

42. **Assertion :** DDT has now become almost ineffective against mosquitoes.
Reason : Introduction of DDT brought a change in the gene frequency with a shift from DDT-sensitive to DDT-resistant mosquitoes.

43. **Assertion:** The theory of special creation states that diversity was always the same since creation.
Reason: The species on present day earth were created as such.

44. **Assertion:** Allele frequencies in a population are stable and is constant from generation to generation.
Reason: In Hardy-Weinberg principle the gene pool remains constant.

45. **Assertion:** Hardy Weinberg principle explains the variations occurring in population and species over a number of generations.
Reason: This principle is applicable only when genetic drift occurs.

46. **Assertion :** As favourable variation are transmitted from generation to generation, successive generation become better adapted to the environment and new adaptations may arise. In this way, adaptive traits preserved by natural selection will gradually change the charactertistics of a species.
Reason : This explains the origin of species.

47. **Assertion:** Evolution of man is the example of progressive evolution.
Reason: Tapeworm is developed due to retrogressive evolution.

48. **Assertion:** Petrified fossils remains consists hard parts of organisms.
Reason: Moulds and casts lack the remains of organisms.

49. **Assertion:** Earliest organisms that appeared on the Earth were non-green and presumably anaerobes.
Reason: The first autotrophic organisms were the chemoautotrophs that never released oxygen.

50. **Assertion :** Human ancestors never used their tails and so the tail expressing gene has disappeared in them.
Reason : Lamarck's theory of evolution is popularly called theory of continuity of germ plasm. **[AIIMS 2005]**

51. **Assertion** : The earliest fossil form in the phylogeny of horse is eohippus.
Reason : Eohippus lived during the early pliocene epoch. **[AIIMS 2007]**

52. **Assertion :** Java Ape-man, Peking man and Heidelberg man are the fossils of *Homo erectus*.
Reason : *Homo erectus* evolved from *Homo habilis*. **[AIIMS 2009]**

53. **Assertion :** Cro-magnon man has more intelligence than the man of present time.
Reason : He is regarded as most recent ancestor of today's man.

54. **Assertion:** Neanderthal man is the intermediate between *Ramapithecus* and *Homo erectus*.
Reason: Neanderthal man, with brain size of 800 cc, used hides to protect their body.

55. **Assertion:** Evolution is not a directed process in sense of determinesm.
Reason: It is not a directed process in sense of determinism.

56. **Assertion:** The chimpanzee is the closest relative of the present day humans.
Reason: The banding pattern in some autosomes of man and chimpanzee is remarkably similar.

57. **Assertion:** Founder effect may lead to formation of new species.
Reason: Founders carry all the parental gene pool to a new location.

58. **Assertion:** The modern horse evolved during pliocene epoch.
Reason: It arose from eohippus.

59. **Assertion:** New world and old world monkeys are alike.
Reason: New world monkeys are closer to man.

60. **Assertion:** All primates have a common ancestry.
Reason: The most primate was shrew like animals.

61. **Assertion:** *Dryopithecus africans* is a common ancestor of man and great apes.
Reason: It gave rise to *Ramapithecus*.

62. **Assertion:** Geographic isolation brings about sympatric speciation.
Reason: Reproductive isolation brings about allopatric speciation.

63. **Assertion:** *Homo habilis* was the first tool maker.
Reason: He was cave-dweller.

64. **Assertion:** Formation of new species is called speciation.
Reason: The deme has a common gene pool.

65. **Assertion:** Atavism is the reappearance of disappered ancestral characters.
Reason: Third molars and hair on body are examples of atavism.

66. **Assertion** : Ponnamperuma proved the synthesis of energy source molecule, ATP.
Reason : ATP is molecule formed from nitrogenous base adenosine.

67. **Assertion :** Ear muscles of external ear in man are poorly developed.
Reason : These muscles are useless.

68. **Assertion :** A sickel-cells anaemia is an example of natural selection in human population.
Reason : It saves Africans from fatal disease of malaria in heterozygous condition.

69. **Assertion :** Industrial melanism of *Biston betularia* is an example adaptation.
Reason : The mutation saved their population.

70. **Assertion :** The immediate ancestor of present day humans was *Australopithecus*.
Reason : The fossils of *Australopithecus* were discovered from Australia, and its cranial capacity was 1150-1300cm^3 which is very close to that of humans 1400-1450 cm^3.

71. **Assertion :** Onychophora is a small group of animals with molluscan and arthropod affinities.
Reason : It represents an early stage of evolution of arthropods.

Solutions

1. (a) Big bang theory explains the origin of universe, according to this hypothesis about 20 billion years ago the universe was the big ball made up of neutrons. Its huge explosion due to its high temperature change in pressure, the universe was formed.
2. (b) Steady State Theory was a theory proposed in twentieth-century cosmology to explain evidence that the universe was expanding, but still retain the core idea that the universe always looks the same. It was first proposed by Sir James Jeans in the 1920s.
3. (d) After the evolution of universe the gases condensed under gravitation and formed the galaxies and Milky Way galaxy is a part of solar system from which the earth was supposed to be formed.
4. (c) The lightest atoms of nitrogen, carbon, *etc.* formed the primitive atmosphere. Hydrogen atoms were most numerous and most reactive in primitive atmosphere. Hydrogen atoms combined with all oxygen atoms to form water leaving no free oxygen. Thus primitive atmosphere was reducing (without free oxygen) unlike the present oxidizing atmosphere (with free oxygen).
   Formation of ozone layer is the consequence of modern oxidizing atmosphere having plenty of free oxygen. As more oxygen accumulated in the atmosphere. Due to photosynthesis, ozone began to appear in the top layers.
5. (b) Organic compounds that first evolved in earth which required for origin of life were protein and nucleic acid. All life forms were in aquatic environment only.
6. (a) The primitive earth conditions were so that they led to the production of organic molecules like proteins, RNA, etc.
7. (b) Louis Pasteur, demonstrated that life comes only from pre-existing life. He observed that in pre-sterilized flasks, life did not come from killed yeast while in another flask open to air, new living organism arose from 'killed yeast'. He showed that the source of the new appearing micro-roganisms was the air and the organisms did not arise from the nutrient media.
8. (a) The interstellar dust from which earth originated was especially rich in hydrogen. It readily combine with nitrogen forming ammonia, with carbon forming methane, and with oxygen forming water leaving no free oxygen. Thus, early atmosphere of primitive earth was strongly reducing, it contains hydrogen, methane, ammonia and water vapours.
9. (a) The Miller-Urey experiment, conducted by chemists Stanley Miller and Harold Urey in 1953, is the classic experiment on the origin of life. It established that the early Earth atmosphere, as they pictured it, was capable of producing amino acids, the building blocks of life, from inorganic substances.
10. (a) Darwin finches are an excellent example of the way in which the species gene pools have adapted in order for long term survival via their offspring. Finches were formed due to divergent evolution (Adaptive radiation) to avoid interspecific competition.
    The common birds of Galapagos islands, the finches were markedly different from the finches of main land. The closely related species of finches had beak of different shapes and sizes, and adapted for feeding on completely different diets. Darwin also found that fossils of Galapagos islands are most similar to living species of South America. The food supply increases in arithmetic ratio but the population increases in geometric ratio. With the study of this theory it struck to Darwin that there is struggle for existence among plants and animals.
11. (d) Coacervates are large colloidal aggregates formed due to intermolecular attraction from large organic molecules synthesized abiotically on primitive earth. It mainly consists of proteins, polysaccharides and water. They do not fulfill the requirement for probable precursors of life.

A coacervate is a tiny spherical droplet of assorted organic molecules which is held together by hydrophobic forces from a surrounding liquid. Coacervates possess osmotic properties and form spontaneously from certain dilute organic solutions. They were even once suggested to have played a significant role in the evolution of cells and, therefore, of life itself. They are interesting not only in that they provide a locally segregated environment but also in that their boundaries allow the selective absorption of simple organic molecules from the surrounding medium. Coacervates do not have lipid outer membrane, hence they cannot reproduce.

12. **(b)** The RNA world is proposed as the first stage in the evolution of life in which RNA catalysed all molecules necessary for survival and replication. If the first cells used RNA as their hereditary molecule, DNA evolved from an RNA template. DNA probably did not evolve as a hereditary molecule until RNA based life became enclosed in a membrane. Once cells evolved, DNA probably replaced RNA as the genetic material for most organisms.

13. **(a)** The first molecules formed for replicating cells were RNA. It was proved by T.Cech in Tetrahymena thermophyla. He discovered that an unprocessed RNA molecule could splice itself.

14. **(c)** We have lost all the direct evidences of origin of life only due to destruction of fossils on account of climatic changes and not due to any person/(s).

15. **(b)** The earliest organisms that appeared on the earth were heterotrophic because of reducing atmosphere and the first autotrophs were chemoautotrophs.

An anaerobic organism does not require oxygen for growth and may even die in its presence. Chemoautatrophs are the first organisms that appeared on earth & obtain energy by the oxidation of electron donating molecules in their environments. These molecules can be organic (organotrophs) or inorganic (lithotrophs). The chemotrophs utilize solar energy and can be either autotrophic or heterotrophic.

16. **(a)** With the help of radioactive carbon dating, the inference was made that earth is billions of years old.

17. **(c)** Divergent evolution gives rise to homology.

18. **(c)** The organs which have the same fundamental structure but are different in functions are called homologous organs. These organs follow the same basic plan of organisation during their development. For example, in plants, the homologous organs are thorns of *Bougainvillea* or a tendril of *Curcurbita*, both arising at the axillary position. This represents divergent evolution.

19. **(d)** Industrial melanism is the increase of melanic (dark) forms of an animal in the areas darkened by industrial pollution. The most common example is of peppered moth which existed in two strains (forms) : light coloured (white) and melanic (black). In the past, bark of trees was covered by whitish lichens, so white moths escaped unnoticed from predatory birds. After industrialisation bark got covered by whitish lichens, so white moths escaped unnoticed from predatory birds. After industrialisation, bark was covered by smoke, so the white moths were selectively picked up by birds, but black moths and so they managed to survive resulting in more population of black moths and less population of white moths. Thus, industrial melanism supports evolution by natural selection.

20. **(a)** The early embryos in all the vertebrates exhibit remarkable similarity and it is not easy to differentiate a human embryo from that of the embryo of a chick, lizard, frog or fish in early stages. This can be explained by 'biogenetic law'given by Haeckel. It states ontogeny recapitulates phylogeny'. Ontogeny is the life history of the individual starting from ovum and phylogeny is the series of adult ancestors of the individual which must have incurred in the evolution of the group of this individual. It means that an individual during its development briefs its ancestral history.

21. **(b)** Oparin reported that if a mixture of a large protein and a polysaccharides is shaken, coacervates are formed. The core of these coacervates was majorly formed of protein, polysaccharides and some water and was partially isolated from the surrounding aqueous solution having lower amount of

proteins and polysaccharides. Coacervates could grow by absorbing materials from outside and could increase in number by budding.

22. (d) The human gestation period cannot be shortened unless there is really a problem. Complete development will not take place before the gestation period of 270 – 290 days in humans.

23. (a) The Darwin's theory of Natural Selection can be generalised as the change in species by the survival of an organism exhibiting a natural variation that gives it an adaptive advantage in an environment. Thus, leading to a new environmental equilibrium. The idea of the survival of the fittest explains the above evolution by natural selection. According to survival of the fittest, some of the variations exhibited by living things make it easier for them to survive and reproduce. Thus, more adaptive forms increase. Those which are not fit (or less adaptive) are eliminated.

24. (a) Polluted areas show less growth of lichens.

25. (b) Natural selection is a process in which the organisms which have better survival capacity survive in hostile environment.

26. (a) Development of different functional structures from a common ancestral form is called adaptive radiation. Homologous organs show adaptive radiation. Darwin's finches of the Galapagos Island had common ancestors but now have different types of modified beaks according to their food habits. Darwin differentiated thirteen species of finches and grouped them into six main types.

27. (d) Disruptive type of selection favours both small-sized and large-sized individuals. It eliminates most of members with mean expression, so produces two peaks in the distribution of the trait that may lead to development of two different populations. This kind of selection is rare in nature but is very important in bringing about evolutionary change.

28. (d) Organs which have the same essential structure, which they inherit from common ancestors though they may be very differently modified in adaptation to different functions are homologous. Analogous organs are structurally different organs which get modified to perform similar functions.

29. (a) *Ginkgo biloba*, belong to the Ginkgoales evolved during the Jurassic period and is still existing without any morphological or anatomical changes. Hence, both assertion and reason are correct.

30. (b) Adaptation is an important feature of animals by which they adopt to different strategies to survive in a hostile environment. The stick insect or praying mantis with green body colour exhibits close resemblance with wings and foliages. It is an adaptation known as protective mimicry.

31. (a) Analogous organs have different structures but perform similar functions.

32. (c) Mutations are sudden changes, which brings about a sudden variation in the organism.

33. (b) Microspheres are believed to be the precursors of life. The microspheres contain mainly proteins, polysaccharides and some water. As coacervates do not have lipid outer membrane hence they cannot reproduce.

34. (b) Genetic drift refers to the elimination of the genes of certain traits when a section of population migrates or dies of natural calamity. It alters the gene frequency of the remaining population. Hence genetic drift is a mechanism of evolution that acts in concern with natural selection to change species characteristics over time. Gene frequency in small populations changes by chance. In small populations some genes may be lost or reduced and others may increase by sheer chance irrespective of their selective advantage or disadvantage. Genetic drift may fix some nonadaptive traits in small populations. It tends to preserve or eliminate genes without distinction (opposite to natural selection which selects and favours genes of adaptive value).

35. (b) The continuous change of the characters within an evolving lineage is called evolutionary trend. A lineage is an evolutionary sequence, arranged in linear order from an ancestral group to descendant group. A trend may be progressive (a general increase in size of organs) or retrogressive (a general degeneration and loss of organs).

36. (a) A species composed of only a few organisms has limited genetic variation and mating possibilities. It conditions for survival change and should some of these organisms die due to their lack of characteristics that could accommodate that change, the species would become smaller over time and could eventually die out.

37. (b) Mutation theory of Hugo de Vries states that evolution is a jerky process where new varieties and species are formed by mut tions that functions as raw material of evolution. A number of mutations have appeared in the past. Mutations are also induced. Ancon sheep is a short legged variety which appeared suddenly in Massachusetts in 1971. Hornless cattle developed as mutation from the horned cattle in 1889.

38. (a) About 3.6 billion years ago oxidizing atmosphere came into existence. Fossils stromatolites have suggested the oxygenic cyonobacteria in that stage.

39. (a) Sometimes mutation become favourable for species. Those species which are able to suppress mutation process might gain a temprorary change in an unchanged environment.

40. (b) Allopatric speciation are most common form of speciation that occurs when species population are geographically isolated.

41. (a) The reproductive isolation established is an event of biological significance. Its absence can merge back into single population.

42. (a) This is an example of natural selection of DDT resistant mosquitoes in pesticide rich environment suggesting evolution is still occuring.

43. (b) The theory of special creation states the life was always same and will remain so forever.

44. (a) Hardy Weinberg principle states that the frequencies of alleles in a population are stable and constant from generation to generation, thus total genes and their alleles remains constant, which is also known as genetic equilibrium.

45. (d) The relative frequencies of various kinds of genes in a large and randomly mating, sexually active population tend to remain constant from generation to generation in the absence of mutation, selection and gene flow. This is called Hardy-Weinberg principle or Hardy-Weinberg equilibrium. It is random in gene (allele) frequency and occurs only by chance. It is non-directional. Genetic drift can cause elimination of certain alleles or fixation of the other in the population leading to a change in the population of alleles in the gene pool. So genetic drift must not occur to maintain the equilibrium.

46. (a) Variations evolved in species get transferred from generation to generation and the successive generation arise becomes better and adapt themselves in new environment, like this the adaptive traits are preserved by natural selection will gradually change the characteristics of species. Hence new organism is evolved.

47. (b) Progressive evolution is the formation of more complex specialized organisms from simple and less elaborate forms. Examples: evolution of amphibians from fish like ancestors and evolution of birds and mammals from reptile-like ancestors. Retrogressive evolution is the formation of simple and less elaborate forms from more complex and specialized ones. Example of evolution of many parasitic organisms like tape worm which does not have digestive system. It absorbs food through body surface.

48. (b) Replacement of organic parts by mineral deposits is called petrification. Fossils formed through petrification are termed petrified fossils. These fossils consist of only the hard part of extinct organisms. Moulds of hardened and fossilized mud that surround over an extinct individuals have been found. In most cases the buried individuals have been completely destroyed, but the moulds have retained true copies of their shapes. Sometimes. a mould is found with petrified fossil of the individual also. Such fossils are termed as casts.

49. (b) Primitive earth was devoid of any oxygen, so only those organism that were able to survive within the anaerobic conditions developed. All those were heterotrophic organisms. Then after autotrophic

organisms were developed that used inorganic sources such as H_2S, NH_3, CH_4 as source of energy. These organism were called chemoautotrophs.

50. (c) According to Lamarck's theory, continuous disuse of organs makes them weak. The theory of continuity of germplasm was given by Weismann.
If humans share ancestry with other primates such as prosimian, monkeys *etc*, then remnants of that common ancestory should be present in our genes.

51. (c) Eohippus is the earliest fossil form in the phylogeny of horse. Origin of horse took place in the Eocene period. The first fossil of horse was found in North America which was named Eohippus or "Dawn Horse. ", that later renamed as hyracotherium. It was found during Eocene period not during Pliocene.

52. (b) The fossil of Java Ape-man was discovered from pleistocene rocks in central Java. The fossil of Peking man was discovered from the lime stone caves of Choukoution near Peking while that of Heidelberg man was discovered in mid pleistocene. All these three fossils come under the category of *Homo erectus*. *Homo erectus* appeared about 1.7 million years ago in the middle pleistocene. *H. erectus* evolved from *Homo habilis*. He was about 1.5-1.8 metres tall. He had erect posture. His skull was flat than that of the modern man. He had protruding jaws, projecting brow ridges, small canines and large molar teeth. He made more elaborate tools of stones and bones, hunted big animals and perhaps knew the use of fire.

53. (b) Cro-Magnon man emerged about 34000 years ago. Thus it is regarded as most recent ancestor of today's man. It has, therefore, been called as *Homo sapiens fossilis*. The Cro-Magnon man was like us, about 1.8 meters, tall well-built body. Its face was perfectly orthognathous with an narrow, elevated nose, broad and arched forehead, moderate brow-ridges, strong jaws with man-like dentition and a well developed chin. Its cranial capacity was, however somewhat more than ours, being about 1650 cc(ours is 1400 cc). The Cro-Magnon man was the direct ancestor of the living man.

54. (d) The Neanderthal man with a brain size of 1400cc lived in near East and Central Asia between 1,00,000-40,000 years back. They used hides to protect their body and bury their dead body. It is established that, neanderthal man appeared later than *Ramapithecus* and *Homo erectus*.

55. (a) Evolution by anthropogenic action, such as excessive use of pesticides and antibiotics may lead to appearance of resistant organisms in a span of months and years, and not centuries. This shows that evolution is not a directed process, it is rather based on chance event and mutations occurring in nature and organisms respectively.

56. (a) It has been observed that the banding pattern of some human chromosomes is very similar to the banding pattern of the corresponding chromosomes in apes. It shows common origin of man and chimpanzee and their close relatedness.

57. (c) When a few individuals or a small group of individuals from some large population invades a new or isolated geographical region, these become the founders or founder memebres. These founders carry on a limited portion of the parental gene pool. Their gene pool may contain certian alleles in a very low frequency or may lack a few alleles. The descendants of the founder i.e. the founder population or marginal isolates in a new area will tend to have ratios similar to the founders rather than the source population. Sometimes they form a new species.

58. (d) The modern horse is *Equus* which arose from *Pliohippus* in pleistocene epoch. *Pliohippus,* the pliocene horse, evolved from *Merychippus* in pliocene epoch about one crore years ago.

59. (d) The new world monkey's have a flat nose with widely separated and outwardly directed nostrils. Their tail is long, sensitive and prehensile for grasping the branches of trees, but their limbs cannot be used for grasping the branches of trees, because of non-opposable thumbs and mostly clawed digits. The old world monkeys posses a narrow nose with closely placed and downwardly directed nostrils. Their tail is generally short and not prehensile, but their limbs having opposable thumbs and nailed digits, are well adapted for grasping.

They are closer to man as they have better developed brain, smaller ear pinnae, sensitive finger tips, presence of both rods and cones in the retina of eyes, etc.

60. (b) All primates have a common ancestry (monophytic origin). Primate evolution began 80-100 million years ago. The evolutionary history of eutherian mammals dates back to early cretaceous period. The earliest eutherians were shrew-like terrestrial insectivores. They were small, ground dwelling mammals.

61. (b) Cro-Magnon man emerged about 34000 years ago. Thus it is regarded as most recent ancestor of today's man. It has, therefore, been called as *Homo sapiens fossilis.* The Cro-Magnon man was like us, about 1.8 meters tall and well-built body. Its face was perfectly orthognathous with a narrow elevated nose, broad and arched forehead, moderate brow-ridges, strong jaws with man-like dentition and a well developed chin. Its cranial capacity was, however somewhat more than ours, being about 1650 cc(ours is 1400 cc). The Cro-Magnon man was the direct ancestor of the living man.

62. (d) In allopatric speciation (species formation), a part of the population becomes geographically isolated from the main population. The population becomes entirely separated and finally constitutes a new species. In sympatric speciation, a small segment of the original population becomes isolated reproductively. As the isolating mechanism comes into force, a new subspecies emerges. In due course of time a new species i formed.

63. (b) *Homo habilis* was the first tool maker and used tools of chipped stones extensively. It is also called handy man because heaps of tools found with these fossils included sharpened stones which indicates that *Homo habilis* was capable of "making tools". He also led community life in caves and greatly cared for the young ones.

64. (b) The phenomenon of development of a new species from pre-existing one is called speciation. A species is a collection of demes. The deme is a groups of populations with a common gene pool.

65. (c) Atavism is the appearance of certain ancestral characters which had either disappeared or were reduced. There are present some examples of atavism in human being, viz., the power of moving pinna in some persons, greatly deveLoped canine teeth, exceptionally long dense hairs, short tail in some babies and presence of additional mammae in some individuals. Third molars and hair on the body are examples of vestigial organs.

66. (b) Cyril Ponnamperuma with the help of simple laboratory equipment artificially produced ATP, the source of energy for all forms of life. ATP stands for Adenosine Tri-Phosphate, and is the energy used by an organism in its daily operations. It consists of an adenosine molecule and three inorganic phosphates.

67. (c) The outer i.e. pinna or external ear are useful that detects sound and focuses on ear drum.

68. (a) The allele (S) for sickle-cell anemia is a harmful autosomal recessive and is caused by a mutation in the normal allele (A) for hemoglobin (a protein on red blood cells). While malaria is a deadly tropical disease and is common in many African populations. Heterozygotes (AS) with the sickle-cell allele are resistant to malaria. Therefore, they are more likely to survive and reproduce. This keeps the S allele in the gene pool. Thus it saves Africans from fatal disease malaria.

69. (d) Industrial melanism in Biston betularia is the example of natural selection. The mutation caused due the industrialization decreased its population size.

70. (d) Both are wrong because Australopithecus is apeman with cranial capacity of 450 to 600 c.c.

71. (d) Onychophora are commonly known as velvet worms. These are more ambiguously as Peripatus and are a phylum of elongate, soft-bodied, many-legged panarthropods. Velvet worms are considered close relatives of the Arthropoda and Tardigrada, through which the taxon Panarthropoda is formed.

Chapter

30

Human Health & Disease

Directions: In the following questions, a statement of assertion is followed by a statement of reason. Mark the correct choice as:

(a) If both Assertion and Reason are true and Reason is the correct explanation of Assertion.

(b) If both Assertion and Reason are true but Reason is not the correct explanation of Assertion.

(c) If Assertion is true but Reason is false.

(d) If both Assertion and Reason are false.

1. **Assertion:** *Streptococcus pneumoniae* and *Haemophilus influenzae* are responsible for causing infectious diseases in human beings.
   Reason: A healthy person acquires the infection by inhailing the droplets/aerosols released by an infected person.

2. **Assertion** : Paroxysms are regular and daily in Quotidian malaria.
   Reason : Recurrence of fever is after 48 hours if the infection is caused by *Plasmodium malariae.*

3. **Assertion:** There is no chance of malaria to a man on the bite of male *Anopheles* mosquito.
   Reason: It carries a non-virulant strain of *Plasmodium*. **[AIIMS 1998]**

4. **Assertion** : *Plasmodium vivax* is responsible for malaria.
   Reason : Malaria is caused by polluted water. **[AIIMS 2001]**

5. **Assertion** : *Escherichia coli, Shigella sp.* and *Salmonella sp.* are all responsible for diarrhoeal diseases.
   Reason : Dehydration is common to all types of diarrhoeal diseases and adequate supply of fluids and electrolytes should be ensured. **[AIIMS 2008]**

6. **Assertion** : Rabies is an infection of mammals, it involves central nervous system which may result in paralysis and finally death.
   Reason : This is caused by neurotropic bacteria in saliva of rabies animal. **[AIIMS 2000]**

7. **Assertion:** Pork should be properly cooked to avoid *Taenia* infection.
   Reason: It contains hexacanth and cysticeric larvae.

8. **Assertion** : Tapeworm, roundworm and pinworm are endoparasites of human intestine.
   Reason : Improperly cooked food is the source of all intestinal infections.

9. **Assertion** : Stool test is done to detect giardiasis.
   Reason : Giardia is enteric flagellate protozoan.

10. **Assertion** : Severe Acute Respiratory syndromes is common in China.
    Reason : China is the most populated country of the world.

11. **Assertion** : β-cells work chiefly by secreting substances called antibodies into the body fluids.
    Reason : Antibodies ambush foreign antigen circulating in the blood stream.

12. **Assertion** : Interferons help in the elimination of viral infections.
    Reason : Interferons released by infected cells, reach nearby unaffected cells and make them resistant to viral infection.

13. **Assertion** : An antibody is represented by H_2L_2.
    Reason : Each antibody is made of four peptide chains.

14. **Assertion** : Innate immunity is non-specific defence.
    Reason : It consists of four types of barriers.

15. **Assertion** : T-lymphocytes mediate CMI response.
    Reason : The above response makes it easy to transplant organs.

16. **Assertion:** Inspite of exposure to large number of infectious agents, humans are resistive to diseases.
    Reason: Humans are able to defend against most of the foreign agents due to the ability to fight disease- causing organisms.

17. **Assertion:** Subsequent encounter with the same pathogen elicits a highly intensified anamnestic response.
Reason: This is based on the fact that our body appears to have memory of the first encounter.

18. **Assertion:** Mucous membrane immobilises the micro-organisms in the body.
Reason: Micro-organisms and dust particles entering the respiratory tract are trapped in the mucus.

19. **Assertion:** Virus-infected cells secrete proteins known as interferons.
Reason: Interferons protect the non-infected cells from bacterial infection.

20. **Assertion:** Cornea is considered as an immunologically privileged site.
Reason: A transplanted cornea is rarely rejected.

21. **Assertion:** Artificially acquired passive immunity results when antibodies or lymphocytes produced outside the host are introduced into a host.
Reason: A bone marrow transplant given to a patient with genetic immunodeficiency is an example of artificially acquired passive immunity.

22. **Assertion:** All immunoglobin molecules have a basic structure composed of four polypetide chains.
Reason: The polypeptide chains consists two identical heavy and light chain connected by disulphide bonds.

23. **Assertion:** IgG is the most abundant class of IGs in the body.
Reason: IgG is mainly found in sweat, tears, saliva, mucus, colostrum and gastrointestinal secretions.

24. **Assertion:** Mucus associated lymphoid tissues are specialised immune barriers located on skin.
Reason: These lymphoid tissues are located within tonsils, adenoids and peyer's patches.

25. **Assertion:** Immunisation is achieved by the successful delivery of vaccines.
Reason: Vaccine is a preparation of one or more microbial agents used to induce protective immunity.

26. **Assertion :** Myasthenia gravis is an autoimmune disease.
Reason : Immune system rejects the transplant muscles.

27. **Assertion :** SCID is a primary immunodeficiency.
Reason : It is a serious congenital immunodeficiency.

28. **Assertion:** Histamine is related with allergic and inflammatory reactions.
Reason: Histamine is a vasodilator.
[AIIMS 2002]

29. **Assertion :** Organ transplantation patients are given immunosuppressive drugs.
Reason : Transplanted tissue has antigens which stimulate the specific immune response of the recipient. **[AIIMS 2005]**

30. **Assertion :** A person who has received a cut and is bleeding needs to be given anti-tetanus treatment.
Reason : Anti-tetanus injection provides immunity by producing antibodies for tetanus.
[AIIMS 2006]

31. **Assertion** : Antigen can be easily recognized because it has antigenic determinants.
Reason : The recognition ability is innate.
[AIIMS 2007]

32. **Assertion :** Interferons are a type of antibodies produced by body cells infected by bacteria.
Reason : Interferons stimulate inflammation at the site of injury. **[AIIMS 2004]**

33. **Assertion:** Morphine is very effective and sedative.
Reason: It is very useful for the patients who have depression.

34. **Assertion :** Interferons are effective against viruses.
Reason : Proteins which can be synthesized only by genetic engineering are effective against viruses.

35. **Assertion:** Artificially acquired passive immunity results when antibodies or lymphocytes produced outside the host are introduced into a host.
Reason: A bone marrow transplant given to a patient with genetic immunodeficiency is an example of artificially acquired passive immunity.

36. **Assertion :** Mast cells in the human body release excessive amounts of inflammatory chemicals, which cause allergic reactions.
Reason : Allergens in the environment on reaching human body stimulate mast cells in certain individuals. **[AIIMS 2003]**

37. **Assertion:** STDs are also called silent diseases.
Reason: These remain asymptomatic during early stages.

38. **Assertion:** Chlamydiosis is most common bacterial sexually transmitted disease.
Reason: It can be easily differentiated from gonococcal urethritis.

39. **Assertion :** The antibodies separted from serum are homogenous.
Reason : Monoclonal antibodies are homogenous immunological reagents.
[AIIMS 2013]

40. **Assertion:** Interferons are a type of antiboides produced by body cells infected by bacteria.
Reason: These stimulate inflamm-ation at the site of injury.

41. **Assertion:** Many visitors of hills suffer from skin and respiratory allergy problem.
Reason: Conifer trees produce a large quantitiy of wind-borne pollen grains.

42. **Assertion:** AIDS is a disorder caused by HIV.
Reason: HIV is a virus that damages the immune system of its host.

43. **Assertion:** HIV infected person are prone to opportunistic diseases.
Reason: Immune system weakens during HIV infection. **[AIIMS 2011]**

44. **Assertion :** HIV infection can be avoided by use of condoms.
Reason : Condoms secrete anti-viral interferons.

45. **Assertion:** AIDS spreads more rapidly than hepatitis.
Reason: HIV has shorter incubation period than that of HBV.

46. **Assertion:** Anti-AIDS vaccines are being developed in USA.
Reason: These vaccines may be used to control HIV infection in India.

47. **Assertion:** Antiretroviral drugs are very effective in treatment against AIDS.
Reason: AIDS virus is a retrovirus with Ss DNA as genetic material.

48. **Assertion :** AIDS is a disorder caused by HIV.
Reason : HIV is a virus that damages immune system of its host.

49. **Assertion :** Intake of potato chips and french fries may induce cancer development.
Reason : On heating, their carbohydrate changes into a carcinogenic chemical called acrylamide.

50. **Assertion:** Epstein– Barr virus is an oncovirus.
Reason: It stimulates the growth of cancer.
[AIIMS 2011]

51. **Assertion :** Cancer cells are virtually immortal until the body in which they reside dies.
Reason : Cancer is caused by damage to genes regulating the cell division cycle. **[AIIMS 2006]**

52. **Assertion :** Cocaine has a potent stimulating action on central nervous system, producing a sense of euphoria and increased energy.
Reason : Injecting the microbes intentionally during immunisation or infectious organisms gaining access into body during natural infection induces active immunity. **[AIIMS 2016]**

53. **Assertion:** The phenomenon where tumour cells detach and migrate to other parts of the body where they give rise to secondary tumors is called metastasis.
Reason: Abnormal antigens on the surface of cell and unusual number of chromosomes cause metastasis.

54. **Assertion:** Genital herpes cannot be cured.
Reason: Genital herpes can be inhibited by Acyclovir.

55. **Assertion:** Surgery has been found highly effective in lung cancer.
Reason: Resection is possible after the thoracotomy.

56. **Assertion:** UV-rays are carcinogenic in nature.
Reason: UV-rays rupture DNA strands and induce mutations to cause cancers.

57. **Assertion:** Adenoma is a sarcoma.
Reason: It is located in the adipose tissue.

58. **Assertion:** Dye workers generally suffer from bladder cancer.
Reason: These are more exposed to a carcinogenic chemical benzopyrene.

59. **Assertion:** Sometimes nonsmokers are prone to lung cancer.
Reason: Nonsmokers are also called passive smokers.

60. **Assertion:** Bacteria and other particles pass down the wind pipe and enter the lungs, causing damage to the tissue.
Reason: Smoking reduces ciliary effectiveness.

61. **Assertion:** Benign tumors are called neoplastic cells.
Reason: Malignant tumors remain in place to form a compact mass by a process known as metastasis.

62. **Assertion:** Proto-oncogenes are cellular genes required for normal growth.
Reason: Under normal conditions they could lead to the oncogenic transformation of the cell.

63. **Assertion** : The normal range of TLC is 4000-11000 per cubic mm of blood. It can be used to test-various diseases.
Reason : An increase in TLC indicates diseases are tuberculosis, typhoid etc.

64. **Assertion:** A person experiences chills and high fever recurring every three to four days in malaria.
Reason: This is caused by the release of haemozoin with rupture of liver cells.

65. **Assertion:** Opioids help to enhance respiratory activity.
Reason: Opioids are the drugs which bind to specific opioid receptors present in the respiratory tract.

66. **Assertion:** Alcoholics may show deficiency symptoms of Wernicke's and Korsakoff's syndromes.
Reason: Alcohol acts as depressant.

67. **Assertion:** Alcohol along with other stimulants or narcotic drugs is extremely harmful.
Reason: Alcohol damages digestive system only.

68. **Assertion:** Tobacco contains a large number of alkaloids including nicotine.
Reason: Nicotine stimulates adrenal gland which decreases blood pressure and increase heart rate.

69. **Assertion** : Alcohol acts as diuretic.
Reason : Sweating is enhanced by alcohol and so it is endothermic.

70. **Assertion** : There is addiction in case of stimulants.
Reason : Withdrawal symptoms are psychological.

71. **Assertion** : Withdrawal symptoms of caffeine are less prominent.
Reason : Caffeine is a mild stimulant.

72. **Assertion** : Cannabinoids is a class of diverse chemical compounds that activates cannabinoid receptors present principally in brain.
Reason : Cannabinoids are known for their effects on cardiovascular system of the body.

73. **Assertion** : Heroin is also called smack.
Reason : Heroin is an opium alkaloid.

74. **Assertion:** LSD and marijuana are clinically used as analgesics.
Reason: LSD and marijuana suppresses the brain function.

75. **Assertion:** Consumption of alcohol during pregnancy is harmful.
Reason: Alcohol causes physical and mental defects in the offspring called Foetal Alcohol Syndrome (FAS).

76. **Assertion:** Repeated use of drugs, increases the tolerance level of receptors in our body.
Reason: Receptors respond only to higher doses of drugs.

77. **Assertion:** Tobacco belongs to solanaceae.
Reason: It was called as pipe of piece.

78. **Assertion:** Nicotine is an alkaloid found in tobacco.
Reason: It has several uses.

79. **Assertion:** Charas is a psychoactive drug.
Reason: Charas contains THC of 25 to 60%.

80. **Assertion:** ISD is the most powerful psychedelic.
Reason: Psychedic drugs cause hallucination.

81. **Assertion:** Good atheletes avoid amphetamine.
Reason: Amphetamine brings about increased activity and alertness.

82. **Assertion:** Caffeine is a CNS stimulant.
Reason: Excessive use of caffeine adversely affects the brain.

83. **Assertion:** Brown sugar is morphine derivative.
Reason: Morphine is the principal opium alkaloid.

84. **Assertion:** Hypnotic drugs induce sleep.
Reason: Central nervous system is sensitive to hypnotic drugs.

85. **Assertion:** Tranquillizers are called antipsychosis drug.
Reason: Tranquillizers are used to treat psychosis.

86. **Assertion** : *Cannabis sativa* is a powerful anti-depressant.
Reason : Hashish and Marijuana are derived from it.

87. **Assertion** : Dope test is used to estimate the level of blood alcohol by analyzing the breath of persons drinking alcohol.
Reason : A drunken person usually feels tense and less talkative. **[AIIMS 2004]**

88. **Assertion** : Bordeaux mixture is able to eradicate many fungal diseases.
Reason : It is a fungicide which has proved to be effective for control of disease.

Solutions

1. **(b)** A healthy person acquires the infection by inhaling the droplets/aerosols released by an infected person or even by sharing glasses and utensils with an infected person.
2. **(d)** Paroxyms a sudden attack or outburst of a particular emotion or activity. Quotidian malaria in which the febrile paroxysms occur daily. In *P. malariae* infection, the relapses occur once every 72 hours and it is called Quartan malaria.
3. **(c)** Male *Anopheles* mosquito do not have piercing and sucking type of mouth parts. So, they can not inject malarial parasite into man.
4. **(b)** Malaria is caused by *Plasmodium* whose sexual phase occurs in the mosquito *Anopheles*. When female *Anopheles* feed on blood, they can serve as vector host for malarial parasite.
5. **(b)** Diarrhoeal disease conditions include frequent and excessive discharge of watery material from the bowel. Such diseases mostly result from ingestion of harmful germs with food and water. *E. coli*, *Shigella sp.* & *salmonella sp.* causes diarrhoea. Diarrhoea caused by virus, bacteria or parasites possesses two characteristics- firstly, the offending organisms colonise the intestine and as a consequence cause inflammation of the intestine or enteritis; and secondly, they upset the balance of intestinal fluid absorption and secretion mechanism, often enhancing the latter very considerably, which is then manifested as watery stool discharged frequently in large volumes. *Shigella sp*, *Salmonella sp.* are quite closely related genera that are responsible for diarrhoeal diseases. Dehydration is common to all types of diarrhoeal diseases & adequate supply of fluids & electrolytes that provides ions, should be ensured.
6. **(c)** Rabies (hydrophobia) is caused by rabies virus. Its vectors are raboid animals especially dogs. It leads to encephalitis, fear of water (hydrophobia), high fever, severe headache, spasm of throat & chest, leading to death.
7. **(c)** Human infection is direct and oral. It occurs by eating raw or under-cooked measly pork (Pig muscle with cysticerus larvae of *Taenia*). Infection in vegetarians occurs through improperly washed vegetable. So proper cooking of pork and properly washed vegetable to avoid *Taenia* infection.
8. **(a)** Endoparasite lives inside its host. Bovine endoparasites may be divided into three categories: nematodes, or roundworms; cestodes, or tapeworms; and trematodes, or flukes.
9. **(a)** If a giardia infection is present, the parasite or its cysts can be seen when the stoolis looked at under a microscope. If giardiasis is suspected, an antigen test may be done on the stool or a sample of the fluid from the small intestine (duodenal contents). Giardia is a genus of anaerobic flagellated protozoan parasites of the phylum Sarcomastigophora that colonise and reproduce in the small intestines of several vertebrates, causing giardiasis.
10. **(b)** On November 16, 2002, an outbreak of what is believed to be severe acute respiratory syndrome (SARS), began in the Guangdong province of China, which borders on Hong Kong. China is the most populated country in the World.
11. **(a)** B-cells work chiefly by secreting soluble substances called antibodies into the body's fluids or humors. Antigens are proteins that are found on the surface of the pathogen. Antigens are unique to that pathogen. When an antigen enters the body, the immune system produces antibodies against it.
12. **(a)** Virus infected cells secrete proteins called interferons, which protect non-infected cells from further viral infection.
13. **(a)** Immunoglobulins, also known as antibodies, are glycoprotein molecules produced by plasma cells (white blood cells). The Ig monomer is a "Y"-shaped molecule that consists of four polypeptide

chains; two identical heavy chains and two identical light chains connected by disulfide bonds.

14. (b) Innate immunity refers to nonspecific defense mechanisms that come into play immediately or within hours of an antigen's appearance in the body. Four barriers are physical, physiological, cellular and cytokine barriers.

15. (c) Cell-mediated immunity (CMI) is an immune response that does not involve antibodies, but rather involves the activation of phagocytes, antigen-specific cytotoxic T-lymphocytes, and the release of various cytokines in response to an antigen. The immune response to a transplanted organ consists of both cellular(lymphocyte mediated) and humoral (antibody mediated) mechanisms. Although other cell types are also involved, the T cells are central in the rejection of grafts.

16. (a) Humans are exposed to large number of infectious agents, However, only a few of these exposures result in disease due to the fact that the body is able to defend itself from most of these foreign agents. This overall ability of the host to fight the disease-causing organisms conferred by the immune system is called immunity.

17. (a) Acquired immunity is pathogen specific, it is characterised by memory. When our body encounters a pathogen for the first time it produces a response called primary response which is of low intensity. Subsequent encounter with the same pathogen elicits a highly intensified secondary or anamnestic response. This is ascribed to the fact that our body appears to have memory of the first encounter.

18. (a) Innate immunity is non-specific type of defence, that is present at the time of birth. This is accomplished by providing different types of barriers to the entry of the foreign agents into our body. Skin on our body is the main barrier which prevents entry of the micro-organisms. Mucus coating of the epithelium lining the respiratory, gastrointestinal and urogenital tracts also help in trapping microbes from entering our body.

19. (c) Virus-infected cells secrete proteins called interferons which protect non-infected cells from further viral infection. Interferons are a group of related low molecular weight regulatory cytokines produced by certain eukaryotic cells in response to a viral infection. Besides defending against viruses, they also help to regulate the immune response.

20. (a) Some transplanted tissues do not stimulate an immune response. For example a transplanted cornea is rarely rejected because lymphocytes do not circulate into the anterior chamber of the eye. Thus, this site is considered as immunologically privileged site.

21. (b) Artificially acquired passive immunity results when antibodies or lymphocytes that have been produced outside the host are introduced into a host. This type of immunity is immediate and short lived, lasting only a few weeks to a few months. An example is bone marrow transplant given to a patient with genetic immunodeficiency.

22. (b) The antibodies are proteins which are produced by the B-lymphocytes in response to pathogens into our blood to fight with them. Each antibody molecule consists of identical light chains and two identical heavy chains held together by disulphide bonds.

23. (c) IgA is the second most abundant class, constituting about 10 to 15 per cent of antibodies of serum. It is mainly found in sweat, tears, saliva, mucus, colostrum (first milk secreted by a mother) and gastrointestinal secretions. IgG is the most abundant class of Ig in the body constituting approximately 8% of the total lgs. It is found in the blood, lymph and intestine.

24. (c) Physical and mechanical barriers are the first line of defence against microorganisms. Like skin lymphoid tissue located within the lining of the major tracts (respiratory, digestive and urogenital tracts) called mucosal-associated lymphoid tissue in human body. The MALT includes the tonsils, adenoids diffused lymphoid areas along the gut and specialised regions

in the intestine called Peyer's patches.

25. (a) A vaccine is a preparation of one or more microbial antigens used to induce immunity. It may consists of killed living, weakened microorganisms, inactivated bacterial toxins (toxoids), etc. Immunization is achieved by the successful delivery of vaccines.

26. (c) Autoimmunity is a type of disorder when the immune system of an individual starts rejecting its own body cells or self. This leads to a variety of disease called autoimmune diseases. If the self antigens are muscle cells, then immune system destroys own muscles cells and causes myasthemia gravis characterized by severe weakness.

27. (a) Severe combined Immuno - deficiency (SCID) is the most serious congential immuno-deficiency of children so called primary immunodeficiency.

28. (a) Histamine is produced by mast cells in response to the allergy and inflammatory reaction. When histamine is released from mast cells, it causes vasodilation and an increase in permeability of the blood vessel walls. These effects, in turn cause the common symptoms of allergy including a running nose and watering eyes.

29. (a) Success of organ transplant depends on proper matching of histocompatibility of antigens that occurs in all cells of the body. As there are antigens which are likely to be attacked by recipient's T-cells and antibodies, the recipient of organ transplant is always given immunosuppressants to prevent immune rejection of the transplanted tissue.

30. (c) Anti tetanus is a disinfectant *i.e.* it prevents the infection due to the entry of bacteria through wounds.

31. (b) Antigen is a substance that when introduced in the body, stimulate the production of antibody. They are mostly proteins but may be carbohydrates, lipids, nucleic acids etc. One antigen can bind with many antibodies. Every antigen has many antigenic determinants called epitopes.
The recognition ability of antibody is innate and develops without exposure to the antigen.

32. (d) Interferons are natural proteins produced by the cells of the immune system in response to challenges by foreign agents such as viruses, parasites and tumor cells. Interferons belong to the large class of glycoproteins known as cytokines. Interferons are produced by a wide variety of cells in response to the presence of double-stranded RNA, a key indicator of viral infection. Interferons assist the immune response by inhibiting viral replication within host cells, activating natural killer cells and macrophages, increasing antigen presentation to lymphocytes, and inducing the resistance of host cells to viral infection. When the antigen is presented to matching T and B cells, those cells multiply and strategically and specifically wipe out the foreign substance. That is why antigen presentation is so important to the immune response.

33. (c) Morphine is a very effective sedative and painkiller, and is very useful in patients who have undergone surgery.

34. (c) Interferons are proteins that are effective against most viruses. They are naturally produced by virus infected cells. The proteins interact with adjacent cells and make them resistant to virus attack. Now interferons are also being manufactured through genetic engineering.
Interferons control the multiplication of virus particles by inhibiting their protein synthesis.

35. (b) Artificially acquired passive immunity results when antibodies or lymphocytes that have been produced outside the host are introduced into a host. This type of immunity is immediate short lived, lasting only a few weeks to a few months. An example is bone marrow transplant given to a patient with genetic immunodeficiency.

36. (a) A mast cell contains many granules rich in histamine serotonin and heparin. Although best known for their role in allergy and anaphylaxis, mast cells play an important protective role as well, being intimately involved in wound healing and defense against pathogens. The symptoms of an allergic reaction develop in response to histamine. Mast cells release a large amount of histamine into the blood stream & it also act as initiator of the inflammatory response, which aids the arrival of leucocytes at a site of infection. Histamine stimulates capillary dilation increased capillary permeability, closure of bronchial tubes, mucus secretion, pain & swelling.

37. (a) STDs are detected only when they become highly aggravated

38. (c) Chlamydiosis is a common, sexually transmitted infection that may not cause symptoms. Urethritis is defined as infection-induced inflammation of the urethra. It is urethral inflammation caused by an STD, and the condition is normally categorized into either Gonococcal Urethritis (GU) or Nongonococcal Urethritis (NGU). Non-gonococcal urethritis (NGU) describes inflammation of the urethra, for which the cause is unknown. NGU is most often caused by chlamydia, a common infection in men and women.

39. (d) From hyperimmunized animals, the blood serum may be taken and antibodies may be isolated from this serum. However, the antibodies, whenever separated from serum after induction due to an antigen, are usually heterogenous, because the cells keep on producing a variety of antibodies. Monoclonal antibodies (Mabs), on the other hand are homogeneous immunological reagents of defined specificity so that these can be utilized for diagnosis and screening of disease.

40. (d) Interferon is a glycoprotein, where production is induced within virally infected cells. Interferon induces an antiviral state within adjacent cells.

41. (a) Gymnosperm like *Pinus* usually grow on the slopes of hills and form dense forests of evergreen trees. The pollination of these plants takes place through wind and during peak hours, the microspore of *pinus* are liberated as clouds of yellow dust (sulphur shower). On inhalation, these microspores (pollens) cause various allergies like dermatitis, asthma, allergic rhinitis, hay fever, ete., in human beings.

42. (a) HIV or human immunodeficiency virus is a causative agent of AIDS. It damages the immune system of the human body. HIV belongs to the family retroviruses.

43. (a) Usually, person shows symptoms of HIV infection within 2 to 6 weeks of exposure to the virus. But in some persons, the virus may remain silent for long periods (upto 10 years) before symptoms of full blown AIDS are observable. The symptoms of HIV infection include fever, lethargy, pharyngitis, nausea, headache, rashes etc. Persons suffering from AIDS have a weakened immune system due to depletion of T- helper cells. Such persons show opportunistic infections, *i.e.*, infection by those fungi, bacteria and viruses to which a person with normal immune system is expected to be resistant. Therefore, persons prone to opportunistic infections may be suspected to be infected by HIV, particularly, if the count of T helper cells in 200/ ml or lower.

44. (c) The use of condoms has been shown to decrease the transmission of AIDS because condoms is contraceptic.

45. (d) Incubation period of different viruses is different.

46. (c) Anti AIDS vaccines are being developed in USA. These vaccines are not being used to control the HIV infection in India.

47. (d) Treatment of AIDS with anti-retroviral drugs is only partially effective. They can only prolong the life of the patient but cannot prevent death .AIDS virus is a retro virus with ssRNA as a genetic material.

48. (a) HIV or human immunodeficiency virus is a causative agent of AIDS. It damages the immune system of the human body. HIV belongs to then family retroviruses.

49. (a) Recently Dr. Leif Busk of sweden reported that when high carbohydrate food like potato chips and french fries are heated then a carcinogenic chemical called acrylamide, us formed.

50. (a) Oncoviruses are cancer – causing viruses and may be DNA or RNA virus *e.g.*, Epstein – Barr – Virus, *Herpes simplex* type 2 virus etc. This shows that the development of cancerous tumour is associated with certain genes.

51. (b) Cancerous cells divide and redivide mitotically and is due to the activation of pro-oncogenes.

52. (c) Cocaine is obtained from the cocaplant, erthyroxylum coca. Cocaine is commonly called as coke or crack which is usually snored. It has a potent stimulating action of euphoria and increased energy. It interferes with the transport of the neurotransmitter dopamine. Its increased dosages cause hallucinations.

53. (a) A phenomenon in which cancer cells are spread to distant sites through body fluids to develop secondary tumour is called metastasis. Abnormal antigens on the surface of the cell and unusual number of chromosomes causes metastasis.

54. (b) Genital herpes and oral herpes are only treatable, not curable. Herpes behaves in a way that makes it very difficult to attempt a cure. It is possible to prevent outbreaks with suppressive therapy and people can reduce the pain of an outbreak with conventional or alternative treatments, but developing treatments is very different than knocking the virus entirely out of a person's body.

55. (d) Resection is the medical term for surgically removing part or all of a tissue, structure or organ. Pulmonary complications are a major cause of morbidity and mortality in the post-operative period after Thoracotomy.

56. (d) Ionising radiation's like X-rays, gamma - rays and particulate radiations from radio active substance are known to rupture DNA strands and induce mutations to cause cancers.

57. (d) Sarcoma are malignant growths of the connective tissue. Adenoma is cancer of gland adenoma is located in various glands.

58. (c) Bladder cancer is caused by certain dyes. It is most commonly reported in the worker who work in industries such as dyeing and printing where these are exposed to aniline.

59. (b) Indoor atmospheres and other confined spaces are oftern contaminated by tobacco smoke which is involuntarily inhaled by both smokers and nonsmokers. It is called involuntary smoke inhalation or passive smoking. It is now recognized as a cause of lung cancer in nonsmokers.

60. (a) Cilia, in the respiratory tract of humans sweep invading bacteria and particles up the trachea and away from the lungs. If ciliary effectiveness is reduced because of smoking or invading organisms particles could pass down the windpipe and enter the lungs, causing damage to the delicate lung tissue that might result in the disease.

61. (d) Cancer cells have lost the property of contact inhibition. The cancerous cells just continue to divide giving rise to masses of cells called tumors. Tumors are of two types: benign and malignant. Benign tumors normally remain confined to their original location and do not spread to other parts of the body and cause little damage. The malignant tumors, on the other hand are mass of proliferating cells called neoplastic or tumor cells. These cells grow very rapidly, invading and damaging the surrounding normal tissues. As these cells actively divide and grow they also starve the normal cells by competing for vital nutrients. Cells sloughed from such :umors reach distant sites through blood, and wherever they get lodged in the body, they start a new tumor there. This property called metastasis is the most feared property of malignant tumors.

62. (c) Proto-oncogenes are cellular genes required for normal growth. If they are mutated or overexpressed, they may become oncogenes and their products contribute to the malignant transformation of the cell.

63. (a) The normal result for TLC for Total Count - WBC is 4,000-11,000 cells/ cumm for Unisex gender and for All age groups. It is used to examine various diseases like tuberculosis, typhoid, etc.

64. (c) Malignant malaria caused by *Plasmodium falciparum* is the most serious one and can even be fatal. The parasites initially multiply within the liver cells and then attack the red blood cells (RBCs) resulting in their rupture. The rupture of RBCs is associated with release of a toxic subtance, haemozoin, which is responsible for the chill and high fever recurring every three to four days.

65. (d) Opioids are the drugs, which bind to specific opioid receptors present in our central nervous system and gastrointestinal tract. Opiates have narcotic, analgesic, astringent (that causes

contraction of body parts), and sedative effect. They slow down respiratory activity, cause constriction of the pupil of eye, decrease glandular secretions, impair the digestion, produce nausea, vomiting and sterility.

66. (b) Alcohol act as a depressant of nervous system and acts as sedative and reduces the efficiency of body organs by reducing blood supply. Deficiency of nutrients such as minerals, proteins and vitamins are found in alcoholics. Thiamine (B_1) deficiency causes Wernicke's and Korsakoff' syndromes. Wernicke's syndrome is characterized by mental disturbance, paralysis of eye movements and ataxia of gait. Korsakoff's syndrome is characterized by confusion and severe impairment of memory.

67. (c) Effect of alcohol is enhanced by taking some other substances, e.g., Tobacco, hashish, acids of badly prepared wines. Exhaustion or hunger also make alcohol more dangerous. The nervous system and digestive system are most markedly affected.

68. (c) Tobacco has been used by human beings for more than 400 years. It is smoked, chewed or used as a snuff. Tobacco contains a large number of chemical substances including nicotine, an alkaloid. Nicotine stimulates adrenal gland to release adrenaline and nor-adrenaline into blood circulation, both of which raise blood pressure and increase heart rate.

69. (c) A diuretic is any substance that promotes diuresis, that is, the increased production of urine. Excess alcohol consumption can cause dehydration in a variety of ways. Firstly, alcohol decreases the body's production of anti-diuretic hormone, which is used by the body to reabsorb water. With less anti-diuretic hormone available, your body loses more fluid than normal through increased urination.

70. (b) Abusing stimulants can have major short- and long-term effects on a person's health. Withdrawal symptoms are not psychological. Heavy users may also experience hallucinations, paranoia and panic. Symptoms of stimulant withdrawal usually last about seven days.

71. (a) Caffeine Withdrawal Symptoms: Headache, sleepiness, irritability, lethargy, constipation, depression, muscle pain, stiffness, cramping, lack of concentration, etc. Caffeine is no longer just a mild stimulant.

72. (b) Cannabinoids is a group of chemicals, which interact with cannabinoid receptors present principally in the brain. Natural cannabinoids are obtained from the inflorescences of the plant *Cannabis sativa*. The flower tops, leaves and the resin of cannabis plant are used in various combinations to produce marijuana, hashish, charas and ganja. They are generally taken by inhalation and oral ingestion. These are known for system of the body.

73. (c) Heroin, also known as diamorphine is an opioid most commonly used as a recreational drug for its euphoric effects. Heroin is also known by many street names including dope, H, smack, junk, horse, and brown.

74. (d) LSD (Lysergic Acid Diethylamide), is obtained from *Claviceps purpurea* (Fungus), while marijuana is obtained from *Cannabis sativa* (plant). Both these drugs are hallucinogens.

75. (a) High alcohol consumption can be harmful during pregnancy. Foetal Alcohol Syndrome (FAS) is the name given to a group of physical and mental defects caused by fetal exposure to alcohol in the womb.

76. (b) There are receptors present in the body that respond to drugs. If drugs are taken for a longer period of time they increase the number of receptors at neuronal junctions.

77. (b) Tobacco is obtained from the dried and cured leaves of young branches of *Nicotiana tobaccum* and *Nicotiana nustica*. These plants belong to the family solanaceae. In early days, tobacco was often called the pipe of piece, as it reduces alertness and gives feeling of tranquility.

78. (a) Tobacco contains an alkaloid, nicotine which can be used as a raw material for preparation of the antipellagra vitamin, nicotinic acid (niacin). Nicotin is also used

in physiological and pharmacological investigation and as insecticide and a fumigant.

79. (a) Charas is the dried resinuous extract from the flowering tops and leaves of *Cannabis sativa*. in some countries like America, charas is called hashish. Liquid hashish is called hash oil, which may contain a THC (Tetrahydrocannabinol) of 25 to 60 percent.

80. (a) Psychedelic drugs change a person's mood, behaviour, thoughts, feeling and perceptions, without any true sensory stimulus. They cause hallucinations. LSD causes horrible dreams,emotional outbursts, hallucination, chronic psychosis and severe damage to the central nervous system. It also brings about chromosomal and foetal abnormalities. An LSD addict can be easily recognised from incoherence in writing and drawing.

81. (b) Amphetamine is one of the drugs included in the 'dope test' for athletes. Amphetamines are found in the urine soon after ingestion. Since metabolism of amphetamines is slow, the drug is found in the urine for several subsequent days. If the drug is found in the urine test of athletes, they are debarred to participate. Amphetamines are synthetic activators of sympathetic nerves bringing about increased activity and alertness. They are used by some persons to work continuously for hours or to reduce weight. They reduce mental capability. The drugs are addictive.

82. (c) Caffeine is a stimulant of CNS (Central Nervous System). Its addiction is psychological. Higher doses of caffeine causes nervousness, restlessness, panic, insomnia (lack of sleep) and excitement. Excessive intake of caffeine also causes addiction and indigesion and disturbs renal functions.

83. (b) Morphine is a derivative of opium. It is the principal opium alkaloid and a strong analgesic. Diacetyl morphine hydrocloride is brown sugar/smack and is more powerful analgesic than morphine.

84. (a) Hypnotic drugs induce sleep. They are more or less general depressants of central nervous system. They are used as antianxiety drugs.

85. (a) Some tranquilizers are also called antipsychotic drugs (major tranquillizers) as they have profound effect in all types of psychosis (patients having severe psychiatric illness, schizophrenic patients). They reduce aggressiveness. Thought and behaviour are gradually normalised and anxiety is relieved. Examples of antipsychotic drugs are Phenothiazines, Butyrophenones, Pimozide, Reserpine, etc.

86. (d) *Cannabis sativa* or Hemp is an annual herb of cannabaceae family. It is mainly the source of fibre. *Cannabis sativa* is not an antidepressant. Antidepressant is a psychiatric medication used to alleviate mood disorders such as major depression. Hashish and Marijuana are drugs derived from it. Preparations of flowers of *Cannabis* is called marijuana while preparations of the resinous extract is called hashish. Both are consumed by smoking, vapourising and oral ingestion and are hallucinogen drugs that cause acute panic anxiety reaction.

87. (d) Blood alcohol test measures the amount of alcohol (ethanol) in the body. Alcohol is quickly absorbed into the blood and can be measured within minutes of having an alcoholic drink. The amount of alcohol in the blood reaches its highest level about an hour after drinking. But food in the stomach may increase the amount of time it takes for the blood alcohol to reach its highest level. About 90% of alcohol is broken down in the liver. The rest of it is passed out of the body in urine and your exhaled breath. Symptoms of alcohol intoxication include confusion, lack of coordination, unsteadiness that makes it hard to stand or walk, or erratic or unsafe driving. Dope test is not related to alcohol. Dope test is a blood test to know whether a person used any drug to improve their performance.

88. (a) Fungal disease like mycosis and thrush can be controlled by using Bordeaux mixture (having copper sulphate).

Chapter 31

Strategies for Enhancement in Food Production

Directions: In the following questions, a statement of assertion is followed by a statement of reason. Mark the correct choice as:

(a) If both Assertion and Reason are true and Reason is the correct explanation of Assertion.
(b) If both Assertion and Reason are true but Reason is not the correct explanation of Assertion.
(c) If Assertion is true but Reason is false.
(d) If both Assertion and Reason are false.

1. **Assertion:** The essential methods for livestock production are breeding, weeding, feeding and heeding.
 Reason: Livestock management deals with processes and systems that increase yield and improve quality of products.
2. **Assertion:** Hisardale is new cross breed of sheep.
 Reason: It is developed by crossing Bikaneri ewe and Marino ram.
3. **Assertion:** Light is essential in poultry farm management.
 Reason: 14-16 hours of light including day light is required for optimum production of eggs.
4. **Assertion :** The behaviour of honey bee to come out of the hive in large number is called swarming.
 Reason : It relieves the crowding and provides a means of founding new colonies.
5. **Assertion:** Beehives are kept in crop field during flowering period.
 Reason: Bees are pollinating agents.
6. **Assertion :** The honey bee queen copulates only once in her life time.
 Reason : The honey bee queen can lay fertilized as well as unfertilized eggs.
7. **Assertion :** Fish meal is a rich source of protein for cattle and poultry.
 Reason : Fish meal is produced from non-edible parts of fishes like fins, tail etc.
8. **Assertion:** Cattle breeds can be improved by superovulation and embryo transplantaion.
 Reason : Superovulation in high milk-yielding cows is induced by hormonal injection.
9. **Assertion:** In MOET, hormones with progesterone like activity are given to the cow to induce superovulation.
 Reason: After mating, the embryos at 4-6 celled stage are recovered and transferred to surrogate mothers.
10. **Assertion :** The depth of sowing has an important effect on some pathogens, notably those which attack seedlings.
 Reason : By delaying the emergences of seedlings, deep sowing may help to increase the resistance of a susceptible crop to a pathogen.
11. **Assertion :** Mass selection is useful in homozygous plants.
 Reason : Mass selection does not work with cross-pollinated plants.
12. **Assertion :** In case of vegetatively propagated crops, pure-line selection is not required.
 Reason : Hybrid vigour is mostly used in vegetatively propagated plants.
13. **Assertion :** Use of fertilizers greatly enhances crop productivity.
 Reason : Irrigation is very important in increasing crop productivity. **[AIIMS 2003]**
14. **Assertion:** Wild varieties of crop plants must be conserved.
 Reason: Genome of wild plants serve as important resource for selection of desired genes like genes for pest resistance.
15. **Assertion:** Removal of male parts is called emasculation.
 Reason: Bagging is not required for emasculated flowers.

16. **Assertion:** A single outcross often helps to overcome inbreeding depression.

Reason: Out- crossing is best breeding method of increasing milk productivity.

17. **Assertion:** Single cell protein is best breeding method for increasing milk productivity.

Reason: SCP now, can be produced in high amount commercially, using low cost substrates.

18. **Assertion:** Allopolyploidy involves numerical increase of the same genome.

Reason: Autopolyploidy develops through hybridization between two species followed by doubling of chromosomes.

19. **Assertion:** Hybrid vigour is the phenotypic superiority of hybrid over either of its parents in one or more traits.

Reason: Suppression of expression of recessive harmful genes occurs in hetero zygotes.

20. **Assertion:** Inbreeding or loss of vigour depression occurs when inbreeding is continued for many generations.

Reason: Quarantine can be done to overcome the harmful effects of inbreeding depression.

21. **Assertion:** Haploids can be produced artificially.

Reason: Morphologically they are similar to diploids.

22. **Assertion:** Hybridization is done between two genetically different types of plants.

Reason: Hybridization is intraspecific.

23. **Assertion:** Aneuploidy may be of hypoploidy or hyperploidy type.

Reason: Monosomy lacks one pair of chromosomes.

24. **Assertion:** Normal embryos are often not formed in interspecific hybridization.

Reason: Such embryos can germinate in culture conditions.

25. **Assertion :** Lac is produced from an in isect.

Reason : Lac is a complex substance having large amount of resins, together with sugar, water and other alkaline substances.

26. **Assertion :** The term 'cross-protection' is used specifically for the protection of a plant by pre-infecting the host with a mild strain of the pathogens.

Reason : Breakdown of resistant genes in plants is responsible for the occurence of disease in a previously resistant variety of a crop.

27. **Assertion :** Diseases reduce the vitality of plants, inhibit their development and cause different morphological and physiological aberrations.

Reason : The diseases can therefore result in the death of a plant.

28. **Assertion :** Indiscriminate exploitation of economically important plants may lead to their extinction.

Reason : Conservation of the germplasm is responsible for extinction of the species.

29. **Assertion :** Man will flourish in all fronts if pests are destroyed.

Reason : The elimination of pests would increase the yield in agricultural production.

30. **Assertion :** Bordeaux mixture is an inorganic fungicide.

Reason : Bordeaux mixture contains copper lime dust.

31. **Assertion:** Bird flu disease is the disease of poultry.

Reason: It is caused by a bacteria.

32. **Assertion:** Biofortification is the most practical aspect to improve health of the people.

Reason: It is the breeding crops with higher levels of vitamins or minerals or higher proteins and healthier fats.

33. **Assertion:** Hydrated artificial seeds have to be planted soon after they are produced.

Reason: These seeds soften, due to absorption of moisture from air.

34. **Assertion:** In tissue cultrue, whole plant can be produced from any plant cell.

Reason: Any viable plant cell can differentiate into somatic embryos that gives rise to different cells of plants.

35. **Assertion:** Virus-free plants can be produced by meristem tissue culture.

Reason: The virus fails to grow during the growth of the host tissue in the artificial medium.

36. **Assertion:** Protoplast fusion is one of the major technique of tissue culture.

Reason: The naked protoplast of the two different plants fuses to form a hybrid.

37. **Assertion :** Protoplast culture is an important technique of genetic engineering.
Reason : Protoplast culture technique results in the production of genetically modified crops.

38. **Assertion :** Multiplication of plants *in vitro* condition from the explants is called micropropagation.
Reason : Micropropagation occurs either in the form of multiple shoot formation or somatic embryos.

39. **Assertion :** In plant tissue culture somatic embryos can be induced from any plant cell.
Reason : Any viable plant cell can differentiate into somatic embryos. **[AIIMS 2003]**

40. **Assertion :** Somatic embryos can be induced from any cell in plant tissue culture.
Reason : Any living plant cell is capable of differentiating into somatic embryos.
[AIIMS 2017]

41. **Assertion :** A major advantage of tissue culture is protoplast fusion.
Reason : A hybrid is formed by the fusion of naked protoplasts of two plants.
[AIIMS 2017]

42. **Assertion:** Using tissue culture, artificial seeds can be produced.
Reason: Artificial seeds can be stored and propagated just like natural seeds.

Solutions

1. **(b)** Livestock refers to farm animals (domesticated animals) such as cow, sheep, etc. kept by humans for a commercial purpose. Its management aims to increase yield and improve the quality of products they generate. Four essential methods for livestock improvement are breeding, weeding, feeding and heeding. (i) Both the male and female animals selected for breeding should be of superior quality. (ii) Weeding aims that uneconomic animals must be prevented from reproducing. (iii) Feeding is also very important for animals. Each animal should be fed on a balance diet. (iv) Heeding implies good animal management and general supervision including housing care and maintenance of proper cleanliness and hygiene.

2. **(a)** Hisardale is a new breed of sheep developed in Punjab by crossing Bikaneri ewe and Marino ram. In cross-breeding method, superior males of one breed are mated with superior females of another breed. Cross-breeding allows the desirable qualities of two different breeds to get combined. The progeny may be used for commercial production. Many new animal breeds have been developed by this approach.

3. **(a)** Light management is essential for high egg production in poultry birds. 14 to 16 hours of light including daylight is required for optimum production.

4. **(a)** Swarming is the process by which a new honey bee colony is formed when the queen bee leaves the colony with a large group of worker bees.

5. **(a)** Bees are the pollinators of many crop species such as sunflower, *Brassica,* apple and pear. Keeping beehives in crop fields during flowering period increases pollination efficiency and improves the yield which is beneficial for both crop and honey yield.

6. **(b)** It is said that the queen gets mated only in her life but in a single chance of mating. After mating the queen lays eggs in one brood cell. The larvae emerge out from both the fertilized as well as unfertilized eggs. Thus the larvae from the unfertilized eggs form the drones while the worker are developed from the larvae of fertilized eggs.

7. **(c)** Fish meal is prepared from the wastes of fish oil or canning industry or from the whole fish of nol-oil-type. Wastes of cod industry are known as white 'fish meal'. The protein content of this meal is highly digestible, nutritive and is of biological importance. This fish meal also contains calcium phospholipids, and iodine, fish meal is also used as major food of domestic animals like pigs, poultry and cattle.

8. **(b)** Superovulation is induced by hormone injection. Superovulation and embryo transplantation techniques have been used in India for cattle improvement.

9. **(d)** In multiple ovulation embryos transfer technology (MOET), hormones (with FSH-like activity) are given to the cow for inducing follicular maturation and super ovulation. Instead of one egg, they produce 6-8 eggs per cycle. The cow is either mated with a best bull or artificially inseminated. The embryos at 8-32 cell stage are recovered and transferred to surrogate mothers. The genetic mother is available for another superovulation. MOET has been done in cattle, sheep, rabbits, buffaloes, mares, etc.

10. **(a)** **Sowing practices**, such as changing time, depth and direction of sowing, and changing the density of the crop can protect plants from pathogens to which they are susceptible only at certain stages of their development. Changing the time of sowing can exploit weather conditions

that are unfavourable to the pathogen, thus reducing crop losses. This might require the use of a specific cultivar that is adapted to the selected growing period, but might also be susceptible to different pathogens. The depth of sowing can have a bearing on the chance of infection, as the seedling's pre-emergence stage, which is usually more susceptible to attack, is longer when seeds are planted deeper. However, deeper planting can stimulate germination.

11. (b) Mass selection is useful in self pollinated plants since they are usually homozygous and retains the selected traits in the progeny. However, cross pollinated plants are usually heterozygous. Their phenotypic expression is largely due to their hybrid vigour or heterozygous nature. Mass selection of such plants fails in subsequent generations.

12. (b) In case of vegetatively propagated crops, pure line selection is not required. Pure-line selection is useful only for sexually reproducing plants. Hybrids vigour is most profitably used in vegetatively propagated crops because they do not involve sexual reproduction and hence loss of hybrid superiority.

13. (b) Irrigation relates to the supply of water to the crops. Fertilizers which are mainly NPK are required to increase the harvest of crops.

14. (a) Plant breeding involves selection of parents with desired characters, their crossing and selection of hybrid progeny with desired character. Wild varieties of crop plants have better resistance to insects, pests, diseases, etc. During plant breeding these wild varieties serve as germplasm resource where genes for disease resistance, etc., can be searched and selected. The wild varities with desired character can be crossed with crop plants to obtain desired set of characters in the progeny. Therefore, wild varieties of crop plants must be conserved, otherwise large amount of germplasm will be lost.

15. (c) In case of bisexual flowers, the anthers of the proposed plant are removed before they dehisce. The process is called emasculation. The emasculated flowers are immediately covered by paper or polythene bags by the process called bagging. It prevents unwanted pollen to come in contact with emasculated flowers.

16. (b) Out-crossing is the mating of animals within the same breed but with no common ancestors on either side of their pedigree up to 4-6 generations. The offspring of such a cross is called as an outcross. Outcrossing is the best breeding method for animals that are below average in productivity in milk, growth rate in beef cattle, etc. Sometimes only one outcross helps to overcome inbreeding depression.

17. (a) Single Cell Proteins (SCP) are proteins produced using bacteria, fungi, algae, etc. SCP is a misnomer term because these are not always produced by single celled organisms. Multicellular algae and fungi may also be used. SCP can help to meet increasing demands of population because of high rate of biomass production and facility to produce it commercially throughout the year. Agricultural crops require large fields and yield is dependent upon the various conditions. This problem is not there in SCP production. SCP also produces biomass at a higher rate. It has been estimated that a 250 kg cow produces 200 g of protein per day. In the same period 25 g of microorganisms like *Methylophilus methylotrophus* can produce about 25 tonnes of protein.

18. (d) Polyploidy is the phenomenon of having more than two sets of chromosomes or genomes which occur in nature due to failure of chromosomes disjunction at the time of division. It can be of three types - autopolyploidy, allopolyploidy and autoallopolyploidy. In autopolyploidy there is a numerical increase of the same genomeo, Allopolyploidy develops through hybridization between two species followed by doubling of chromosomes.

Autoallopolyploidy is the type in which genome is in more than diploid state.

19. (a) Plant breeding exploits the phenomenon of hybrid vigour or heterosis. It is the phenotypic superiority of the hybrid over either of its parents in one or more traits. These hybrids generally have greater strength and resistance to disease and larger life span than either parents. This may be due to suppression of expression of harmful recessive genes that are expressed only in homozygous conditions.

20. (c) Inbreeding is mating of individuals closely related individually. It produces loss of vigour when continued for several generations in plants and animals. This loss of vigour, called inbreeding depression, appears because of increased homozygosity and results in expression of harmful effects of recessive alleles. Quarantine is careful examination of all organisms being introduced into a new area for the presence of weeds, insects and disease causing organisms. Quarantine cannot overcome inbreeding depression.

21. (c) Haploids can be artificially produced by any one of the following methods. (i) X-ray treatment, (ii) delayed pollination, (iii) temperature shocks, (iv) colchicine treatment, (v) distant hybridization, (vi) anther or pollen culture. Haploids are characterised morphologically by a reduction in size of all vegetative and floral parts.

22. (b) Hybridization is the obtaining of progeny after crossing two or more types of plants which differ genetically from one another in one or more traits. Hybridization may be intravarietal, intervarietal, interspecific and intergeneric. Interspecific hybridization is rare because species are genetically and reproductively isolated.

23. (c) Aneuploidy can be either due to loss of one or more chromosomes (hypoploidy) or due to addition of one or more chromosomes to complete the chromosome complement (hyperploidy). Hypoplodiy is mainly due to loss of a single chromosome, monosomes ($2n - 1$) or due to loss of one pair of chromosomes, nullisomes ($2n - 2$).

24. (b) Interspecific hybridization often fails because the embryo dies quite early or fails to reach maturity. In such cases, the embryo is taken out of the fertilized ovule and cultured in nutrient medium under controlled conditions.

25. (b) The lac insect (*Laccifer lacca*) secretes a sticky, resinous material called lac, from which shellac and a red dye are produced.

26. (b) Cross-protection is a natural phenomenon whereby tolerance or resistance of a plant to one virus strain is induced by systemic infection with a second.

27. (a) A disease reduces a plant's overall vitality, inhibits its growth, or limits the ability of the plant to survive and reproduce. Plant disease agents are bacteria, fungi, viruses, nematodes, abiotic and oomycetes.

28. (c) Germplasm is living genetic resources such as seeds or tissues that are maintained for the purpose of animal and plant breeding, preservation, and other research uses. The conservation of germplasm involves the preservation of the genetic diversity of a particular plant or genetic stock. It can be used at any time in future.

29. (a) The elimination of pests would increase the yield in agriculture production. Man will flourish in all fronts if they are vanished.

30. (a) Bordeaux mixture (also called Bordo Mix) is a mixture of copper(II) sulfate ($CuSO_4$) and slaked lime, $Ca(OH)_2$ used as a fungicide. It is used in vineyards, fruit-farms and gardens to prevent infestations of downy mildew, powdery mildew and other fungi.

31. (c) Bird flu is a disease of poultry caused by a virus H_5N_1. The virus enters man through chicken.

32. (a) Biofortication is a measure of improving food quality with the help of breeding techniques. The main objectives of biofortification include improving protein content and quality, oil content and quality, vitamin content and micronutrient and

mineral content of the crop plant. It will help the human race to have adequate food to meet their daily food and nutritional requirements. Biofortified plants reduce the risk for diseases, increase life span and increase mental abilities.

33. (c) In the hydrated system, the beads become hardened as calcium alginate is formed, after about 20-30 minutes the artificial seeds are removed, washed with water and are used for planting. Hydrated artificial seeds become rapidly dry in the open air. Therefore, hydrated artificial seeds have to be planted soon after they are produced.

34. (a) In tissue culture, somatic embryos or embryoids are non-zygotic embryo like strucutres that develop in invitro cultures from somatic cells of any type of tissue, but it is easier to raise them from culture of immature embryos. Thus, reason is the correct explanation of assertion.

35. (c) Virus-free plants can be produced from the virus infected plants by means of meristem tissue culture. By removing the meristem and growing in vitro, virus free plants can be obtained. Some plants developed by meristem culture are banana, sugarcane, potato, etc.

36. (b) Protoplast cuture is an important technique of tissue culture and this technique results in the production of somatic hybrid plants. In this case, scientists have even isolated single cells from the plants and after digesting their cell walls, they have been able to isolate naked protoplasts (surrounded only by plasma membranes).

37. (b) Protoplast culture is an important technique of tissue culture and this technique results in the production of somatic hybrid plants.

38. (b) The part of plant which is cultured is called explant. Micropropagation is the rapid vegetative multiplication of plants in artificial media under aseptic conditions from the explants. Multiple shoot production is used in rapid multiplication of pathogen free plants, rare hybrids, sterile plants, multiple copies of one sex. Somatic embryos or embryoids are non zygotic embryo-like structures that develop *in vitro* cultures from somatic cells of callus raised from an embryo.

39. (a) Any living plant cell which is viable can be used to culture somatic embryos. These embryos have the characteristic features of the parent plant. The somatic cultures are viable from the stem, root or leaves and the most viable part is the meristematic cell.

40. (a) Somatic embryos are non- zygotic embryo like structures that develop into from any type of tissue in plant tissue culture.

41. (b) An important technique of tissue culture, somatic hybridization results in the production of somatic hybrid plants. Two different plant varieties each with a desirable character can be made to undergo protoplast fusion, which further can be grown into a new plant.

42. (b) An artificial seed is a bead of gel containing a somatic embryo (or shoot bud) and the nutrients, growth regulators, pesticides, antibiotics, etc., needed for the development of a complete plantlet from the enclosed somatic embryo or shoot bud. Somatic embryos are formed using plant tissue culture techniques and in some plant species e.g., oil palm, date palm, etc., they are the only route available for micro propagation. Artificial seeds can be directly sown in the soil and stored upto a year without loss of viability.

Chapter 32

Microbes in Human Welfare

Directions: In the following questions, a statement of assertion is followed by a statement of reason. Mark the correct choice as:

(a) If both Assertion and Reason are true and Reason is the correct explanation of Assertion.
(b) If both Assertion and Reason are true but Reason is not the correct explanation of Assertion.
(c) If Assertion is true but Reason is false.
(d) If both Assertion and Reason are false.

1. **Assertion:** Besides curdling of milk, LAB also improve its nutritional quality by increasing vitamin-B_{12}.

   Reason: LAB, when present in human stomach, check disease causing microbes.

2. **Assertion:** *Streptococcus thermophilus* increases nutritional value of milk.

   Reason: Milk has lesser vitamin content than curd and yoghurt.

3. **Assertion :** Vitamins B_2 is found in cereals, green vegetables, brewer's yeast, egg white, milk and liver.

   Reason : It can be commercially produced by some yeasts.

4. **Assertion :** Lichen is important for chemical industries.

   Reason : Litmus and Orcein are formed from lichens. **[AIIMS 2009]**

5. **Assertion :** Yeasts such as *Saccharomyces cerevisiae* are used in baking industry.

   Reason : Carbon dioxide produced during fermentation causes bread dough to rise by thermal expansion. **[AIIMS 2003, 2011]**

6. **Assertion:** Rennet and fruit extract of *Withania somnifera* have antagonistic functions.

   Reason: Rennet is obtained from calf's liver and is used for curdling of milk.

7. **Assertion:** After 24 hours, toddy becomes unpalatable.

   Reason: The fermentation of toddy is continued by naturally occurring yeasts.

8. **Assertion:** Beer and wine are called soft liquors while gin, rum, etc. are hard liquors.

   Reason: Beer and wine are made without distillation.

9. **Assertion:** Griseofulvin extracted from *P. griseofulvum* is used for ringworm treatment.

   Reason: Trichophyton, Epidermophyton, etc. cannot grow well in presence of *Penicillium griseofulvum*.

10. **Assertion:** Acetic acid production involves both aerobic and anaerobic processes.

    Reason: Production of alcohol from glucose is an aerobic process and production of acetic acid from alcohol is an anaerobic process.

11. **Assertion:** An organ transplant patient if not provided with cyclosporin A may reject the transplanted organ.

    Reason: Cyclosporin A inhibits activation of T-cells and interferes with destruction of non-self cells.

12. **Assertion:** The kneaded flour shows leavening, when yeast is added to it.

    Reason: Enzymes secreted by yeast cause leavening.

13. **Assertion :** *Saccharomyces* species are utilized for making alcoholic beverages.

    Reason : Yeast has an enzyme, zymase responsible for fermentations.

14. **Assertion:** Secondary treatment of sewage is also called biological treatment while primary treatment is called physical treatment.

    Reason: Primary sewage treatment depends only upon sedimentation properties of materials present in sewage and filteration.

15. **Assertion:** Energy value of biogas is lower than that of organic matter.

    Reason: Biogas minimises the chances of spread of fecal pathogens.

16. **Assertion:** Biogas is used as fuel for cooking and lighting.
 Reason: It is considered as ecofriendly and pollution free source of energy.

17. **Assertion :** Bioenergy is the energy available from biological sources.
 Reason : Fossil fuels are examples of bioenergy.

18. **Assertion:** Most orchid seedlings cannot develop well in the absence of fungal mycelium.
 Reason: Fungal mycelium increases efficiency of absorption only.

19. **Assertion:** Nucleic acid complexes alone cannot cause diseases.
 Reason: Only nucleoproteins can function as infectious agents.

20. **Assertion:** Dragonflies can be used to decrease occurrence of diseases like malaria, dengue, etc.
 Reason: Baculoviruses are effective in controlling many insects and other arthropods.

21. **Assertion:** Integrated pest management (IPM) programme at the same time deals with conservation of insects and destruction of insects.
 Reason: IPM programmes are specially used in dealing with ecologically sensitive areas.

22. **Assertion:** Disadvantages of synthetic pesticides can be overcome by the use of natural biopesticides.
 Reason: Biopesticides are harmless agents which are used to control weeds and pest without causing any damage.

23. **Assertion:** Chemical pesticides are more hazardous as compared to biopesticides.
 Reason: Chemical pesticides are mostly non-specific, expensive, hazardous and pollute the atmosphere.

24. **Assertion:** Leguminous plants are best preferred in rotation of crops.
 Reason: They have root nodules, which have nitrogen-fixing bacteria *Clostridium*.

25. **Assertion:** Use of fertilisers greatly enhances crop productivity.
 Reason: Irrigation is very important in increasing crop productivity.

26. **Assertion :** Use of fertilisers greatly enhances productivity.
 Reason : Irrigation is very important to increase crop productivity.

27. **Assertion:** Biofertilizers are preferred to chemical fertilizers.
 Reason: Chemical fertilizers are generally more expensive and hazardous to environment.

28. **Assertion:** Nitrogenase enzyme gets inactivated in presence of oxygen yet N_2 fixation occurs in aerobic cells of legume nodules.
 Reason: Leghaemoglobin allows presence of oxygen just sufficient for cellular respiration only.

29. **Assertion :** Leguminous plants are nitrogen fixers.
 Reason : Leguminous plants have *Rhizobium* in their root nodules. **[AIIMS 1997]**

30. **Assertion :** Nitrogen-fixing enzyme in legume root nodules function at low oxygen concentration.
 Reason : Low oxygen concentration is provided by leghaemoglobin. **[AIIMS 2004]**

31. **Assertion:** Extraction and purification of enzymes is laborious and expensive.
 Reason: Protein engineering can be used to produce enzymes at large scale.

32. **Assertion:** Enzyme application in industry is enhanced by its immobilization.
 Reason: Immobilization provides protection to enzymes without affecting their activity.

33. **Assertion :** Due to increasing concern about contamination of environment by herbicides, safer and biodegradable pesticides are used.
 Reason : This has neccessitated the development of resistance in crop plants against safe herbicides.

Solutions

1. **(b)** Curd is more nutritious than milk as it contains a number of organic acids and vitamins including B_{12}. LAB present in curd also checks growth of disease causing microbes in stomach and other parts of digestive tract.

2. **(a)** Microbes have been used for long time in production of dairy products like curd, yoghurt, cheese, etc. Yoghurt is produced by curdling milk with the help of *Streptococcus thermophilus* and *Lactobacillus bulgaricus.* Yoghurt has higher nutritional value than milk thus, it can be said that *Streptococcus thermophilus* increases nutritional value of milk.

3. **(b)** Besides cereals, green vegetables, brewer's yeast, egg white, vitamin B_2 is also produced by intestinal bacteria. The vitamin was first obtained in 1938 using wild strain of mould *Ashbhya gossypii.* Vitamin B_2 is essential for normal growth and reproduction in a number of laboratory animals.

4. **(a)** Litmus is an important and widely used dye in chemical laboratories as an acid-base indicator. It is obtained from *Rocella montaignei.* Orcein, a biological stain, is obtained from *Rocella tinctoria.*

5. **(a)** Yeast is a fermentation agent. It is a known fact that yeast raises bread dough to rise and hence, Yeast is also used to increase the volume, making the dough porous and the product soft. It is the yeast that helps the dough to rise.

6. **(d)** Rennet is obtained from calf's stomach and is a commercially available form of enzyme rennin. Rennet is used from curdling of milk to initiate the process of cheese formation. The same function can be carried out with the help of fruit extract of *Withania somnifera.* Thus, rennet and fruit extract of *Withania somnifera* have similar functions and are not antagonistic.

7. **(a)** Toddy is a traditional drink of some parts of South India which is made by fermentation of sap of palms. Toddy left for few hours undergoes fermentation with the help of naturally occurring yeast to form beverage containing about 6% alcohol. But after about 24 hours, toddy becomes unpalatable because fermentation is carried on. At this time, it can be used for production of vinegar.

8. **(b)** Beer, wine, gin, rum, vodka, etc. are fermentation products but beer and wine are formed without distillation. However, distillation of fermented broth is carried out in case rum, gin, etc. Distillation increases the alcohol concentration of the beverage. Thus, gin with 40% alcohol, rum with 40% alcohol and brandy with 60-70% alcohol are more alcoholic than beer (3-6% alcohol) and wine (9-12% alcohol).

9. **(a)** Antibiotics are chemical substances produced by some microbes which in small concentration can kill or retard the growth of harmful microbes without adversely affecting the host. Griseofulvin is an antibiotic produced by *Penicillum griseofulvum* and is antifungal in nature, especially effective against ringworm. Ringworm is caused by dermatophytic fungi like *Epidermophyton, Trichophyton, Microsporium, etc.* which cannot grow in presence of *P. griseofulvum* because of the antagonistic effect of antibiotic griseofulvin secreted by it.

10. **(c)** Acetic acid is prepared from fermented alcohols with the help of acetic acid producing bacteria, *Acetobacter aceti.* Alcoholic fermentation of sugars is an anaerobic process but the conversion of alcohol to acetic acid is an aerobic process. This reactions occurring can be summarised as: Anaerobic formation of alcohol:

$$C_6H_{12}O_6 \xrightarrow{\text{Zymase complex}} \underset{\text{ethyl alohol}}{2C_2H_5OH} + 2CO_2$$

Aerobic formation of acetic acid

$$C_2H_5OH + O_2 \longrightarrow \underset{\text{acetic acid}}{CH_3COOH} + H_2O$$

Acetic acid is either used as vinegar after ripening or in pharmaceuticals, colouring agents, insecticides, plastics, etc.

11. **(a)** Cyclosporin is cyclic oligopeptide obtained-through fermentative activity of fungus *Trichoderma polysporum.* It has immunosuppressive properties and inhibits activation of T-cells. T cells of immune system mainly function to kill non-self cells. Because cyclosporin A inhibits T cells function, it causes immunosuppression and chances of rejection of transplanted organ are reduced. Thus, organ transplant patients are provided with cyclosporin A.

12. **(a)** A small quantity of yeast is added to wheat flour and is kneaded. The kneaded flour is kept at a warm temperature for few hours. It swell up. This phenomenon is called leavening. Leavening is caused by secretion of three types of enzymes by yeast. These are amylase, maltase and zymase.

13. **(a)** *Sacharomyces cerevisiae* produces an enzyme called zymase which can cause fermentation to produce alcohol.

14. **(a)** Sewage treatment is divided into primary treatment and secondary treatment. Primary treatment involves filtration of the sewage and then sedimentation of the debris present on filtrate. No microbes are used.

The sediment of primary treatment, called primary sludge, is treated by aerobic microbes and then by anaerobic microbes to reduce its organic components during secondary treatment. Secondary treatment involves microbes, thus it is also called biological treatment.

15. **(b)** Biogas is an excellent example of beneficial functions of microbes. It is a mixture of CH_4, CO_2, H_2S, etc. and is produced by the action of methanogenic bacteria on fecal organic matter. It has wider applications than the direct burning of organic wastes (as dungcakes) and it is an easily storable form of energy which can be used more efficiently and economically. The energy value of biogas is lower than that of organic matter but due to more efficient handling, the net energy output is roughly equal to direct burning of organic wastes. Besides biogas production minimises the chances of spread of fecal pathogens and produces manure which has fertilizer value similar to that of manure formed directly from organic wastes.

16. **(b)** Gases present in bio-gas produce energy by combustion or oxidation which can be used for heating purpose or for generation of power through gas engines. Biogas is used as fuel for heating and cooking, lighting, power for irrigation and other purposes as an alternative of firewood, kerosene, dung cakes or even electricity and pollution free source of energy.

17. **(c)** Bioenergy is the energy extracted from biological sources, both living and their immediate remains e.g. wood, gobar gas. It does not include fossil fuels (coal, petroleum, natural gas etc.)

18. **(c)** Some fungi form a mutually beneficial or symbiotic association with the roots of higher plants. In seedling stage of most orchids, the fungal hyphae not only increase absorption frequency but also provide nourishment by forming nutrient rich cells.

19. **(d)** Microbes are extensively used in human welfare but they sometimes prove harmful too. Most of the human, animal and plant diseases occur because of infections caused by micro-organisms. Viruses are nucleoprotein complexes that cause disease. But nucleic acid alone and proteins alone can also cause diseases. Disease causing nucleic acid complexes are termed viroids while prions are proteinaceous infectious agents.

20. (b) Baculoviruses and dragonflies act as biocontrol agents. Biocontrol agents are organisms that control population of some harmful organisms.
Dragonflies prey upon mosquito larvae and thus, check mosquito population. Hence, they serve to control spread of mosquito borne diseases like malaria, dengue, etc. Baculoviruses are effective narrow spectrum bioinsecticides which are specific for their target insects and do not have side effects on plants, mammals, birds, fish and non-target insects. Thus, these are widely used in fields.

21. (b) In an ecosystem, many insects are present. Some of them may be harmful but generally most of them are beneficial and have important roles in the ecosystem maintenance. Chemical insecticides, when applied, kill all insects whether they are beneficial or harmful. Integrated pest management programmes are designed specially to kill only the harmful organisms but in a manner that beneficial organisms can be conserved. IPM programmes are necessary for ecologically sensitive areas where loss of ecosystem can occur very rapidly in response to changes in the ecosystem balance.

22. (b) Biopesticides are better and safer than chemical pesticides. biopesticides can be produced locally with cheap materials and simple equipment.

23. (a) Biopesticides are better and safer than chemical pesticides. biopesticides can be produced locally with cheap materials and simple equipment. While, chemical pesticides are expensive, non-specific, hazardous and pollute the atmosphere.

24. (c) In the rotation of crops, leguminous crops like pulses beans, peas, groundnut and Bengal gram are sown in between the seasons of cereal crops like wheat, maize and pearl millet. The leguminous plants are grown alternately with non-leguminous plants to restore the fertility of the soil.
When the cereal crops like rice, wheat, maize are grown in the soil, it uses up lot of nitrogenous salts from the soil. If another crop of cereal is grown in the same soil, the soil becomes nitrogen deficient.
So by rotation a leguminous crop is grown. These plants have the ability to fix atmospheric nitrogen to form nitrogen compounds through the help of certain bacteria (*Rhizobium*) present in their root. Genus *Clostridium* includes about 100 sps., most of them are either free-living or pathogenic.

25. (b) Among the sixteen essential plant nutrients nitrogen, phosphorus and potash are the most common nutrients found deficient in Indian soil. Supply of these nutrients to soil artificially through fertilisers is necessary to keep the soil rich in plant nutrients for achieving maximum yield. Irrigation practices are also helpful in enhancing the crop yield. In this way, both fertiliser and irrigation are equally important for high crop yield.

26. (b) Among the sixteen essential plant nutrients nitrogen, phosphorus and potash are the most common nutrients found deficient in India soil. Supply of these nurtients to soil artificially through fertilisers is necessary to keep the soil rich in plant nutrients for achieving maximum yield. Irrigation practices also helpful in enhancing the crop yield. In this way both fertilisers and irrigation are equally important for high crop yield.

27. (a) Biofertilizers are micro-organisms that are used for increasing fertility of soil. For example, free-living bacteria and cyanobacteria that fix nitrogen increase soil productivity. Biofertilizers are preferred over chemical fertilizers because chemical fertilizers are more expensive, disturb soil fauna and flora and affect soil pH. Although chemical fertilizers initially show better response than the biofertilizers however they decrease soil fertility in the long run.

28. (a) Nitrogenase enzyme is the enzyme responsible for nitrogen fixation in leguminous plants inside nodules infected by *Rhizobia*. This enzyme undergoes

irreversible damage in presence of oxygen and N_2 fixation is stopped but the eukaryotic cells of nodules respire aerobically thus, requiring oxygen so proper balance of oxygen amount is maintained by oxygen scavanger protein called leghaemoglobin which maintains oxygen level just sufficient for cellular respiration so the cells do not die and also removes extra oxygen in order to produce anaerobic atmosphere for proper functioning of nitrogenase enzyme.

29. (a) The *Rhizobium* bacteria converts the atmospheric nitrogen into soluble nitrates that is absorbed by the plants.
Soyabean root nodules, contain billions of *Bradyrhizobium* bacteria.

30. (a) Leghaemoglobin is the oxygen scavenger and it protects nitrogen fixing enzyme nitrogenase from oxygen.

31. (b) Although thousands of proteins have been characterized in prokaryotes and eukaryotes, only few became commercially important. This is due to the high cost of isolating and purifying enzymes in sufficient quantities. Through recombinant DNA technology, a protein can be obtained in abundant quantity. The objectives of protein engineering are to create superior enzymes to catalyze production of high value specific chemicals and to produce enzymes for large scale use.

32. (a) An immobilized enzymes is physically entrapped or covalently bonded by chemical means to an inert and usually insoluble matrix, where it can act upon its natural substrate. The matrix is usually a high molecular weight polymer such as polyacrylamide, cellulose, starch, glass, beads, etc. Because of its binding with a matrix the immobilized enzyme has better stability in many cases. Efficiency of immobilized enzyme is better. The enzyme can be recovered at the end of the reaction and can be used repeatedly.

33. (a) Biopesticides are certain types of pesticides derived from such natural materials as animals, plants, bacteria, and certain minerals. For example, canola oil and baking soda have pesticidal applications and are considered biopesticides. Some pesticides are non-biodegradable, also called recalcitrant pesticides. The longest-lived pesticide materials include parathion, aldrin, chlordane, DDT and endrin, which survive in soil for 15 years or more.

Chapter 33

Biotechnology: Principles and Processes

Directions: In the following questions, a statement of assertion is followed by a statement of reason. Mark the correct choice as:

(a) If both Assertion and Reason are true and Reason is the correct explanation of Assertion.

(b) If both Assertion and Reason are true but Reason is not the correct explanation of Assertion.

(c) If Assertion is true but Reason is false.

(d) If both Assertion and Reason are false.

1. **Assertion:** Restriction enzymes recognize palindromic sequence.
Reason: Palindromic sequences read same in both directions of the two strands.

2. **Assertion:** Restriction enzymes Hind II and Hpa are produced from two different genera of bacteria.
Reason: Hind II is produced from *Haemophilus* while Hpa is produce from *Hematococcus*.

3. **Assertion :** Restriction enzymes of different organisms that recognize the identical sequences are called isoschizomers.
Reason : They are present only in eukaryotes.

4. **Assertion:** Restriction digestion is a process of cutting DNA by restriction enzyme.
Reason: DNA ligase joins two DNAs.

5. **Assertion:** Restriction endonucleases are also called 'molecular scissors'.
Reason: When fragments generated by restriction endonucleases are mixed, they join together due to their sticky ends.

6. **Assertion:** A bacterial cell with no restriction enzymes will be easily infected and lysed by bacteriophages.
Reason: Restriciton enymes catalyse synthesis of protective coat around bacterial cell that prevents bacteriophage attack.

7. **Assertion :** Restriction enzymes cut the strand of DNA to produce sticky ends.
Reason : Stickiness of the ends facilitates the action of the enzyme DNA polymerase.
[AIIMS 2009]

8. **Assertion:** The matrix used in gel electrophoresis should have controllable pore size.
Reason: Agarose concentration can be changed to change pore sizes.

9. **Assertion:** Foreign DNA and vector DNA cut with the help of ligase.
Reason: Ligase act on sugar phosphate backbone of DNA.

10. **Assertion:** In gel electrophoresis, DNA fragments are separated.
Reason: DNA is negatively charged, so it moves towards anode under electric field.

11. **Assertion :** All endonuclease cut DNA at specific sites.
Reason : Endonucleases are found in viruses.

12. **Assertion:** Genetic engineering requires both nucleases and ligases.
Reason: Ligases produce the nick in the recombinant DNA molecule.

13. **Assertion :** Enzyme application in industry is enhanced by its immobilization.
Reason : Immobilization provides protection to enzymes without affecting their activity.

14. **Assertion :** The uptake of DNA during transformation is an active, energy requiring process.
Reason : Transformation occurs in only those bacteria, which possess the enzymatic machinery involved in the active uptake and recombination.

15. **Assertion :** In recombinant DNA technology, human genes are often transferred into bacteria (prokaryotes) or yeast (eukaryote).
Reason : Both bacteria and yeast multiply very fast to form huge population which express the desired gene.

16. **Assertion :** Plasmids are extrachromosomal DNA.
Reason : Plasmids are found in bacteria and are useful in genetic engineering. **[AIIMS 2011]**

17. Assertion: Plasmids are single-stranded extra chromosomal DNA.
Reason: Plasmids are usually present in eukaryotic cells. **[AIIMS 2002]**

18. Assertion : Insertion of recombinant DNA within the coding sequence of β-galactosidase results in colourless colonies.
Reason : Presence of insert results in inactivation of enzyme β-galactosidase known as insertional inactivation. **[AIIMS 2017]**

19. Assertion: Asexual reproduction is more important with regard to biotechnology.
Reason: Asexual reproduction preserves the genetic information while sexual reproduction permits variations.

20. Assertion: Recognition site should be preferably single and responsive to commonly used restriction enzyme.
Reason: In *pBR*322 alien DNA is ligated generally in the area of *Bam-HI* site of tetracycline resistance gene.

21. Assertion: A piece of DNA inserted into an alien organism generally does not replicate if not inserted into a chromosome.
Reason: Chromosomes have specific sequences called 'ori' region where DNA replication is initiated.

22. Assertion: Genetic engineering can overcome the drawbacks of traditional hybridization.
Reason: Genetic engineering can create desired DNA sequences to meet specific requirements.

23. Assertion: All expression vectors are cloning vectors and vice versa.
Reason: Expression vectors have at least the regulatory sequences i.e., promoters, operators, ribosomal binding sites, etc. having optimum function in the chosen control but not origin of replication.

24. Assertion: *E.coli* having pBR322 with DNA insert at BamHI site cannot grow in medium containing tetracycline.
Reason: Recognition site for Bam HI is present in tet^r region of pBR322.

25. Assertion: Special methods are used for transformation *i.e.*, incorporation of recombinant DNA into molecule.
Reason: DNA is a hydrophilic molecule.

26. Assertion: Origin of replication is an essential part of a vector.
Reason: Ori is responsible for initiating replication.

27. Assertion: Phagemid vector is made of plasmid and bacteriophage.
Reason: These vectors accomodate 300-350 kb of foreign DNA.

28. Assertion: Ori is a sequence from where replication starts.
Reason: A prokaryotic DNA has a single origin of replication.

29. Assertion : Plasmids are tools of genetic engineering.
Reason : Virculence plasmids provide pathogenicity to bacteria.

30. Assertion: Electroporation uses electric pulses for making competent host.
Reason: The electrical pulses induce transient pores in the plasmalemma through which DNA molecules are incorporated.

31. Assertion: Ethidium bromide (EtBr) under UV radiation gives bright orange coloured bands.
Reason: The separated DNA fragments can be seen after staining the DNA with compound EtBr.

32. Assertion: *Agrobacterium tumefaciens* is a pathogen of several monocot plants.
Reason: Retroviruses in plants have ability to transform normal cells into cancerous cell.

33. Assertion: In recombinant DNA technology, human genes are often transferred into bacteria or yeast.
Reason: The selected vectors multiply very fast to form huge population which can express the desired gene.

34. Assertion: *Agrobacterium tumefaciens* is popular in genetic engineering because this bacterium is associated with roots of all cereals and pulse crops.
Reason: A gene incorporated in the bacterial chromosomal genome gets automatically transferred to the crop with which the bacterium is associated. **[AIIMS 2005]**

35. Assertion: A gene from *Bacillus thuringiensis* is incorporated in plant genome to increase yield.
Reason: It is *Bt* toxin producing gene which kills larvae of insects.

36. Assertion: Biotechnology deals with techniques that use living organism to produce products useful for humans.
Reason: Biotechnology uses only a unicellular organism.

37. **Assertion:** Maintenance of sterile environment is essential for manufacture of biotechnological products.
Reason: This is to enable growth of only desired products.

38. **Assertion:** Clones are produced by sexual reproduction.
Reason: These are prepared by group of cells descended from many cells or by inbreeding of a heterozygous line. **[AIIMS 2002]**

39. **Assertion :** "DNA finger printing" has become a powerful tool to establish paternity and identity of criminals in rape and assault cases.
Reason : Trace evidences such as hairs, saliva and dried semen are adequate for DNA analysis. **[AIIMS 2010]**

40. **Assertion :** Extraction and purification of enzymes is laborious and expensive.
Reason : Protein engineering can be used to produce enzymes at large scale.

41. **Assertion :** The antibodies separted from serum are homogenous.
Reason : Monoclonal antibodies are homogenous immunological reagents.

42. **Assertion :** Interferons are effective against viruses.
Reason : Proteins which can be synthesized only by genetic engineering are effective against viruses.

43. **Assertion:** In a chemical engineering process, it is necessary to prepare sterile ambience.
Reason: Sterile ambience inhibits the growth of undesirable microbes during manufacture of products like antibiotics, vaccines and enzymes.

44. **Assertion:** Use of chitinase enzyme is necessary for isolation of DNA from yeast cells but not in case of *Spirogyra.*
Reason: Fungal cell wall is made up of fungal cellulose or chitin.

45. **Assertion:** PCR primers must not have self complementary regions.
Reason: Self comeplementary regions result in hairpin structures adversly affecting the PCR.

46. **Assertion:** Downstream processing is generally considerd more difficult and costlier in plants than that in microbes.
Reason: Rhizosecretion is used as a method to facilitate easier recovery of recombinant proteins from plants.

47. **Assertion :** Superbug gas been biopatented on name of Prof. A Chakrabarty.
Reason : Superbug was created by him with exceptional degradative plasmid to degrade toxic substances.

48. **Assertion :** One application of genetic engineering is the production of human insulin by microbes.
Reason : Gene for production of human insuling can be transferred to Escherichia coli by recombinant DNA technique.

49. **Assertion :** All GM organisms are rich in chimeric DNA (rDNA).
Reason : Chimeric DNA constitutes genes of two different organisms.

Solutions

1. **(b)** The palindrome in DNA is a sequence of base pairs that reads same on the two strands when orientation of reading strand is kept same. Restriction enzymes cut the strand of DNA a little away from the centre of the palindrome sites, but between the same two bases on opposite strands.

2. **(d)** In nomenclature of restriction enzymes, the first letter of the name of the genus in which given enzyme is discovered is written first in capital. It is followed by the first two letters of species name of the organism and these three letters are generally written in italics. Hind II and Hpa, both are produced from a single genus *Haemophilus* but from two different species i.e., *H. influenzae* and *H. parainfluenza* respectively.

3. **(c)** Isoschizomer are pairs of restriction enzymes specific to the same recognition sequence. e.g., SphI (CGTAC/G) and BbuI (CGTAC/G) are isoschizomers of each other. These are isolated from different strains of bacteria.

4. **(b)** DNA ligase joins complementary sticky ends to two DNAs.

5. **(b)** Restriction endonuclease are molecular scissors, which cut a DNA molecule within certain specific site called restriction site. Common restriction endonucleases are Eco RI, Bam II, Hind III, etc.

6. **(d)** Restriction enzymes were named due to the phenomenon of host restriction of bacterial phages. Restriction enzymes produced in a bacterial cell, recognize and cleave foreign DNA introduced (such as from bacteriophage) into the cell. Thus, bacterial cell cannot be infected and lysed by bacteriophage and hence a bacterial cell lacking restriction enzymes is easily susceptible to infection of phages. The DNA of the host bacterial cell is protected from its own restriction endonucleases by methylation (usually of A and C) within their recognition sites.

7. **(c)** Restriction enzyme, a type of endonuclease, functions by "inspecting" the length of a DNA sequence. Once it finds a recognition sequence, it binds and cut each of the two strands of the double helix at specific point leaving single stranded portions at the ends. This results in overhanging stretches called sticky ends. These are named so because they form hydrogen bonds with their complementary counter parts i.e., they can join similar complementary ends of DNA fragment from some other source with the help of DNA ligase. This stickness of the ends facilitates the action of the enzyme DNA ligase, not DNA polymerase.

8. **(b)** Agarose is a polysccharide obtained from red algae. Agarose dissolves in hot water and when it is cooled, it forms gel. Pore size depends upon agarose concentration. In general, a 1% (w/v) gel will have a pore size of 150 nm. While a 0.16% gel has pore size of 500 nm.

9. **(d)** In formation of rDNA, restriction endonucleases cut both foreign DNA and vector DNA and act on sugar phosphate backbone of DNA.

10. **(a)** DNA fragments can be isolated with the help of gel electrophoresis, where DNA moves towards the anode (+vely charged).

11. **(d)** Restriction endonuclease is a type of endonuclease which cut DNA at specific sites, not all endonuclease cut DNA at specific sites. These are not found in virus. There were discovered from bacteria.

12. **(c)** Nucleases are the enzymes that remove nucleotides or produce nick in the DNA strand. Exonucleases remove nucleotides from the free ends of DNA while endonucleases produce internal nick in DNA. Now, the desired gene is inserted and the cut ends are sealed with the help of DNA ligase. Ligases are also called molecular glue as they join together two strands by forming phosphodiester bonds between adjacent nucleotides.

13. (a) An immobilized enzymes is physically entrapped or covalently bonded by chemical means to an inert and usually insoluble matrix, where it can act upon its natural substrate. The matrix is usually a high molecular weight polymer such as polyacrylamide, cellulose, starch, glass, beads, etc. Because of its binding with a matrix the immobilized enzyme has better stability in many cases. Efficiency of immobilized enzyme is better. The enzyme can be recovered at the end of the reaction and can be used repeatedly.

14. (a) Transformation does not involve passive entry of DNA molecules through permeable cell walls and membranes. It does not occur 'naturally' in all species of bacteria, only in those species possessing the enzymatic machinery involved in the active uptake and recombination processes. Even in these species, all cells in a given population are not capable of active uptake of DNA. Only competent cells, which possess a so called competence factor are capable of serving as recipients in transformation.

15. (a) Bacteria and yeast are easily grow in culture medium and multiply very fast so it is best for making the many copies of recombinant DNA, and express character of desired gene.

16. (b) Plasmids are the extrachromosomal part in the bacteria and are useful in recombinant DNA technology.

17. (c) Plasmid is an extra chromosomal DNA present in prokaryotes e.g., bacteria.

18. (a) Alternative markers have been developed that can differentiate recombinants from non-recombinants based upon their ability to produce colour in presence of a chromogenic substrate. The plasmid in the bacteria, lacking an insert produces blue coloured colonies, while those plasmids with an insert do not produce any colour due to insertional inactivation of the enzyme, β-galactosidase.

19. (a) Biotechonology studies need a quick growing population of genetically uniform individuals so that similar changes may be produced in all the genetically engineered organisms. Hence, asexual reproduction, which is a quicker and faster method of reproduction that preserves genetic information of individuals, is better suited for biotechnological experiments. For example, if an organism that has been incorporated with a gene for disease resitance reproduces sexually, then recombination and segregation of genes will occur during gamete formation. Hence, some of the progeny may lose the gene of disease resistance incorporated into the parent. On the other hand, if the genetically engineered organism reproduces asexually, then all its progeny will invariably contain the gene for disease resistance.

20. (b) Recognition site or site where alien DNA can be inserted should be single because occurrence of more than one recognition site will cause DNA fragmentation and disturb gene cloning.

21. (a) 'Origin of replication' is a sequence from where replication starts by binding of polymerase enzyme. An isolated piece of DNA without origin of replication or 'ori' site cannot replicate and is gradually lost during nuclear divisions. But if it is inserted within a chromosome, it is replicated along with the chromosome as a result of the replication process initiated by the 'origin of replication' site of the chromosome. This is the reason why recombinant vectors used in genetic engineering must contain origin of replication so that they can replicate themselves during cell division in order to ensure presence of recombinant gene in all the progeny.

22. (a) Traditional hybridization procedures involve mating of organisms to be modified with another individual of the same species having desired characters and screening the progeny for expression of desired set of characters. These procedures often lead to inclusion and multiplication of

undesirable genes alongwith desired genes. Besides inter-specific hybridization are generally not very successful. Genetic engineering can overcome all these drawbacks because use of recombinant DNA technology, gene cloning and gene transfer allow us to isolate and introduce only one or a set of desirable genes without introducing undesirable genes into the target organism that too from any distant organism.

23. (d) All vectors used for propagation of DNA inserts in a suitable host are called cloning vectors. But when a vector is designed for the expression *i.e.*, production of the protein specified by the DNA insert, it is termed as expression vector. Expression vectors need regulatory machinery suitable for the host, *e,g.*, if an eukaryotic gene is to be expressed in prokaryotes, the expression vectors should contain gene without introns because prokaryotes lack intron removal machinery for transcripts. But all vectors, including expression vectors must contain 'origin of replication' so that they can replicate when the host cell divides and their presence is ensured in all progeny.

24. (a) pBR322 has recognition sites for several commonly used restriction enzymes. Recognition site for *Bam* HI is present in tet^r region *i.e.*, region responsible for tetracycline resistance. When an insert is added at the *BamHI* recognition site the gene for tetracycline resistance becomes non-functional and the recombinant bacteria with plasmid pBR322 that has DNA insert at *BamHI* loses tetracycline resistance.

25. (a) Transformation is permanent heritable change in a cell, particularly a bacteria cell, that occurs as a result of its acquiring foreign DNA. But cells normally do not take up foreign DNA molecule because DNA is a hydrolic macromolecule and its passage through lipid membrane is opposed special methods such as $CaCl_2$ treatment, electroporation, particle delivery method, etc., are used to make host cells competent *i.e.*, able to take up foreign DNA.

26. (a) Ori is the DNA sequence that signals for the origin of replication, sometimes referred to simply as origin.

27. (c) Phagemid vector carries large DNA sequences.

28. (b) Ori is origin of replication. It is a sequence, where any piece of DNA when linked can be made to replicate within the host cells.

29. (b) Plasmids are most commonly found in bacteria as small circular, double-stranded DNA molecules. These are sometimes present in archaea and eukaryotic organisms. They are used in genetic engineering. There are five main classes of Plasmids. Virulence plasmids which turn the bacterium into a pathogen.

30. (a) Electroporation involves low or high voltage pulses which open pores of membrane making cell competent.

31. (a) Ethidium Bromide (EtBr) is a compound which stain DNA followed by exposure to UV radiation and seen as bright orange coloured bands.

32. (d) *Agrobacterium tumefaciens* is pathogen of dicot plants. Retroviruses are vectors for cloning genes in animals.

33. (a) Multiple copies of its gene will increase the yield of the desired product.

34. (d) *Agrobacterium tumefaciens* infects certain plants, (dicots) in which T_i-plasmid causes the formation of tumour like growth called a crown gall. *Agrobacterium* does not infect grasses (i.e. cereals).

35. (a) Strains of the Bacillus thuringiensis produce different Bt toxins, each harmful to different insects. Most notably, Bt toxins are insecticidal to the larvae of moths and butterflies, but are harmless to other forms of life. The gene coding for Bt toxin has been inserted into cotton as a transgene, causing it to produce this natural insecticide in its tissues.

36. (c) Biotechnology is the use of biological processes, organisms, or systems to manufacture products intended to improve the quality of human life.

37. (a) There are two core techniques that enabled birth of modern biotechnology
(i) Genetic engineering
(ii) Chemical engineering (maintaining sterile environment). Sterile environment ensures growth of only microbe cell of interest.

38. (d) Cloning is a shortcut method to amplify the number of organisms with a desirable constitution. No sex is involved in their production. Members of clone are genetically identical as they are derived from single parent.

39. (a) DNA finger printing has become a powerful tool due to its ability in tracing evidences of crime and to establish the paternity. These evidences can be collected from hairs, semen and saliva.

40. (b) Although thousands of proteins have been characterized in prokaryotes and eukaryotes, only few became commercially important. This is due to the high cost of isolating and purifying enzymes in sufficient quantities. Through recombinant DNA technology, a protein can be obtained in abundant quantity. The objectives of protein engineering are to create superior enzymes to catalyze production of high value specific chemicals and to produce enzymes for large scale use.

41. (d) From hyperimmunized animals, the blood serum may be taken and antibodies may be isolated from this serum. However, the antibodies, whenever separated from serum after induction due to an antigen, are usually heterogenous, because the cells keep on producing a variety of antibodies. Monoclonal antibodies (Mabs), on the other hand are homogeneous immunological reagents of defined specificity so that these can be utilized for diagnosis and screening with ease and certainty.

42. (c) Interferons are proteins that are effective against most viruses. They are naturally produced by virus infected cells. The proteins interact with adjacent cells and make them resistant to virus attack. Now interferons are also being manufactured through genetic engineering.

Interferons control the multiplication of virus particles by inhibiting their protein synthesis.

43. (a) During sterilization, the equipments, etc., are made free of any micro-organisms before the addition of desired microbe or cell. Now, this desired organism does not get any competition from other organisms and expresses all its characters thus, growing effectively. Hence, sterilization enables growth of only the desired microbe. It is also evident that along with genetic engineering, sterilization is also essential for successful biotechnological experiments.

44. (a) In order to use the DNA for genetic engineering processes, it must be in pure form, free from other macromolecules. This is termed DNA isolation and is the pioneer step. Since the DNA is enclosed within the membranes, it is required to break open the cell to release DNA a long with other macromolecules such as RNA, proteins, polysaccharides, lipids, etc. and from this mixture DNA is purified. Release of DNA from a cell is achieved by treating the cells with enzymes such as lysozyme (bacteria), cellulose (plant cells), chitinase (fungus), etc. These enzymes degrade cell wall while plasma membrane degrading enzymes like lipase, etc., are also needed. Since yeast is a fungus and fungal cell wall is made of chitin (fungal cellulose), isolation of DNA necessarily requires use of chitinase.

45. (a) Primers are nucleotide sequences that serve as the base for formation of new DNA strands. In PCR, primers are added at the ends of DNA strand to be copied and the primers are extended towards each other so that the DNA segment lying between the two primers is copied. If self complementary bases are present in primers than hydrogen bonds are formed

between them and hairpin-like structure is formed. It makes the primers unsuitable for PCR.

46. (b) Purification of desired biochemicals from the biomass or the culture medium is called downstream processing. It is generally more difficult and costlier in plants mainly due to low concentration of recombinant protein in the total biomass. Rhizosecretion is one of the methods that overcomes this problem. In this method the transgene is driven by a root specific promoter and an appropriate signal sequence is added to it to ensure the secretion of recombinant protein from the root. Hence, the recombination product is obtained very easily.

47. (a) Prof. Chakrabarty genetically engineered a new species of Pseudomonas bacteria ("the oil-eating bacteria") in 1971. Microbes resistant to multiple antimicrobials are called multidrug resistant (MDR); or sometimes superbugs. Ananda Mohan Chakrabarty demonstrates a very diverse metabolism, including the ability to degrade organic solvents such as toluene. This ability has been put to use in bioremediation, or the use of microorganisms to biodegrade oil. Use of P. putida is preferable to some other Pseudomonas species

48. (a) Recombinant DNA technology is used in genetic engineering where the tool is plasmid of *Escherichia coli* therefore, reason is correct explanation to assertion.

49. (a) Recombinant DNA molecules are sometimes called chimeric DNA, because they can be made of material from two different species. A transgenic, or genetically modified, organism is one that has been altered through recombinant DNA technology, which involves either the combining of DNA from different genomes or the insertion of foreign DNA into a genome.

Chapter 34

Biotechnology and its Applications

Directions: In the following questions, a statement of assertion is followed by a statement of reason. Mark the correct choice as:

(a) If both Assertion and Reason are true and Reason is the correct explanation of Assertion.

(b) If both Assertion and Reason are true but Reason is not the correct explanation of Assertion.

(c) If Assertion is true but Reason is false.

(d) If both Assertion and Reason are false.

1. **Assertion:** '*Cry*' proteins are named so because they are crystal proteins.
Reason: In acidic environment of insect midgut '*Cry*' proteins are solubilized and then release toxic core fragments after proteolytic action.

2. **Assertion:** *Cry* gene expressing crop is resistant to a group of insects.
Reason: *Cry* proteins produced from *Bacillus thuringiensis* are toxic to larvae of certain insects.

3. **Assertion** : Transgenic plant is a product of plant tissue culture.
Reason : An organism that contains and expresses a transgenic organism.

4. **Assertion** : A crop expressing a cry gene is usually resistant to a group of insects.
Reason : *Cry* proteins produced from *Bacillus thuringiensis* is toxic to larvae of certain insects.

5. **Assertion** : FlavrSavr, a transgenic tomato which remains fresh and retains their flavour for long time.
Reason : Production of polygalacturonase enzyme, which degrades pectin, is blocked in FlavrSavr.

6. **Assertion:** GMO tomato i.e., 'flavr Savr' has increased shelf life and better nutrient quality.
Reason: This is achieved by reducing the amount of cell wall degrading enzyme 'polygalacturonase' responsible for fruit softening.

7. **Assertion:** By insertion of gene encoding complementary RNA only the RNAi can be introduced in an organism.
Reason: In vitro there are no methods by which synthesised complementary RNA can be inserted in an organism to induce RNAi (RNA interference).

8. **Assertion:** Cellular defence mechanism in eukaryotes is RNAi.
Reason: RNAi is silencing of a specific *t*RNA.

9. **Assertion:** Tobacco plant yield is highly reduced because of damage to roots.
Reason: Nematode *Meloidogyne incognita* infects the root.

10. **Assertion:** Biotechnology produces transgenic micro-organisms that acts as microfactories for proteins.
Reason: To produce proteins of human use like insulin. Transgenic microorganisms can be developed.

11. **Assertion:** Using biotechnology human insulin can be produced into bacterial cells.
Reason: To produce human insulin the A, B and C polypeptides of the human insulin are produced in the bacterial cells, separately extracted and combined by creating disulfide bonds.

12. **Assertion:** Due to excessive synthesis of gene for adenosine deaminase ADA deficiency disorder is caused.
Reason: It affects the human digestive system.

13. **Assertion:** The ADA gene gives instruction for producing the enzyme adenosine deaminases.
Reason: Throughout the body this enzyme is found but is most active in lymphocytes.

14. **Assertion:** *Via* recombinant DNA technology transgenic plant production can be achieved.
Reason: Transgenic organism are an organism that contains and expresses a transgene is called.

15. **Assertion:** The first transgenic animal was GM salmon for performing vaccine safety tests.
Reason: Genetically modified ova were fused with normal sperms of the same species. For the production of GM salmon.

16. **Assertion:** In human beings the transgenic food may cause toxicity and product allergy.
Reason: The bacteria present in alimentary canal of human beings may become resistant to the antibiotics by taking up the antibiotic resistant gene that is present in the GM food.

17. **Assertion:** Transgenic mouse is also known as 'super mouse' because it is twice big in size than the normal mouse.
Reason: The gene for human growth factor has been introduced and expressed in 'super mouse'.

18. **Assertion:** To make them tolerant to abiotic stresses many crops are induced with foreign genes.
Reason: Many plant genomes are manipulated or altered by combining them with other genes in order to get desired traits.

19. **Assertion:** Hirudin is a type of protein that prevents blood clotting.
Reason: The gene that encodes hirudin is transferred into *Brassica napus,* where hirudin is accumulated in the seeds .

20. **Assertion :** Humulin is better than conventional insulin.
Reason : Conventional insulin produces many side effects.

21. **Assertion :** Second generation vaccines are safer to use.
Reason : They are produced by genetic engineering.

22. **Assertion:** Unwanted immunological responses cannot be induced by Recombinant therapeutics.
Reason: The human body do not recognise them as foreign elements.

23. **Assertion:** Animal antibodies produced in plants are plantibodies.
Reason: Plantibodies are just a theoretical concept.

24. **Assertion:** To cure SCID, the first clinical gene for ADA therapy was given.
Reason: Using retroviral vector the normal gene was delivered into the patient's cells.

25. **Assertion:** Transgenic plants consisting virus coat protein gene express resistance to that virus and other related varieties.
Reason: Inside the plant cells coat protein gene interferes with uncoating of viruses.

26. **Assertion:** To diagnose presence of a specific DNA segment in a mixture, complementary pairing between nucleotides is exploited.
Reason: DNA probes having radioactive isotopes help to detect DNA by autoradiography.

27. **Assertion:** ELISA test is a technique based on antigen-antibody interactions where a pathogen can be detected by the presence of antibodies (proteins, glycoproteins etc) on it.
Reason: The pathogen antibody to be identified is immobilised on the surface of specially constructed ELISA plates and is then tested.

28. **Assertion:** Colon bacilli can be used to produce glycoproteins that can be used for treatment of hepatitis-B.
Reason: Hepatitis B is a viral disease and using interferons its spread in body can be checked.

29. **Assertion:** *Bacillus anthracis* exemplifies how biotechnology can be used for destructive processes.
Reason: Anthrax bacterium spores were spread via letters in the form of powder.

30. **Assertion :** Protein engineering can be used to produce enzymes at large scale, which is used for synthesis of monoclonal antibodies.
Reason : Monoclonal antibodies are homogeneous immunological reagents.

31. **Assertion :** The term hybridoma is applied to fused cells.
Reason : They are formed by the fusion of lymphocyte cell and myeloma cell.

32. **Assertion :** Hybridoma cells are shifted to a medium deficient in nutrient which cannot be synthesised by myeloma cells.
Reason : This medium allows selection of hybridoma cells.

33. **Assertion:** Organisations like GEAC are necessary to monitor GM researches and test the safety of introducing gM organisms for public services.
Reason: When genetically modified organisms are introduced into the ecosystem. GM researches can have unpredictable results which even can be disastrous.

34. **Assertion:** In developing world, Green revolution was comparatively less effective where farmers were dependent on conventional breeding.
Reason: In developing world, inability to buy expensive agro-chemicals forced farmers to rely on conventional breeding.

35. **Assertion:** An example of biopiracy is USA's patent of brazzein.
Reason: Brazzein a protein that was obtained from West African plant, *Pentadiplandra brazzenana* and the gene encoding it has been patented by USA.

36. **Assertion:** For gene transfer in plant cells *Ti* plasmid obtained from *Agrobacterium tumefaciens* is effectively used as a vector.
Reason: The part of Ti plasmid transferred into the DNA of plant cells is called as T-DNA.

37. **Assertion:** In genetic engineering *Agrobacterium tumefaciens* is popular because this bacterium is associated with the stems of all cereal and pulse crops.
Reason: A gene incorporated in the bacterial chromosomal genome automatically get transferred to the crop with which bacterium is associated.

Solutions

1. (c) The *cry* gene of *Bacillus thuringiensis* produces a protein, that forms crystalline inclusions *i.e.*, is crystal in nature in the bacterial spores. Due to their crystal nature these proteins are named 'cry' proteins and are responsible for the insecticidal activities of the bacterial strains. In alkaline environment of insect midgut 'Cry' proteins are solubilized. Then to release core toxic fragments these proteins undergo proteolytic digestion. These toxins bind to receptors in brush border of midgut epithelial cells. As a result, brush border, membrane develop pores, most likely non-specific in nature and cause influx of ions and water into the cells resulting in their swelling and eventual lysis.
2. (b) A soil bacterium *Bacillus thuringiensis (Bt)* produces a *Cry* protein (crystal protein). This protein is toxic to the larvae of certain insects. There are several kinds of *Cry* proteins, which are is toxic to a different group of insects. The gene encoding *Cry* protein, that is *cry* gene has been isolated and transferred into several crops. A crop expressing a cry gene is usually resistant to the groups of insects.
3. (b) Plant tissue culture has various applications in the different fiields of biology. An example of this is the production of transgenic plants and animals. Transgenic organisms contain genes, which are transferred into them through the genetic engineering. These genes are known as transgenic.
4. (b) *Bacillus thuringiensis (Bt)*, a soil bacterium produces a *Cry* protein (crystal protein). This protein is toxic to the larvae of certain insects. There are several kinds of *Cry* proteins. Each *Cry* protein is toxic to a different group of insects. The gene encoding *Cry* protein, i.e., *cry* gene has been isolated and transferred into several crops. A crop expressing a *cry* gens is usually resistant to the groups of insects.
5. (a) FlavrSavr is a transgenic tomato variety. Fruits of this variety remain fresh and retain their flavour for much longer than normal fruits. It happens due to the blockage of the production of pectin degrading enzyme polygalacturonase.
6. (a) Genetically modified tomato i.e., flavr savr show delayed ripening. By the use of antisense RNA technology the enzyme polygalacturonase, that causes damage to pectin is deactivated and for longer duration the tomato is kept fresh.
7. (d) RNAi (RNA interference) occurs in all eukaryotic organisms as a method of cellular defense. This method involves silencing of a specific *m*RNA due to a complementary dsRNA molecule that binds to specific mRNA and prevents translation of the *m*RNA. To induce RNA interference in any organism *in vitro* there are two methods, the complementary RNA can be synthesized and then annealed to produce dsRNA and inserted into cells or the cells are genetically modified to produce the two complementary RNA strands or duplex form *in vivo* by transcription. However, the first method *i.e., in vitro* insertion of synthesized complementary RNA stops target gene expression for only 4-6 days and their re-introduction is required. But the second method *i.e.,* the vector DNA construct once transfected into the cells, will keep on generating RNA interference and hence, cause a permanent inhibition of the damage.
8. (c) RNAi is the silencing of a specific *m*RNA.
9. (a) *Meloidogyne incognita* infects the root of tobacco plant that leads to the degradation of cell walls of the roots and reduce the yield.
10. (b) By inserting genes (or desired protein products transgenic micro-organisms can be developed using recombinant DNA technology. These transgenic organisms acts as living microfactories that produce proteins like human insulin, human growth hormone, etc. Production of proteins from such organisms is easier, more efficient and cost effective.

11. (c) Adult onset diabetes management is possible by taking insulin at regular time intervals, but insulin from other animals could elicit immune response in body. Biotechnology has helped to overcome this problem. Transgenic bacteria have been produced that translate the constituting polypeptide chains of human insulin from the bacterial cells. These polypeptides can be extracted and combined to produce human insulin, by creating disulfide bonds. In humans, insulin is produced as a prohormone with three polypeptides A, B and C. After processing, the C peptide is removed and mature insulin is formed. When transgenic bacteria are used, instead of producing extra stretch of C peptide, only A and B polypeptides are produced and then linked directly to produce mature insulin.

12. (d) ADA disorder is caused because of lack of gene for adenosine deaminase. It affects the human immune system.

13. (b) The ADA gene gives instructions for producing the enzyme adenosine deaminase. In all cells this enzyme is produced, but the highest levels of adenosine deaminase takes place in immune system cells called lymphocytes, that develop in lymphoid tissues. Lymphocytes form the immune system, that defends the body against potentially harmful invaders, such as viruses or bacteria.

14. (b) Transgenic organisms contain genes, that are transferred into them through the genetic engineering. These genes are called transgenes. Using recombinant DNA technology transgenic organisms can be produced.

15. (d) Those organisms that have their genetic material modified to meet some desired conditions are genetically modified (GM) organisms. They generally carry a foreign gene in their DNA. GM salmon was the first transgenic animal for food production. It was produced by fusion of normal ova (eggs) with genetically modified sperms. The zygotes with modified gene developed into embryos that gave rise to much bigger adults than either parent thus have greater food value. It is achieved by addition of a gene that codes for the growth hormone that allows the fish to grow larger more rapidly than the non-transgenic salmon.

16. (b) Several animal studies indicate serious health risks associated with genetically modified (GM) food including infertility, immune problems,accelerated aging, faulty insulin regulation, and changes in major organs and the gastrointestinal system. The bacteria in the alimentary canal become resistant to antibiotic by taking up the resistant gene present in GM foods.

17. (a) Palmiter and Brinster (1981) developed the first transgenic animal 'supermouse'. It has human growth hormone gene. It has been intoroduced and expressed. Size of supermouse is big in size than the normal mouse.

18. (a) Improved resistance to drought, salinity and extreme temperatures has been observed in transgenic plants that express/ over express genes regulating osmolytes, specific proteins, antioxidants, ion homeostasis, transcription factors and membrane composition. Many plants genome are altered by combining them with other genes in order to get desired traits.

19. (b) Hirudin is a protein that prevents blood clotting. The gene responsible for the production of blood clotting preventing protein have been chemically synthesised and then transferred into *Brassica napus* (Brassicaceae). Hirudin protein accumulates in the seeds of this plant.

20. (a) Humulin is the first genetically engineered pharmaceutical product. It is better than conventional insulin because conventional insulin produces many side effects over a long period.

21. (b) Second generation vaccines were developed to reduce the risks from live vaccines. These are subunit vaccines, consisting of specific protein antigens (such as tetanus or diphtheria toxoid) or recombinant protein components (such as the hepatitis B surface antigen). They are produced through genetic engineering.

22. (a) The recombinant therapeutics are identical to human proteins they do not induce unwanted immunological responses and are free from risk of infection as is commonly observed in case of similar products isolated from non-human sources.

23. (c) The term 'plantibody' is derived from fusion of plant and antibody. Transgenic plants plantibodies are produced that express the animal antibody genes transferred into them. In 1989 the first plantibody was produced by expressing mouse antibody gene in tobacco. So far only sIgA (secretary IgA) has been produced in the plant systems. Plantibodies have two applications (i) treatment of human and animal diseases and (ii) protection of plants from nematodes and viruses.

24. (b) SCID (severe combined immuno-deficiency disease) is an immune disorder caused due to ADA (adenosine deaminase) deficiency. The patient has defective ADA gene thus ADA enzyme becomes deficient. Normal ADA gene that could function normally is inserted into the patient's cell. Such process of introduction of a normal functional gene into cells, that contains the defective allele of concerned gene with the objective of correcting a genetic or acquired disorder is called gene therapy. To cure SCID first gene therapy was done and the normal gene was introduced using retroviral vector.

25. (a) In many crop plants transgenic plants having virus coat protein gene linked to a strong promoter have been produced *e.g.,* tobacco, tomato, alfalfa, sugar beet, potato etc. In 1986, the first transgenic plant of this type was tobacco produced, which contained coat protein gene of tobacco mosaic virus (TMV) strain U_1. Most likely the resistance generated by coat protein gene is due to the blocking of the uncoating process of virus particles, that is necessary for viral genome replication as well as expression. However, other effects seem to be involved in producing coat protein mediated virus resistance.

26. (b) DNA probes are ss DNA molecules of known sequences that consists radioactive isotopes. They are used to detect presence of a specific DNA segment complementary to their base sequences. Here, the complementary pairing between base nucleotides proves useful as the probe DNA and DNA to be detected being complementary to each other form hydrogen bonds between base pairs and form double stranded DNA molecule by autoradiography. This double stranded DNA can be easily detected due to radioactiviey isotopes present in DNA probe.

27. (d) ELISA (enzyme linked immuno-sorbant assay) is a technique based on the principle of antigen-antibody interactions. On their surface pathogens have specific antigens like protein, glycoproteins, etc. Thus, by using the antibodies specific to bind with those antigens their infection can be detected. In process antigens are immobilized on ELISA plates. Then antibody specific to the antigen is added and allowed to react with the adsorbed antigen. A complex procedure is followed.

28. (b) Interferons are the antiviral glycoproteins that function as immune regulators or Iymphokines and are produced by the infected cells in response to viral infections. Until recently the only source of interferons was human white blood cells or virus infected human cells that is grown in tissue culture. Nowadays colon bacilli can be genetically engineered to produce human interferons. These interferons (particularly IFNa) are significantly used for the hepatitis B treatment. They are also being tested for the treatment of cancer and some viral diseases including AIDS.

29. (b) In welfare of human race biotechnology has extensively used but it can used for destructive purposes too. One such use of biotechnology are bioweapons. War which is fought by bioweapons against human and or their crops and animals is called biowar. Viruses, bacteria and some other harmful organisms can be used as biological weapons. Bioweapons take much less space than traditional weapons and can be far more disastrous. One such example is *Anthrax* bacterium which was sent through letters after September 2001.

30. (a) Protein engineering is the design of new enzymes or proteins with new or desirable functions. It is based on the use of recombinant DNA technology to change amino acid sequences. Applications range from biocatalysis for food and industry to environmental, medical and nanobiotechnology applications.

Monoclonal antibodies are homogeneous immunological reagents of defined specificity and they are produced by hybridoma technology.

31. (a) A hybridoma cell, is produced by the injection of a specific antigen into a mouse, procuring the antigen-specific plasma cells (antibody-producing cell) from the mouse's spleen and the subsequent fusion of this cell with a cancerous immune cell called a myeloma cell.

32. (a) Fused cells are incubated in HAT medium (hypoxanthine-aminopterin-thymidine medium) for roughly 10 to 14 days. Aminopterin blocks the pathway that allows for nucleotide synthesis. Hence, unfused myeloma cells die, as they cannot produce nucleotides by the denovo or salvage pathways because they lack HGPRT. Removal of the unfused myeloma cells is necessary because they have the potential to outgrow other cells, especially weakly established hybridomas. Unfused B cells die as they have a short life span. In this way, only the B cell-myeloma hybrids survive, since the HGPRT gene coming from the B cells is functional. These cells produce antibodies (a property of B cells) and are immortal (a property of myeloma cells).

33. (a) By the human race manipulation of living organisms *i.e.,* genetic modification of organisms cannot go on continuously without regulation. The outcomes may pose threat to our ecosystem. Some ethical standards (termed bioethics) are needed to evaluate the morality of all human activities that might help or harm living organisms. GEAC (Genetic Engineering Approval Committee) is an organization set up by Indian government to ensure that bioethics are being followed in all GM researches being carried on in India.

34. (a) The phase of enormous increase in the agricultural production, when high yielding improved varieties of crop plants were used was known as green revolution. But the increased yield was partly due to use of improved crop varieties but mainly due to use of better management practices and agrochemicals (chemicals and fertilizers). Generally these practices and agrochemicals were very expensive in developing world that the farmers could not afford. Hence, the farmers of developing world relied mainly on cheaper methods of conventional breeding thus green revolution could not become as productive or effective as it was in developed world.

35. (a) The use of bio-resources by multinational companies and other organisations without proper authorisation from the countries and people concerned without compensatory payment is known as Biopiracy. Brazzein is produced by *Pentadiplandra brazzeana* and is approximately 2,000 times as sweet as sugar. It is used as a low calorie sweetener. Local people have been using the super sweet berries from their plants for centuries but protein brazzein and 'tre' gene coding it is patented in U.S.A. It has been proposed to transfer the brazzein gene into maize and express it in maize kernels from where it can be easily extracted. This is an example of biopiracy.

36. (b) *Agrobacterium* is natural genetic engineer of plants. It is a pathogen of several dicot plants can transfer a piece of DNA called (T-DNA) to transform normal plant cells into a tumor cells. Ti plasmid of *Agrobacterium tumefaciens* and Ri plasmid of A. *rhizogens* are best known plant cloning vectors.

37. (d) *Agrobacterium tumefaciens* is a pathogenic bacterium which produces crown galls or tumours in plants on infection. It contains a large Ti-plasmid (tumour inducing plasmid) and it can transfer a part of its plasmid DNA to the host plant. Therefore, the bacterium can be used in the transfer of genes in biotechnological techniques.

Chapter 35

Organisms and Populations

Directions: In the following questions, a statement of assertion is followed by a statement of reason. Mark the correct choice as:

(a) If both Assertion and Reason are true and Reason is the correct explanation of Assertion.

(b) If both Assertion and Reason are true but Reason is not the correct explanation of Assertion.

(c) If Assertion is true but Reason is false.

(d) If both Assertion and Reason are false.

1. **Assertion :** Tropical rain forests are disappearing fast from developing countries such as India.
   Reason : No value is attached to these forests because these are poor in biodiversity.
   [AIIMS 2015]
2. **Assertion :** Flora contains the actual account of habitat and distribution of plants of a given area.
   Reason : Flora helps in correct identification.
   [AIIMS 2016]
3. **Assertion :** Species are groups of potentially interbreeding natural populations which are isolated from other such groups.
   Reason : Distinctive morphological characters are displayed due to reproductive isolation.
   [AIIMS 2017]
4. **Assertion:** "The Biological Species" concept helps us to ask how species are formed.
   Reason: The concept of biological species focuses our attention on the question of how reproductive isolation comes about.
5. **Assertion :** Cold deserts too exist. e.g., Tibet, Gobi.
   Reason : Desert can be hot, e.g., Thar, Sahara.
6. **Assertion :** Biotic community has higher position than population in ecological hierarchy.
   Reason : Population of similar individuals remains isolated in the community.
7. **Assertion :** Indo-Gangetic plains have high population density.
   Reason: These have favourable climate and fertile soil.
8. **Assertion :** Living organisms are regarded as open systems.
   Reason: Energy of living organisms can be lost or gained from external environment.
9. **Assertion :** Ecological equivalents possess similar types of adaptations.
   Reason : Ecological niche is the total interaction of a species with environment.
10. **Assertion :** Heliophytes, generally have low photosynthetic, respiratory and metabolic activities.
    Reason : This is an adaptation of heliophytes to high intensity of light.
11. **Assertion :** Leaf butterfly and stick insect show mimicry to dodge their enemies.
    Reason : Mimicry is a method to acquire body colour blending with the surroundings.
    [AIIMS 2003]
12. **Assertion :** Animals adopt different strategies to survive in hostile environment.
    Reason : Praying mantis is green in colour which merges with plant foliage. **[AIIMS 2004]**
13. **Assertion :** Thick cuticle is mostly present in disease resistant plants.
    Reason : Disease causing agents cannot grow on cuticle and cannot invade the cuticle.
14. **Assertion:** *Daphnia* populations in a water body, at different seasons of a year showed marked variations in their body morphology.
    Reason: Cyclomorphosis in some organisms is influenced by the variations in temperatures prevailing in their water-bodies at different seasons.

15. **Assertion:** The prickly pear cactus introduced into Australia in early 1920s caused havoc by spreading rapidly into millions of hectares of land range.
Reason: When certain exotic species are introduced into a geographical area, they become invasive and start spreading fast because the invaded land does not have the natural predators.

16. **Assertion:** Plants need the help of insects and animals for pollinating their flowers and dispersing their seeds.
Reason: Plants offer rewards in the form of pollen and nectar for pollinators and juicy and nutritious fruits for seed dispersers.

17. **Assertion:** The aquatic organisms in which the osmotic concentration and temperature of body change according to the ambient conditions of water are referred to as conformers.
Reason: These organisms are able to maintain homeostasis through thermoregulation and osmoregulation by physiological or behavioural means.

18. **Assertion:** Small sized animals are scarce in polar regions.
Reason: Small sized animals have larger surface area relative to their volume and they have to spend much energy to generate body heat through metabolism.

19. **Assertion:** The community of an ecotone commonly contains the organisms of each of the overlapping communities and in addition the organisms which are restricted to the ecotone.
Reason: The tendency for increased variety and density at community junctions is known as the edge effect.

20. **Assertion:** In deep water bodies, variations in temperature of water at different depths results in thermal stratification.
Reason: In temperate lakes, cooling of surface water during autumn and warming of it during spring results in circulation of nutrients as well as oxygen, twice a year.

21. **Assertion:** Coral reefs are not found in the regions from West Bengal to Andhra Pradesh but are found in Tamil Nadu and on the East coast of India.
Reason: Corals require low siltation, low fresh water inflow by rivers, high salinity and optimal temperature to colonize.

22. **Assertion:** Aerenchyma is present in the leaves and petioles of hydrophytes.
Reason: It imparts buoyancy to the hydrophytes.

23. **Assertion:** Many mangrove plants possess high levels of organic solutes.
Reason: This is an adaptation to cope with the conditions of high salt concentration and osmotic potential.

24. **Assertion:** True xerophytes do not store water in the form of mucilage which helps to withstand prolonged period of drought.
Reason: Vascular and mechanical tissues are well developed in true xerophytes.

25. **Assertion:** It drains off oxygen from water and is seen growing in standing water with respect to *Eichorrnia.*
Reason: It is an indigenous species of our country.

26. **Assertion:** The rate at which a population can be expected to grow in the future can be assessed graphically by means of a population pyramid.
Reason: A triangular population pyramid is characteristic of a country whose population is stable, neither growing nor shrinking.

27. **Assertion:** A population growing in a habitat with limited resources shows initially a lag phase, followed by phases of acceleration and deceleration and finally an asymptote, when the population density reaches the carrying capacity.
Reason: This type of population growth is called Verhulst Pearl Logistic growth, in which a plot of N (population density) at time (t) results in a sigmoid curve.

28. **Assertion:** Bell shaped age pyramid represents a stable population.
Reason: Proportion of individuals in reproductive age group is higher than the individuals in pre-reproductive age group.

29. **Assertion :** In sigmoid growth curve, population finally stabilizes itself.
Reason : Finally, the death rate increases than the birth rate.

30. **Assertion :** With increase in population size, environmental resistance tends to increase.
Reason : This is a nature's way to check the expression of biotic potential.

31. Assertion : Removal of keystone species doesnot cause any serious disruption in the functioning of the community

Reason: Keystone species are high in abundance (or biomass) than the dominant species.

32. Assertion : The sex ratio of Kerala is highest in India.

Reason : In countries like India the population is increasing at a rapid rate. **[AIIMS 2005]**

33. Assertion : Natural populations are capable of rapid number increase, but remain constant in size.

Reason : Human interference has led to constancy of size of natural populations.

34. Assertion: Plant-animal interactions do not generally involve co-evolution of the mutualist organisms.

Reason: Evolution of the plants and animals can never happen side by side.

35. Assertion : Predation is an interspecific interaction with a feeding strategy.

Reason: Predation and their prey maintain fairly stable population through time and rarely one population become abundant or scarce.

36. Assertion: Predators not only take the old, sick and young individuals but also the healthy individuals.

Reason: If predators kille only the old, sick and young prey individuals, then there would be no evolution of antipredatory traits in the prey population.

37. Assertion : Sometimes one population adversely affects the other by direct attack but yet depends upon them.

Reason : In predation the contact is instant.

38. Assertion : Predation is an interspecific interaction with a feeding strategy.

Reason : Predator and their prey maintain fairly stable population through time and rarely one population become abundant or scarce.

39. Assertion : No two species can occupy the same ecological niche in a habitat.

Reason: A habitat can contain only on ecological niche.

40. Assertion: Prolonged intraspecific competition causes an increase in the size of the niche of a population.

Reason: In such a population, use of a new type of resource will increase through the generations.

41. Assertion: Competitive exclusion principle is the tendency for competition to bring about an ecological separation of closely related, or otherwise similar species.

Reason: If two species compete for the same resources, they could avoid competition by choosing different times for feeding or different foraging patterns.

42. Assertion : Interspecific competition is the only potent force in organic evolution.

Reason : Unexceptionally two closely related species competing for the same resources cannot co-exist indefinitely.

43. Assertion: External parasitism is generally marked by much more extreme specialization than internal parasitism.

Reason: The structure of an internal parasite is usually very complex possessing suckers, reproductive organs, etc.

44. Assertion : The relationship between sucker fish and shark is considered to be an example of commensalism.

Reason : Sucker fish gets food and shelter from shark.

45. Assertion : Relationship between sea anemone and hermit crab is said to be an example of obligate mutualism.

Reason: Obligate mutualism is a negative harmful interaction between two species.

46. Assertion: The epiphytes use the trees only for attachment and manufacture their own food by photosynthesis.

Reason: This type of interaction is a type of negative interaction which results in negative effects on the growth and survival of one or both of the populations.

47. Assertion: Mycorrhizae represent a mutually beneficial interspecific interaction of fungi with roots of higher plants.

Reason: In this relationship both the organisms are involved in some sort of physiological exchange.

48. Assertion : In mutualism both the population are benefitted and neither can survive under natural condition without other.

Reason : Both populations are benefitted by the association but their relationships are not obligatory.

Solutions

1. (c) Tropical rain forests have disappeared mainly due to man's activities. Due to over population in countries like India, rain forests are cut to make place available for man to live and build houses. To build buildings and factories man has incessantly cut down trees. This has caused the depletion of rain forests.
2. (b) Flora contains the actual account of habitat and distribution of plants of a given area. It provides the index to the plant species found in particular area.
3. (b) A group of individuals resembling each other in morphological, physiological, biochemical and behavioural characters constitute a species. Such individuals can breed among themselves but cannot breed with members other than their own to produce fertile offsprings. New species are formed mainly due to reproductive isolation.
4. (a) Ernst Mayr proposed the biological species concept, which defines species as groups of actually or potentially inter-breeding natural populations which are reproductively isolated from other such groups.
5. (b) Desert can be cold (e.g., Tibet, Gobi) and hot (e.g., Thar, Sahara). The true desert is a place that has a rainfall of less than 12 cm/yr while in extreme desert is less than 7 cm/yr.
6. (c) The organisms of all the species that live in a particular area and interact in various ways with one another form biotic community. Biotic community is a grouping that is higher than population. It is an assemblage of all the populations of different organisms occurring in an area. The different populations of a community do not remain isolated. They show interactions and inter-dependence.
7. (a) Soils of Indo-Gangetic plains and the Indus valley are highly fertile and suitable for agriculture, so these areas have high population density. Favourable climate increases population density of a geographical area because it favours increase in population growth. High soil fertility favours population density.
8. (d) Living organisms are regarded as open system as they can gain or loose energy from external environment. All living organisms restore their energy either directly from sunlight or indirectly from food.
9. (b) Organisms occupying similar ecological niches but living in different regions are called ecological equivalents. Ecological equivalents possess similar types of adaptations but belong to different taxonomic groups. For example; succulents of American deserts are cacti while those of African desert are euphorbias.
10. (d) Plants have special traits that help them to enlarge their tolerance limits to light regimes. Heliophytes are the sun adapted plants which are adapted to high intensity of light, and have higher temperature optima for photosynthesis, as well as have high rate of respiration. On the other hand, shade adapted plants also called as sciophytes generally have low photosynthetic, respiratory and metabolic activities. Plants such as ferns and several herbaceous plants growing on the ground under the dense canopy of trees, are shade tolerant plants.
11. (a) Leaf butterfly is green in colour and stick insect also mimics in order to escape from the enemies and also to catch prey. The camouflaging mechanism helps the organism to get adapted to its surroundings. The Leaf butterfly is seen more near the leaves while the stick insect camouflages with its surroundings by living on the branches.
12. (a) Animals blend with the surroundings or back ground to remain unnoticed for

protection and aggression.

13. **(a)** Disease resistant plants possess thick cuticle. Infectious organisms can not grow or invade cuticle.

14. **(a)** In *Daphnia* the cyclomorphosis (cyclic change in morphology) is seen. The morphology depends upon the temperature variation in water. So at different seasons of the year the *Daphnia* shows different morphology.

15. **(a)** The introduction and spread of exotic plant and animal species in Australia has impacted on the environment, native biodiversity and local communities, transforming the landscape. The most widespread invasive weed in Queensland was a group of cactus species from the Americas, collectively known as prickly pear.

16. **(b)** Pollination is the act of transferring pollen grains from the male anther of a flower to the female stigma. The goal of every living organism, including plants, is to create offspring for the next generation. Flowers must rely on vectors to move pollen. These vectors can include wind, water, birds, insects, butterflies, bats, and other animals that visit flowers called "pollinators". However, in general, plants that rely on pollen vectors tend to be adapted to their particular type of vector, for example day-pollinated species tend to be brightly coloured, but if they are pollinated largely by birds or specialist mammals, they tend to be larger and have larger nectar rewards than species that are strictly insect-pollinated.

17. **(a)** The aquatic organisms in which the osmotic concentration and temperature of body change according to the ambient conditions of water are called conformers.About 99 percent of animals and nearly all plants are included in the category of conformers, which do not have a mechanism to maintain a constant internal body environment. Their body temperature changes with the surrounding temperature. Some organisms (*e.g.,* birds and mammals) on the other hand, are able to maintain a constant body temperature and constant osmotic concentration despite changes in the external environment. They are called as regulators. They perform homeostasis mostly through thermoregulation and osmoregulation by physiological or behavioural means.

18. **(a)** Thermoregulation is an energetically expensive process for many organisms. Heat loss or heat gain is a function of surface area. Small sized animals (such as shrews, humming birds etc.), have a larger surface area relative to their volume, they tend to lose body heat very fast when it is cold outside; thus they have to expand much energy to generate body heat through metabolism. This is the main reason why very small animals are rarely found in polar regions.

19. **(b)** An ecotone is a transition between two or more diverse communities as, for example, between forest and grassland or between a soft bottom and hard bottom marine community. It is a junction zone or tension belt which may have considerable linear extent but is narrower than the adjoining community areas themselves. The ecotonal community commonly contains many of the organisms of each of the overlapping communities and, in addition, organisms which are characteristic of and often restricted to the ecotone. Often, both the number of species and the population density of some of the species are greater in the ecotone than in the communities flanking it. The tendency for increased variety and density at community junctions is known as the edge effect.

20. **(b)** In deep water bodies, variations in temperature of water at different depths result in thermal stratification. There are three thermal strata -Epilimnion (upper stratum of water), Metalimnion (middle stratum of water) and the Hypolimnion (lower stratum of water). During summer, temperature of the surface water is higher and is separated from the cooler hypolimnion zone by a thermocline. During winter season, temperature of surface water

is at freezing temperature in the temperate lake whereas hypolimnion stratum of the lake has a temperature of about 4°(, In temperate lakes, cooling of surface water during autumn and warming of it during spring results in circulation of nutrients as well as oxygen twice a year.

21. (a) Coral reefs are abundantly found in the regions of Tamil Nadu and the East coast of India. It is because these areas provide the suitable conditions required for colonization of corals such as low siltation, low fresh water inflow by rivers, high salinity and optimal temperature.

22. (a) Plants which remain permanently immersed in water are called hydrophytes. They may be submerged or partly submerged and show the presence of aerenchyma (large air space) in the leaves and petioles. Aerenchyma helps to transport oxygen produced during photosynthesis and permits its free diffusion to other parts, including roots located in anaerobic soils. These tissues also impart buoyancy to the plants. Presence of inflated petioles in Eichhornia (water hyacinth) keeps the plants floating on the surface of water.

23. (a) Mangroves are found in marshy conditions of tropical deltas and along ocean edges. For coping with conditions of high salt concentration and osmotic potential, many mangrove plants have high levels of organic solutes, such as proline and sorbitol. Dunaliella species (green and halophytic algae found in hyper saline lakes) can tolerate saline conditions by accumulating glycerol in the cells, which helps in osmoregulation. Some species of mangroves can excrete salts through the salt glands on the leaves. Some mangroves can exclude salts from the roots by pumping excess of salts back into soil.

24. (a) True xerophytes are the non-succulent perennials which suffer dryness externally as well as internally, e.g., *Calotropis*, *Acacia*, *Zizyphus*, *Nerium*, etc. These possess thick, waxy cuticle, multilayered epidermis and well developed mechanical tissue etc.

25. (c) The aquatic plant Water hyacinth (Eicchornia) is one of the most invasive weeds found growing wherever there is standing water. It drains oxygen from the water, which leads to death of fishes. This plant was introduced in India because of its beautiful flowers and shape of leaves.

26. (c) The rate at which a population can be expected to grow in the future can be assessed graphically by means of a population pyramid-a bar graph displaying the numbers of people in each age category. Males are conventionally shown to the left of the vertical age axis and females to the right. A human population pyramid thus displays the age composition of a population by sex. In general, rectangular pyramids are characteristic of countries whose populations are stable, their numbers neither growing nor shrinking. A triangular pyramid is characteristic of a country that will exhibit rapid future growth, as most of its population has not yet entered the child-bearing years. Inverted triangles are characteristic of populations that is shrinking.

27. (b) A population growing in a habitat with limited resources shows initially a lag phase, followed by phases of acceleration and deceleration and finally an asymptote, when the population density reaches the carrying capacity. A plot of population density (N) in relation to time (t) results in a sigmoid curve. This type of population growth is called Verhulst-Pearl logistic growth and is described by the following equation:

$$\frac{dN}{dt} = rN\left(\frac{K-N}{K}\right)$$

Where N = Population density at time t
r = Intrinsic rate of natural increase
and K = Carrying capacity.

28. (c) In a bell-shaped age pyramid, the number of pre-reproductive and reproductive individuals is almost equal. Post-reproductive individuals are comparatively fewer. It represents a stable population.

29. (c) In sigmoid growth curve, finally, growth rate becomes stable because mortality and natality rates become equal to each other and finally the population shows zero growth rate as birth rate equals death rate.

30. (a) The inherent maximum capacity of an organism to reproduce or increase in number is termed biotic potential (designated by the symbol r). Biotic potential is realised only when the environmental conditions are non-limiting, so that natality rate (birth-rate) is maximum and mortality rate (death -rate) is minimum. Under these conditions, population size increases at the maximum rate. However, nature keeps a check on the expression of biotic potential. For example, if a pair of flies is allowed to reproduce unchecked, the fly population may outweigh the earth in a few years. The environmental check on population size, or its biotic potential is called environmental resistance. With increase in population size, the environmental resistance (against the population) tends to increase.

31. (d) Only one or few species in a community are in sufficient abundance (having high density) to dominate and influence other species in terms of numbers and biomass production. Such species are called dominant species. But there are other species which have much greater influence on community characteristics, relative to their low abundance or biomass. Such species are called keystone species. These species play a vital role in controlling the relative abundance of other species. Removal of keystone species causes serious disruption in the functioning of the community.

32. (b) Kerala has a six ratio of 1058 Indian population is growing with 1.2% animal change.

33. (c) Human interference has not led to constancy in the size of the natural population.

34. (d) Plant-animal interactions often involve co-evolution of the mutualists, that is, the evolution of the flower and its pollinator species are closely linked with one another. This is because plants need the help of animals for pollinating their flowers and dispersing their seeds. Animals get rewards in the form of pollen and, nectar for pollinators and juicy and nutritious fruits for seed dispersers.

35. (a) Predation is an interspecific interaction with a feeding strategy *i.e.*, one species (prey) is eaten up by another (predator). The number of predator usually depends upon the population of prey, but the later is also controlled by predators. Thus, predatory and the prey maintains fairly stable population through time and rarely one population becomes abundant or scarce.

36. (a) If predators kill only the old, sick, and young prey animals, then there would be no evolution of antipredatory traits in the prey population. The most conspicuous traits of prey animals are anti predatory traits. Sensory capacities, body size, running speed, pattern of flight, camouflage, startle behaviour, poisonous body fluids, and mimicry are all traits that help a prey evade its predator. There are strong evidences that predators take not only the old, sick, and young, but also healthy individuals that, because of gene-based traits, are more easily captured than others in the population.

37. (a) In an ecosystem, predation is a biological interaction where a predator (an organism that is hunting) feeds on its prey (the organism that is attacked).

38. (a) Predation is an interspecific interaction with feeding strategy. The number of predator usually depends upon the population of prey, but later is also controlled by predators.

39. (c) The place where an organism lives is called its habitat. Habitats are characterised by conspicuous physical features, which may include the dominant forms of plant and animal life. Habitat may also refer to the place occupied by an entire biological community. For example, a large number of

species are found in a forest habitat. On the other hand, the ecological niche of an organism represents (i) the range of conditions it can tolerate (ii) the resources it utilises, and (iii) its functional role in the ecological system. A habitat can contain many ecological niches and support a variety of species. Each species has a distinct niche, and no two species are believed to occupy exactly the same niche.

40. (a) Prolonged intraspecific competition causes an increase in the size of the niche of a population. A population at its carrying capacity does not have enough of the limiting resources to go around, and any individual who makes use of a new type of resource will experience less competition and would be able to produce more offsprings. Use of the new resources will increase through the generations and the niche thus will become larger.

41. (b) The tendency for competition to bring about an ecological separation of closely related, or otherwise similar species is known as the competitive exclusion principle (Hardin, 1960).This phenomenon is also called as Gause's principle. Thus, Gause's 'Competitive Exclusion Principle' states that two closely related species competing for the same resources cannot co-exist indefinitely and the competitively inferior one is eliminated eventually. This may be true if resources are limiting, but not otherwise. Mechanism of 'Resource partitioning' states that if two species compete for the same resource, they could avoid competition by choosing, for instance, different times for feeding or different foraging patterns.

42. (d) Darwin was convinced that interspecific competition is a potent force in organic evolution. It is generally believed that competition occurs when closely related species compete for the same resources that are limiting, but it is not entirely true. Totally unrelated species could also compete for the same resource. Gause's Competitive Exclusion Principle states that two closely related species competing for the same resources cannot co-exist indefinitely and the competitively inferior one will be eliminated eventually. This may be true if resources are limiting. but not otherwise.

43. (d) Internal parasitism is generally marked by much more extreme specialization than external parasitism, as shown by many protists and invertebrate parasites that infect humans. The more closely the life of the parasite is linked with that of its host, the more its morphology and behaviour are likely to have been modified during the course of its evolution. Conditions within the body of an organism are different from those encountered outside and are apt to be much more constant. Consequently, the structure of an internal parasite is often simplified, and unnecessary ornaments and structures are lost as it evolves.

44. (a) The relationship between sucker fish and shark is an example of commensalism and not parasitism. Commensalism is a positive beneficial interaction between two species where one species is benefitted, while the other neither gets any benefit, nor is adversely affected under normal conditions. Some organisms live inside or outside the bodies of larger animals in order to protect themselves from the enemies and adverse environment. The sucker fish attaches to shark surface with the help of its dorsal fin, which is modified into a holdfast. The sucker fish is dispersed to distant areas with better food supply. Besides, the fish gets protection from predators due to its association with shark. However, the shark does not get any benefit from sucker fish and it is also not affected adversely.

45. (d) The interactions between populations of species in community are broadly categorised into positive (beneficial) and negative (inhibitory) interactions, depending upon the nature of effect on the interacting organisms. An association of two species, in which both species are benefitted, is called mutualism. Mutualism is a functional association, not merely living together. Mutualism may be obligate in which species are completely dependent upon each other, for example, in the case of coral reef, coelentrates and algae live in obligate relationship, or mutualism can be facultative in which one species may survive even in the absence of the other partner species. The relationship between sea anemone and hermit carb is an example of facultative mutualism. The sea anemone grows on the back of the crab, providing camouflage and protection (the sea anemone has stinging cells) and, in turn, the sea anemone is transported about reaching new food sources. This type of mutualism is also called protocooperation.

46. (c) Epiphytes which grow on the branches and in the forks of some trees, cite an example of commensalism. Commensalism is a type of positive interaction in which, two organisms (of different species) live together without any physiological dependence between them, and one gets the benefit from the association while the other is neither benefitted nor harmed.

47. (a) Mycorrhizae is the symbiotic association of fungal hyphae with the roots of higher plants. In this association, the two symbionts are in close contact and are physiologically interdependent on each other. Mycorrhizae increase the ability of the plant to extract minerals from the soil. In return, fungi are provided with shelter and photosynthate by the plant. Plants having such associations show other benefits also, such as resistance to root-borne pathogens, tolerance to salinity and drought, and an overall increase in plant growth and development.

48. (c) Mutualism is the way two organisms of different species exist in a relationship in which each individual benefits from the activity of the other.

Chapter 36

Ecosystem

Directions: In the following questions, a statement of assertion is followed by a statement of reason. Mark the correct choice as:

(a) If both Assertion and Reason are true and Reason is the correct explanation of Assertion.
(b) If both Assertion and Reason are true but Reason is not the correct explanation of Assertion.
(c) If Assertion is true but Reason is false.
(d) If both Assertion and Reason are false.

1. **Assertion :** Net primary productivity is gross primary productivity minus respiration.
Reason : Secondary productivity is produced by heterotrophs.

2. **Assertion:** Despite occupying about 70% of the earth's surface. Oceans are a low productivity ecosystems.
Reason: In aquatic ecosystems, productivity is limited by light that decreases with increasing water depth.

3. **Assertion:** During the *process* of *photosynthesis* amount of organic matter synthesized by producers per unit time and per unit area is referred to as net primary productivity.
Reason: Due to abundance of sunlight. Primary productivity is usually high and sustained throughout the year in temperate areas.

4. **Assertion :** Primary productivity is shown by green plants only.
Reason : Primary productivity is also shown by chemosynthesizers.

5. **Assertion :** Biotic and abiotic components constitute ecosystem.
Reason : Change in living forms will affect non-living things.

6. **Assertion :** There is no loss of water by transpiration below the forest canopy.
Reason : Forest canopy is exposed to sunlight and wind fury and acts as effective wind and light barrier.

7. **Assertion :** The flora of Tundra consists of lichens, mosses and conifers.
Reason : Temperature and water supply to plants are limiting factors.

8. **Assertion :** The collective ecosystem of plants and animals is called biome.
Reason : Coral reefs have richest biomes.

9. **Assertion :** Ecosystem can be defined as the community of organism together with the environment in which they live.
Reason : It includes both biotic and abiotic factors.

10. **Assertion :** Bacteria and fungi are micro consumers.
Reason : Bacteria and fungi consume only a little part of living plants and animals.

11. **Assertion :** A light is the energy which is stored as chemical energy in the form of food during photosynthesis.
Reason : Light also influences various other activities of the organism as photoperiodism, etc.

12. **Assertion :** Food web consists of several food chains.
Reason : Food web decreases the stability of an ecosystem.

13. **Assertion :** The conversion of productivity at next trophic level is 10%.
Reason : Energy is lost in the respiration process.

14. **Assertion :** Biomes are the major ecosystem of the world.
Reason : Tundra is an example of biome.

15. **Assertion :** Chaparral is also called "shrub forest".
Reason : Trees are totally absent in chaparral.

16. **Assertion :** Coral reefs are equivalent to tropic rain forest.
Reason : Maximum diversity of biota occurs in the reefs.

17. **Assertion :** Tropical rain forests are disappearing fast from developing countries such as India.

Reason : No value is attached to these forests because these are poor in biodiversity.

18. **Assertion :** In a food chain members of successive higher levels are fewer in number.

Reason : Number of organisms at any trophic level depends upon the availability of organisms which serve as food at the lower level.

19. **Assertion :** A network of food chains existing together in an ecosystem is known as food web.

Reason : An animal like kite cannot be a part of a food web. **[AIIMS 2006, 2008]**

20. **Assertion :** Pyramid of energy may be upright or inverted.

Reason: Only 20% of energy goes to next trophic level. **[AIIMS 2011]**

21. **Assertion:** Ecological pyramids are also known as Eltonian pyramids.

Reason: An ecological pyramid is always upright.

22. **Assertion:** The important climatic factors that regulate the process of decomposition are temperature and soil moisture.

Reason: Warm and moist environments favour decomposition whereas low temperature and anaerobiosis inhibit decomposition.

23. **Assertion:** The consequence of the second law of thermodynamics is the loss of biologically useful energy as heat with *every* energy transfer in a food chain

Reason: Energy does not permanently remain trapped in any organism, it is either passed on to a higher trophic *level* or becomes available to detrivores and decomposers after the organism dies.

24. **Assertion:** In a marine aquatic ecosystem, at any given time, the biomass of phytoplanktons (producers) is lower than the biomass of zooplanktons (primary consumers).

Reason: Phytoplanktons are consumed almost as rapidly as they are formed and thus have shorter life spans.

25. **Assertion:** As compared to terrestrial herbivores. aquatic *herbivores* are usually more productive.

Reason: Because of their smaller size and lack of structural tissues, the phytoplanktons_achieve faster growth rates and are more nutritious to heterotrophs than their terrestrial counterparts.

26. **Assertion:** The number of species increases, the community biomass increases and the community's ratio of respiration to photosynthesis also increases. During an ecological succession.

Reason: The rate of photosynthesis of a community is almost equal to the rate of respiration, respiration, at climax community of an ecological succession.

27. **Assertion:** Herbivores are also known as key industry animals because they convert plant matter into animal matter.

Reason: In an ecosystem decomposers play a vital role and they indirectly support the producers.

28. **Assertion:** An interaction between biotic and abiotic components is an ecosystem.

Reason: The term ecosystem is coined by AG Tansley.

29. **Assertion:** Microconsumers are microscopic organism such-as bacteria and fungi.

Reason: Bacteria and fungi are a very little part of living plants and animals.

30. **Assertion:** Herbivores are also known as first order consumers.

Reason: Directly from plants herbivores obtain their food.

31. **Assertion:** The pyramid of energy is always upright.

Reason: Maximum number of autotrophs is present in the pyramid of energy.

32. **Assertion:** Pond ecosystem is upright in the pyramid of number.

Reason: Phytoplanktons are maximum and secondary consumers are lesser in number.

33. **Assertion:** A food web is a network of food chains existing together in an ecosystem.

Reason: An animal like kite cannot be a part of a food web.

34. **Assertion :** Green plants only show primary productivity.

Reason : Chemosynthesizers are responsible for primary productivity also.

35. **Assertion** : Primary consumers are plant eating animals.
Reason : Micro consumers break down the dead protoplasm into simpler ones. They are last in the sequence of a food chain.

36. **Assertion** : The example of primary consumers includes herbivores.
Reason : The driving force of any ecosystem is its producers.

37. **Assertion** : The pyramid of biomass indicates the decrease in biomass at each trophic level from base to apex.
Reason : Parasites have inverted pyramid for biomass.

38. **Assertion** : The excess of organic matter is stored by green plants for the utilization by the herbivores.
Reason : Work energy put by man in agriculture is used in the ecosystem.

39. **Assertion** : Trophic levels are only observed in the plant and animal kingdom.
Reason : Food chains and webs are formed due to linked organisms on the basis of their nutrition.

40. **Assertion** : The pyramid of energy is always upright.
Reason : Number of autotrophs in the pyramid of energy are maximum.

41. **Assertion** : The pyramid of number of pond ecosystem is upright.
Reason : Phytoplanktons are maximum and secondary consumers are least in number.

42. **Assertion** : A big fish eats small fish which eats water fleas and water fleas in turn eat phytoplanktons. In this chain, water fleas are primary consumers.
Reason : Secondary consumers will be phytoplanktons.

43. **Assertion** : Maximum contribution of oxygen is from phytoplankton.
Reason : 90% of the photosynthesis with oxygen evolution is contributed by them.

44. **Assertion** : A lake can undergo ecological succession and become a forest over time.
Reason : A bare rock can become a forest through ecological succession.

45. **Assertion** : Oceans acts as a global sink for CO_2.
Reason : Human activities are increasing CO_2 concentration in the air.

46. **Assertion** : Every biological system resists a change and wants to remain in state of equilibrium.
Reason : Climax communities of an ecosystem are produced after several changes it has under gone through succession.

47. **Assertion:** The nitrification process involves the decomposition of proteins of dead plants and animals, and nitrogenous wastes like urea, uric acid etc. of animals to ammonia.
Reason: Nitrification is carried out by putrefying bacteria for example *Bacillus ramosus, B. vulgaris,* etc.

48. **Assertion:** Phosphorus cycle is an imperfect cycle as a sufficient amount of phosphorus combines with Al^{3+}, Fe^{2+} and Ca^{2+} to form insoluble and unavailable salts.
Reason: Phosphate circulates in abiotic environment in both lithosphere and in atmosphere.

49. **Assertion:** With time ecological succession can turn a lake into a dryland forest.
Reason: Through ecological succession a bare rock can become a forest.

50. **Assertion:** The cycling of glucose or reserved food material within the plant body is nutrient cycle.
Reason: Biogeochemical cycle is transfer of biogenetic nutrients between living and non-living components.

51. **Assertion:** Primary succession takes place over a primarily bare area where there was no *living* matter from *the very* beginning.
Reason: Reproductive structures of the previous occupants give rise to a new seral community as soon as the conditions become favourable, during primary succession.

52. **Assertion:** In a lithosere, crustose lichens, secrete organic acids causing weathering of rocks so that minerals essential for proper growth of lichens are released.
Reason: In a primary succession early colonists are usually lichens, which suggests that colonization is easier when an organism has a mutualistic association.

53. **Assertion:** Secondary succession always involves a predictable species sequence and ends up with the same climax community as existed prior to the disturbance.
Reason: A pond never be considered as a self-sustained ecosystem as it lacks all the structural and functional components that work as a unit in an ecosystem.
54. **Assertion:** Mosses and lichens are said to form the pioneer community in xerarch succession.
Reason: It is because during the course of succession these species get established later.
55. **Assertion:** The recycling of carbon is essentially a self regulating feedback system in nature.
Reason: In the atmosphere the reservoir pool of carbon consists of free CO_2.
56. **Assertion:** Nitrogen is an important structural and functional constituent of living protoplasm.
Reason : Plants and animals mostly depend upon atmospheric nitrogen.
57. **Assertion :** Hydrological cycle is a perfect one.
Reason : The cycling of water is a fast process.
58. **Assertion :** Gaseous cycle is faster than the cycle of matter.
Reason : Sedimentary cycles are very slow.
59. **Assertion:** Sedimentary nutrient cycles of phosphorus, calcium, magnesium etc. are considered as imperfect cycles.
Reason: These cycles caused by local disturbances get more easily disrupted as the bulk of material remains in the relatively inactive and immobile reservoir on the earth's crust.
60. **Assertion:** Between hypolimnion and epilimnion thermocline exists.
Reason: Between the two layers. Thermocline acts as a barrier.
61. **Assertion:** Insectivorous habitat of plants is to cope up N_2 deficiency.
Reason: Insectivorous plants are partly autotrophic and partly heterotrophic.
[AIIMS 1998]
62. **Assertion** : A biotic community has higher position than population in ecological hierarchy.
Reason : Population of similar individuals remains isolated in the community.
[AIIMS 2012]
63. **Assertion :** Ecotone shows more diversity.
Reason : Ecotone is a sharp transition zone between two or more diverse communities.
64. **Assertion** : Phosphorus cycle does not involve microorganisms.
Reason : Microorganisms are mainly associated with nitrogen cycle.
65. **Assertion** : Biogeochemical cycling means cycling of nutrients in an ecosystem.
Reason : Decomposers play a major role in biogeochemical cycling.

Solutions

1. (b) Net primary productivity is the rate of organic matter built up or stored by producers in their bodies per unit time and area. Net productivity is equal to gross primary productivity minus loss due to respiration and other reasons. Rate of increase in energy containing organic matter or biomass by heterotrophs or consumers per unit time and area is known as secondary productivity.
2. (a) Ecosystem productivity levels of an depends upon plant species inhabiting a particular area, their photosynthetic capacity, sunlight, moisture, availability of nutrients, and a variety of other environmental factors. The annual net primary productivity of the whole biosphere is approx. 170 billion tons (dry weight) of organic matter. Of this, despite occupying about 90% of earth's surface, oceans contribute only 32% of the total productivity (55 billion tons out of 170 billion tons). Thus, oceans are low productivity ecosystems.
3. (d) Gross primary productivity (GPP) is the total amount of organic matter synthesized by producers per unit time and per unit area in the process of photosynthesis, in tropical areas primary productivity is high and sustained throughout the year while it is limited in temperate areas by cold climate and small growing period. Maximum sunlight is available in tropics whereas poles receive minimum sunlight. Because of this, photo synthesis is maximum and net primary productivity (NPP) is highest (>20 t $ha^{-1} year^{-1}$) in tropics against average (8 t ha^{-1} $year^{-1}$) in temperate forests.
4. (b) Green plants and chemosynthesizers act as producers.
5. (a) An ecosystem includes all of the living things (plants, animals and organisms) in a given area, interacting with each other, and also with their non-living environments (weather, earth, sun, soil, climate, atmosphere).
6. (a) In forest ecology, canopy also refers to the upper layer or habitat zone, formed by mature tree crowns and including other biological organisms (epiphytes, lianas, arboreal animals, etc.). The canopy layer provides protection from strong winds and storms, while also intercepting sunlight and precipitation, leading to a relatively sparsely vegetated understory layer.
7. (a) In physical geography, tundra is a type of biome where the tree growth is hindered by low temperatures and short growing seasons. In tundra, the vegetation is composed of dwarf shrubs, sedges and grasses, mosses, and lichens.
8. (b) Biomes are very large ecological areas on the earth's surface, with fauna and flora (animals and plants) adapting to their environment. The largest coral reef biome in the world is found in the Northeast of Australia. It is called the Great Barrier Reef.
9. (a) An ecosystem is a community of living organisms in conjunction with the nonliving components of their environment (things like air, water and mineral soil), interacting as a system. These biotic and abiotic components are regarded as linked together through nutrient cycles and energy flows.
10. (c) Microconsumers are microscopic organisms such as bacteria and fungi. These microorganisms breakdown the complex organic compounds of dead bodies of both plants and animals and absorb some of the decomposed products, while release most of inorganic compounds into the environment. From there, these are used by the plants. These are biotic components of an ecosystem.
11. (b) Photosynthesis is the process by which green plants and some other organisms use sunlight to synthesize nutrients from carbon dioxide and water. Photoperiodism refers to the response of plants to the lengths of dark and light periods. Many

angiosperms, or flowering plants, have a protein that can sense seasonal changes in light. A plant will flower depending on these changes in light levels.

12. (c) Food web is a network of food chains which become interconnected at various trophic levels so as to form a number of feeding connections amongst the different organisms of a biotic community. Food web is meant for increasing the stability of an ecosystem by providing alternate source of food and allowing the endangered population to grow in size.

13. (a) Ten percent law put forth by Lindemann states that while transferring organic food from one trophic level to the next, about ten percent of the organic matter is stored as flesh, the remaining is lost during transfer or broken down in respiration. The net productivity of the next higher trophic level shall be 10% of the first one.

14. (b) A biome is defined as a large natural ecosystem which is distinct in its climate conditions and has its specific type of plant and animal life. Biomes are two types - terrestrial and aquatic. The major terrestrial biomes are - tundra, taiga, deciduous forest, tropical rain forest, chaparral, tropical savannah, grassland and desert.

15. (c) Chaparral is a broad - leaved evergreen shrub forest of hard and thick leaved small trees and shrubs which usually contain resin but are resistant to fires.

16. (a) Coral reefs are the specialized ecosystem of ocean which are among the most productive of all ecosystem anywhere, with a diversity equalled only by tropical rainforest. The amount of oxygen is very high. During the day it may reach 250 percent of saturation because of the production of O_2 by algae in the reef structure. The productivity of reefs is also caused by quickly and efficient running of nutrients cycle between the components of reef ecosystem. No organic matter is incorporated permanently into the sedimentary portion of reef. The condition of rapid nutrient cycling allow a mechanism by which the natural paucity of nutrients in the ocean can be effectively circumvented. All these conditions favour the high biodiversity in coral reef.

17. (c) Tropical rain forests are located in the equatorial regions where the annual rainfall exceeds 140 cm. They are also called jungles and cover one twelveth of earth's surface but contain more than half of the earths flora and fauna (*i.e.*, rich in biodiversity). Now-a-days these forests are disappearing due to excessive use in domestic purposes like fuel, furnitures, accomodations, cloths, resin, gum, etc.

18. (a) Each food chain contains many levels like producers, herbivores, primary carnivores and so on. Each step of the food chain is called trophic level. Number of organisms at any trophic level depends upon the availability of food. In grassland ecosystem the maximum number of organisms are found in lower trophic level but in forest ecosystem and parasitic food chain it is reverse.

19. (c) In the food web, different food chains are interconnected. Each chain is interconnected and consists of different trophic levels i.e. producers, consumers and detrivores. So, kite can also be a part of food web.

20. (d) Energy flow in the ecosystem is in a unidirectional manner. There is a decline in the amount of energy passing from one trophic level to the next. Thus the pyramid of energy is always upright. According to Lindemann, only 10% of energy goes to the next trophic level.

21. (c) Ecological pyramids were developed by Charles Elton and are, therefore, also known as Eltonian pyramids. Tehy can be upright, inverted or spindle shaped depending upon criteria of formation of pyramid(like energy, biomass or number) and the type of food chain involved: parasitic, aquatic or terrestrial.

22. (b) Decomposition is largely an oxygen-requiring process. Chemicals control the rate of decomposition. The most important climatic factors are temperature and soil moisture that regulate decomposition through their effects on the activities of soil microbes. Warm and moist environments favour decomposition whereas low temperature and anaerobiosis (due to excessive moisture) inhibit decomposition that results in the build up of organic materials.

23. (b) According to second law of thermodynamics, every activity involving energy transformation is accompanied by dissipation of energy. In other words, the consequence of the second law of thermodynamics is the loss of biologically useful energy as heat with every energy transfer in a food chain. Every time energy is transferred from one place to another some of it is converted into heat. An organism transfers chemical energy from glucose or fatty acids to ATP (cellular respiration) and then to the chemical bonds of new molecules (during molecular synthesis), and transforms chemical energy into motion during active transport, muscle contractions, and a variety of other activities, that are essential to life. Energy does not permanently remain trapped in any organism. It is either passed on to the higher trophic level or becomes available to detrivores and decomposers after the organism dies. Death of organism is the beginning of the detritus food chain/web.

24. (a) In a marine aquatic ecosystem, the biomass of zooplanktons (primary consumers) is larger than that of phytoplanktons (producers) and the biomass of zooplanktons is smaller than that of secondary consumers. This forms inverted pyramid of biomass in an aquatic ecosystem. This shape is the consequence of the very short life spans of phytoplanktons, that are consumed almost as rapidly as they are formed.

25. (a) By terrestrial herbivores, most plant material is not consumed or is not digested because plants have so much structural material most algal material (phytoplanktons) is consumed by aquatic herbivores and digested because algae have very little structural material. Moreover, turn over by phytoplanktons is much more rapid than terrestrial plants, so at any given time biomass is low as compared to the productivity. Phytoplanktons grow and reproduce rapidly, so a small mass can have a faster rate of primary production. In contrast, terrestrial primary producers grow and reproduce slowly. Thus, terrestrial herbivores are less productive than aquatic herbivores.

26. (b) The number of species increases, the community biomass increases and the community's ratio of respiration to photosynthesis increases during an ecological succession. At climax, the rate of photosynthesis is almost equal to the rate of respiration.

27. (b) According to Elton (1939), herbivorous animals are key industry animals because they can convert plant matter into animal matter and all other consumers' or higher animals' lives are dependent upon these primary consumers.
Decomposers are also known as transformers. It transforms organic compounds into simple inorganic compounds. Saprophytic fungi and bacteria belong to this category. They act upon dead remains of plants and animals and decomposes them to their elemental stage. These in turn can be used by producers for their growth and photosynthetic activity. In this way, decomposers indirectly support the producers and play a vital role in ecosystem.

28. (b) The term ecosystem was coined by AG Tansley. It is an integrated natural system resulting from the interaction of living and non-living factors of the environment.

29. (c) Microconsumers are microscopic organisms such as bacteria and fungi. These microorganisms breakdown the complex organic compounds of dead remains of both plants and animals and absorb some of the decomposed products, while releasing most of inorganic compounds into the environment. These are biotic components of an ecosystem.

30. (a) This group of organisms are consumers of first order and include the herbivores which directly feed upon green plants (producers).

31. (c) Pyramid of energy is always upright due to unidirectional the flow of energy. All the energy stored by the autotrophs in the form of food is available to the herbivores as food.

32. (a) In the graphical representation pyramid of number shows the arrangement of number of individuals (population size) of different trophic levels in a food chain in an ecosystem.

The pyramid of pond ecosystem is upright, because the base of this pyramid is occupied by the maximum number of phytoplanktons (autotrophs) and number of individuals gradually decreases towards the primary and secondary consumers side respectively.

33. (c) A food chain is a linear sequence of organisms through which nutrients and energy pass as one organism eats another. In a food chain, each organism occupies a different trophic level, defined.

34. (b) In ecology, productivity refers to the rate of generation of biomass in an ecosystem. Primary productivity is the rate at which energy is converted by photosynthetic and chemosynthetic autotrophs to organic substances.

35. (c) Plants and algae make their own food and are called producers. Level 2: Herbivores eat plants and are called primary consumers. Micro-consumers, mainly bacteria and fungi, which feed by breaking down complex organic compounds in dead protoplasm, absorbing some of the decomposition products, and at the same time releasing inorganic and relatively simple organic substances to the environment.

36. (b) Herbivores eat plants and are called primary consumers. Producers are organisms that make their own food; they are also known as autotrophs. They are the driving force of any ecosystem.

37. (b) The Pyramid of Biomass is a graphical representation that depicts the extent of biomass per unit area within different trophic levels in an ecological system. The primary producers will lie at the bottom of the biomass pyramid.

38. (b) Man power utilized in agriculture is used in the ecosystem. When herbivores eat the plants, they acquire the carbon stored in plant tissues. Much of the food (carbon compounds) eaten is used up for the herbivore's life processes and given off as carbon dioxide in respiration but some is stored in animal tissues.

39. (b) A trophic level is the group of organisms within an ecosystem which occupy the same level in a food chain. A food web consists of many food chains. A food chain only follows just one path as animals find food. A food web shows the many different paths plants and animals are connected.

40. (c) Pyramid of energy is a graphical representation of amount of energy trapped per unit time and area in different levels of a food chain. Pyramid of energy is always upright because the flow of energy is unidirectional. All of the energy stored by the autotrophs in the form herbivores as food.

Herbivores can store only 10% of this energy in their energy in their biomass and remaining 90% is used by them in metabolic activities. In the same trophic way, only 10% of energy of lower trophic levels can be captured by the organisms of next higher trophic level. This, this pyramid depends upon energy and not the number of individuals, in a trophic level.

41. (a) Pyramid of number is the graphical representation showing the arrangement of number individuals (population size) of different trophic levels in a food chain in an ecosystem. The pyramid of number in a pond ecosystem is upright because base of this pyramid is occupied by the maximum number of phytoplanktons (autotrophs) and number of individuals gradually decreases towards the primary and secondary consumers side respectively.

42. (c) A pond's ecosystem food chain has three basic trophic levels. The first trophic level represents the producer and autotrophs. The second trophic level consists of herbivores, such as insects, crustaceans, and invertebrates that inhabit the pond and consume the plants. The third trophic level comprises of carnivores, such as various sizes of fish, which feed on both the plants and herbivores atop the first and second trophic levels. Saprotrophic organisms, also known as decomposers located on the bottom of the food chain, help decompose dead organic matter.

43. (a) Phytoplanktons account for almost half of the photosynthetic activity on earth. Thus they are responsible for maximum (about 90%) of the oxygen present on the earth while the rest is because of the other plants.

44. (b) Ecological succession means the natural development of a series of biotic communities, one after the other, in some area till a permanent climax community is established. A lake can become a dryland forest through ecological succession. Ecological succession can turn a bare rock into a forest with time.

45. (b) Carbon dioxide is almost certainly being absorbed by the oceans, which acts as a global 'sink' for CO_2, It is not clear how much more CO_2 the ocean can hold. Human activities like deforestation massive burning of fossil fuel for energy and transport has caused an increase in the amount of CO_2 in atmosphere.

46. (b) In ecology, climax community, or climatic climax community, is a historic term for a biological community of plants, animals, and fungi which, through the process of ecological succession in the development of vegetation in an area over time, have reached a steady state.

47. (d) The decomposition process of proteins of dead plants and animals, and nitrogenous wastes like urea, uric acid etc., of animals to ammonia is referred to as ammonification. Ammonification is a part of nitrogen cycle and it is carried out by decay causing organisms, that act upon nitrogenous excretions and proteins of dead bodies of living organisms *e.g., Bacillus ramosus, B. vulgaris, B. mesentericus* etc. Proteins are first broken down into amino acids, the latter are deaminated, for their own metabolism. Organic acids released in the process are used by microorganisms.

$$\text{Proteins} \xrightarrow{+H_2O} \underset{\text{Amino acid}}{R-NH_3} \xrightarrow{H_2O} \underset{\text{Organic acid}}{ROH} + \underset{\text{Ammonia}}{NH_3}$$

48. (c) Phosphorus cycle is an example of sedimentary cycle. In the world greatest reservoir of phosphate is relatively insoluble ferric and calcium phosphate in rocks. Cyclic pool is soil for terrestrial ecosystems (lithosphere) and water for aquatic ecosystems (hydrosphere). Phosphate circulates in the abiotic environment in both lithosphere and hydrosphere. Atmosphere or gaseous cycle is absent. Inside soil through leaching. some phosphorus is lost Similarly, a sufficient amount of phosphorus combines with calcium, iron or aluminium and becomes insoluble. It settles down at the bottom of lake or ocean as sediment. Bone and teeth may also remain undegraded. Such phosphorus becomes part of lithosphere. After a very long interval it is released when the rocks containing them are exposed to weathering agencies or are mined. Thus, phosphorus cycle is an imperfect cycle.

49. (b) Natural development of biotic communities, one after the other, in some area till a permanent climax community is establ ished is ecological succession. A lake can become a dryland forest through ecological succesion. Ecological succession can tum a bare rock into a forest with time.

50. (d) Recycling of biogenetic nutrients through abiotic and biotic components of an ecosystem is called biogeochemical cycle or nutrient cycle.

51. (c) The biotic succession that occurs on a previously sterile or primarily bare area is primary succession. Newly exposed sea floor, igneous rocks, sand dunes, new cooled lava sediments or newly submerged areas are some of the examples of primary bare area. At the beginning of primary succession soil and humus is absent and reproductive structures of any previous community are absent. Thus, the environment is very hostile for pioneer community and primary succession takes a long time for completion.

52. (b) In a lithosere the pioneer community (biotic succession on bare rock) is constituted by lichens. The pioneer lichens are usually crustose lichens for example *Graphis, Rhizocarpon* etc. Lichens can tolerate desiccation. They produce organic acids that causes weathering of rocks so that minerals essential for proper growth of lichens are released. Lichens hold the fine particles of rock and initiate soil formation, it paves the way for growth of next seral community. Lichens are dual organisms which contain a permanent symbiotic association of a fungus and an alga. Earlier colonization by lichens suggests that colonization is easier when the organism has mutualistic association.

53. (d) Secondary succession does not always involve a predictable species sequence and does not always end up with the same climax community as existed prior to the disturbance. Chance factors may play a role when species not normally a part of the succession happen to colonize, and so alter the normal sequence. If these aberrant species prevent colonization in the normal sequence by later species the process is called 'inhibition'. If they appear in the sequence but have little effect on later colonization, the process is known as 'tolerance'. Succession will not follow a predictable sequence if the climax community was a relict of soil and past climatic conditions. Instead, a new form of community that is more appropriate to the new conditions appear after destruction of the relict community. Similarly, where human activities have modified the climate or soil or have removed potential colonists by destroying adjacent communities, the same climax community may not reappear. All the components of an ecosystem function as a unit with a number of delicately balanced and controlled processes. Pond is a self-sustained ecosystem that is present in a shallow water body. It has all the structural components (biotic and abiotic) that work as a unit and show all the functional aspects of the ecosystem.

54. (c) The plants that invade the base land initially, are called pioneer community. In xerarch succession species, lichens and mosses form the pioneer community. The assemblage of pioneer species forms the pioneer. Lichens form a crust over the base rocks and begin to form soil from their organic remains and by stimulating chemical breakdown of the rocks. Lichens are normally followed by mosses, that speed up the process of soil accumulation by trapping wind blown particles. Mosses grow together with lichens, in bunch, make a mat over the substratum. In this way, lichens and mosses get established on barren rock as pioneer species forming the pioneer community.

55. (c) Biogeochemical cycle of carbon is a gaseous cycle. In the atmosphere, its cycling pool consists of 6×10^{14} kg (29%) of free CO_2 and 1.45×10^{15} kg (71%) of dissolved CO_2 in the oceans. Oceans also regulate the amount of CO_2 in the atmosphere. Reservoir pool of carbon is lithosphere. Lithosphere contains 2.8×10^{21} kg of carbon. Natural exchange between lithosphere and hydrosphere or atmosphere is a very slow process. Major exchange in carbon cycle takes place between organisms and the atmosphere or hydrosphere. This cycling is a self-regulated feed back system but has recently been upset because of rapid deforestation and increasing combustion of fossil fuels.

56. (c) Nitrogen is a component of amino acids, proteins, enzymes, nucleotides and nucleic acids, which form important constituents of living protoplasm. The atmosphere contains approximately 80% nitrogen gas which cannot be directly utilized by most

organisms except certain nitrogen fixers. Animals mostly depend upon the organic nitrogen provided by plants. The inorganic nitrogen picked up by plants is mostly in the form of nitrate and to some extent ammonium ions.

57. **(b)** Unlike most other nutrient or material cycles, the hydrological cycle involves the movement of a chemical compound water. The hydrologic cycle is one of the most nearly perfect cyclical processes. *i.e.*, the cycle rotates in hydrosphere, lithosphere and atmosphere efficiently. The cycling of water in the atmosphere is a fairly rapid process, the average residence time being only about 10 days, but possibly less in the humid tropics.

58. **(b)** Gaseous cycles are quick and take little time to complete beyond the stay of matter in the food chain. Sedimentary cycles are usually very slow. They operate *via* sea food chain or coastal sprays. A still slow process is the formation of rocks and their exposure.

59. **(a)** As compared to sedimentary cycles, gaseous nutrient cycles are rapid and more perfect. It is because in gaseous nutrient cycles, *e.g.*, carbon, hydrogen, oxygen, nitrogen, remains of nutrients in circulation are more or less uniform. In these cycles, nutrients quickly self-adjust because of large reservoir pool (atmosphere or hydrosphere other hand, sedimentary nutrient cycles, *e.g.*, phosphorus, calcium, magnesium are less perfect (or imperfect) as by local disturbances they get more easily disrupted as the bulk of material remains in the relatively inactive reservoir on the earth's crust (lithosphere).

60. **(a)** Epilimnion or the warmer upper part of the lake becomes temporarily isolated from the colder lower water or hypolimnion by a thermocline zone (temperature stratification) which acts as a barrier to exchange of materials. Consequently, the supply of oxygen in the hypolimnion and nutrients in the epilimnion may run short.

61. **(a)** Insectivorous plants are those plants which capture and digest live prey (normally insects) to obtain nitrogen compounds that are lacking in its usual marshy habitat. These plants are partly autotrophic and partly heterotrophic.

62. **(c)** The organisms of all the species that live in a particular area and interact in various ways with one another form biotic community. Biotic community is a grouping that is higher than population in ecological hierarchy. It is an assemblage of all the populations of different organisms occurring in an area. The different populations of a community do not remain isolated. They show interactions and inter-dependence.

63. **(a)** A sharp transition between two or more diverse communities, for example, between forest and grassland, is known as ecotone. The ecotonal community commonly contains many of the organisms of each of the overlapping communities and in addition, organisms are characteristic of and often restricted to ecotone. The tendency for increased variety and density at community junctions is known as the edge effect.

64. **(b)** Phosphorus moves in a cycle through rocks, water, soil and sediments and organisms. Over time, rain and weathering cause rocks to release phosphate ions and other minerals. This inorganic phosphate is then distributed in soils and water. Plants take up inorganic phosphate from the soil. Phosphorous cycle does not involve microorganism.

65. **(a)** Biogeochemical cycle is a pathway by which a chemical substance moves through both the biotic (biosphere) and abiotic (lithosphere, atmosphere, and hydrosphere) components of Earth. Decomposers take the dead and decaying material and break it down (decomposition) so that the components can be recycled through the biogeochemical cycles.

Chapter 37

Biodiversity and its Conservation

Directions: In the following questions, a statement of assertion is followed by a statement of reason. Mark the correct choice as:

(a) If both Assertion and Reason are true and Reason is the correct explanation of Assertion.
(b) If both Assertion and Reason are true but Reason is not the correct explanation of Assertion.
(c) If Assertion is true but Reason is false.
(d) If both Assertion and Reason are false.

1. **Assertion :** Alpha diversity is said· to be higher if the dissimilarity between communities is higher.
Reason : Alpha diversity is a measure of diversity between the communities.

2. **Assertion:** The species diversity present in a given community or habitat is referred to as alpha diversity.
Reason: Alpha diversity is usually expressed by species richness and species evenness in that community habitat.

3. **Assertion :** Diversity observed in the entire geographical area, is called gamma diversity.
Reason : Bio-diversity decreases from high altitude to low altitude.

4. **Assertion :** A biosphere reserve is a specified area.
Reason : No restriction on human activities has been imposed in biosphere reserve.

5. **Assertion :** In tropical rain forests. O-horizon and A-Horizon of soil profile are shallow and nutrient-poor.
Reason : Excessive growth of micro-organisms in the soil depletes its organic content.
[AIIMS 2006]

6. **Assertion:** Communities that comprise of more species tend to be more stable.
Reason: A higher number of species results in less animal variation in total biomass.
[AIIMS 2017]

7. **Assertion:** Community with more species tends to be more stable than those with less species.
Reason: More will be the species, less will be year to year variation in total biomass.

8. **Assertion:** A stable community should not show too much variation in productivity from year to year.
Reason: A stable community must be resistant to invasions by the alien species.

9. **Assertion:** Decrease in species diversity occurs as we ascend a high mountain.
Reason: Decrease in species diversity occurs with increase in altitude due to rise in temperature.

10. **Assertion :** Most common forest type in India is tropical dry deciduous forests.
Reason : They are common in West Bengal.

11. **Assertion :** Tropical latitudes have greater biological diversity then temperate latitudes.
Reason : Tropical regions remain relatively undisturbed for millions of years.

12. **Assertion:** If the species-area relationships are analyzed among very large areas like the entire continents, the value of Z *i.e.,* slope of line lies in the range of 0.1 to 0.2.
Reason: The value of Z *i.e.,* slope of line of species area relationships lies in the range of 0.6 to 1.2 when analysis is done among small areas.

13. **Assertion:** Speciation is a function of time and tropical regions had got a long evolutionary time for species diversification as compared to temperate regions.
Reason: Temperate regions have undergone frequent glaciations in the past whereas tropical regions have remained relatively undisturbed for millions of years.

14. **Assertion:** Taiga is also called North coniferous forest.
Reason: The ground flora is absent in Taiga.

15. **Assertion:** Temperate deciduous forest is two – storeyed forest.
Reason: Two stories are formed of soft wood and hard wood trees.

16. **Assertion:** When the rain forest is removed, grasslands appear.
Reason: In rain forest, nutrient cycling is slow.

17. **Assertion:** Chaparral is also called "shrub forest".
Reason: Trees are totally absent in chaparral.

18. **Assertion:** Savannahs show rich species diversity.
Reason: The biome is prone to fires.

19. **Assertion:** Biomes are the major ecosystem of the world.
Reason: Tundra is an example of biome.

20. **Assertion :** Tropical rain forests are disappearing fast from developing countries such as India.
Reason : No value is attached to these forests because these are poor in biodiversity.
[AIIMS 2012, 2013]

21. **Assertion:** The presently occurring species extinction is different from the earlier mass extinction.
Reason: Present species extinction is due to natural causes, whereas the earlier extinction was due to man made causes.

22. **Assertion:** In case, a species becomes extinct, the plant and animal species associated with it in an obligatory way also become extinct.
Reason: When a host fish species becomes extinct, its unique assemblage of parasites also become extinct.

23. **Assertion:** Over-exploitation of a species reduces the size of its population eventually leading to its extinction.
Reason: Steller's sea cow is a large, herbivorous, terrestrial mammal which is on the verge of extinction due to over exploitation.

24. **Assertion:** 'Critically endangered' category includes the species which have sufficient population at present but is undergoing depletion due to some factors.
Reason: 'Vulnerable' category includes the species which are posing very high risk of extinction in the wild and can become extinct any moment.

25. **Assertion:** The Nile perch introduced into lake Victoria in East Africa to the extinction of an ecologically unique assemblage of more than 200 species of cichlid fish in the lake.
Reason: When alien species are introduced deliberately for economic or other uses, they often become invasive and cause extinction of indigenous species.

26. **Assertion:** Species with low genetic variability are generally at greater risk of extinction than the species with more genetic variability.
Reason: Species with low genetic variability are more vulnerable to diseases, predators or other environmental challenges.

27. **Assertion:** Genetic variation shown by the plant *Rauwolfia vomitoria* growing in different himalayan ranges is very important economically.
Reason: The amount and variety of alkaloids present in this plain change both between the *Rauwolfia* species and between the different strains of *R. vomitoria.*

28. **Assertion:** Excess of sulphur reaches to reservoir pool.
Reason: *Thiobacillus* and *Desulpho vibrio* convert elemental sulphur into the sulphate.

29. **Assertion:** The whole of biogenetic nutrients donot always show circulation.
Reason: Biogeochemicals cycles operate in the biosphere.

30. **Assertion :** If the forest cover is reduced to half, what is most likely to happen on a long term basis is that tribals living in these areas will starve to death.
Reason : Forests are essential as they conserve wild plants so their lack will affect crop breeding programmes due to non availability of germplasm.

31. **Assertion:** Broadly utilitarian arguments say that we should conserve biodiversity because biodiversity plays a major role in many ecosystem services that nature provides.
Reason: Exploration of molecular, genetic and species level diversity to obtain the products of economic importance is included under broadly utilitarian category.

32. **Assertion :** A sanctuary is formed for the conservation of animals only.
Reason : Restricted human activities are allowed in sanctuaries.

33. **Assertion :** National parks are meant for the welfare of the wild life.
Reason : National parks are controlled by State Governments.

34. **Assertion :** Tiger is not an endangered animal in India.
Reason : Project Tiger was launched to improve tiger population.

35. **Assertion :** Indian elephants are confined to Terai and the foot hills.
Reason : Elephants are herbivores and needs plenty of water.

36. **Assertion :** Red data book has a record of only those animals which are known to be in danger.
Reason : Endangered species no need to be noticed.

37. **Assertion :** Great Indian Bustard is a rare species.
Reason : Vulnerable species are rare species.

38. **Assertion:** Jim Corbett National Park is the first National Park of India which is famous for tigers.
Reason: Though the main focus is protection of wildlife, the reserve management has also encouraged ecotourism in this national park.

39. **Assertion:** In a wildlife sanctuary, collection of timber, harvesting of minor forest products and private ownership rights are allowed.
Reason: A sanctuary is a protected area meant for the conservation of both flora and fauna where cultivation of land is permitted.

40. **Assertion:** Offsite collections can be used to restock depleted populations, reintroduce species in the wild and restore degraded habitats.
Reason: *In situ* conservation refers to the conservation of endangered species in their natural habitats.

41. **Assertion:** One of the most important traditional uses of sacred groves was that they acted as a repository for various ayurvedic medicines.
Reason: In modern times, sacred groves have become biodiversity rich areas, as they provide refuge to various plant and animal species of conservation significance.

42. **Assertion:** Biodiversity hotspots are the regions which possess high levels of species richness, high degree of endemism and no loss to habitats.
Reason: Total number of biodiversity hotspots in the world is 32 with two of these hotspots found in India.

43. **Assertion:** Threatened species are those living species which have been greatly reduced in their number and are liable to become extinct if the causative factors continue.
Reason: IUCN is an international organisation which maintains the IUCN red list of threatened species, to assess the conservation status of different species.

44. **Assertion:** Bird ringing was carried in Harike Pattan Sanctuary.
Reason: Bird ringing was helpful in bird census.

45. **Assertion:** Pitti island of Lakshadweep is a sanctuary.
Reason: Lions are protected in Pitti island.

46. **Assertion :** The National bird of New Zealand is Apteryx.
Reason : Flightless birds are native of New Zealand.

47. **Assertion :** Role of biological productivity in human welfare programme was carried out under IBP.
Reason : IBP stands for International Biological program.

48. **Assertion :** Bharatpur and chilka sanctuaries are very famous.
Reason : They are associated with migratory birds.

49. **Assertion :** Rann of Kutch has breeding grounds for flamingos.
Reason : Rann of Kutch is a natural reserve for wild ass also.

50. **Assertion :** Biological conservation under natural conditions is in situ conservation.
Reason : Increase of Manipur deer from 17 animals to 150 in Calcutta and Delhi zoos is one of an example of in situ conservation.

51. **Assertion :** The largest serpentarium in India is located in south.
Reason : Madras is famous for its snake park.

52. **Assertion :** A number of natural reserves have been created to conserve specific wild life species.
Reason : Kaziranga is one of these conserving rhinoes.

Solutions

1. (d) Alpha diversity (within-community diversity) refers to the diversity of organisms sharing the same community/habitat. A combination' of species richness and equitability/evenness is used to represent diversity within a community or habitat. Generally, greater the species richness, greater is the species diversity. Species frequently change when habitat or community changes. The rate of replacement of species along a gradient of habitats or communities is called beta diversity between-community diversity. Higher the heterogeneity in the habitats in a region or greater the dissimilarity between communities, higher is the beta diversity. Diversity of the habitats over the total landscape or geographical area is called gamma diversity.
2. (a) Alpha diversity within community diversity is species diversity in a given community or habitat. It is dependent upon species richness and species evenness/equitability. There is a lot of competition, adjustments and interrelationships amongst members of the same community. The number of species per unit area is called species richness. Number of individuals of different species represent species evenness or species equitability.
3. (c) Biodiversity is not uniform on the earth. It varies with change in latitude or altitude. Biodiversity increase, when we move from high to low latitude (*i.e.* from the poles to the equator).
4. (c) A biosphere reserve is a specified area in which multiple use of the land is permitted by dividing it into zones, each for a particular activity. These zones are
   (i) Core (no human activity is there),
   (ii) Buffer (limited human activity is permitted),
   (iii) Manipulation zone (several human activities can occur in this zone).
5. (c) O-horizon occupies the topmost soil and is rich in mineral and decomposed organic matter (humus). A-horizon is dark coloured and has abundant minerals mixed with humus.
6. (a) Communities with higher number of species are more stable as it can resist occasional disturbances. A stable community should show less variation in productivity from year to year and resistance towards alien species.
7. (a) Communities with more species tend to be more stable than those with less species. It is able to resist occasional disturbance. A stable community should not show too much variation in productivity from year to year; it must be resistant to invasions by alien species. David Tilman's long term experiments showed the plots with more species, experience less year to year variation in total biomass.
8. (b) A stable community should not show too much variation in productivity from year to year; it must be either resistant or resilient to occasional disturbances (natural or man-made), and it must also be resistant to invasions by alien species.
9. (c) Barring arid/semiarid and aquatic habitats, biodiversity shows a latitudinal and altitudinal gradient.
   A decrease in species is observed as we ascend a high mountain due to drop in temperature (lapse temperature being 6.5°C for 1 km or 1000 m) and greater seasonal variability.
10. (c) The tropical monsoon deciduous forests are found in areas receiving an annual rainfall of 100 to 200cms in India, with a distinct dry and rainy season and minimum temperature. The south western ghats moist deciduous forests are a tropical moist broad leaf forest ecoregion of southern India. It covers the southern portion of the Western Ghats range and

the Nilgiri Hills between 250 and 1000 meters elevation in Kerala, Karnataka and Tamil Nadu states.

11. (a) Tropical latitudes have greater biological diversity. It is quite true. Ecologists and evolutionary biologists have proposed various hypothesis in support of this. Speciation is generally a function of time and unlike temperate regions, subjected to frequent glaciations. In the past, tropical latitudes remained undisturbed for millions of years, where species continued to flourish.

12. (d) Alexander von Humboldt observed that within a region, species richness (number of species per unit area) increases with increasing explored area, but only upto a limit. The relationship between species richness and area turned out to be rectangular hyperbola for a wide variety of taxa such as birds, bats, fresh water fishes or flowering plants. On a logarithmic scale, the relationship is a straight line. $\log S = \log C + Z \log A$ Here, S is species richness, Z is slope of line or regression coefficient, C is Y intercept while A is area. The value of Z *i.e.*, slope of line (regression coefficient) of species-area relationships is similar and lies in the range of 0.1 to 0.2 when analysis is done among small areas. If the species area relationship is for very large areas like entire continent, the slope of the line is much steep with value of Z in the range of 0.6 to 1.2, *e.g.*, frugivorous birds and mammals of tropical forests of different continents with a steeper line of 1.15. Thus, larger the explored area, more is steepness of the slope of line.

13. (a) Speciation is a function of time. Temperate regions have undergone frequent glaciations in the past, due to which many species had been killed. However, tropical latitudes have remained relatively undisturbed for millions of years and thus, had a long evolutionary time for species diversification.

14. (c) Taiga biome occurs just South of tundra across North America, Europe and Asia. It is also found in the Southern hemisphere (*e.g.*, – parts of New Zealand). Dominant vegetation consists of evergreen conifers which are able to tolerate wide fluctuation of temperature, light and soil. They are pine, fir, hemlock, spruce, jumper, yew, larch, deodar. The ground flora consists of herbs, ferns, mosses and lichens.

15. (d) Temperate deciduous forest are four – storeyed. The top stratum is occupied by trees reaching a height of 30–40 m. There is an understorey of small trees, an intermediate stratum of shrubs and a ground stratum made of herbs, grasses, ferns, mosses and lichens. Vines are found here and there. A few soft wood trees conifers may occur at places interspersed with hard wood trees.

16. (d) When the rain forest is removed, a secondary forest often develops that includes soft wood trees such as *Musanga* (Africa), *Cecropia* (America) and *Macoranga* (Malaysia). Efficient direct nutrient cycling by mutualistic micro – organisms is a remarkable property of rain forests that enable them to be as luxuriant on poor soils as on more fertile sites.

17. (c) Chaparral is a broad – leaved evergreen shrub forest of hard and thick leaved small trees and shrubs which usually contain resin but are resistant to fires. Crop land is man made ecosystem. Man has been doing his best in modifying the cropland to get maximum benefit out of them. A cropland ecosystem may be illustrated by crops like wheat, maize, rice, sugarcane, etc.

18. (a) Tropical savannahs are grasslands with scattered trees or clumps of trees. The areas of tropical savannah have one or two prolonged dry seasons when fires are an important part of the environment. Since both trees and grass must be resistant to drought and fire, the number of species in the vegetation is not large.

19. (b) A biome is defined as a large natural ecosystem which is distinct in its climate conditions and has its specific type of plant and animal life. Biomes are of two types – terrestrial and aquatic. The major terrestrial biomes are – tundra, taiga, deciduous forest, tropical rain forest, chaparral, tropical savannah, grassland and desert.

20. (c) Tropical rain forests are located in the equatorial regions where the annual rainfall exceeds 140 cm. They are also called jungles and cover one twelveth of earth's surface but contain more than half of the earth's flora and fauna (i.e., rich in biodiversity). Now-a-days these forests are disappearing due to excessive cutting of forests for domestic purposes like fuel, furnitures, accomodations, cloths, resin, gum, etc.

21. (c) From a study of the history of life on earth through fossil records, we learn that large scale loss of species like the one we are currently witnessing have also happened earlier, even before human appeared. During the long period (>3 billion years) since the origin and diversification of life on the earth, there were five episodes of mass extinction of species, the sixth extinction is in progress. The present occurring species extinction is different from the earlier mass extinction as the present species extinction is due to man made causes, whereas the earlier extinction was due to the natural causes.

22. (b) Coextinction is one of the causes of the loss of biodiversity. When a species becomes extinct, the plant and animal species associated with it in an obligatory way also become extinct. This is called coextinction, e.g. when a host fish species becomes extinct, its unique assemblage of parasites also becomes extinct.

23. (c) Over exploitation or over-harvesting of a plant or an animal species reduces the size of its population leading to its extinction. Over-exploitation is one of the major causes threatening global biodiversity. Steller's sea cow *(Hydrodamalis gigas)* was a large, herbivorous, marine mammal (largest member of the order-Sirenia) which had been discovered in 1741 and became extinct by 1768. It is one of the few megafaunal mammal species to have died out during the historical period. It was over-harvested for food, for skin, for its valuable subcutaneous fat, etc.

24. (d) 'Critically endangered' is the highest risk category assigned by the IUCN red list for wild species. Critically endangered species are those that are facing a very high risk of extinction in the wild and can become extinct any moment in the immediate future. 'Vulnerable' species are those whose population is sufficient at present but is undergoing depletion due to some factors so that it is facing the risk of becoming extinct in medium term future. In other words, a taxon is vulnerable when it is not critically endangered or endangered but is facing a high risk of extinction in the wild in the medium-term future.

25. (a) When non-native or alien species are introduced in advertently for their economic or other uses, they often turn invasive and cause decline or extinction of native species. Alien species invasion is considered to be one of the major causes of biodiversity losses. Nile Perch (a predator fish) was introduced in lake victoria of East Africa. It killed and eliminated ecologically unique assemblage of over 200 native species of small cichlid fish.

26. (a) Species with low genetic variability are generally at significantly greater risk of extinction than the species with more genetic variability, simply because they have limited arsenal with which these respond to the various environmental changes. Species with extremely low genetic variability are particularly vulnerable towards a new disease, predator or other environmental challenges, *e.g.*, lack of genetic variability in the African cheetah *(Acinonyx jubatus)* has been considered to be a significant factor contributing towards decline of cheetah population.

27. (a) *Rauwolfia vomitoria* is a medicinal plant used in modern medicines because of the presence of certain alkaloids in its plant parts. This plant reveals genetic variation in different himalayan ranges in terms of the potency and concentration of an active chemical. The amount and variety of these chemicals change both between the *Rauwolfia species* and between the different strains of *R. vomitoria.*

Because of the increasing demand and decreasing natural resources, there is an attempt to develop new strains suitable for agricultural production.

28. (c) Some bacteria and fungi can change H_2S and elemental sulphur to sulphate state (*e.g., Beggiotoa, Thiobacillus, Penicillium, Neurospora*). Reverse can also occur (*e.g., Aerobacter, Desulpho vibrio*). *Delsulpho vibrio* bacteria are ecologically important, because they give SO_4 in deep segments and in anoxic waters, such as the Black Sea to H_2S gas and precipitation of sulphur takes out some sulphur from circulating pool converting it into part of reservoir pool.

29. (b) Circulation of biogenetic materials between the living and the non-living world is called cycles of matter of biogeochemical cycling. The important biogeochemical cycles that operates in biosphere are carbon cycle, sulphur cycle, O_2 cycle, N_2 cycle, etc. The whole of biogenetic nutrients are not always in circulation. For example, rocks from which nutrients are very slowly transferred to the cycling pool.

30. (b) If the forest cover is reduced to half, these are most likely to happen. Tribals living in these areas will starve to death. Cattle in these and adjoining areas will die due to lack of fodder. Large areas will become deserts. Crop breeding programmes will suffer due to a reduced availability of variety of germplasm.

31. (c) The reasons for why should we conserve biodiversity have been included under three categories-narrowly utilitarian, broadly utilitarian and ethical. The broadly utilitarian arguments for conserving biodiversity say that biodiversity plays a major role in many ecosystem services that nature provides, *e.g.,* replenishing O_2 of atmosphere by plants, nutrient cycling, aesthetic value etc. Bioprospecting (*i. e.,* exploring molecular, genetic and species level diversity for products of economic importance) is included under narrowly utilitarian category, which is concerned with the countless direct economic benefits obtained from nature.

32. (a) A sanctuary is an area which is reserved for the protection of wild animals only. The activities like harvesting of timber, collection of minor forest products and private ownership rights are allowed, however, such activities should not have any adverse effect on animals.

33. (c) A National park is an area which is strictly reserved for the welfare of wild life. No human activities are allowed there. Central Government control them but are administered by state government.

34. (a) There are 21 Tiger reserves in India. To save the tiger from extinction in India Project Tiger was launched on April 1, 1973. This project planned to create Tiger reserves in selected areas of India. Due to this effort considerable improvement has been observed in tiger population.

35. (a) Indian elephants (*Elephas maximus*) is the largest terrestrial mammal and is confined to the Terai and the foot hills because of its dependence on succulent grass, bamboo and plenty of water.

36. (c) Red data book contains a record of species of an area which are known to be in danger. Endangered species need to be noticed because only after that the planning for their protection and improving their population can be given the proper direction.

37. (d) Rare species are those which have small population in the world. They are usually confined to limited areas or are thinly scattered over a more wide area. Great Indian Bustard are the species which are in danger of extinction, hence are endangered species. Black buck population is likely to be in danger of extinction, hence vulnerable.

38. (b) Jim Corbett National Park (District Nainital, Uttrakhand) is the first national park of India, established in 1936. The park was the first to come under the 'Project Tiger' initiative. Tourism activity is allowed only in the selected areas of the park so that people get an opportunity to see its splendid landscape and diverse wildlife.

39. (c) A wildlife sanctuary is a protected area which is meant for the conservation of only fauna. Human activities like harvesting of timber, collection of minor forest products and private ownership rights are allowed as long as they do not interfere with the well-being of animals.

40. (b) *In situ* conservation is the conservation of endangered species in their natural habitats. Hot spots and protected areas are the methods of *in situ* conservation. Offsite collections are a part of ex *situ* conservation *i.e.* conservation of endangered species outside their natural habitats. Offsite collections refer to the live collections of wild and domesticated species in botanical gardens, zoological parks, wildlife safari parks, arboreta, etc. Many of the botanical gardens have seed banks, tissue culture facilities and other *ex-situ* technologies. Similarly, most of the zoological gardens have well managed captive breeding programmes. As a result many animals which have become extinct in the wild continue to be maintained in zoological parks. Captive breeding is also resorted to those cases where the number of surviving individuals is so small that there is no realistic chance of *in situ* survival. As the number increases in captive breeding, the individuals are selectively released in the wild. *E.g.*, Californian Candor *(Gymnogyps californicus)* and Black-Footed Ferret *(Mustela nigripes)* have been saved from extinction by this method Therefore, offsite collections can be used to restock depleted populations, reintroduce species in the wild and restore degraded habitats.

41. (b) Sacred groves are relic forest patches traditionally protected by communities in reverence of a diety. In many cultures, tracts of forest were set aside, and all the wildlife within were venerated and given total protection. One of the most important traditional uses of sacred groves was that they acted as a repository for various ayurvedic medicines. Other uses involved a source of replenishable resources like honey and fruits. The groves are often associated with ponds and streams, which meet water requirements of local communities, these sometimes help in recharging aquifers as well. In modern times, sacred groves have become biodiversity rich areas, as various species seek refuge in these areas due to progressive habitat destruction and hunting. Sacred groves often contain plant and animal species that have become extinct in neighbouring areas.

42. (d) Biodiversity hotspots are the regions characterized by very high levels of species richness, high degree of endemism and are also the regions of accelerated habitat loss. Initially 25 biodiversity hotspots were identified but subsequently nine more have been added to the list, bringing the total number of biodiversity hotspots in the world to 34. Three of these hotspots *i.e.*, Western Ghats -Sri Lanka, Indo-Burma and Himalayas - cover our country's exceptionally high biodiversity regions.

43. (b) IUCN (International Union of Conservation of Nature and Natural Resources) is an international organisation, which is now called World Conservation Union (WCU). It has its headquarters at Morges, Switzerland. It maintains a red data book or red list which is a catalogue of taxa facing risk of extinction. Threatened species is the one which is liable to become extinct if not allowed to realise its full biotic potential by providing protection from alien species, human exploitation, habitat destruction, depletion of food etc.

44. (a) Bird ringing or banding is fixing an identifying ring or band to a bird's leg indicating the time and place of the bird's visit. It is useful in bird census. It was carried out at Harike by Bombay Natural History Society from 1980 to 1985.

45. (c) The Pitti island in Lakshadweep has been declared as a protected bird sanctuary under its wildlife act. It is populated by exotic birds.

46. (b) Kiwi is a national symbol and icon of New Zealand. The name of the bird - Kiwi comes from the language of Maori (indigenous

NZ people). It means "hidden bird". Kiwi is flightless - their Latin species name is Apteryx, which means wingless. New Zealand has more species of flightless birds - both living and extinct - than any other country. They include kiwi, kakapo, takahe, penguin, weka, moa, three flightless wrens and two adzebills.

47. **(b)** The International Biological Program (IBP) was an effort between 1964 and 1974 to coordinate large-scale ecological and environmental studies for human welfare.

48. **(a)** Keoladeo National Park formerly known as the Bharatpur Bird Sanctuary in Bharatpur, Rajasthan, India is a famous avifauna sanctuary that hosts thousands of birds during the winter season. Chilika Wildlife Sanctuary is one of the most visited wildlife sanctuaries in Odisha. This wildlife sanctuary is home to various migratory and local birds such as Flamingo, White Bellied Sea Eagle, Brahminy Kite, etc.

49. **(c)** The most famous wildlife of the region includes the Indian Wild Ass, as well as the chinkara, desert fox, jackal, desert cat, caracal, nilgai, wolf, blackbuck, and striped hyena. Asses are the prominent attractions and the animal found in large numbers in the region.

50. **(c)** In-situ conservation is a set of conservation techniques involving the designation, management and monitoring of biodiversity in the same area where it is encountered. Examples of In situ Conservation are national parks, wild life sanctuaries, biosphere reserves and gene sanctuaries.

51. **(c)** Serpentarium is a place where snakes are housed, especially for exhibition. The largest serpenterium is located in South.

52. **(a)** National parks are often made to protect the animals that live inside them or the land itself. Kaziranga National Park - A world heritage site, the park hosts two-thirds of the world's Great One-horned rhinoceros. It is situated in Assam state of India.

Chapter 38

Environmental Issues

Directions: In the following questions, a statement of assertion is followed by a statement of reason. Mark the correct choice as:

(a) If both Assertion and Reason are true and Reason is the correct explanation of Assertion.
(b) If both Assertion and Reason are true but Reason is not the correct explanation of Assertion.
(c) If Assertion is true but Reason is false.
(d) If both Assertion and Reason are false.

1. **Assertion** : Pollution is always caused by human activities.
Reason : Pollution is not different from contamination. **[AIIMS 2007]**

2. **Assertion:** Through the use of catalytic converters, unburnt hydrocarbons are changed into carbon monoxide which in turn is changed into nitrogen oxides and water.
Reason: Motor vehicles equipped with catalytic converters should use leaded petrol to protect the catalyst from degradation.

3. **Assertion :** Suspended particulate matter (SPM) is an important pollutant released by diesel vehicles.
Reason : Catalytic converters greatly reduce pollution caused by automobiles.

4. **Assertion:** Bharat stage IV emission norms have been in place since April 2010, for 4 wheelers in 13 mega cities of India.
Reason: Green muffler scheme refers to the plantation of trees and shrubs along road sides and is effective to control noise pollution only.

5. **Assertion:** Compressed natural gas (CNG) is natural gas under pressure and mainly composed of methane.
Reason: One of the advantages of using CNG as a fuel in automobiles is that it requires very less space for storage as compared to that of petrol or diesel.

6. **Assertion:** Photochemical smog is mainly composed of nitrogen oxides, volatile organic compounds, ozone and peroxyacetyl nitrates.
Reason: Photochemical smog develops in cold weather conditions by the interaction of secondary pollutants.

7. **Assertion** : Smog is commonly formed at places having low temperature and high pollution of aerosol.
Reason : It is very common in metropolis cities of India.

8. **Assertion :** Methylmercury is a highly persistent kind of pollutant that accumulates in food chains.
Reason : Mercury pollution is responsible for Minamata disease.

9. **Assertion :** Water pollutants are measured by BOD.
Reason : If BOD is more, the water is polluted.

10. **Assertion :** Eutrophication shows increase in productivity in water.
Reason : With increasing eutrophication, the diversity of the phytoplankton increases.

11. **Assertion :** Excess of nitrates in drinking water are harmful for infants.
Reason : Nitrates are responsible for blue baby syndrome. **[AIIMS 2009]**

12. **Assertion :** Eutrophication shows increase in productivity in water.
Reason : With increasing eutrophication, the diversity of the phytoplankton increases. **[AIIMS 2013, 2017]**

13. **Assertion:** There is a sharp decline in dissolved oxygen downstream from the point of sewage discharge.
Reason: Microorganisms involved in biodegradation of organic matter in the receiving water body consume a lot of oxygen.

14. **Assertion:** Cultural eutrophication is nutrient enrichment of water bodies due to human activites like passage of sewage, industrial effluents etc.
Reason: The prime contaminants from sewage and industrial effluents are nitrates and phosphates, which act as plant nutrients and overstimulate the growth of algae.
15. **Assertion:** Sewage, industrial effluents and waste waters are non points sources of water pollution.
Reason: Surface runoff is point source of water pollution.
16. **Assertion** : The major pollutants in big and industrialised cities are carbon monoxide and oxides of sulphur.
Reason : CO is inhibitor of cytochrome oxidase.
17. **Assertion** : Water pollution is caused by 2, 4-D and pesticides.
Reason : 2, 4-D acts as a strong weedicide in high concentrations.
18. **Assertion** : Inhabitants close to very busy airports are likely to experience health hazards.
Reason : Sound level of jet aeroplanes usually exceeds 160 dB.
19. **Assertion:** A brief exposure to extremely high sound level, 150dB or more generated by take off of a jet plane or rocket, may damage ear drum or dislocate ear ossicles and permanently impair the hearing ability.
Reason: In India, the Air (prevention and control of pollution) Act came into force in 1981, but was amendedes in 1987 to include noise as an air pollutant.
20. **Assertion:** Heavy metals and persistent pesticides pass into the food chain and increases in amount per unit weight of the organism at successive trophic levels.
Reason: Such heavy metals and persistent pesticides can be easily metabolized by the organism's body.
21. **Assertion** : Organochlorine pesticides are organic compounds that have been chlorinated.
Reason : Fenitrothion is one of the organochlorine pesticides. **[AIIMS 2003]**
22. **Assertion** : Agricultural output increased several times after introduction of DDT.
Reason : DDT was the first insecticide used on a wide scale. **[AIIMS 2004]**
23. **Assertion:** A particle from flowing air use the force of an induced electrostatic charge.
Reason: An ESP is a higly efficient device as it removes 99 per cent of particulate matter present in the exhaust from a thermal power plant.
24. **Assertion** : Plants when exposed to excess fluoride develop necrosis and chlorosis of leaf tips and margin.
Reason : Fluorides cause diseases in human beings in excess as well as deficient conditions.
25. **Assertion** :α,β and γ rays are emitted by disintegration of atomic nuclei of radioactive elements.
Reason : Nuclear fall out is shown by radioactive elements.
26. **Assertion:** Evences refers to a scientific method of treating e-wastes in an environment friendly manner.
Reason: Recycling of e-wastes in developed countries often involves manual participation and exposes the workers to toxic substances present in e-wastes.
27. **Assertion** : Persons exposed to Chernobyl disaster suffered with leukaemia.
Reason : Exposure of human body to radiation causes leukaemia.
28. **Assertion** : CO_2 causes green house effect.
Reason : Other gases do not show such effect.
29. **Assertion** :Presently, the global atmosphere is warming up.
Reason : The depletion of stratospheric ozone layer has resulted in increase in ultraviolet radiations reaching the earth.
30. **Assertion** : Deforestation is one main factor contributing to global warming.
Reason : Besides CO_2, two other gases methane and CFCs are also included under green house gases. **[AIIMS 2006]**
31. **Assertion** : UV radiation causes photo-dissociation of ozone into O_2 and O, thus causing damage to the stratospheric ozone layer.
Reason : Ozone hole is resulting in global warming and climate change.

32. **Assertion :** The concentration of methane in the atmosphere has more than doubled in the last 250 years.
Reason : Wetlands and rice fields are the major sources of methane. **[AIIMS 2006]**

33. **Assertion :** Chlorofluorocarbons are responsible for ozone depletion.
Reason : Ozone level decreases by as much as 67% every year. **[AIIMS 2007]**

34. **Assertion :** Methane, component of green house gases, contributing to global warming is about 20 percent.
Reason : Introduction of multi-point fuel injection engines in automobiles has decreased methane content in the exhausts.
[AIIMS 2005, 2015]

35. **Assertion:** Ozone layer present in the stratosphere protects the living organisms from harmful UV-rays coming from sun by absorbing nearly all of them.
Reason: Ozone formed in the troposphere by photochemical reactions as a result of human activities is harmful for all living organisms.

36. **Assertion:** Deforestation increases carbon dioxide concentration in the atmosphere.
Reason: Deforestation may lead to desertification generally.

37. **Assertion:** An equilibrum is established between generation and destruction of ozone, leading to a steady state concentration of ozone layer in the stratosphere at an altitude of 20-30 km. above sea level.
Reason: The thickness of the ozone layer is generally larger above the equator and smaller above the poles.

38. **Assertion:** Contribution of CO_2, CH_4, CFCs and N_2O towards green house effect is respectively 60%, 6%, 14% and 20%.
Reason: Green house gases are radioactively active gases and which prevent the short wavelength radiations emitted by earth to escape into space.

39. **Assertion :** Chlorofluorocarbons deplete ozone.
Reason : Chlorofluorocarbons contain chlorine, bromine and fluorine.

40. **Assertion :** Ozone is a powerful oxidizing agent in comparison to O_2.
Reason : Ozone is diamagnetic but O_2 is paramagnetic.

41. **Assertion :** Major cause of ozone depletion is CFCs but other greenhouse gases also have a negative effect on ozone layer.
Reason : Greenhouse gases increases the temperature of troposphere but decreases the temperature of stratosphere which facilitate the ozone depletion.

42. **Assertion :** Global warming (Green house effect) occurs due to penetrability of low wavelength radiation through ozone layer.
Reason : CFC is green house gas which results in impenetrability of long wave length radiation through CO_2 of the atmosphere.

43. **Assertion :** Human regulated environment is also called noosphere.
Reason : Man is the main cause for polluting in our ecosystem due to exploitation of natural resources.

44. **Assertion:** Green-house effect is due to thick layer of carbon dioxide.
Reason: The glass panels of a green-house allowing the sunlight to filter through but preventing the beat from being re-radiated in outer space.

45. **Assertion:** Montreal protocol, was signed at Montreal (Canada) in 1987 to control the emission of ozone depleting substances.
Reason: Kyoto protocol, held in Kyoto (Japan) in 1997, has specified the commitments of different countries to mitigate climate change.

46. **Assertion :** Emphysema disease is very common in Kanpur and Calcutta.
Reason : It is disease of respiratory tract occuring due to pollution.

Solutions

1. (d) Pollution may be defined as an undesirable change in physical, chemical or biological characteristics of air, water and land causing harmful effects on living organisms. Pollution can be natural or man made. Natural pollution includes volcanic eruptions, soil erosion, UV- rays, *etc.* Pollution is different from contamination. Contamination is the presence of harmful organisms causing disease.

2. (d) A catalytic converter is a vehicle emissions control device that converts toxic pollutants of the exhaust gas into less toxic pollutants by catalyzing a redox reaction. Catalytic converters, having expensive metals namely platinum, palladium and rhodium as catalysts, are fitted into automobiles for reducing emission of poisonous gases. Rhodium is used as reduction catalyst, palladium is used as an oxidation catalyst, and platinum is used both for oxidation and reduction. As the exhaust passes through the catalytic converter, unburnt hydrocarbons are converted into carbon dioxide and water, and carbon monoxide and nitric oxide are changed to carbon dioxide and nitrogen gas, respectively. Motor vehicles equipped with catalytic converter should use unleaded petrol because lead in the petrol inactivates the catalyst.

3. (b) SPM (Suspended Particulate Matter) is defined as particles floating in the air with a diameter below 10 μm. Studies have shown that high SPM concentrations in the air can have a detrimental impact on respiratory organs. SPM generation from natural sources (*e.g.*, volcanoes or dust storms) and human activities (vehicles, incinerators and industrial plants).

   Catalytic converters is a devices designed to reduce the amount of emissions from automobiles. The current (so-called three-way) systems use a heated metal catalyst to reduce the emissions of carbon monoxide (CO), hydrocarbons, and nitric oxide (NO), all of which contribute to the formation of photochemical smog.

4. (c) Bharat stage emission standards are emission standards issued by the Government of India to regulate the emission of air pollutants from internal combustion of engine equipments of motor vehicles. Bharat Stage IV norms have been in place for 4-wheelers in 13 mega cities of India since April 2010. Green muffler or green belt vegetation is rows of trees and shrubs grown and maintained to serve as noise absorbers. It also reduces air pollution because the trees and shrubs absorb pollution gases and cause settling of suspended particulate matter.

5. (c) Compressed natural gas (CNG), made by compressing natural gas mainly composed of methane, CH_4, it is a better fuel than petrol or diesel as its combustion produces fewer undesirable gases than petrol or diesel. The cost and placement of fuel storage tanks is the major barrier to wider adoption of CNG as a fuel. CNG vehicles require a great amount of space for fuel storage than conventional gasoline-powered vehicles. Laying down pipelines to deliver CNG through distribution points/ pumps is another difficulty faced in switching over to CNG as an automobile fuel.

6. (c) Photochemical smog is a condition that develops when primary pollutants (such as oxides of nitrogen and volatile organic compounds) interact under the influence of sunlight to produce a mixture of secondary pollutants. Thus photochemical smog is mainly composed of oxides of nitrogen volatile organic compounds (pr. pollutants), ozone and peroxyacetyl nitrate PAN (sec. pollutants). It was first reported over Los Angeles in 1940s. Photochemical smog is formed at high temperature over cities and towns due to still air, emission of

nitrogen oxides and hydrocarbons from automobile exhausts and solar energy. Nitrogen dioxide splits into nitric oxide and nascent oxygen. Nascent oxygen combines with molecular oxygen to form ozone. Ozone reacts with carbohydrates to form aldehydes and ketones. Reaction inside engine

$$N_2 + O_2 \longrightarrow 2NO$$

Reaction in atmosphere

$$2NO + O_2 \longrightarrow 2NO_2$$

Photochemical reactions

$$NO_2 \xrightarrow{UV} NO + [O]$$

$$O_2 + [O] \longrightarrow O_3$$

$$NO + HC + O_2 \longrightarrow NO_2 + PAN$$

7. (a) Smog is a kind of air pollution, originally named for the mixture of smoke and fog in the air. It is very common in metropolitan cities. Classical smog occurs in cool humid climate. It is a mixture of smoke, fog and sulphur dioxide.

8. (b) Mercury pollution has been responsible for several deaths in Sweden and Japan and has caused the Minamata disease in Japan, chlor alkali plants seem to be chief sources of mercury containing effluents. Mercury is persistent in water it gets changed into water soluble dimethyl form $[(CH_3)_2Hg]$ and enters the food chain accompanied by biological or ecological amplification.

9. (a) Water pollutants are commonly measured by their main common denominator, called BOD (Biochemical Oxygen Demand), *i.e.*, the amount of free oxygen absorbed by extraneous substances from water. If water is polluted, it will consume more oxygen, thereby enhancing the BOD of water.

10. (b) Eutrophication is a natural process which literally means well nourished or enriched. It is a natural state in many lakes and ponds which have a rich supply of nutrients. Eutrophication become excessive, however when abnormally high amount of nutrient from sewage, fertilizers, animal wastage and detergent, enter streams and lakes causing excessive growth or blooms of microorganisms. With increasing eutrophication, the diversity of the phytoplankton community of a lake increases and the lake finally becomes dominated by blue - green algae.

11. (a) Excess of nitrates in drinking water are harmful for human health and may be fatal for infants. Excessive use of fertilizers often leads to accumulations of nitrates in water. In infants, excess nitrate reacts with haemoglobin to form nonfunctional methaemoglobin that impairs oxygen transport. This condition is termed as methaemoglobinemia or blue baby syndrome. This disease can damage respiratory and vascular systems and even cause suffocation.

12. (a) Eutrophication is a gradual increase in biological productivity of an aquatic ecosystem with time. Direct and indirect ecological impacts of nutrient enrichment include increased primary productivity, increased phytoplankton biomass, reduction in water clarity, increased incidences of low oxygen events (hypoxia and anoxia), and changes in the trophic structure, and trophodynamics of phytoplankton, zooplankton, and benthic communities.

13. (a) Domestic sewage is rich in biodegradable organic matter and the decomposition of this organic matter by microorganisms requires oxygen. Microorganisms involved in biodegradation of organic matter in the receiving water body consume a lot of oxygen, and as a result there is a sharp decline in dissolved oxygen downstream from the point of sewage discharge. If sewage quantity is large, the whole of dissolved oxygen may be consumed leaving nothing for respiration for fish and other clean water organisms. They, therefore, get killed. However, as sew age is decomposed, there is a gradual rise in dissoved oxygen downstream. Fish and other clean water organisms reappear indicating the recovery of river from sewage discharge.

14. (a) Cultural or accelerated eutrophication is nutrient enrichment of water bodies due to human activities like passage of sewage, industrial effluents and run off from fertilized fields rich in nitrates and phosphates. Nutrients present in sewage, agriculture wastes and fertilizers cause dense growth of plants and planktonic algae. Soon planktonic algae increase in number and impart a characteristic colouration to water depending upon the pigments present in them. The excess growth of planktonic algae that causes colouration of water is called algal bloom.

15. (a) Point source of water pollution is caused by discharge of effluents at one point. Non-point source of water pollution is caused by discharge of pollutants over a wide area. Sewage, industrial effluents and waste waters are point source pollutants while surface runoff is a nonpoint source pollutant.

16. (b) Cyanide, azide, and carbon monoxide all bind to cytochrome c oxidase, thus competitively inhibiting the protein from functioning by preventing the binding of oxygen at the active site, which results in the chemical asphyxation of cells.

17. (b) 2, 4-D is 2, 4-dichlorophenoxyacetic acid is a white to crystalline powder used as a weedicide used in the control of broad leaf weeds. The ethyl hexyl form of the compound is rapidly hydrolyzed in soil and water to form the 2, 4-D acid and pollute the water.

18. (a) Noise level upto 64 dB (decibel) is well tolerated. Prolonged exposure to noise level to 80 dB or more leads to loss of hearing ability, fatigue, nervousness, fever, hypertension, gastric disorder, increase in cholesterol level and dilation of pupil of the eye. As the jet aeroplanes have the noise upto 150-160 dB, the inhabitants in the vicinity of busy airports are likely to experience above health hazards. Maximum noise level is recorded in rockets, *i.e.*, 180dB.

19. (b) In India, the Air (Prevention and Control of Pollution) Act came into force in 1981, but was amended in 1987 to include noise as an air pollutant. A brief exposure to extremely high sound level, 150 dB or more generated by take off of a jet plane or rocket, may damage ear drums thus permanently impairing hearing ability. Even chronic exposure to a low level noise (80 - 100 dB) as found in many industries and metropolitan cities near the roads may permanently damage hearing ability of humans.

20. (c) Heavy metals and persistent pesticides (*e.g.*, organo-chlorine or chlorinated hydrocarbons like DDT) pass into food chain and increase in amount per unit weight of organisms with the rise in trophic level due to their accumulation in fat. The phenomenon is called biomagnification/ bioconcentration/biological amplification. In other words, biomagnification refers to increase in concentration of the toxicant at successive trophic levels. This happens because a toxic substance accumulated by an organism cannot be metabolised or excreted, and is thus passed on to the next higher trophic level. This phenomenon is well-known for mercury and DDT. High concentrations of DDT disturbs calcium metabolism in birds, which causes thinning of eggshell and their premature breaking, eventually causing decline in bird populations. These chlorinated hydrocarbons affect CNS, cause softening of brain, cerebral haemorrhage, liver cirrhosis, hypertension, also affect an organism's reproductive system.

21. (c) Organochlorine are persistent pesticides (*e.g.* DDT) which pass into food chain and increase in amount per unit weight of organisms with the rise in trophic level. Fenitrothion is organophosphate.

22. (a) DDT (dichloro diphenyl trichloroethane) is a organochlorine contact insecticide that kills by acting as a nerve poison. DDT was originally used during world war II to control typhus which was spread by body louse. Since then it has been used to control mosquito borne malaria and was used extensively as a general agricultural insecticide.

23. (b) Electrostatic precipitators (ESPs) are very efficient devices which remove 99% of particulates present in the industrial and thermal plant exhausts. An ESP has electrode wires that are maintained at several thousand volts, which produce a corona that releases electrons. These electrons attach to dust particles giving them a net negative charge. The collecting plates are grounded and attract the charged dust particles. The velocity of air between the plates must be low enough to allow the dust to fall.

24. (b) The symptoms of fluoride toxicity in plants are necrotic regions, especially at the tips and along margins of leaves. Various studies of fluoride-exposed workers, primarily from the aluminium smelting industry, showed an increased incidence of lung and bladder cancer and increased mortality due to cancer. The prevalence and severity of dental fluorosis within the population increases with the concentration of fluoride in drinking water.

25. (b) The elements that give radiation are called radioactive elements. The radioactive materials are transformed into gases and fine particles which are carried to distant places by wind. When rain drops, the radioactive particles fall on the ground, it is called nuclear fall - out.

26. (c) Irreparable computers and other electronic goods are known as electronic wastes (e-wastes). E-wastes are buried in landfills or incinerated. Over half of the e-wastes generated in the developed world are exported to developing countries, mainly to China, India and Pakistan, where metals like copper, iron, silicon, nickel and gold are recovered during recycling process. A scientific method of treating e-wastes in an environment friendly manner has been developed. It is called evences.

27. (a) The Chernobyl disaster, also referred to as the Chernobyl accident, was a catastrophic nuclear accident. It occurred on 26 April 1986. The Chernobyl Research Unit at the Radiation Epidemiology Branch of the National Cancer Institute describes the increased risks of leukemia among these workers between 1986 and 2006.

28. (c) Green house effect is due to the occurrence of high carbon dioxide content, high vapour content and glass walls. Gases like CO_2 are called green house gases because they are transparent to solar radiations (wavelength 0.15 - 4.00 μm) but are strong absorbers of long wave or infra red radiations emitted by the surface of the earth.

29. (b) The warming up of global atmosphere in present time is due to the increase in green house effect. Green house effect (GHE) describe the roles of water vapour, CO_2 and other trace gases in keeping the Earth's surface warmer than it would be otherwise. There is concern that increasing concentration of the green house gases including CO_2, CH_4, and man made chlorofluorocarbons (CFC), may enhance the green house effect and cause global warming.

Ozone layer present in the stratosphere is depleted by the aerosols and chloroflurocarbons. Ozone protects the earth from high energyultra violet radiation.

30. (b) Deforestation results in increase in green house gases which retains more and more UV radiations and leads to global warming. Global warming is the warming/heating up of the earth's atmosphere due to depletion of ozone in the stratosphere.

31. (c) Ozone in stratosphere is responsible for the protection of earth from high energy UV rays *i.e.* it acts as life saving screen. Ozone layer found in troposphere protects from warming effect of earth.

Due to human activities, the ozone layer in the stratosphere starts thinning, which is also called ozone hole. Ozone hole is resulting in rain failure, increase in radiation, cancer (skin) and reduction in crop production.

32. (a) Wetland and rice fields are the major sources of methane. It is a green house gas whose concentration is double now than it was 250 years ago.

33. (b) Stratosphere zone of Earth's atmosphere contains a layer of ozone which protects us from harmful ultraviolet radiations of the sun.A group of chlorine containing compounds called chlorofluoro carbon (CFCs) used as coolants in air conditioners and refrigerators are primary chemicals responsible for ozone depletion. After their release into troposphere, CFCs go to stratosphere where they are broken down by UV radiations releasing chlorine.In presence of sunlight, chlorine breaks O_3 into O_2. Due to ozone depletion, its levels decreases by 67% every year causing higher levels of UV radiations reaching earth which may cause eye cataracts, skin cancer, etc.

34. (b) Methane is produced by incomplete biomass combustion, incomplete decomposition mostly by anaerobic methanogens.

Carbon dioxide contributes about 60% of the total global warming and share of methane (CH_4) and chlorofluoro carbons (CFCs) is 20% and 14% respectively. N_2O also contributes 6% in total global warming. Efficient engine such as multi point fuel injection engine can reduce the unburnt hydrocarbon (methane) in auto-emissions.

35. (b) Good ozone is formed in the stratosphere and absorbs harmful UV-radiations from the sun. Bad ozone is formed in the troposphere and is harmful to plants and animals.

$$O_3 \xrightarrow{\text{UV-radiations}} O_2 + [O]$$

36. (c) Deforestation is the conversion of forested areas to non-forested ones.One of the major effects of deforestation is enhanced carbon dioxide concentration in the atmosphere because trees that could hold a lot of carbon in their biomass are lost with deforestation. Deforestation also causes loss of biodiversity due to habitat destruction, disturbs hydrological cycle, causes soil erosion and may lead to desertification in extreme cases.

37. (a) Ozone a or shield is present in the stratosphere. It is also called ozonosphere. Ozonosphere lies at altitude of 23-25 km over equator and at slightly lower altitude elsewhere with 11 -16 km height over poles. 90% of atmospheric ozone is present in ozonosphere. Thickness of ozone is measured in Dobson units (D.U). An equilibrium is estable is hed between generation and destruction of ozone, leading to a steady state concentration of ozone layer in the stratosphere.

$$O_3 \xrightleftharpoons{\text{UV}} O_2 + [O]$$

Of late, this equilibrium (or balance has been disrupted due to enhancement of ozone deg radation ozone depleting substances (ODS). Ozone layer present in stratosphere (good ozone) is vitally important to life as it absorbs harmful UV radiations is proportional to thickenss of ozone layer. Therefore, maximum amount of UV radiations passing through the atmosphere reaches the earth's surface in the tropiccs (i.e., near the equator) and this amount decrease towards the poles.

38. (d) The gases which are transparent to solar radiation but retain and partially reflect back long wave heat radiations are called green house gases (GHGs). Green house gases are essential for keeping the earth warm and hospitable. The various green house gases are CO_2 (warming effect 60%), CH_4 (effect 20%), chlorofluorocarbons or CFCs (14%) and nitrous oxide (N_2O, 6%). Others of minor significance are water vapours and ozone.

39. (c) Chlorofluorocarbon (CFC) is an organic compound that contains carbon, chlorine, and fluorine, produced as a volatile derivative of methane and ethane. It depletes ozone layer.

40. (b) Ozone acts as powerful oxidizing agent because it can easily decompose to give an atom of nascent oxygen which is more reactive than oxygen. Ozone's ground state is a singlet. All electrons there in are paired so it is diamagnetic.

41. (a) Greenhouse gases lower the temperature of stratosphere and lower temperature facilitates the ozone depletion so greenhouse gases indirectly affects the ozone layer or ozone depletion.

42. (a) Global warming occurs when carbon dioxide (CO_2) and other air pollutants and greenhouse gases collect in the atmosphere and absorb sunlight and solar radiation that have bounced off the earth's surface. Normally, this radiation would escape into space-but these pollutants trap the heat and cause the planet to get hotter, known as the greenhouse effect. Many greenhouse gases occur naturally in the atmosphere, such as carbon dioxide, methane, water vapor, and nitrous oxide, while others are synthetic (man-made) include the chlorofluorocarbons (CFCs), hydrofluorocarbons (HFCs) and sulfur hexafluoride (SF_6).

43. (b) The noosphere is the sphere of human thought. The majority of air pollution is the result of human activities. For example, increased fossil fuel combustion from motor vehicles, industrial factories and power plants all pump large quantities of air pollutants, such as carbon monoxide, ozone and nitrous oxides, into the atmosphere.

44. (b) CO_2 in troposhpere behave like the glass panels of a green-house and allowing the sunlight to filter through but preventing the heat from being re-radiated in outer space. This is so called green-house effect. Carbon dioxide and water vapours absorb most heat present in atmosphere and add it to the heat which is already present. Thus, the net result is the warming up of the earth's atmosphere.

45. (b) The Montreal Protocol is an international treaty governing the protection of stratospheric ozone, originally signed in 1987 and substantially amended in 1990 and 1992. The Kyoto Protocol is an international agreement on the reduction of greenhouse gas emissions and on mechanisms aimed at cutting the costs of reducing emissions, in order to address possible changes in the climate. The Protocol was adopted by COP_3 of UNFCCC on 11 December 1997 in Kyoto, Japan.

46. (a) Emphysema is a lung condition that causes shortness of breath. In people with emphysema, the air sacs in the lungs (alveoli) are damaged. Smoking is the most common cause, but emphysema can also be genetic. Air pollution in Kolkata and Kanpur are too much all because of industrialization.